SAMUEL Z. GOLDHABER, M.D.
Assistant Professor of Medicine
Harvard Medical School
Associate Physician
Cardiovascular Division and Channing Laboratory
Department of Medicine
Brigham & Women's Hospital
Boston, Massachusetts

# Pulmonary Embolism and Deep Venous Thrombosis

1985
W. B. SAUNDERS COMPANY
PHILADELPHIA • LONDON • TORONTO • MEXICO CITY • RIO DE JANEIRO • SYDNEY • TOKYO

W. B. Saunders Company: West Washington Square
Philadelphia, PA 19105

1 St. Anne's Road
Eastbourne, East Sussex BN21 3UN, England

1 Goldthorne Avenue
Toronto, Ontario M8Z 5T9, Canada

Apartado 26370—Cedro 512
Mexico 4, D.F., Mexico

Rua Coronel Cabrita, 8
Sao Cristovao Caixa Postal 21176
Rio de Janeiro, Brazil

9 Waltham Street
Artarmon, N.S.W. 2064, Australia

Ichibancho, Central Bldg., 22-1 Ichibancho
Chiyoda-Ku, Tokyo 102, Japan

**Library of Congress Cataloging in Publication Data**

Main entry under title:

Pulmonary embolism and deep venous thrombosis.

1. Pulmonary embolism. 2. Thrombosis. I. Goldhaber, Samuel Z. [DNLM: 1. Pulmonary embolism. 2. Thrombophlebitis. WG 420 G618p]

RC776.P85P824 1985 616.2′49 84–1394

ISBN 0–7216–4151–2

Pulmonary Embolism and Deep Venous Thrombosis ISBN 0–7216–4151–2



Last digit is the print number: 9 8 7 6 5 4 3 2 1

In honor of Dr. Lewis Dexter, who has inspired generations of physicians to strive to be caring, astute practitioners of medicine. He has been germinal in arousing my interest in pulmonary embolism and deep venous thrombosis.

# CONTRIBUTORS


ADLER, DALE S., M.D.

Clinical and Research Fellow in Cardiology, Harvard Medical School; Associate Physician, Brigham and Women's Hospital, Boston, Massachusetts

*Nonthrombotic Pulmonary Embolism*

BURING, JULIE E., Sc.D.

Instructor, Department of Preventive Medicine and Clinical Epidemiology, Harvard Medical School; Adjunct Assistant Professor in Public Health (Epidemiology and Biostatistics), Boston University School of Public Health; Associate Epidemiologist, Brigham and Women's Hospital, Boston, Massachusetts

*Epidemiologic Concepts and Strategies*

EZEKOWITZ, MICHAEL D., M.R.C.P., D.Phil.

Associate Professor of Medicine and Diagnostic Radiology, Yale University School of Medicine; Attending Cardiologist, Yale–New Haven Hospital, New Haven, and West Haven VA Medical Center, West Haven, Connecticut

*Indium-111 Platelet Imaging*

FULTON, DAVID R., M.D.

Assistant Professor of Pediatrics, Tufts University School of Medicine; Assistant Cardiologist and Associate Director, Intensive Care Unit, The Floating Hospital for Infants and Children, Boston, Massachusetts

*Venous Thromboembolism in Children*

GODLESKI, JOHN J., M.D.

Assistant Professor of Pathology, Harvard Medical School; Pulmonary Pathologist, Brigham and Women's Hospital, Boston, Massachusetts

*Pathology of Deep Venous Thrombosis and Pulmonary Embolism*

GOLDHABER, SAMUEL Z., M.D.

Assistant Professor of Medicine, Harvard Medical School; Associate Physician, Cardiovascular Division and Channing Laboratory, Department of Medicine, Brigham and Women's Hospital, Boston, Massachusetts

*Epidemiologic Concepts and Strategies;*
*Strategies for Diagnosis; Strategies for Management;*
*Prevention of Venous Thromboembolism*

HECHTMAN, HERBERT B., M.D.

Associate Professor of Surgery, Harvard Medical School; Senior Associate in Surgery, Brigham and Women's Hospital, Boston, Massachusetts

*Vasoactive Humoral Factors*

HENNEKENS, CHARLES H., M.D.

Associate Professor of Medicine, Harvard Medical School; Associate in Medicine, Brigham and Women's Hospital, Boston, Massachusetts

*Epidemiologic Concepts and Strategies*

HOAGLAND, PETER M., M.D.

Clinical and Research Fellow in Cardiology, Harvard Medical School; Associate Physician, Brigham and Women's Hospital, Boston, Massachusetts

*Massive Pulmonary Embolism*

MANNY, JONAH, M.D.

Associate Professor of Surgery, Hadassah University Medical School; Senior Associate in Surgery, Hadassah University Medical Center, Jerusalem, Israel

*Vasoactive Humoral Factors*

MARKISZ, JOHN A., M.D., Ph.D.

Assistant Professor of Radiology, Cornell University Medical College; Assistant Attending Radiologist, The New York Hospital, New York, New York

*Radiologic and Nuclear Medicine Diagnosis*

POPE, CHRISTOPHER F., M.B., Ch. B.

Resident in Radiology, Yale University, New Haven, Connecticut

*Indium-111 Platelet Imaging*

SHURE, DEBORAH, M.D.

Assistant Professor of Medicine, University of California School of Medicine; Chief, Division of Pulmonary and Critical Care Medicine, San Diego Veterans Administration Medical Center, San Diego, California

*Pulmonary Angioscopy*

SMITH, EILEEN O., B.S.

Chief Technician, Human Cell Labelling Laboratory, Yale University School of Medicine, New Haven, and West Haven VA Medical Center, West Haven, Connecticut

*Indium-111 Platelet Imaging*

STEAD, RICHARD B., M.D.

Medical Staff Fellow, Laboratory of Molecular Biology, National Cancer Institute, Bethesda, Maryland

*Regulation of Hemostasis; Clinical Pharmacology; The Hypercoagulable State*

UTLEY, JOE R., M.D.

Clinical Professor of Surgery, Medical University of South Carolina, Charleston; Chief of Division of Cardiac Surgery, Spartanburg General Hospital, Spartanburg, South Carolina

*Pulmonary Thromboendarterectomy*

# FOREWORD

Over 500,000 persons are afflicted with pulmonary thromboembolism each year in the United States. In probably more than 10 per cent of cases, it is the cause of death. In hospitalized patients, pulmonary embolism (PE) may be the most common form of acute lung disease and is an important cause of sudden, unexpected death. Pulmonary emboli are detected during more than one fourth of all routine autopsies, and clinical-pathological correlations indicate that the antemortem diagnosis of PE is made correctly in probably less than one fourth of these patients. Although PE often goes unrecognized in the chronically ill, it is often overdiagnosed in previously normal patients.

Despite extensive basic and clinical research in this area during the past two decades, our understanding of PE is still far from complete. Nevertheless, some important recent developments make this a propitious time to pull together the many threads of information about PE that have come to light in the last few years. In this book, Dr. Goldhaber has succeeded admirably in weaving these threads into a fabric that provides a clear, comprehensive, and contemporary picture of PE.

Although much has been written about the causes of venous thrombosis and pulmonary embolism, debate persists in the literature on this subject because of confusing and often inadequate observations on disparate patient populations. In the first chapter of this book, Dr. Goldhaber and his associates place the epidemiology of PE in its proper perspective. This is followed in Chapter 2 by Godleski's review of the pathology of and pathogenetic mechanisms underlying venous thrombosis and PE. Many important insights have been gained concerning normal function of the hemostatic system and how it may go awry to cause intravascular thrombosis, and these are presented by Stead in Chapter 3.

To arrive at an accurate diagnosis of venous and pulmonary thromboembolism, the clinician must rely heavily on the results of a number of available laboratory tests. These include venous and pulmonary angiography, ventilation-perfusion lung scanning, Doppler ultrasound to detect blood flow in the veins of the lower extremities, radionuclide venography, $^{125}I$ fibrinogen scanning, and impedance plethysmography. The advantages and limitations of each of these methods are discussed by Markisz in Chapter 4, and the manner in which these test results may be evaluated in conjunction with clinical findings is the subject of Chapter 5 by Goldhaber. Here, he develops a logical strategy for investigating patients suspected of having pulmonary thromboembolism—one that balances sensitivity and specificity and can provide accurate diagnosis without overutilization of expensive or invasive tests, such as pulmonary angiography.

Treatment of PE is no less complex than diagnosis and requires an understanding of the pharmacology of anticoagulants, of fibrinolytic agents, and of platelet-active drugs. These pharmacologic agents are described in Chapter 6 by Stead, while in Chapters 7 and 8 Goldhaber outlines a useful approach incorporating these agents in the management and prevention of PE and deep venous thrombosis.

A variety of hypercoagulable syndromes may play underlying roles in the etiology of pulmonary embolism. In Chapter 9, Stead presents the clinical and pathophysiologic features of these syndromes as well as laboratory tests to aid in their recognition. Pulmonary embolism not only is a consequence of mechanical obstruction of the pulmonary vascular bed but also depends on the release of a variety of vasoactive humoral factors, including serotonin; their role is outlined in Chapter 16 by Manny and Hechtman.

Massive pulmonary embolism is a dramatic, often lethal condition characterized by certain clinical, electrocardiographic, and hemodynamic abnormalities. These features as well as management approaches to this life-threatening condition, such as thrombolytic therapy, vena caval interruption, and pulmonary embolectomy, are reviewed in Chapter 10 by Hoagland. Pulmonary hypertension secondary to chronic pulmonary emboli occurs rarely; in Chapter 15, Utley describes the value and limitations of pulmonary thromboendarterectomy for patients with this unusual condition.

Many substances other than thrombi may embolize to the lungs—including parasites, catheters, bullets, amniotic fluid, air, fat, tumors, and the like. Although these events are uncommon, it is vitally important to recognize these complications. The approach to detecting and managing nonthrombotic PE is described in Chapter 11 by Adler. Venous thrombosis and pulmonary embolism frequently remain undetected in children; the diagnosis and treatment of these conditions in the pediatric age group are outlined in Chapter 12 by Fulton. Of late, a number of new techniques for diagnosing PE have begun to emerge, including the use of $^{111}$In-labeled platelets, discussed by Ezekowitz and associates in Chapter 13, and—perhaps even more exciting—fiberoptic angioscopy described in Chapter 14 by Shure.

Because pulmonary thromboembolism is such a common condition, it is important that it be recognized, understood, and properly treated by generalists as well as a wide variety of specialists such as internists, pulmonologists, cardiologists, surgeons, obstetricians, hematologists, and pediatricians—all of whom should find this book of interest. Dr. Goldhaber and his colleagues are to be congratulated for providing such a complete, well-written, and lucid summary of current knowledge about this important disorder, and W. B. Saunders is to be congratulated for having the foresight to select Dr. Goldhaber to be the editor of this important volume.

EUGENE BRAUNWALD, M.D.
*Boston*

# PREFACE

Pulmonary embolism (PE) and deep venous thrombosis (DVT) are common but elusive illnesses that can cause suffering and death if unrecognized. If diagnosed in a timely and accurate manner, they can usually be treated successfully. Approaches to the management of these conditions are highly varied and constantly evolving. Most recent information on venous thromboembolism is scattered among journals in many areas, including internal medicine, surgery, radiology, pathology, and obstetrics and gynecology, and the articles logically tend to focus narrowly on a specific aspect of a particular problem. The few current textbooks that exist are usually oriented toward specialized audiences such as hematologists, vascular surgeons, or pathologists. However, the clinical management of patients with PE and DVT requires a truly interdisciplinary effort.

This book is designed to assist *all* who participate in the clinical care and investigation of venous thromboembolic disorders. In particular, we have sought to provide information necessary for *clinical* decision making, thus rendering this book especially valuable to the physician engaged in the community or academic-based *clinical* practice of medicine, surgery, obstetrics and gynecology, or pediatrics. For radiologists and pathologists, this text should afford an important clinical perspective that can help to enhance their diagnostic insights. In addition, for those in training—medical students, interns, residents, and fellows—this extensively referenced text should be an important resource.

The book has been divided into four parts. Part I compiles knowledge from the disciplines of epidemiology, pathology, hematology, and radiology in order to provide a foundation for clinical management. Although these chapters review fundamental principles and mechanisms, the presentation is oriented toward the clinician. Part II constitutes the "clinical core" of the book and comprises detailed discussions of diagnosis, clinical pharmacology, management, and prophylaxis. Special clinical topics not often given sufficient emphasis in the venous thromboembolism literature are presented in Part III and include the hypercoagulable state, massive PE, nonthrombotic PE, and venous thromboembolism in children. Part IV highlights several areas of active and exciting research that may have important clinical implications in the near future. These areas are $^{111}$In-labeled platelet imaging, pulmonary angioscopy, pulmonary thromboendarterectomy, and vasoactive humoral factors.

Throughout the text, one finds that tables, diagrams, and photographs have been utilized extensively. Virtually all the photographs in the pathology (Chapter 2), radiology (Chapter 4), diagnosis (Chapter 5), and pediatrics (Chapter 12) chapters comprise original case material, previously unpublished. Similarly, the diagrams of hematologic pathways (Chapters 3, 6, and 9) for the most part represent original efforts to illustrate clearly and simply subject matter that is fairly complex. In Part IV (Chapters 13 to 16), the authors have included graphic material derived from their own research efforts. With the help of the publisher, we have been able to cite the most recent original reports available just prior to publication. Often, no definitive answer can be given to a particular management issue. In such situations, we present practical approaches based on our own experience but call attention to limitations in our current knowledge.

I wish to thank those individuals who helped to make this book possible: Ms. Diane Q. Forti urged me to undertake this project, and her encouragement and editorial suggestions have been invaluable. Dr. Thomas W. Smith, Chief of the Cardiovascular Division; Dr. Charles H. Hennekens, Associate Professor of Medicine; and Dr. Eugene Braunwald, Chief of the Department of Medicine, have given their ongoing support to this project. The efforts of the contributing authors have been outstanding, and I have found their enthusiastic dedication most heartening. Ms. Donna Gordon provided most competent assistance in preparing many of the chapter manuscripts and in assisting with a large volume of editorial correspondence. It has been a pleasure to work with the professional and always cooperative staff of the W. B. Saunders Company. Ms. Lisette Bralow, Medical Editor, guided this project from outline to final form. Ms. Elizabeth Gittens copy edited the text most expeditiously. Mr. Robert Butler supervised the book's production and was extremely helpful to me. Ms. Terri Siegel designed the cover, transforming ideas into art.

Finally, I wish to offer special thanks to my family. My parents, Paul and Ethel, and my brother Joshua were continuing sources of encouragement. My wife Reeve and my daughter Alissa endured my frequent absence. Reeve was extraordinarily patient, understanding, and supportive, for which I will always be appreciative.

SAMUEL Z. GOLDHABER

# CONTENTS

# PART I

# FUNDAMENTALS

CHAPTER 1

# EPIDEMIOLOGIC CONCEPTS AND STRATEGIES

*SAMUEL Z. GOLDHABER, M.D.*
*JULIE E. BURING, Sc.D.*
*CHARLES H. HENNEKENS, M.D.*

## INTRODUCTION

To evaluate clinical studies of pulmonary embolism (PE) and deep venous thrombosis (DVT), it is important to understand the epidemiologic concepts of *association* and *causation*, as well as the different epidemiologic strategies that can be utilized to formulate and test hypotheses. For example, although the association between prior surgery and the development of PE may be statistically significant, this association may not be causal. Specifically, PE may result from immobilization rather than from the surgery itself. Thus, guidelines are needed to judge whether an observed association is one of cause and effect. Furthermore, potential risk factors for PE and DVT may be identified from many different types of study designs, each with its particular strengths and limitations. The goal of this chapter is to discuss these basic epidemiologic concepts and strategies, with examples from studies of PE and DVT.

## ASSOCIATION AND CAUSATION

### Association

A statistical association between an exposure and a disease is defined as the probability of a disease occurring in the presence of an exposure being different from the probability of the same disease occurring in the absence of such an exposure. A *valid* statistical association between an exposure and disease is present after the roles of chance, bias, and confounding as alternative explanations have been excluded (Table 1–1).[1]

#### CHANCE

The evaluation of chance involves the performance of a statistical test of significance and calculation of a p-value. This p-value is a conditional probability, namely that the observed data are due to chance, given that there is no association between the exposure and disease (i.e., the null hypothesis is true).

If this p-value is low, conventionally chosen as equal to or less than 0.05, it is concluded that chance is an unlikely explanation of the result, that the null hypothesis can be rejected, and that there is a statistically significant association between the exposure and the disease. This arbitrary cutoff point for defining statistical significance is referred to as the alpha level. If the alpha or significance level is greater than the specified value, conventionally p greater than 0.05, then we conclude that there is no statistically significant association, and we do not reject the null hypothesis. This would mean that chance cannot be excluded as an explanation of the observed association.

By definition, the smaller the alpha level (or Type I error), the smaller the probability

***Table 1–1.*** Interpretations of Cause-Effect Relationships in Epidemiologic Studies: Association vs. Causation

I. Noncausal associations
  A. Can occur by chance alone
  B. Can occur due to bias
    1. Selection bias
    2. Observation bias (including recall bias and misclassification bias)
  C. Can occur due to confounding
II. Causal associations: positive criteria
  A. Strong association (e.g., high relative risk)
  B. Biologic credibility
  C. Consistency of the observed association

of rejecting the null hypothesis when there really is no association. Another source of possible error is the probability of failing to reject a null hypothesis that is, in fact, false. This latter type of error is known as the beta or Type II error. The power of a study to detect a significant association is defined as (1–Type II error). The smaller the sample size, the larger the Type II error and thus the smaller the power of the study to detect a significant association. This consideration is crucial in interpreting findings of no statistically significant association in studies of small sample size.[2]

The p-value, or alpha value, depends on both the magnitude of the association and the size of the sample. Thus, a small difference, even if clinically meaningless or irrelevant, will be statistically significant if the sample size is sufficiently large. Conversely, a large and clinically important difference may not reach statistical significance if based on a small sample. Because interpretation of the p-value has this limitation, estimating the magnitude of an association is as important as testing its statistical significance. In addition, whether or not the statistical association between an exposure and disease is likely to be due to chance, the possibilities of bias and confounding must also be considered.

### BIAS

Bias may be defined as any source of error in the estimation of the association between an exposure and disease. In any study, there may be various potential sources of bias, and the degree to which any of these may be distorting the estimate of the association should be ascertained.

*Selection bias* results when the subjects in the study are enrolled differentially. This can be a special problem in a case-control study, in which the cases and controls may be selected on the basis of whether they were exposed to the factor under investigation. For example, in studying only women hospitalized for thromboembolism, an overestimate of the true association with use of oral contraceptives would be reported if physicians were more likely to hospitalize users of oral contraceptives with symptoms of thromboembolism compared with nonusers who had the same clinical syndrome.

*Observation bias* results from the differential recording of information on exposure status or disease outcome among the groups under study. For example, observation bias may occur in studies of PE when the interpretation of a diagnostic test is made on the basis of exposure status. To avoid this source of bias, it is necessary to define in advance reproducible and objective criteria for interpreting various diagnostic tests. There are several particular types of observation bias. *Recall bias* results from the tendency of those who are sick to remember antecedent events differently from those who are well. *Misclassification* is another type of observation bias that can occur when an illness such as PE is underdiagnosed or overdiagnosed. This is a special problem in studies of PE and DVT, since underdiagnosis can occur because the symptoms, signs, and available noninvasive screening tests for PE are often nonspecific and can simulate myocardial infarction, pneumonia, or congestive heart failure. In addition, Robin[3] has stated that PE has often been overdiagnosed and overtreated in previously normal young women using oral contraceptives. He believed that nondiagnostic lung scans were often systematically being misclassified as diagnostic of PE. He also observed that viral syndromes such as pleuritis might mimic PE and cause minor nondiagnostic abnormalities on the perfusion lung scan. Such over- or underdiagnosis of PE would tend to dilute any exposure-disease association if the misclassification were unrelated to the exposure under study (random misclassification). However, if the misclassification were differential, that is, related to exposure status, then the estimate of the effect might be artificially increased or decreased.

### CONFOUNDING

Confounding, simply defined, is an undesired mixing of effects. A confounding factor is a variable that is associated with the exposure under study but is also an independent risk factor for the disease. This confounding factor may account totally or in part for the observed association. When confounding occurs but is not controlled, one may fail to observe real differences between study groups or, conversely, one may observe apparent differences between study groups when such differences do not truly exist.

For example, in reviewing previous trials of inferior vena cava (IVC) interruption by clip or filter, it becomes apparent that uncontrolled confounding limits their interpretability. Usually, because of poor prognosis and poor overall medical condition, a higher proportion of patients with cancer undergoes filter insertion rather than IVC clipping. When a higher mortality rate is reported with filters, this may be due at least in part to either the malignancy or to the poor overall general medical condition rather than to the therapeutic modality.[4]

### Causation

Once a valid statistical association is established, the likelihood of a causal relationship is a matter of judgment. Belief in causality is enhanced when the strength of the association is large, when there is biologic credibility, and when multiple types of studies done by different investigators show consistent results[1] (Table 1–1).

#### Strength of Association: Concept of the Relative Risk

The *relative risk* measures the strength of association between an exposure (e.g., oral contraceptives) and a disease (e.g., pulmonary embolism). Relative risk is defined as the ratio of the rate of disease in those exposed to the rate of disease in those not exposed. The relative risk is calculated directly for cohort and intervention studies, but must be estimated as the cross-product or odds ratio for case-control studies. A relative risk of 1.0 implies no association, whereas a relative risk less than 1.0 implies an inverse association. When a relative risk is greater than 1.0, there is a positive association. The stronger the association (either positive or inverse), the less likely the observed relationship is due to additional uncontrolled confounding variables, and the more likely the exposure is to cause (if the association is positive) or prevent (if inverse) the disease.[1]

#### Biologic Credibility

A second positive criterion supporting a judgment of causality is the biologic credibility of the association between the exposure and the disease. For instance, it is known that antithrombin III deficiency predisposes to venous thrombosis. Furthermore, oral contraceptives consistently induce a decrease in antithrombin III levels in clinically healthy women.[5] Thus, a causal association between use of oral contraceptives and development of PE has biologic credibility.

#### Consistency of Findings

The likelihood that an observed association is causal increases when different investigators using varying study methodologies report similar results. Consistency is an important consideration, because it includes variations among populations, investigators, and study protocols. As an example, a consistent association between use of oral contraceptives and development of DVT and PE has been found by many different groups of investigators in Europe, Scandinavia, and the United States, using many different strategies of epidemiology.

## STRATEGIES OF EPIDEMIOLOGY: TYPES OF STUDIES

Many epidemiologic strategies can be employed to formulate and test hypotheses. Each has inherent strengths and limitations. *Descriptive* studies include *correlational studies* of populations as well as *case reports, case series,* and *cross-sectional surveys* of individuals. These are useful only for hypothesis formulation. *Analytic studies* of individuals can be divided into *observational* (cohort and case-control) and *intervention* studies and are suitable for hypothesis testing[1] (Table 1–2).

### Descriptive Studies

*Correlational studies* describe the relationship between exposure variables and disease outcomes among populations. For example, such studies have indicated a positive correlation between increased use of oral contraceptives and increased mortality from venous thromboembolism. In England and Wales,[6] the estimated frequency of use of oral contraceptives increased from 1963 to 1967. During this time period, the estimated number of

***Table 1–2.*** Epidemiologic Strategies: Types of Studies

I. Descriptive: to formulate hypotheses
   A. Correlational studies
   B. Case reports
   C. Case series
   D. Cross-sectional surveys
II. Analytic: to test hypotheses
   A. Observational
      1. Cohort
      2. Case-control
   B. Intervention
      1. Randomized
      2. Nonrandomized
         a. Concurrent
         b. Historical

deaths from venous thromboembolism also increased. This raised the question of whether use of oral contraceptives was responsible for the increased deaths due to venous thromboembolism. However, correlational studies evaluate populations; they cannot determine whether those who died from venous thromboembolism were those who took oral contraceptives. In addition, one cannot control for other changes over time such as possible differences in treatment or diagnosis of PE or other changes in health-related practices aside from the use of oral contraceptives.

Individual *case reports* may also generate hypotheses, but because the observation is in a single affected individual, the inferences from this strategy are obviously quite limited. *Case series* have a larger sample size but lack a comparison group.

The association between oral contraceptives and pulmonary embolism is an example of a hypothesis formulated from case reports. For example, in 1961, Jordan reported that a 40-year-old surgical nurse sustained a PE without DVT.[7] She was healthy except for endometriosis. Five weeks prior to her PE, she had begun treatment with oral contraceptives for an exacerbation of endometriosis. The drugs provoked severe nausea, which was treated with antiemetics. Jordan believed the PE occurred "secondary to the dehydration and vomiting" caused by the contraceptive preparation. "Because Enovid (the estrogen preparation) may produce uncontrollable vomiting and provoke pulmonary embolism and infarction, I would counsel caution in the use of this widely advertised drug," Jordan stated.

*Case series* have also contributed to formulation of the hypothesis that an association exists between oral contraceptives and venous thromboembolism. For example, by 1963, the Food and Drug Administration had received approximately 350 reports of thrombosis or embolism in women taking Enovid.[8] Another case series was compiled in the United Kingdom in 1966, when the Committee on Safety of Drugs was informed of 19 thromboembolic deaths among the 400,000 women estimated to have used oral contraceptives that year. Ten of the 19 women had no predisposing conditions.[9] However, because there is no comparison series, it is not possible to determine whether this represents an increased risk of PE associated with use of oral contraceptives *per se.* To test this hypothesis requires the use of analytic studies.

As with case reports and case series, *cross-sectional surveys* have the advantage of studying individuals rather than populations. Although cross-sectional surveys also have a potential comparison group among those not affected by the disease of interest, the temporal sequence of the exposure and the disease is often unclear. This type of epidemiologic strategy is rare in the PE and DVT literature. Like other descriptive studies, cross-sectional surveys are useful only to formulate hypotheses.

## Analytic Studies

### Observational Studies

Observational studies are either *cohort* or *case-control* in design. In a *cohort study,* the study groups are defined on the basis of exposure status (exposed vs. nonexposed), and the subsequent occurrence of diseases of interest is determined. In a *case-control study,* patients with the disease are identified together with a comparably chosen control group that is free from the illness. Data are collected from both groups on exposures that occurred prior to the development of the disease among the cases and for a corresponding time period among the controls.

### Cohort Studies

A cohort study is the optimal design to evaluate the effects of a rare exposure. There are, of course, corresponding limitations to this approach. The necessity of following all enrolled subjects for development of the outcome of interest is expensive and time consuming. If there are losses to follow-up, despite the time and expense involved, the result may be biased.

In England, general practitioners were asked to evaluate the possible association between oral contraceptives and thromboembolism by classifying their patients as users or nonusers of these drugs and following them for possible development of thromboembolic disease. In 1974, the Royal College of General Practitioners reported that those women who used oral contraceptives had 5.7 times the risk of developing DVT as nonusers.[10]

### Case-Control Studies

The case-control study design is optimal for rare diseases and can evaluate the effects of multiple exposures on a single disease. Case-control studies can be conducted quickly, compared with cohort studies. Because long-term follow-up is not necessary, a large case-control study is relatively inexpensive (hundreds of thousands of dollars) compared with a large cohort study (millions of dollars). However, the corresponding limitations of a case-control design are (1) the increased possibility of bias, especially recall bias, because the exposure and disease status are known when the study is performed and (2) insuring that the controls are comparable to the cases with respect to all potential confounding factors.

For example, in 1969, Vessey and Doll[14] reported the results of a case-control study in which the cases were selected from nonpregnant, premenopausal, nonsterilized women hospitalized with DVT, and the controls were nonpregnant, premenopausal, nonsterilized women hospitalized with acute medical or surgical conditions and matched for age, parity, and date of hospitalization.[14] Both cases and controls were interviewed at home after hospital discharge and were questioned about use of oral contraceptives as well as other potential risk factors for DVT. In this study, users of the drugs had a risk of DVT 6.3 times that of nonusers.

There have been multiple case-control studies linking oral contraceptives with venous thromboembolism.[9, 11–19] The consistency of their findings increases the likelihood that the association between use of oral contraceptives and DVT is causal.

### Intervention Studies

In an intervention trial, which we consider a type of cohort study, the investigator determines who is exposed. When this exposure is allocated at random, the randomized trial design provides the most direct evidence of whether an association is causal. The unique strength of randomization is that, on the average, all known and unknown confounding variables are distributed equally between the study groups. With respect to known confounders, if the data on these variables are collected at baseline, it is possible to assess whether they are evenly distributed and, if not, to adjust for imbalances. Of at least equal concern, there will always exist important confounding factors (i.e., variables associated with the exposure and risk factors for the disease) that are unknown to the investigator because of limitations of knowledge at the time any trial is initiated. The utility of randomization, especially when the sample is large, is that it usually assures a degree of comparability between study groups that can never be achieved with any of the strategies of observational epidemiology. Thus, randomized trials are particularly valuable for studying small to moderate effects, especially when the trial is sufficiently large.

Whereas intervention trials have the usual strengths and weaknesses of observational cohort studies, the unique features of randomization make randomized trials the most powerful tool of the epidemiologist. The limitations of randomized trials include ethical considerations, cost, and feasibility. Ethical considerations preclude randomization of hazardous exposures if the risks obviously outweigh the benefits. Further, because of the investigator's control over the allocation of the exposure, the design tends to be even more expensive and less feasible than observational cohort studies. With regard to oral contraceptives and venous thromboembolism, we believe a cause-effect relationship does exist because of the strength of the association, biologic credibility, and consistency of the descriptive and analytic observational findings. It would, therefore, be unethical for us to conduct a randomized clinical trial to test directly whether oral contraceptives are causally associated with venous thromboembolism. In addition to ethical considerations, the cost and feasibility factors would probably preclude use of this strategy.

This strategy, however, has been used in an attempt to advance current knowledge of the epidemiology of deep venous thrombosis. Specifically, results of a randomized clinical trial have been reported in which streptokinase was compared with heparin in phlebographically documented DVT.[20] In one study, Porter and coworkers randomized 50 patients to either streptokinase or heparin. Of 24 patients receiving streptokinase, 13 (54 per cent) achieved phlebographically documented lysis, compared with 8 (31 per cent) of 26 receiving heparin ($p = 0.10$). Thus, the results tended to favor streptokinase over heparin, but the results did not achieve statistical significance, possibly due to the small sample size.

At times, the results of a randomized controlled trial (such as the study by Porter and coworkers) will be reported as "negative" because of an inadequate sample size, even when a small to moderate difference truly exists (the beta or Type II error).[21] In the absence of a single large randomized intervention study, which is optimal, the results of several small trials may be viewed in aggregate to obtain a pooled estimate of relative risk for a particular therapeutic intervention. However, if such trials are not randomized, pooling may not be appropriate. There have been a total of six randomized trials of small sample size in which streptokinase therapy was compared with heparin for phlebographically documented DVT.[20, 22–26] When the results were pooled, clot lysis occurred 3.7 times more frequently among those who received streptokinase than among those treated with heparin[27] (Fig. 1–1). Thus, the pooled results gave a more precise estimate of the relative risk (3.7 versus 1.7 for the single trial) and, owing to this estimate as well as the larger sample size, were highly significant ($p < 0.0001$ versus $p = 0.10$ for the single trial).

Intervention studies can be nonrandomized as well as randomized. The control group for a nonrandomized study can be either *concurrent* or *historical*. Concurrent controls might be allocated by nonrandom methods such as alternating patients or alternating days of the week. However, such a predictable allocation scheme might allow even the best-intentioned physician to influence which group his patient enters. This potential manipulation of the study, in turn, might result in bias. With regard to historical controls, a major problem is that the patient population and methods of diagnosis and

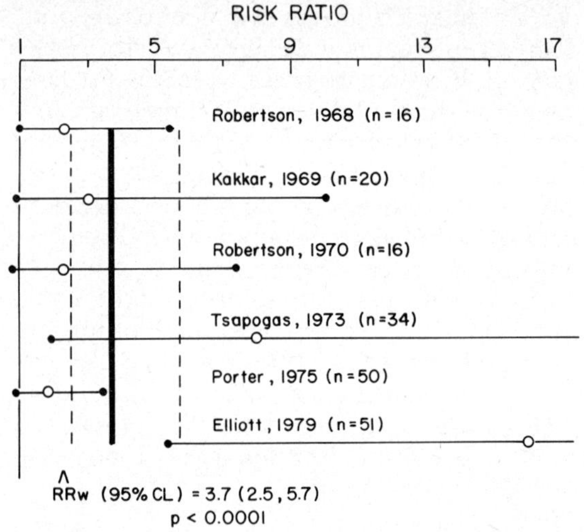


***Figure 1–1.*** Deep leg vein clot lysis. Pooled results from six randomized trials.[20, 22–26] A risk ratio (i.e., relative risk) greater than one signifies that streptokinase lysed the clot more often than heparin. The open circles indicate the risk ratio for each individual trial. The closed circles indicate the 95 per cent confidence limits for each individual trial. The heavy vertical line indicates the pooled risk ratio of 3.7 for the six studies. The hatched vertical lines are the pooled 95 per cent confidence limits (2.5, 5.7).

treatment may have changed over time. Because of changes in medical care, historical controls may have a different outcome than a current intervention group, regardless of the intervention. Thus, the use of nonrandomized concurrent or historical controls may lead to comparisons that are, at best, comparable to observational studies and, at worst, biased.

## CONCLUSIONS

In evaluating the literature, it is important to determine first whether there is a statistical association between an exposure and diseases such as DVT or PE. A valid statistical association is present after chance, bias, and confounding can be excluded as alternative explanations. Once statistical association is established, the belief that the association is one of cause and effect is enhanced by the presence of positive criteria such as strength of association, biologic credibility, and the consistency of the epidemiologic evidence. This evidence can come from many different analytic study designs, including both observational (case-control or cohort) and intervention studies. The latter, when properly randomized and sufficiently large, are the most powerful tool of the epidemiologist.

Each strategy has its particular strengths and limitations. In general, descriptive studies can help to formulate hypotheses, whereas analytic studies are necessary for testing them. In the remainder of this book, the results of additional descriptive and analytic studies will be presented. These studies should be viewed in the context of the principles set forth in this chapter.

## REFERENCES


1. Hennekens, C. H., and Buring, J. E.: Epidemiology in Medicine. Little, Brown and Co., Boston, 1985. (In press.)
2. Colton, T.: Statistics in Medicine. Little, Brown and Co., Boston, 1974, pp. 115–122.
3. Robin, E. D.: Overdiagnosis and overtreatment of pulmonary embolism: The emperor may have no clothes. Ann. Intern. Med., *87*:775, 1977.
4. Goldhaber, S. Z., Buring, J. E., Lipnick, R. J., et al.: Interruption of the inferior vena cava by clip or filter. Am. J. Med., *76*:512, 1984.
5. Fagerhol, M. K., Abilgaard, U., Bergsjo, P., et al.: Oral contraceptives and low antithrombin-III concentration. Lancet, 2:1175, 1970.
6. Vessey, M. P., and Weatherall, J. A. C.: Venous thromboembolic disease and the use of oral contraceptives: A review of mortality statistics in England and Wales. Lancet, 2:94, 1968.
7. Jordan, W. M.: Pulmonary embolism. Lancet, 2:1146, 1961.
8. Food and Drug Administration. Final report on Enovid by the ad hoc committee for the evaluation of a possible etiologic relation with thromboembolic conditions. Department of Health, Education, and Welfare, Washington, D.C., 1963.
9. Inman, W. H. W., and Vessey, M. P.: Investigation of deaths from pulmonary, coronary, and cerebral thrombosis and embolism in women of child-bearing age. Br. Med. J., *2*:193, 1968.
10. Royal College of General Practitioners: Oral contraceptives and Health: An interim report from the Oral Contraception Study of the Royal College of General Practitioners. Pitman Medical Publishing Co., Kent, England, 1974, pp. 43–50.
11. Royal College of General Practitioners: Oral contraception and thromboembolic disease. J. Coll. Gen. Practit., *13*:267, 1967.
12. Medical Research Council: Risk of thromboembolic disease in women taking oral contraceptives: A preliminary communication to the Medical Research Council by a subcommittee. Br. Med. J., 2:355, 1967.
13. Vessey, M. P., and Doll, R.: Investigation of relation between use of oral contraceptives and thromboembolic disease. Br. Med. J., *2*:199, 1968.
14. Vessey, M. P., and Doll, R.: Investigation of relation between use of oral contraceptives and thromboembolic disease. A further report. Br. Med. J., *2*:651, 1969.
15. Sartwell, P. E., Masi, A. T., Arthes, F. G., et al.: Thromboembolism and oral contraceptives: An epidemiologic case-control study. Am. J. Epidemiol., *90*:365, 1969.
16. Vessey, M. P., Doll, R., Fairbairn, A. S., et al.: Postoperative thromboembolism and the use of oral contraceptives. Br. Med. J., *3*:123, 1970.
17. Greene, G. R., and Sartwell, P. E.: Oral contraceptive use in patients with thromboembolism following surgery, trauma, or infection. Am. J. Public Health, *62*:680, 1972.
18. The Boston Collaborative Drug Surveillance Programme: Oral contraceptives and venous thromboembolic disease, surgically confirmed gallbladder disease, and breast tumours. Lancet, *1*:1399, 1973.
19. Stolley, P. D., Tonascia, J. A., Tockman, M. S., et al.: Thrombosis with low-estrogen oral contraceptives. Am. J. Epidemiol., *102*:197, 1975.
20. Porter, J. M., Seaman, A. J., Common, H. H., et al.: Comparison of heparin and streptokinase in the treatment of venous thrombosis. Am. Surgeon, *41*:511, 1975.
21. Freiman, J. A., Chalmers, T. C., Smith, H., Jr., et al.: The importance of beta, the type II error and sample size in the design and interpretation of the randomized control trial. Survey of 71 "negative" trials. N. Engl. J. Med., *299*:690, 1978.
22. Robertson, B. R., Nilsson, I. M., and Nylander, G.: Value of streptokinase and heparin in treatment of acute deep venous thrombosis: A coded investigation. Acta Chir. Scand., *34*:203, 1968.
23. Kakkar, V. V., Flanc, C., Howe, C. T., et al.: Treatment of deep vein thrombosis. A trial of heparin, streptokinase, and arvin. Br. Med. J., *1*:806, 1969.
24. Robertson, B. R., Nilsson, I. M., and Nylander, G.: Thrombolytic effect of streptokinase as evaluated by phlebography of deep venous thrombi of the leg. Acta Chir. Scand., *136*:173, 1970.
25. Tsapogas, M. J., Peabody, R. A., Wu, K. T., et al.: Controlled study of thrombolytic therapy in deep vein thrombosis. Surgery, *74*:973, 1973.
26. Elliot, M. S., Immelman, E. J., Jeffery, P., et al.: A comparative randomized trial of heparin versus streptokinase in the treatment of acute proximal venous thrombosis: An interim report of a prospective trial. Br. J. Surg., *66*:838, 1979.
27. Goldhaber, S. Z., Buring, J. E., Lipnick, R. J., et al.: Pooled analyses of randomized trials of streptokinase and heparin in phlebographically documented acute deep venous thrombosis. Am. J. Med., *76*:393, 1984.

CHAPTER 2

# PATHOLOGY OF DEEP VENOUS THROMBOSIS AND PULMONARY EMBOLISM

*JOHN J. GODLESKI, M.D.*

## INTRODUCTION

Thrombi are formed in large veins; they may dislodge, travel to the lung, and occlude pulmonary vessels. The result of these events can range from sudden death to no perceptible change in well-being. This chapter will present our current understanding of the pathologic changes in this sequence viewed primarily from the anatomic perspective.

The first description of massive occlusion of the pulmonary artery was reported by Tulpius in 1641 (cited by Liebow).[1] Appreciation that emboli originate in the deep veins of the legs emerged in the nineteenth century. Ideas relevant to our current understanding of venous thrombosis also were presented at that time. Virchow[2] emphasized the importance of slowing of the bloodstream as a factor predisposing to coagulation of blood in the veins. Cohnheim[3] and Ribbert[4] showed that injury to the lining of a blood vessel was important in the development of a thrombus. Others showed that a postoperative increase in the number of blood platelets occurred at the same time that thrombosis was most frequently found.[5] Also, infection was noted to play a role in the pathogenesis of some cases.[6] This last observation was followed by many years of controversy over whether venous thrombosis occurred spontaneously, based on the factors noted above, or whether infection, either overt or subclinical, was the underlying cause of all venous thrombi.[7] This controversy began to wane in the 1930s and 1940s as it became clear that the incidence of pulmonary embolism was rising sharply and attention was being focused on the diagnosis.[8]

Classic studies such as those by Hampton and Castleman[9] were important in defining pathologic changes and their clinical correlates. Multiple recurrent emboli causing cor pulmonale were recognized in studies of clinical pathologic correlation.[10] Autopsy studies of the 1940s, 1950s, and 1960s produced increased awareness of the clinical problems presented to the physician in dealing with patients with pulmonary embolism and defined the pathologic changes found in these cases.

## PATHOLOGY OF DEEP VENOUS THROMBOSIS

In autopsy studies in which the lower venous tree was carefully dissected, early microscopic thrombi were found in the pockets of valve cusps, in saccules in the vein wall, and at vein junctions.[11] These were found in the deep veins of the pelvis, thigh, and calf. Six primary sites have been described: (1) the iliac vein, especially the external iliac vein; (2) the common femoral vein, including the medial and lateral circumflex tributaries and the termination of the superficial femoral vein; (3) the termination of the deep femoral vein, usually at a valve cusp at its ostium; (4) the popliteal vein, distal to the adductor ring and at a relatively large valve; (5) the posterior tibial veins; and (6) the intramuscular veins of the calf, particularly the soleal veins. Thrombosis at one site is independent of thrombosis elsewhere, and thrombi may arise in one or more places. Thrombi occur bilaterally, though the location and distribution in the two limbs may differ. Thrombi in calf veins are the most frequent and often the first manifestation of deep venous thrombosis.[12] There is evidence to suggest that independent thigh vein thrombi form later.[11, 12]

Extensive study of the leg veins at autopsy is not routinely done. The minimum study performed by most pathologists is to externally push on the veins of the thigh to "milk" blood back through the transected iliac vein. The flow of blood is observed to determine if the blood flows freely, is obstructed, or contains thrombi. If obstruction and/or thrombi are seen, dissection of the veins may be done. However, in some areas of the United States, special permission must be obtained from the family to perform any dissection of the limbs at autopsy. Local practice of pathology in other areas of the country is less restrained, and if the permission for the autopsy is unrestricted, dissection of leg veins will proceed as indicated. The usual approach involves exploration of the iliacs from within the pelvis, the femorals from an anterior incision at the femoral triangle, and the popliteal from a longitudinal incision through the popliteal fossa. If thrombi are not found at these sites and there is reason to continue to search, the entire length of the venous system can be exposed. In addition to grossly searching for thrombi, samples of veins are taken for histologic study.

Many pulmonary emboli arise in thrombi within the large deep veins of the lower legs.[13] Although thrombi within veins of the calf muscles are most common, they are less likely to cause significant emboli. Similarly, thrombi in superficial varicose veins rarely embolize. Other sites of venous thrombosis, such as the veins of the periprostatic plexus, the broad ligaments, the periovarian veins, and the uterine veins, may embolize but in fact are very uncommon sites of origin of emboli.

Thrombi in the deep leg veins are usually red in color because of the large numbers of trapped red cells.[14, 15] The thrombi have a laminated structure both circumferentially and longitudinally. Figure 2–1 illustrates the

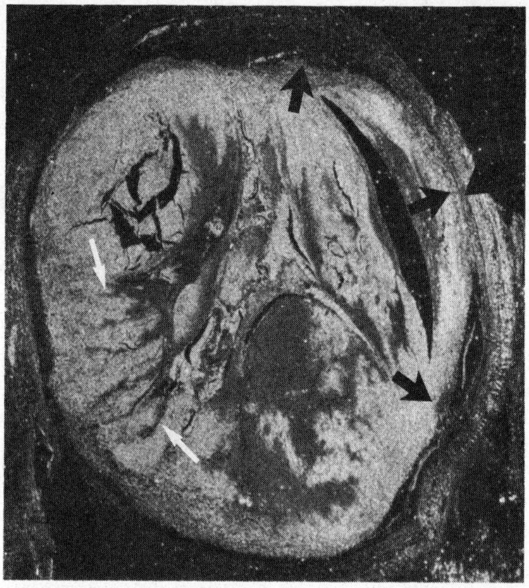

***Figure 2–1.*** Cross section of a recently formed thrombus in a leg vein. Attachment to the vein wall is visible in several areas (black arrows). A layered pattern of buildup of platelets and fibrin (light colored) and red cells (darker layers) can be seen (white arrows). Also note that in this vessel there appear to be three semicircular masses formed and extending from opposite walls of the vessel. Their appearance may be related to propagation of this thrombus from within venous valve cusps.

appearance of a cross section of a recently formed thrombus in a leg vein. This picture of the entire cross section of the vein shows attachment of the thrombus to the wall of the vein in several areas (black arrows). The large darker areas are red cells and the linear dark streaks are layers of red cells. This lamination (white arrows) of fibrin, platelets, and red cells is indicative of clot formation in a vessel with some flow. The overall arrangement of this thrombus suggests agglomeration of three semicircular propagations. It is possible that these began within the valves of the vein and propagated longitudinally. This could account for the somewhat segmented, rather than circumferentially laminated, appearance. Attachment to the wall by granulation tissue as well as the laminar arrangement of red cells, fibrin, and platelets can be better appreciated in the microscopic pictures in Figure 2–2*A*, *B*, *C*. Figure 2–2*A* illustrates a typical recently formed venous thrombus. The wall of the vein is defined by the two black arrows. The endothelium is continuous with newly formed granulation tissue composed of proliferating small vascular channels, connective tissue cells (fibroblasts), and intracellular matrix. The granulation tissue is continuous

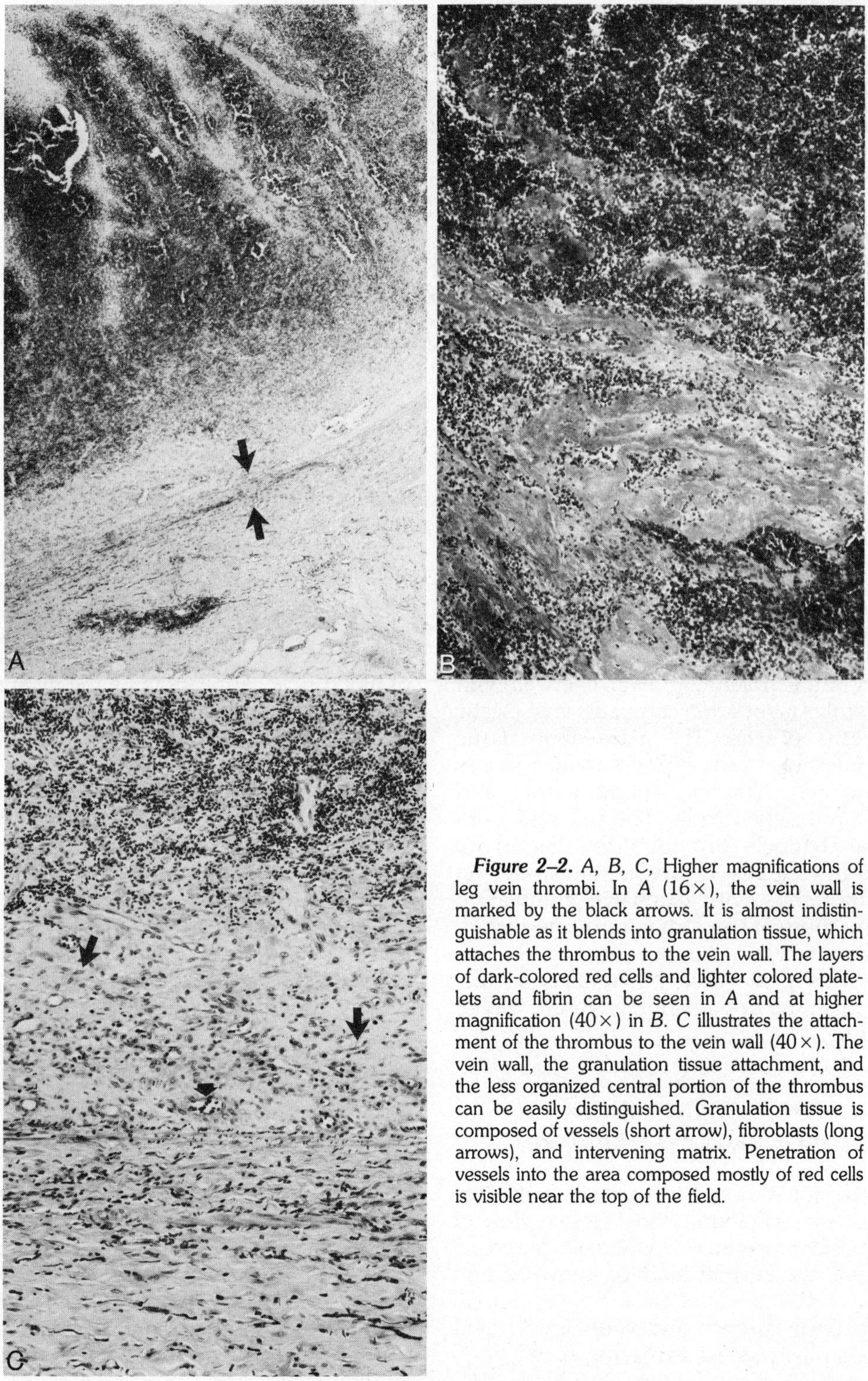


***Figure 2–2.*** *A, B, C,* Higher magnifications of leg vein thrombi. In *A* (16×), the vein wall is marked by the black arrows. It is almost indistinguishable as it blends into granulation tissue, which attaches the thrombus to the vein wall. The layers of dark-colored red cells and lighter colored platelets and fibrin can be seen in *A* and at higher magnification (40×) in *B. C* illustrates the attachment of the thrombus to the vein wall (40×). The vein wall, the granulation tissue attachment, and the less organized central portion of the thrombus can be easily distinguished. Granulation tissue is composed of vessels (short arrow), fibroblasts (long arrows), and intervening matrix. Penetration of vessels into the area composed mostly of red cells is visible near the top of the field.

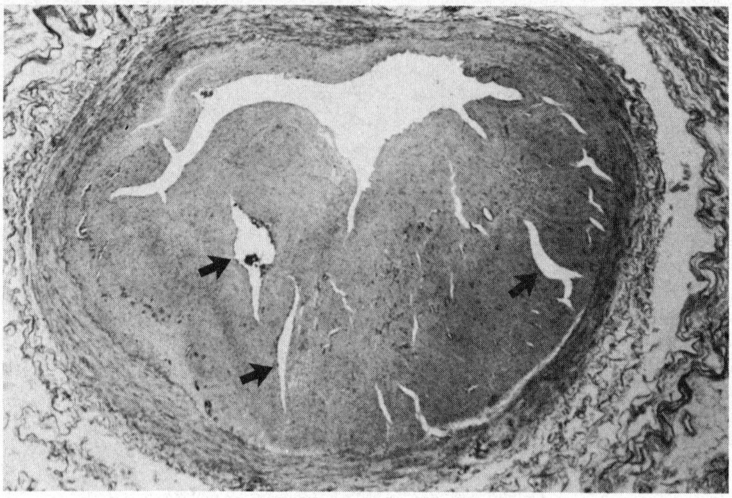

*Figure 2–3.* Cross section of an old venous thrombus. This thrombus is composed of granulation and fibrous tissue with recanalized smaller channels (arrows). A larger channel is present that may have been the original lumen but is more likely a large recanalized channel. The thrombus is attached to the wall around its entire circumference.

with the clot and forms the site of attachment to the wall. The lumen of the vessel is obliterated by the thrombus. The layers of red cells (dark areas) and layers of the more amorphous-appearing fibrin and platelets are easily distinguished. In Figure 2–2*B*, the appearance of the red cells and the fibrin layers can be seen. Figure 2–2*C* is a higher magnification of the attachment site. The wall with its muscular layer and scattered wavy elastic fibers can be seen. The granulation tissue with endothelial cells lining vascular spaces (short arrow), fibroblasts (long arrow), and matrix are easily visible. The red cells with vascular channels forming at the margin are also clearly visible. Figure 2–3 illustrates an older thrombus with extensive granulation tissue in most of the structure of the thrombus. Recanalized channels are visible (arrows). This clot would be unlikely to dislodge, given its firm anchorage to the wall of the vein.

## PATHOGENESIS OF THROMBOSIS—OVERVIEW

The pathogenesis of thrombosis is an area of active investigation. Here, an overview of thrombosis is presented, whereas Chapter 3 will detail the current state of knowledge in this area.

Thrombi in arteries and veins are formed by a complex process involving blood flow, blood vessel walls, platelets, the blood clotting system, and the fibrinolytic system. These factors are important in (1) the formation of a clot to stop blood loss after injury to a vessel, (2) thrombosis in atherosclerotic disease, and (3) venous thrombi. However, the relative importance of each differs in the three situations. Following injury, vasoconstriction occurs and reduces blood loss. Although vasoconstriction does not appear to play a role in venous thrombosis, the change in normal blood flow, i.e., stasis or slowing of blood flow, appears to be the most important factor in the genesis of venous thrombi.[2, 14] An injury usually involves the blood vessel wall and especially the endothelial cells. It exposes thrombogenic subendothelial connective tissue[16] and results in adherence, activation, and aggregation of platelets.[17] However, in venous thrombosis, the role of endothelial injury appears to be minor.[14] Following vascular injury, the plasma coagulation sequence is activated by release of tissue factors as well as by the release of platelet factors.[18] Prostaglandin and derivatives are synthesized by endothelial cells and platelets, and act to control the hemostatic sequence.[9] The production of a permanent hemostatic plug results from the combined activities of endothelial cells, platelets, and the coagulation sequence. The clotting system also appears to play a very important role in venous thrombosis. There is evidence that the intrinsic coagulation sequence may become activated in sites of marked stasis.[20] Hypercoagulability may be involved in the development of some venous thrombi,[21] especially those in patients with abdominal cancers as was first noted by Trousseau.[22] All the preceding factors, which tend toward thrombosis, are balanced to some extent by the fibrinolytic system.[23] Evidence for the roles of blood vessel walls, platelets, coagulation, stasis, and fibrinolysis will be highlighted in the following paragraphs.

**Blood Vessel Walls.** The endothelial lining of all blood vessels resists thrombosis by a number of mechanisms. The luminal surface of the endothelium is covered by an endocapillary layer, the glycocalyx. The glycocalyx is composed of glycoproteins, glycolipids, membrane-associated polysaccharides, and glycosaminoglycans, including heparan sulfate and sialic acid residues. Heparan sulfate has structural similarities to the anticoagulant heparin and may inhibit blood clotting.[24] An alpha-2 macroglobulin protease is also associated with the vascular lining. It inhibits the antiproteases in the coagulation sequence and hence activation of clotting factors in that sequence. Endothelial cells also synthesize plasminogen activators and inhibitors, which favor fibrinolytic activity in the blood, clear fibrin deposits from the endothelial surface, and participate in the resolution of intravascular thrombi.[25] In addition to actions in the coagulation sequence, endothelial cells also inhibit platelet aggregation. Proaggregating adenosine diphosphate (ADP) released from platelets is converted to adenine nucleotide platelet inhibitors by endothelial cells.[26] Endothelial cells actively synthesize prostacyclin, $PGI_2$, which blocks aggregation of platelets.[27, 28]

Despite this large armamentarium to resist thrombosis, the endothelial cell can also promote thrombosis. The extrinsic clotting pathway can be activated by thromboplastin, which is present in latent form in endothelium and may be released by endothelial cell injury.[29] Endothelial cells also synthesize and secrete von Willebrand's factor, which is a component of the coagulant factor VIII.[30] Von Willebrand's factor is necessary for adherence of platelets to subendothelial components.[31] Endothelial cells synthesize basement membrane collagen, fibrillar collagen, elastin, glycosaminoglycans, and fibronectin. These are deposited to form the subendothelial connective tissues, which are highly thrombogenic. Fibrillar collagen appears to be most important in providing a substrate for attachment and activation of platelets[32] and for activation of clotting factors in the extrinsic pathway of blood coagulation. Fibronectin stabilizes cell-to-cell and cell-to-substrate attachments in the normal endothelial lining, is cross-linked to fibrin, and facilitates anchorage of hemostatic plugs.[33] Thus, damage to endothelial cells exposes the thrombogenic subendothelium, which initiates thrombosis.

Although evidence of platelet aggregation at sites of minimal venous endothelial injury has been reported,[34] others have studied newly formed thrombi in femoral veins and found no evidence of underlying endothelial damage.[14] When a small electric charge was used to minimally injure the endothelium of veins, it was found that fibrin was deposited first on the endothelial surface, followed by platelets. Subendothelial elements were not necessary.[35] Malone[36] has suggested that endothelium in areas of stasis could be damaged by impaired nutrition or hypoxia. On balance, however, it appears that the venous endothelium functions to protect against thrombosis, and data strongly supporting a role for endothelial injury in the formation of venous thrombi have not yet been obtained.

**Platelets.** Platelets play a central role in blood clotting and thrombosis.[37] At sites of endothelial injury, "platelet activation" occurs, which includes: (1) adhesion and shape transformation, (2) release reaction, and (3) aggregation. Platelets adhere to sites of endothelial cell injury where subendothelial elements, particularly fibrillar collagen, are exposed. They attach by long pseudopods but then spread broadly to become tightly adherent. The shape changes are mediated by intraplatelet actomyosin microfilaments and microtubules.[38]

The release reaction empties the contents of platelet granules and follows soon after adhesion. Platelets have two major types of granules—alpha granules and dense bodies.[39] Alpha granules contain fibrinogen, fibronectin, platelet growth factor, antiheparin (platelet factor 4), cationic proteins, and beta-thromboglobulin. Beta-thromboglobulin may inhibit $PGI_2$ production and is used as an indicator of platelet activation.[40] Dense bodies contain adenosine diphosphate (ADP), ionized calcium, histamine, epinephrine, and serotonin. Calcium is necessary in the coagulation sequence, and ADP mediates platelet aggregation. With platelet activation, a phospholipid complex (platelet factor 3) appears on the platelet surface and provides a site on that surface where coagulation factors X and V and $Ca^{++}$ can bind to activate factor X.[18, 41] Platelet activation, therefore, contributes to the intrinsic pathway of blood clotting and the formation of thrombin.

Platelet aggregation closely follows platelet adherence and activation. Aggregation is promoted by the formation of thromboxane ($TxA_2$) by activated platelets.[42, 43] The adherent and activated platelets also release ADP, which initiates an autocatalytic reaction to build up the platelet aggregate. The activation of the coagulation sequence through the mediation of platelet factor 3 generates thrombin, a platelet agonist. The combination of thrombin, ADP released from platelets, and $TxA_2$ synthesized by the platelets induces platelet contraction, which creates a fused mass of platelets constituting a definitive hemostatic plug. By this time, fibrin is formed to further stabilize the plug and anchor it via fibronectin to its site of origin.[33]

When endothelial damage precedes venous thrombosis, the platelet activity previously outlined is likely to follow. Similar mechanisms may occur in the formation of platelet aggregates found in venous valve pockets. It is clear that platelets are part of the laminated structure of venous thrombi.

**Blood Clotting System.** The coagulation system, a major contributor to the hemostatic process and also to thrombus formation, will be discussed in detail in the following chapter. The conversion of prothrombin (factor II) to thrombin (factor IIa) is important. Thrombin contributes to the aggregation of platelets and simultaneously converts fibrinogen to fibrin.[44] Thrombin is generated via the intrinsic and extrinsic pathways. In the intrinsic pathway, factor XII (Hageman factor) is activated and converted to a proteolytic enzyme, factor XIIa. Activation of factor XII occurs when fluid blood "contacts" almost any surface except normal endothelium. Within a blood vessel, a platelet aggregate can initiate activation. Additionally, there is conversion of prekallikrein into kallikrein, which participates in a positive feedback loop activating more factor XII.[45] Factor XIIa can also activate the complement system by cleaving the C'1,2,4 and C'3 components. Thus, different but interrelated systems are set in motion with the conversion of factor XII to its activated form. With the formation of factor XIIa, the cascade goes on to the development of factor Xa.

The extrinsic pathway is initiated by a lipoprotein normally present on the surface of most cells, including endothelial cells.[29] This "tissue factor" forms a complex with factor VII that interacts with factor X to form factor Xa.[46] As the two separate pathways of blood clotting converge, prothrombin is converted to thrombin.

The role of the clotting system in the development of venous thrombi has been studied experimentally by Wessler in isolated venous segments.[47] By infusing serum, then causing stasis in the segment, a thrombus was formed. In other studies, Hageman factor,[48] long-chain saturated fatty acids,[49] and endotoxin[50] produced thrombi. The activated forms of factors XII, XI, and IX[51] as well as X[52] were found to be important.

Hypercoagulability has been proposed to explain venous thrombosis in some situations.[21] In patients with abdominal cancers, such as those of the pancreas, a well-defined predisposition to phlebothromboses was first noted by Trousseau.[22] Although the origin of the hypercoagulable state is still poorly understood, a number of procoagulant factors have been identified in cancer cells that could be released into the blood to initiate coagulation.[53] These include tissue factor (analogous to that activating the extrinsic pathway of coagulation); cancer procoagulant A, which activates clotting factor X; and other procoagulants released from tumor cells along with shed plasma membrane vesicles. The best established hypercoagulable state is a genetic deficiency of antithrombin III[54] (see also Chapter 9). Several kindreds have been identified with blood levels of antithrombin III approximately 50 per cent below the normal range. Leg vein thromboses were extremely common in these people.[55, 56]

**Fibrinolysis.** The fibrinolytic system provides an important mechanism for the dissolution of fibrin clots. Several components have been defined, including the precursor plasminogen, plasminogen activators, antiactivators (which block formation of plasmin), and antiplasmins (which inhibit already formed plasmin).[57] Plasminogen, a beta-globulin present in plasma, can be converted to plasmin by factor XIIa or by plasminogen activators within endothelial cells released with cell damage. Plasmin is a proteolytic enzyme that splits fibrin and fibrinogen, thereby delaying the polymerization of fibrin and resulting in a poorly formed fibrin clot.[58] Plasmin also lyses factors V and VIII. Systems are present that block the formation and action of plasmin. The major blocker of plasmin formation is alpha-2 plasmin inhibitor, an antiactivator. Other antiplasmins are alpha-2 macroglobulins, alpha-1 antitrypsin, and a fast reacting alpha-1 globulin—the most potent of the three.[57] Any lack of fibrinolytic function is an important predisposition to thrombosis. The inhibition of activated factor IX by antithrombin III in the presence of exogenous heparin may be the critical reaction in the prevention of venous thrombosis.

**Understanding Venous Thrombosis.** The important roles of stasis, endothelial injury, the coagulation system, platelets, and hypercoagulability in the pathogenesis of venous thrombosis were first proposed many years ago. The continued definition of factors and cofactors in these complex processes will enhance our understanding and hopefully will provide additional sites for therapeutic intervention.

## PATHOLOGY OF PULMONARY EMBOLUS ARISING IN VENOUS THROMBI

When venous thrombi dislodge from their site of formation, they flow with the blood through the venous system to the pulmonary arterial circulation. If the embolus is extremely large, it can stop at the bifurcation of the pulmonary artery, forming a "saddle embolus" as illustrated in Figure 2–4. More commonly, a major pulmonary vessel is occluded, as shown in Figure 2–5. In this illustration, the dark color of the embolus can be seen, as well as the indentations in the surface (arrows), which are thought to represent impressions of the venous valves of the leg veins. This patient died very soon after embolization; therefore, there is minimal attachment to the vessel wall.

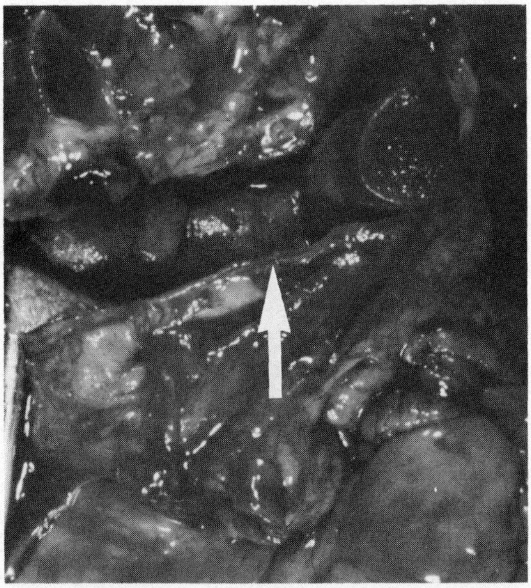

***Figure 2–4.*** Saddle embolus at the bifurcation of the pulmonary artery.

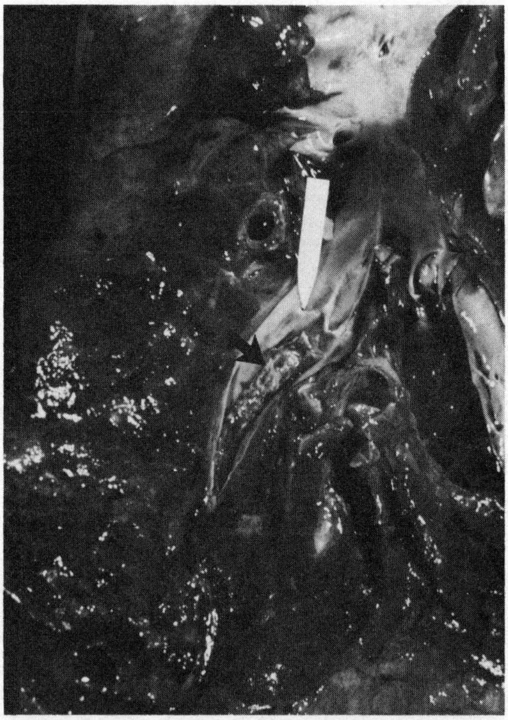

***Figure 2–6.*** Pulmonary embolus in an artery about 5 mm in diameter. This embolus is attached to the wall and has a light-colored surface of granulation tissue.

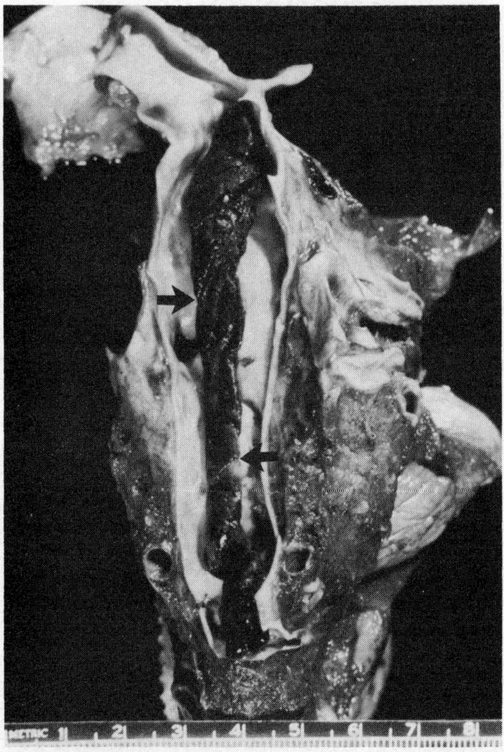


***Figure 2–5.*** Pulmonary embolus in the left lower lobe pulmonary artery. The embolus was dark red, typical of venous thrombi, and had indentations that are thought to represent impressions of the venous valves (arrows). There is minimal attachment to the wall of the pulmonary artery.

The embolus illustrated in Figure 2–6 is in a subsegmental artery of the lower lobe. The majority of emboli lodge in the lower lobes, particularly in the posterior basal and apical segments of these lobes.[60, 61] Two reasons have been suggested to account for this distribution: (1) much greater blood flow through the lower portions of the lungs, and (2) termination of the main axial arteries supplying the lower lobes in these segments.[61, 62] Emboli are also more common to the right than to the left lung. Again, perhaps this is related to blood flow patterns. The embolus shown in Figure 2–6 is adherent to the wall of the artery and has granulation tissue on its visible aspect (black arrow).

Figure 2–7 illustrates a histologic section of a recent embolus in a midsized pulmonary artery. There is minimal attachment, and it has the typical laminated structure with numerous red cells found in venous thrombi. Acute pulmonary emboli must be differentiated from postmortem clots by the pathologist. Postmortem clots can be red or yellow. Yellow clots, often called "chicken fat" clots,

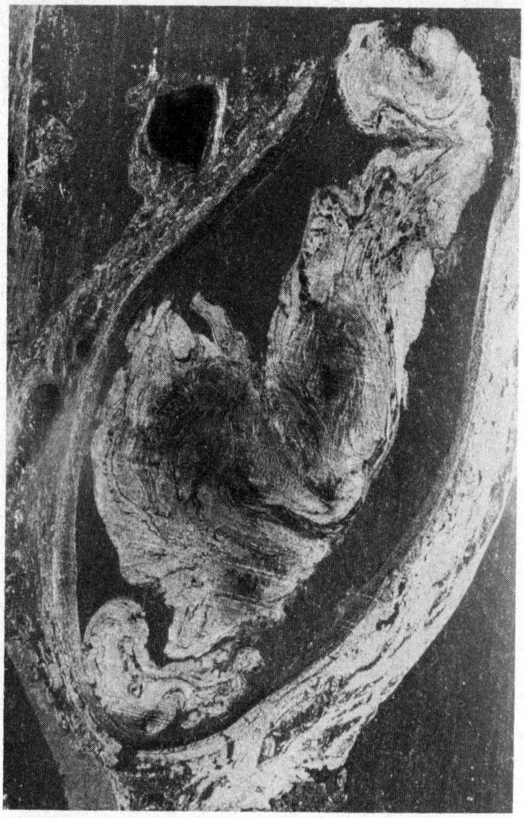

*Figure 2–7.* Histologic section of a recent embolus in a pulmonary artery. There is minimal attachment to the wall, and folding or coiling of the thrombus can be appreciated. Lamination in the structure can also be seen and there are large dark areas of red cells.

lack red cells and are easily distinguished. Red clots, if postmortem, are very soft and rubbery with no lamination of constituents. Emboli have lamination, a granular surface, and a firm consistency; are often coiled in place, indicating displacement from the leg veins; and have branch and/or valve markings, indicating organization or attachment to the pulmonary artery wall.[63] Soon after embolization into the lungs, thrombi become coated with a layer of platelets and fibrin. Elevated fibrin degradation products may be found in the blood.[64] The blood coagulation sequence is activated by the pulmonary embolic process, and thrombin is formed both locally and in the circulation.

Emboli may undergo complete lysis, extend or migrate distally, or organize to form webs or scars in the vessel. Evidence for complete or partial lysis and migration of emboli is based on angiographic data.[65, 66] Based on pathologic studies, nonfatal pulmonary emboli have been known to undergo a healing process by organization.[67] Following the initial fibrin coating described above, connective tissue cells (such as fibroblasts and perhaps smooth muscle cells) and inflammatory cells extend from the endothelium into the embolus and attach the embolus to the site of impaction. The pathogenetic factors of this process have not been specifically studied, but it is likely that some endothelial damage is caused by impaction of the embolus. This endothelial damage initiates many of the factors discussed earlier, resulting in a localized inflammatory reaction.

This pattern of healing is illustrated in Figure 2–8*A, B, C.* The progression from organization and early recanalization to band formation and finally a "web" is seen. This progression from acute embolus to a weblike scar in the vessel lumen was first described in 1962.[67]

## PATHOPHYSIOLOGY OF PULMONARY EMBOLI

The occlusion of more than one third of the major pulmonary arterial flow has been associated with acute right ventricular failure and sudden death.[68] A large embolus in the main pulmonary artery or its primary division into right and left branches may cause sudden death. Emboli to lobar or segmental arteries may be associated with reflex or humoral vasoconstriction and bronchoconstriction[69–73] (see also Chapter 16). Small emboli are less likely to cause sudden death. They travel out into the more peripheral areas of the lung where they may cause no apparent pulmonary parenchymal change or pulmonary hemorrhages or infarcts.[65] The number of emboli are of importance because all contribute to the extent of embolic obstruction.

The cardiac and pulmonary status of the patient prior to embolism will determine the outcome. The occlusion of a pulmonary vessel results in acute mechanical obstruction of blood flow, neurohumorally-mediated vasoconstriction, and bronchoconstriction. If the right ventricle cannot cope with this acute increase in resistance, right ventricular failure ensues. How well the right ventricle deals

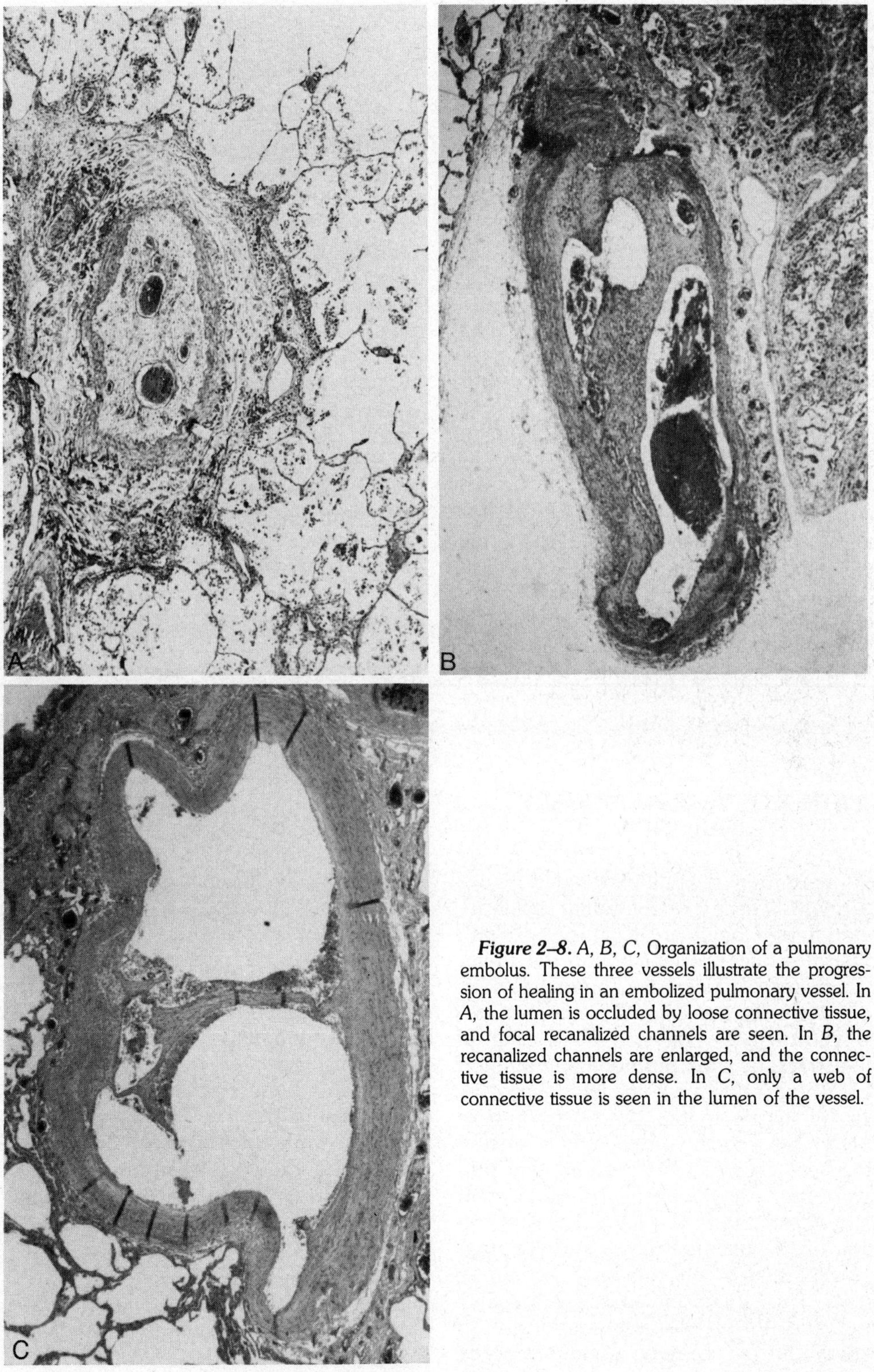


***Figure 2–8.*** *A, B, C,* Organization of a pulmonary embolus. These three vessels illustrate the progression of healing in an embolized pulmonary vessel. In *A,* the lumen is occluded by loose connective tissue, and focal recanalized channels are seen. In *B,* the recanalized channels are enlarged, and the connective tissue is more dense. In *C,* only a web of connective tissue is seen in the lumen of the vessel.

with this increased load is determined by the status of the heart before the embolism occurred. A small embolus in a patient with compromised pulmonary reserve may be fatal.

Similarly, the cardiopulmonary status of the patient influences the likelihood of developing a pulmonary infarction. The important determinants are the size of the vessel occluded, the adequacy of the bronchial circulation, and the patency of the air space. When large central arteries are occluded, infarction is less likely.[74] Apparently, with large emboli, collateral blood flow via the bronchial arteries is preserved and bronchoconstriction is not sufficiently severe to cause local hypoxia. However, with occlusion of smaller arteries, infarction is more likely to occur. This likelihood is increased if there is additional compromise of the air space by preexisting pulmonary edema, infection, or some other pathologic process.

The persistence of the occlusion is also related to prognosis. Sequential angiographic studies have shown that within 24 hours, flow begins to improve and may be completely reestablished in 7 to 30 days. This is usually attributed to fibrinolytic resolution.[66] If resolution does not occur, the embolus will undergo organization as described previously.

## PATHOLOGY OF PULMONARY INFARCTION

Pulmonary infarcts are illustrated in Figure 2–9 (arrows). These are triangular, well-demarcated hemorrhagic areas. This case again demonstrates the propensity for the lower lobe. Pulmonary infarcts are hemorrhagic, as illustrated in Figure 2–10. This infarct occurred within a few days of death. Figure 2–11 illustrates a later pulmonary infarction in which resorption of some blood has occurred, the tissue in the central portion of the infarct has broken down, and a pleural reaction has occurred. The pathology of pulmonary infarcts has been described in great detail by Castleman.[9, 76] Infarcts heal by resorption of the necrotic tissue and scarring. A linear scar is often the only remaining evidence of an infarction. These scars may be small and not visible radiographically. In one study, 50 per cent of angiographically proven pulmonary infarcts had no residual radiographic findings.[77]

## PATHOLOGY OF PULMONARY EMBOLI OF EXTRAVASCULAR ORIGIN

Although we have focused on thrombi formed in the deep veins as the source of most pulmonary emboli, emboli of extravascular origin also occur (Chapter 11). These include malignant cells,[78] air,[79] fat,[80] bone marrow,[81] amniotic fluid,[82] tissues from sites of injury,[83] parasites,[84] and foreign materials.[85] Tumor emboli are illustrated in Figure 2–12. These may be composed entirely of tumor cells (Fig. 2–12*A*) or fibrous tissue with a few scattered tumor cells (Fig. 2–12*D*). Figure 2–12*B* illustrates tumor emboli enmeshed in large amounts of fibrin. This fibrin–tumor cell complex attaches to the endothelium, and the process of organization begins (Fig. 2–12*C*). It is well known that tumor cells can induce a fibrous tissue response, often referred to as the desmoplastic response to malignancy. In the pulmonary vessels, this desmoplastic response also seems to take place, because there is often far more fibrous reaction than tumor.[78] This progression could also represent the natural evolution of an intravascular occlusion as described earlier for emboli arising in venous thrombi.

The reaction pattern to foreign material injected into the venous system and then lodged in the lung is somewhat different. Figure 2–13 illustrates the foreign body giant cell reaction to talc (Fig. 2–13*A*) in an intravenous drug user's lung and to hair (Fig. 2–13*B*) in the lung of a patient with fever of unknown origin. This patient with fever had been injecting herself with excreta to produce the fever.

Fat and bone marrow emboli may occur with skeletal trauma. However, they are usually incidental postmortem findings related to cardiopulmonary resuscitation efforts. A bone marrow embolus from a patient with multiple myeloma is illustrated in Figure 2–14.

Acknowledgment: The contribution and advice of Dr. Stanley L. Robbins in the organization and preparation of this chapter is gratefully acknowledged.

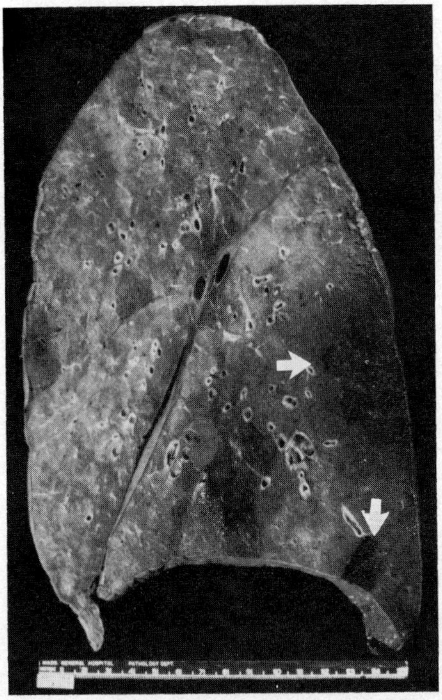

***Figure 2–9.*** Multiple pulmonary infarcts. Pulmonary infarcts are hemorrhagic wedge-shaped areas extending to the pleura.

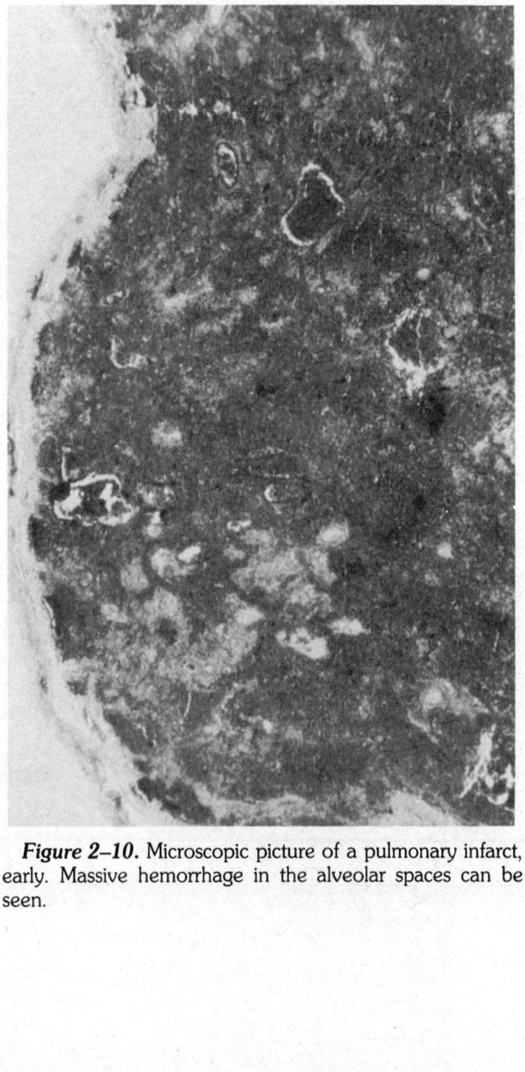

***Figure 2–10.*** Microscopic picture of a pulmonary infarct, early. Massive hemorrhage in the alveolar spaces can be seen.

***Figure 2–11.*** Microscopic picture of a pulmonary infarct at a later stage. There is breakdown of the alveolar tissue and red cells, and organization extending from the pleural surface.

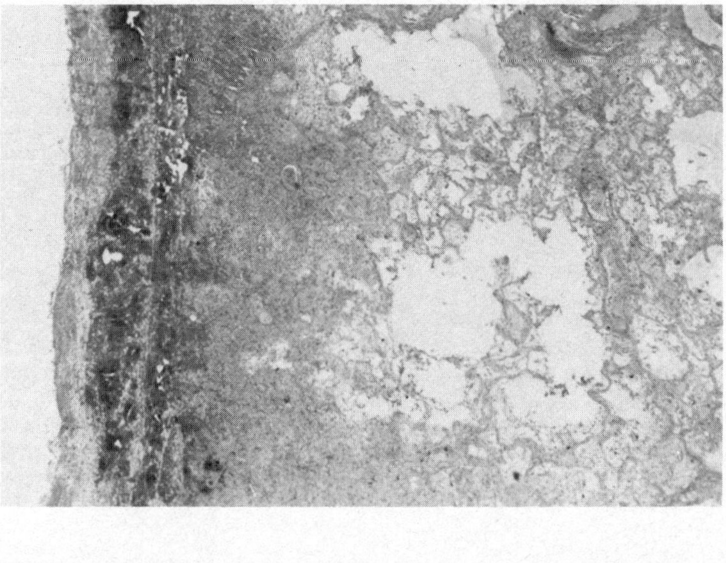

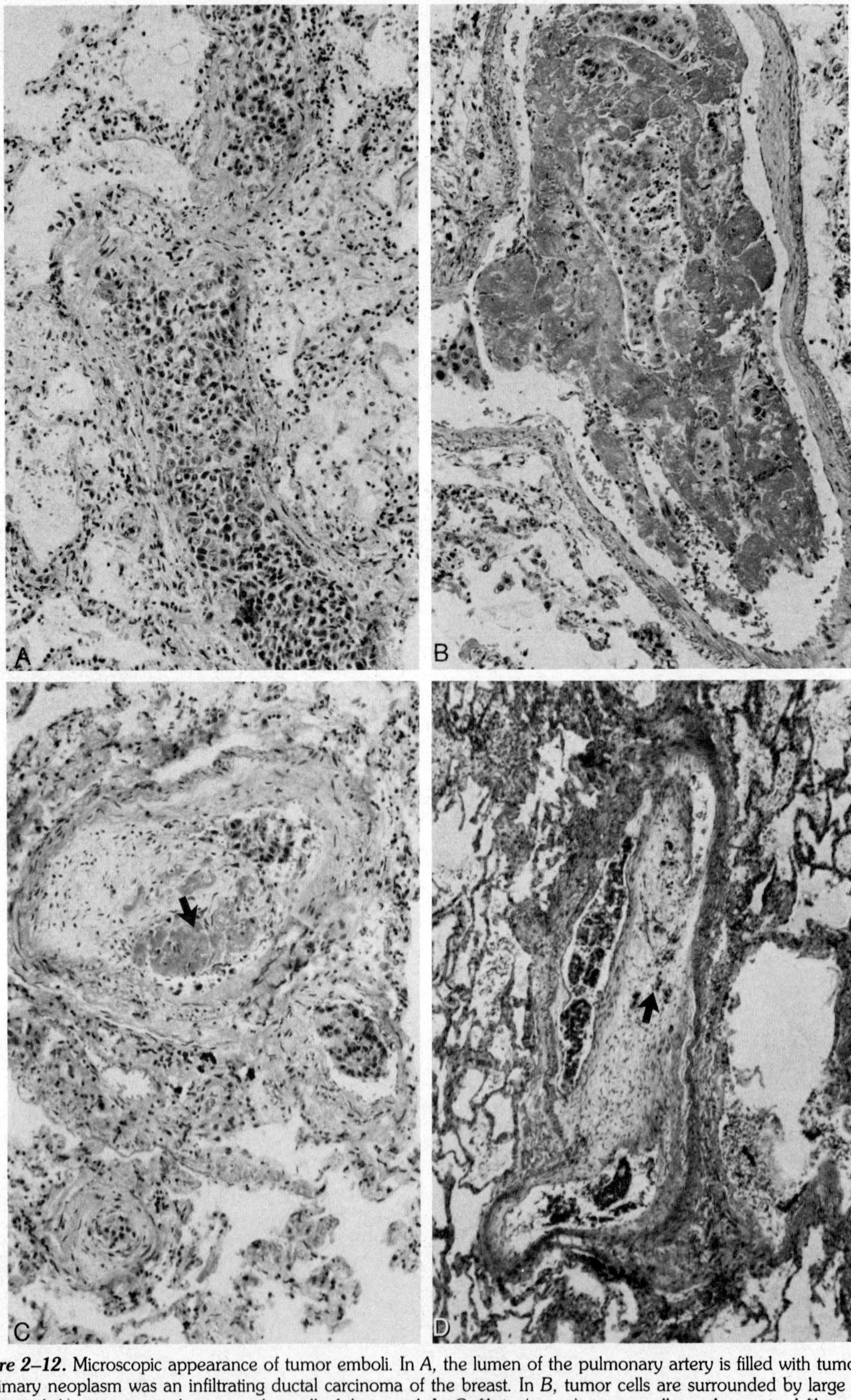

***Figure 2–12.*** Microscopic appearance of tumor emboli. In *A,* the lumen of the pulmonary artery is filled with tumor cells. The primary neoplasm was an infiltrating ductal carcinoma of the breast. In *B,* tumor cells are surrounded by large masses of fibrin, and there is no attachment to the wall of the vessel. In *C,* fibrin (arrow), tumor cells, and organized fibrous tissue that is attached to the vessel wall are all seen in the vessel lumen. Other smaller vessels in this picture have tumor cells alone filling their lumina. In *D,* tumor cells are scattered in dense intravascular fibrous tissue in the vessel lumen (arrow). There are also large recanalized channels filled with tumor cells.

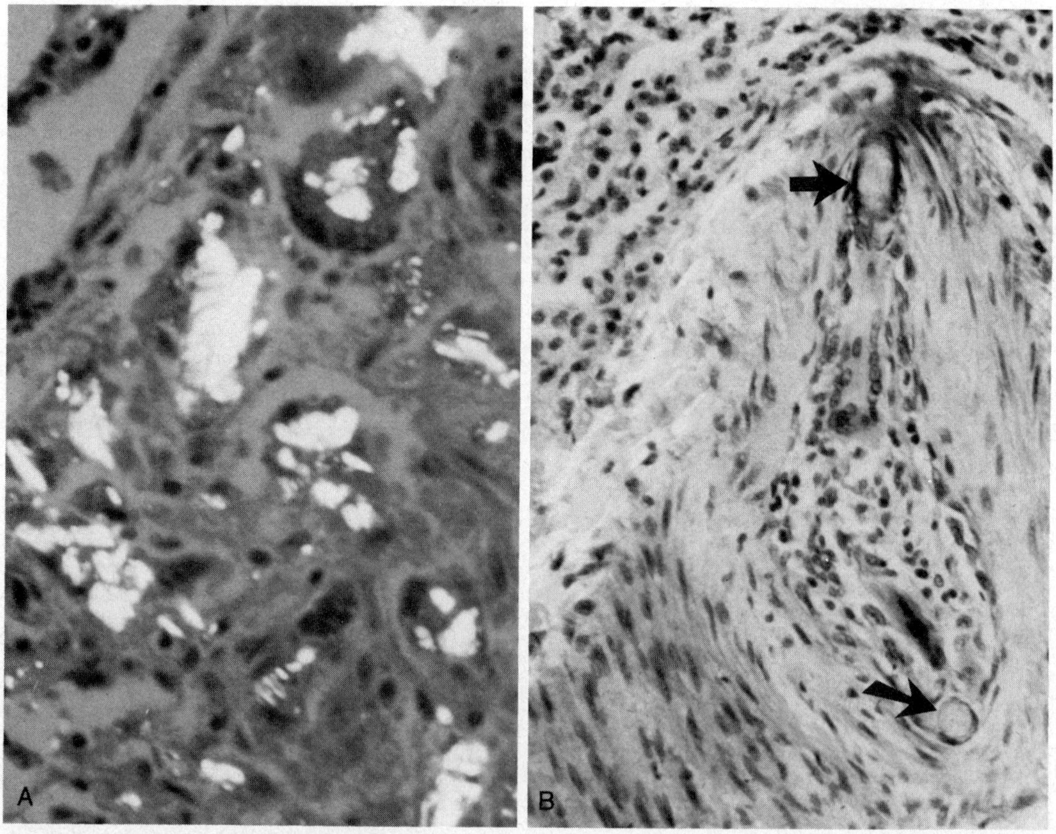


***Figure 2–13.*** Microscopic pictures of foreign material in the pulmonary vasculature. In *A*, there is extensive deposition of talc and other crystalline debris in the pulmonary vessels of a heroin addict. This photograph was taken with polarized light to highlight the foreign material. In *B*, a hair is seen in a pulmonary vessel of a patient with fever of unknown origin. The hair and other debris suggested that the patient was injecting foreign material into her vasculature. A foreign body giant cell reaction is present in the vessel lumen.

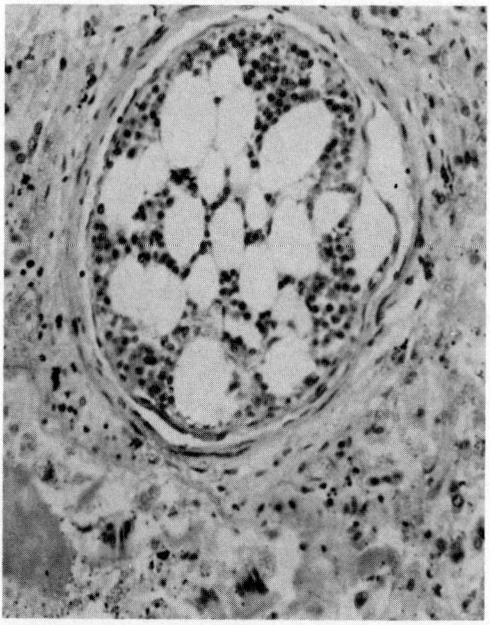

***Figure 2–14.*** Microscopic bone marrow embolus. Bone marrow fills the lumen of this pulmonary vessel. The marrow is filled with plasma cells in this patient with multiple myeloma. (Courtesy Dr. B. Berger.)

## REFERENCES

1. Liebow, A. A.: Cardiopulmonary Disease. *In* Gould, S. E. (Ed.): Pathology of the Heart, 2nd ed. Charles C Thomas Publishers, Springfield, IL, 1960, p. 958.
2. Virchow, R.: Gesammelte Abhandlungen zur Wissenschaftlichen Medizin. Von Meidinger Sohn, Frankfort-am-Main, 1856.
3. Cohnheim, J.: Lectures on General Pathology. Translated by A. B. McKee, New Sydenham Society, London, *1*:172, 1889.
4. Ribbert, H.: Ueber die Thrombose. Deutsche Med. Wchnschr., *38*:1577, 1912.
5. Dawbarn, R. Y., Earlam, F., and Evans, W. H.: The relation of the blood platelets to thrombosis after operation and parturition. J. Path. Bact., *31*:833, 1928.
6. Welch, W. H.: Venous thrombosis as a complication of cardiac disease. Jacobi Festschrift. Knickerbocker Press, New York, 1900, p. 463.
7. Rosenthal, S. R.: Thrombosis and fatal pulmonary embolism. Arch. Path., *14*:215, 1932.
8. Belt, T. H.: Thrombosis and pulmonary embolism. Am. J. Path., *10*:129, 1934.
9. Hampton, A. O., and Castleman, B.: Correlation of post mortem chest teleroentgenograms with autopsy findings with special reference to pulmonary embolism and infarction. AJR, *43*:305, 1940.
10. Owen, W. R., Thomas, W. A., Castleman, B., et al.:

Unrecognized emboli to the lungs with subsequent cor pulmonale. N. Engl. J. Med., *249*:919, 1953.
11. Sevitt, S.: Pathology and Pathogenesis of Deep Vein Thrombi. *In* Moser, K. M., and Stein, M. (Eds.): Pulmonary Thromboembolism. Year Book Medical Publishers, Chicago, 1973, p. 93.
12. Thomas, M. L., and O'Dwyer, J. A.: Site of origin of deep vein thrombosis in the calf. Acta Radiol. [Diagn.], *18*:418, 1977.
13. Sevitt, S., and Gallagher, N. G.: Venous thrombosis and pulmonary embolism. A clinicopathological study in injured and burned patients. Br. J. Surg., *48*:475, 1961.
14. Sevitt, S.: The structure and growth of valve pocket thrombi in femoral veins. J. Clin. Pathol., *27*:517, 1974.
15. Sevitt, S.: Organization of valve pocket thrombi and the anomalies of double thrombi and valve cusp involvement. Br. J. Surg., *61*:641, 1974.
16. Jamieson, G. A., Urban, C. L., and Barber, A. J.: Enzymatic basis for platelet-collagen adhesion as the primary step in haemostasis. Nature (New Biol.), *234*:5, 1971.
17. Shattil, S. J., and Bennet, J.: Platelets in hemostasis. Ann. Intern. Med., *94*:108, 1981.
18. Zwaal, R. F. A.: Membrane and lipid involvement in blood coagulation. Biochim. Biophys. Acta, *515*:163, 1978.
19. Haslam, R. J., Davidson, M. M., Fox, J. E., et al.: Cyclic nucleotides in platelet function. Thromb. Haemost., *40*:232, 1978.
20. Deykin, D., and Wessler, S.: Activation product, factor IX, serum thrombotic accelerator activity and serum induced thrombosis. J. Clin. Invest., *43*:160, 1964.
21. Hirsh, J.: Hypercoagulability. Semin. Hematol., *14*:409, 1977.
22. Trousseau, A.: Phlegmasic alba dolens. Clinique Medicale de L'Hotel Dieu de Paris Balhiere, Paris, 1865, p. 94.
23. Robbins, K. C.: The human fibrinogenic system: regulation and control. Mol. Cell. Biochem., *20*:149, 1978.
24. Gamse, G., Fromme, H. G., and Kresse, H.: Metabolism of sulfated glycosaminoglycans in cultured endothelial cells and smooth muscle cells from bovine aorta. Biochim. Biophys. Acta, *544*:514, 1978.
25. Barlow, G. A., and Robbins, K. C.: Fibrinolytic Agents. *In* Colman, R. W., Hirsch, J., Marder, V. J., et al. (Eds): Hemostasis and Thrombosis. J. B. Lippincott, Philadelphia, 1982.
26. Pearson, J. D., and Gordon, J. L.: Vascular endothelial and smooth muscle cells in culture selectively release adenine nucleotides. Nature, *281*:384, 1979.
27. Moncada, S., Korbut, R., Bunting, S., et al.: Prostacyclin is a circulating hormone. Nature, *273*:767, 1978.
28. Curwin, K. D., Gimbrone, M. A., and Handin, R. I.: In vitro studies of thromboresistance: The role of $PGI_2$ in platelet adhesion in cultured normal and virtually transformed human vascular endothelial cells. Lab. Invest., *42*:366, 1980.
29. Maynard, J. R., Hechman, C. A., Pitlick, F. A., et al.: Association of tissue factor activity with the surface of cultured cells. J. Clin. Invest., *55*:814, 1975.
30. Jaffe, E. A., Hoyer, L. W., and Nachman, R. L.: Synthesis of antihemophilic factor antigen by cultured human endothelial cells. J. Clin. Invest., *52*:2757, 1973.
31. Tschopp, T. B., Weiss, H. J., and Baumgarten, H. R.: Decreased adhesion of platelets to subendothelium in Von Willebrand's disease. J. Lab. Clin. Med., *83*:296, 1974.
32. Stemerman, M. B.: Vascular intimal components: precursors of thrombosis. Prog. Hemost. Thromb., *2*:1, 1974.
33. Birdwell, C. R., Gospodarowicz, D., and Nicolson, G. L.: Identification, localization, and role of fibronectin in cultured bovine endothelial cells. Proc. Natl. Acad. Sci. (*USA*), *75*:3273, 1978.
34. Ashford, T. P., and Freiman, D. G.: Platelet aggregation at sites of minimal endothelial injury. Am. J. Pathol., *53*:599, 1968.
35. Day, T. K., Cowper, S. V., Kakkar, V. V., et al.: Early venous thrombosis. A scanning electronmicroscopic study. Thromb. Haemost. *37*:477, 1977.
36. Malone, P. C.: A hypothesis concerning the aetiology of venous thrombosis. Med. Hypotheses, *3*:189, 1977.
37. Weiss, H. J.: Platelet physiology and abnormalities of platelet function. N. Engl. J. Med., *293*:531, 1975.
38. Crawford, N.: Platelet Microfilaments and Microtubules. *In* Gordon, G. L. (Ed.): Platelets in Biology and Pathology. Elsevier-North Holland Press, Amsterdam, 1976, p. 121.
39. Holmsen, H., and Weiss, H. J.: Secretable storage pools in platelets. Ann. Rev. Med., *30*:119, 1979.
40. Hope, W., Martin, T. J., Chesterman, C. N., et al.: Human β-thromboglobulin inhibits $PGI_2$ production and binds to a specific site in bovine aortic endothelial cells. Nature, *282*:210, 1979.
41. Kane, W. H., Lindhout, M. J., Jackson, C. M., et al.: Factor Va dependent binding of factor Xa to human platelets. J. Biol. Chem., *255*:1170, 1980.
42. Olley, P. M., and Coceani, F.: The prostaglandins. Am. J. Dis. Child., *134*:688, 1980.
43. Moneada, S., and Vane, J. R.: Arachidonic acid metabolites and the interactions between platelets and blood vessel walls. N. Engl. J. Med., *300*:1142, 1979.
44. Mann, K. G., and Lundblad, R. L.: Biochemistry of Thrombin. *In* Colman, R. W., Hirsch, J., Marder, V. J., et al. (Eds.): Hemostasis and Thrombosis. J. B. Lippincott, Philadelphia, 1982, p. 112.
45. Colman, R. W.: Deficiencies of Factor XII and Prekallikrein and High Molecular Weight Kininogen. *In* Colman, R. W., Hirsch, J., Marder, V. J., et al. (Eds.): Hemostasis and Thrombosis. J. B. Lippincott, Philadelphia, 1982, p. 3.
46. Jesty, J., Spencer, A. K., and Nemerson, Y.: The mechanism of action of factor X. J. Biol. Chem., *249*:5614, 1974.
47. Wessler, S., Reimer, L., Freiman, D. G., et al.: Serum-induced thrombosis. Studies of its induction and evolution under controlled conditions in vivo. Circulation, *20*:864, 1959.
48. Botti, R. E., and Ratnoff, O. D.: Studies on the pathogenesis of thrombosis and experimental "hypercoagulable" state induced by the intravenous injection of ellagic acid. J. Lab. Clin. Med., *64*:385, 1964.
49. Connor, W. E., Hoak, J. C., and Warner, E. D.: Fatty Acids and Thrombus Formation. *In* Sasahara, A. A., and Stein, M. (Eds.): Pulmonary Embolic Disease. Grune and Stratton, New York, 1965, p. 50.
50. Thomas, D. P., and Wessler, S.: Stasis thrombi induced by bacterial endotoxin. Circ. Res., *14*:486, 1964.

51. Wessler, S.: Thrombosis in the presence of vascular stasis. Am. J. Med., *33*:648, 1962.
52. Wessler, S., and Yin, E. T.: Experimental hypercoagulable state induced by factor X: comparison of the non-activated and activated forms. J. Lab Clin. Med., *72*:256, 1960.
53. Dvorak, H. F.: Fibrin as a component of the tumor stroma: origins and biologic significance. Cancer Metastasis Reviews, *2*:41, 1983.
54. Stewart, G. J.: The role of hypercoagulability in thrombosis. Br. J. Haematol., *40*:359, 1978.
55. Egeberg, O.: Inherited antithrombin deficiency causing thrombophilia. Thromb. Haemost., *13*:516, 1965.
56. Marciniak, F., et al.: Familial thrombosis due to antithrombin III deficiency. Blood, *43*:209, 1974.
57. Aoki, N.: Natural inhibitors of fibrinolysis. Prog. Cardiovasc. Dis., *21*:267, 1979.
58. Weinstein, M. J., and Doolittle, R. F.: Differential specificities of thrombin, plasmin and trypsin with regard to synthetic and natural substrates and inhibitors. Biochim. Biophys. Acta, *258*:577, 1972.
59. Gitel, S. N., Stephenson, R. C., and Wessler, S.: In vitro and in vivo correlation of clotting protease activity: effect of heparin. Proc. Natl. Acad. Sci. (*USA*), *74*:3028, 1977.
60. Macleod, J. G., and Grant, I. W. B.: A clinical, radiographic and pathological study of pulmonary embolism. Thorax, *9*:71, 1954.
61. Pryce, D. M., and Heard, B. E.: The distribution of experimental pulmonary emboli in the rabbit. J. Path. Bact., *71*:15, 1956.
62. Spencer, H.: Pathology of the Lung, 3rd edition. W. B. Saunders, Philadelphia, 1977, p. 550.
63. Freiman, D. G., Suyemoto, J., and Wessler, S.: Frequency of pulmonary thromboembolism in man. N. Engl. J. Med., *272*:1278, 1965.
64. Cade, J. F., Hirsh, J., and Regoeczi, E.: Mechanisms for elevated fibrin/fibrinogen degradation products in acute experimental pulmonary embolism. Blood, *45*:563, 1975.
65. Dalen, J. E., and Alpert, J. S.: Natural history of pulmonary embolism. Prog. Cardiovasc. Dis., *17*:259, 1975.
66. Urokinase Pulmonary Embolism Trial. Circulation, *47*(Suppl. 2):7, 1973.
67. Korn, D., Gore, I., Blenke, A., et al.: Pulmonary arterial bands and webs: an unrecognized manifestation of organized pulmonary emboli. Am. J. Path., *40*:129, 1962.
68. Smith, G. T., Dammin, G. J., and Dexter, J.: Postmortem arteriographic studies of the human lung in pulmonary embolization. JAMA, *188*:135, 1964.
69. Severinghaus, J. W., Swenson, E. W., Finley, T., et al.: Unilateral hypoventilation produced by occlusion of one pulmonary artery. J. Appl. Physiol., *16*:53, 1961.
70. Gurewich, V., Cohen, J. L., and Thomas, D. P.: Humoral factors in massive pulmonary embolism: An experimental study. Am. Heart J., *76*:784, 1968.
71. Thomas, D., Stein, M., and Tanabe, G.: Mechanisms of bronchoconstriction produced by thromboemboli in dogs. Am. J. Physiol., *206*:1207, 1964.
72. Widdicombe, J. G.: Reflex Mechanisms in Pulmonary Thromboembolism. *In* Koser, K. M., and Stein, M. (Eds.): Pulmonary Thromboembolism. Year Book Medical Publishers, Chicago, 1973.
73. Levy, S. E., and Simmons, D. H.: Mechanism of arterial hypoxemia following pulmonary thromboembolism in dogs. J. Appl. Physiol., *39*:41, 1975.
74. Dalen, J. E., Haffajie, C. I., Alpert, J. S., et al.: Pulmonary embolism, hemorrhage and infarction. N. Engl. J. Med., *296*:1431, 1977.
75. Tsao, M. S., Schraufnagel, D., and Wang, N. S.: Pathogenesis of pulmonary infarction. Am. J. Med., *72*:599, 1982.
76. Castleman, B.: Healed pulmonary infarcts. Arch. Path., *30*:130, 1940.
77. McGoldrick, P. J., Rudd, T. G., Figley, M. M., et al.: What becomes of pulmonary infarcts. AJR, *133*:1039, 1979.
78. Winterbauer, R. H., Eldenbein, I. B., and Ball, W. C.: Incidence and clinical significance of tumor embolization to the lung. Am. J. Med., *45*:271, 1968.
79. Morgan, A. D.: The pathology of subacute cor pulmonale in diffuse carcinogenesis of the lungs. J. Pathol. Bacteriol., *61*:75, 1949.
80. Sevitt, S. S.: Fat Embolism. Butterworth, London, 1962.
81. Garvey, J. W., and Zak, F. G.: Pulmonary bone marrow emboli in patients receiving external cardiac massage. JAMA, *187*:59, 1964.
82. Attwood, H. D.: The histologic diagnosis of amniotic fluid embolism. J. Pathol. Bacteriol., *76*:211, 1958.
83. Moser, K. M.: Pulmonary Vascular Obstruction Due to Embolism and Thrombosis. *In* Moser, K. M. (Ed.): Pulmonary Vascular Diseases. Marcel Dekker, New York, 1979, p. 341.
84. Jawalurz, K. I., and Karpas, C. M.: Pulmonary schistosomiasis: A detailed clinicopathological study. Am. Rev. Respir. Dis., *88*:517, 1963.
85. Tomashefski, J. F., and Hirsch, C. S.: The pulmonary vascular lesions of intravenous drug abuse. Hum. Pathol., *11*:133, 1980.

CHAPTER 3

# REGULATION OF HEMOSTASIS

RICHARD B. STEAD, M.D.

The hemostatic system can be thought of not only in terms of the intrinsic and extrinsic pathways (forming the so-called coagulation cascade) but also more broadly as a dynamic interaction of four major components (Fig. 3–1): (1) the vessel wall, (2) the platelet, (3) the clotting cascade, and (4) the fibrinolytic system. Each of these components is controlled by regulatory elements that may favor clot formation or dissolution, depending on the surrounding physiologic conditions. The factors that determine the exact balance between clot formation (coagulation) and dissolution (fibrinolysis) are not completely understood. Indeed, the hemostatic system has historically been approached by asking the question, "What makes blood clot?," whereas the system may be better understood by asking, "What elements regulate and inhibit clotting to keep the blood fluid?" What follows is a brief description of our current understanding of the main components of the hemostatic system and their physiologic interactions and regulation.

## THE VESSEL WALL AND PLATELETS

Platelet–vessel wall interactions play an important role in this delicate balance. The vessel wall plays key roles in vasoconstriction, formation of the platelet plug, and regulation of coagulation and fibrinolysis. Vasoconstriction is a primary defense mechanism in vessel injury and is controlled by neural, humoral, and local mechanisms. Vasoconstriction may be enhanced by the local release of vasoactive substances from platelets, including serotonin and thromboxane-$A_2$ (Fig. 3–2).[1] Vasoconstriction serves to reduce blood flow and to reduce the area that must be occluded by the hemostatic plug. One of the initial events following vessel injury involves platelet adhesion to the damaged vessel wall. The mechanism of platelet adhesion is uncertain but probably involves platelet membrane receptors for a number of intrinsic platelet and vessel wall proteins. Von Willebrand's factor (VIII/vWF), the large, multimeric[36] portion of factor VIII, plays a critical role in adhesion[2, 3] (Fig. 3–2). In addition to its important role in platelet adhesion, VIII/vWF also serves as a carrier protein for factor VIII procoagulant (VIII-C), the antihemophilic factor.

Once platelet adhesion has occurred, the platelets undergo a complex set of morphologic and biochemical changes comprising the release reaction and *aggregation* (Fig. 3–3). This serves to recruit more platelets, form an initial platelet plug, and accelerate the fluid phase of coagulation to form thrombin. Thrombin, in addition to generating fibrin, is one of the most potent inducers (agonists) of platelet aggregation; platelet aggregation and thrombin formation thus form a positive feedback loop[4] (Fig. 3–3*D*). On aggregation, platelets release a host of platelet-active and vasoactive mediators (Fig. 3–3C). Dense granules release adenosine diphosphate (ADP), which itself induces aggregation and vasoactive substances, including serotonin. Alpha granules release platelet factor 4 ($PF_4$), a heparin-neutralizing protein of uncertain significance, beta-thromboglobulin (βTG) (function unknown), and platelet-derived growth factor—a stimulator of vascular smooth muscle and fibroblast growth believed to be of importance in vascular repair. Radioimmunoassays for $PF_4$ and βTG have been used as

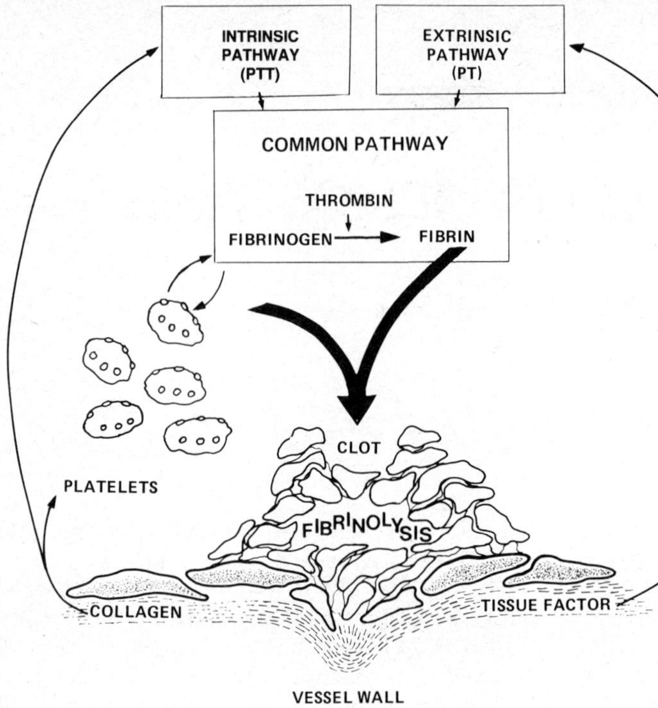


***Figure 3–1.*** Simplified scheme of the hemostatic system, showing interaction of vessel wall platelets, coagulation pathways, and fibrinolytic system. Not shown are regulatory and inhibitory mechanisms.

markers of in vivo platelet aggregation and release.[5] The regulation of aggregation and release at the biochemical level is not well understood but appears to involve rapid fluxes in platelet calcium concentration, which is modulated by levels of prostaglandins and thromboxane vis-à-vis cyclic AMP (cAMP).[6, 7]

## Arachidonic Acid Metabolism: Critical Differences Between Platelets and Endothelial Cells

Platelet agonists, such as thrombin, ADP, collagen, and epinephrine, all activate platelet arachidonic acid metabolism,[8] a crucial component of the aggregation mechanism. The agonists activate membrane-bound phospholipases to generate free arachidonic acid, the precursor of the prostaglandins and thromboxane (Fig. 3–4). Once formed, arachidonate is rapidly metabolized by the nonregenerable platelet enzyme *cyclooxygenase* to form unstable prostaglandin intermediates. Aspirin and other antiplatelet agents inhibit cyclooxygenase,[8, 9] thereby blocking one of the initial steps in prostaglandin and thromboxane production. Once formed in the platelet, the prostaglandin intermediates are converted to thromboxane-$A_2$ ($TxA_2$) by *thromboxane synthetase.* $TxA_2$ is one of the most potent platelet *aggregating agents* and *vasoconstrictors* known[10, 11] (see Fig. 3–2*D*). $TxA_2$ is rapidly degraded to a stable, inactive metabolic product, thromboxane-$B_2$ ($TxB_2$), which can be measured as a marker of platelet activation.

Endothelial cells also contain phospholipase and cyclooxygenase and form prostaglandins but do not contain thromboxane synthetase (Fig. 3–4). They contain the enzyme *prostacyclin synthetase* instead of $TxA_2$ synthetase and produce prostacyclin ($PGI_2$) as the end product. $PGI_2$ directly opposes the action of $TxA_2$; $PGI_2$ is a potent *vasodilator* and *antiaggregatory agent.*[12, 13] $PGI_2$ synthetase is found in the endothelium but not in the platelets. Thus, the end product of parallel metabolic pathways of arachidonate metabolism in the platelet and endothelium exerts opposite effects on platelet aggregation and on vascular smooth muscle (Fig. 3–4).

The physiologic implications of the balance between $TxA_2$ and $PGI_2$ are apparent; it may be possible to modify this balance to therapeutic advantage with antiplatelet agents.[37] Under normal circumstances, the platelet release and aggregation reaction is sustained by the positive feedback loops noted in Fig-

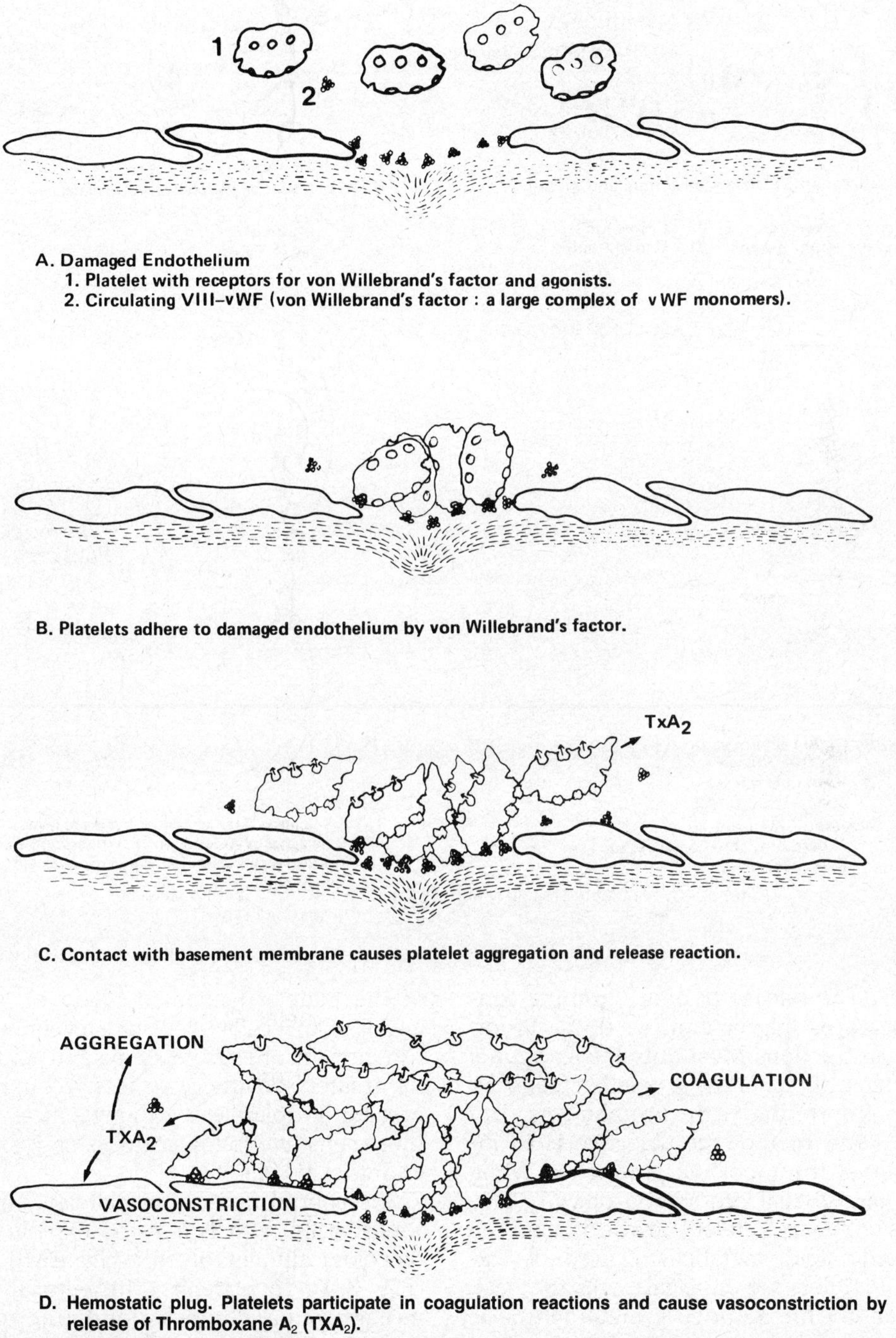


***Figure 3–2.*** Platelet adhesion and aggregation. *A* and *B* depict the role of von Willebrand's factor in initial platelet adhesion to damaged endothelium. *C* and *D* show subsequent platelet release, aggregation, and role in vasoconstriction and coagulation reactions.

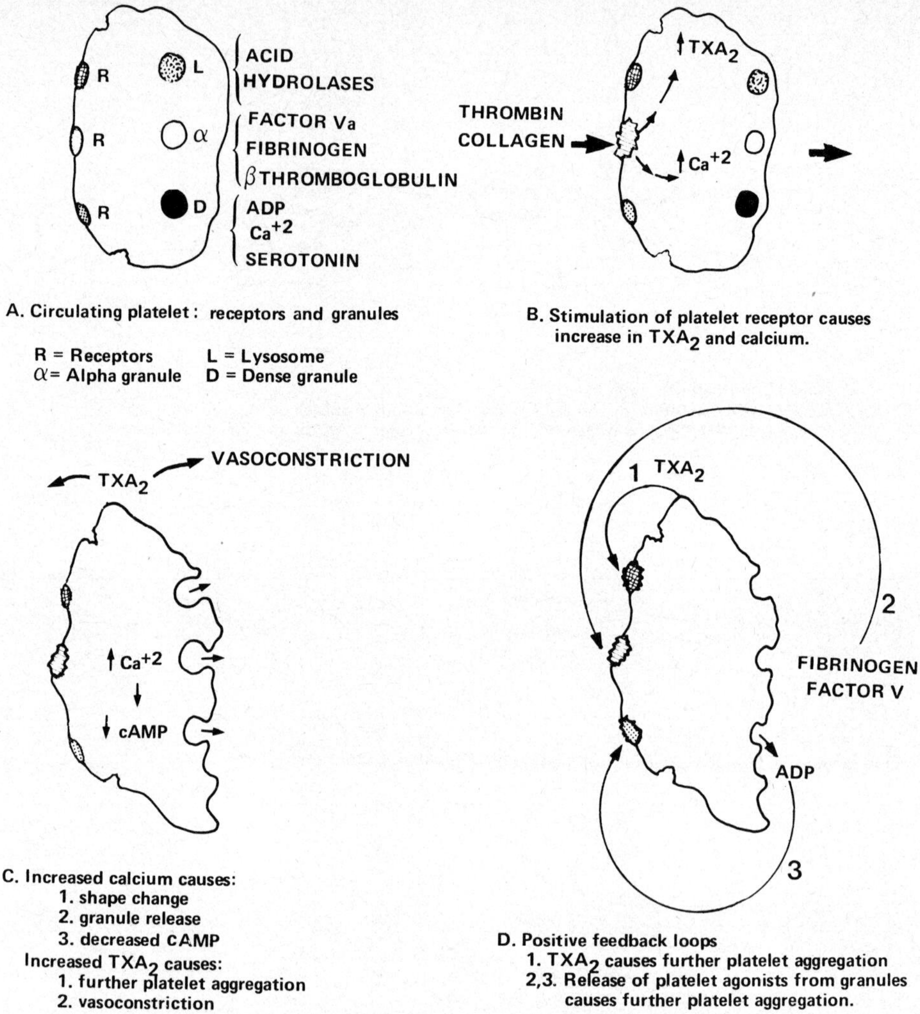


***Figure 3–3.*** Platelet aggregation and release reactions. See text for details.

ure 3–3*D*. The release of dense granule contents increases aggregation as does thromboxane production. Most antiplatelet agents act to interrupt one of these positive feedback loops by interfering with thromboxane production. One therapeutic objective is to inhibit platelet thromboxane production while sparing endothelial production of $PGI_2$. Differences between platelet and endothelial cell arachidonic acid metabolism may be exploited. Platelets are enucleate cells that lack the capability for de novo protein synthesis and therefore cannot regenerate cyclooxygenase once it has been irreversibly inactivated (acetylated) by aspirin.[9] Endothelial cells can synthesize new cyclooxygenase to replace the inactivated enzyme. Platelet cyclooxygenase is inactivated for the lifespan of the platelet (seven to 10 days), whereas endothelial cells recover cyclooxygenase function in one to two days. In addition to its greater sensitivity to less frequent doses of aspirin, platelet cyclooxygenase may be more sensitive to lower doses of aspirin than endothelial cells.[14, 15]

A second difference in platelets and endothelial cells, which may be exploited pharmacologically, involves cyclic AMP (cAMP) (Fig. 3–4). In platelets, thromboxane exerts its aggregatory effects by inhibiting adenylate cyclase to *decrease* cAMP. $PGI_2$, on the other hand, stimulates adenylate cyclase and increases cAMP in platelets and endothelial cells. Thus, drugs that increase cAMP synthesis, such as $PGI_2$ or analogs, may be clinically useful in blocking platelet aggrega-

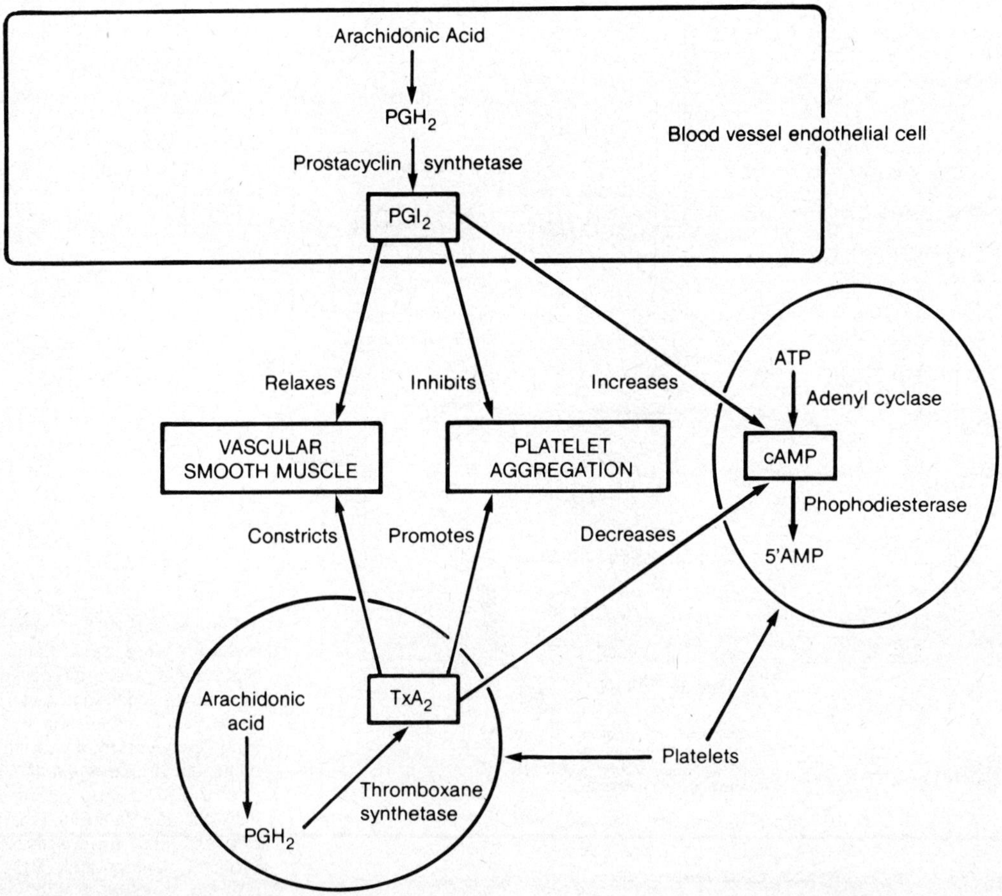


***Figure 3–4.*** A schematic representation of the thomboxane $A_2$/prostacyclin ($TxA_2$:$PGI_2$) balance within the circulation. An endothelial cell of the blood vessel wall is on top; the blood vessel lumen below contains two platelets. In the endothelial cell, arachidonic acid is converted to $PGH_2$ (a cyclic endoperoxide) and then to $PGI_2$ (prostacyclin), which increases intracellular cAMP levels, relaxes vascular smooth muscle, and inhibits platelet aggregation. In contrast, in the platelet, arachidonic acid is converted to $PGH_2$ and then to $TxA_2$, which decreases intracellular cAMP levels, constricts vascular smooth muscle, and promotes platelet aggregation. (From Hirsh, P. D., et al.: Prostaglandins and ischemic heart disease. Am. J. Med., *71*:1009, 1981.)

tion. Analogs that specifically block thromboxane synthetase, while sparing $PGI_2$ synthetase, are being developed. Finally, agents that specifically block platelet membrane receptors for agonists may hold promise for inhibiting platelet function.

Thus, via adhesion, release, and platelet aggregation, a platelet plug rapidly forms the initial mechanical barrier to prevent further hemorrhage, promotes vasconstriction, and catalyzes the fluid phase of coagulation by providing the surface on which key coagulation reactions take place. This surface displays many important receptors and cofactors that serve both to activate and to localize the coagulation reactions.

## THE FLUID PHASE: COAGULATION AND FIBRINOLYSIS

The fluid phase of the hemostatic system serves two interrelated and opposing functions. The *coagulation system* generates and stabilizes fibrin clot, and the *fibrinolytic system* dissolves the polymerized fibrin clot. Fibrinogen is cleaved by *thrombin* to form fibrin, the substance of clot. Thrombin occupies a central position in the hemostatic system (see Fig. 3–1); it is involved in platelet aggregation, fibrin formation, and the modulation of fibrinolysis. Thrombin can itself be generated by two interrelated mechanisms—the extrinsic and intrinsic pathways (Fig. 3–5). For

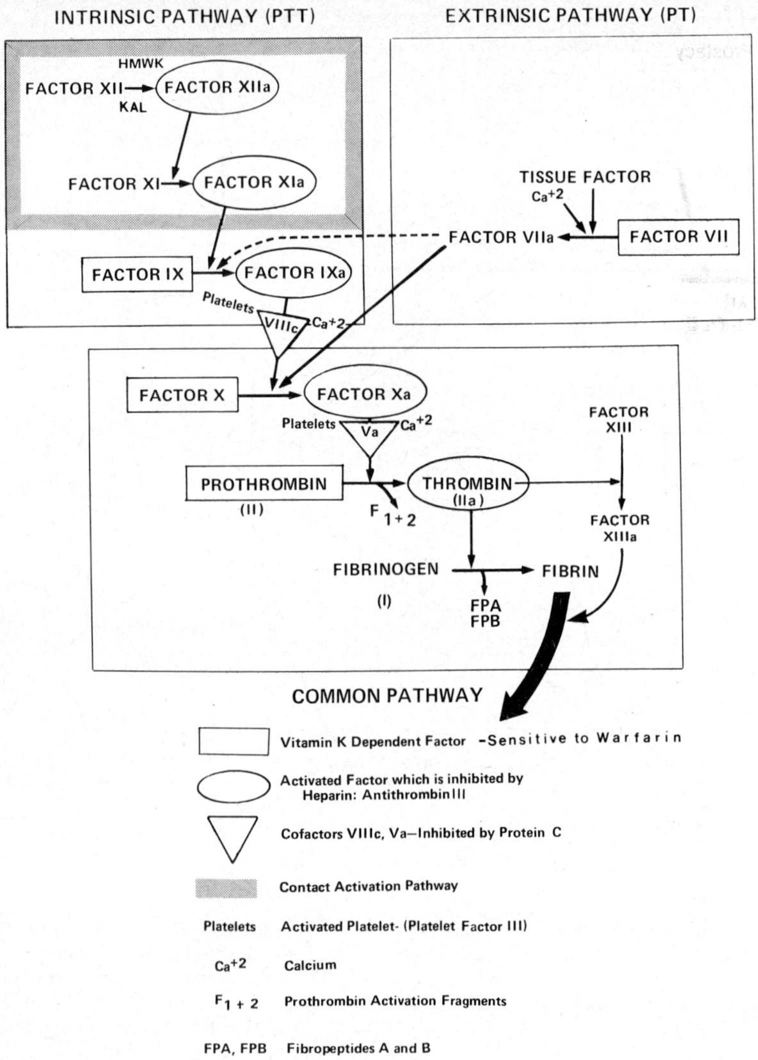


***Figure 3–5.*** The coagulation pathways. Important features include the contact activation phase, vitamin K–dependent factors (affected by warfarin), the activated serine proteases that are inhibited by heparin:antithrombin III, and the role of platelets and calcium. Factors VIIIc and Va are nonenzymatic cofactors that are inactivated by Protein C. The protime (PT) measures the function of the extrinsic and common pathways; the partial thromboplastin time (PTT) measures the function of the intrinsic and common pathways. HMWK = high molecular weight kininogen; KAL = kallikrein.

historic reasons, the factors are not numbered in the order of discovery or in their relative positions in the coagulation pathways; the numbers VI, IV, and III are not assigned to specific proteins. Table 3–1 summarizes some properties of the human clotting factors.

Before turning to the individual pathways, it is useful to discuss some general mechanisms of the coagulation system. Coagulation factors as well as key enzymes in the fibrinolytic system generally circulate as *inactive* forms (zymogens) in vast excess of physiologic requirements. They must be activated in high concentrations, locally, at the site of clot formation. This activation may be accomplished by proteolytic cleavage of a small peptide activation fragment allowing the enzymatically active form of the clotting factors (designated by lower case "a," such as Xa) to participate in the subsequent coagulation reactions. The activated clotting factors, XIIa, XIa, Xa, IXa, VIIa, IIa (thrombin), and plasmin are enzymes that cleave specific proteins by a trypsinlike mechanism and contain a serine at their active center—they are designated serine proteases.

Other clotting factors may be activated by a cofactor that induces a conformational change in the three-dimensional structure. Factors, notably high molecular weight kininogen, Va, and VIIIc, act by nonenzymatic mechanisms, facilitating a specific reaction by positioning the necessary constituents in the proper three-dimensional arrangement. For example, factor Va induces a conforma-

*Table 3–1.* Properties of Human Clotting Factors

| Clotting Factor | Normal Plasma Concentration (μg/ml) | $T_{1/2}$ Elimination (Hours) | Active Form Function | Sensitivity to Warfarin (W) and Heparin/ Antithrombin (H) |
|---|---|---|---|---|
| *Intrinsic System* | | | | |
| Factor XII (Hageman factor) | 29 | 60 | Serine protease | H |
| Prekallikrein | 50 | ? | Serine protease | |
| High molecular weight kininogen (Fitzgerald factor) | 70 | ? | Cofactor | |
| Factor XI (plasma thromboplastin antecedent) | 4 | 65 | Serine protease | H |
| Factor IX (Christmas factor) | 4 | 20 | Serine protease | H, W |
| Factor VIIIc (antihemophilic factor) | <.1 | 10 | Cofactor | |
| Factor VIII—vWF (von Willebrand factor) | 7 | ? | Cofactor (high molecular weight multimer) | |
| *Extrinsic System* | | | | |
| Factor VII (proconvertin) | 1 | 5 | Serine protease | H(?), W |
| Tissue factor | — | — | Cofactor | |
| *Common Pathway* | | | | |
| Factor X (Stuart-Prower factor) | 5 | 65 | Serine protease | H, W |
| Factor V (proaccelerin) | 5–12 | 25 | Cofactor | |
| Prothrombin (Factor II) | 100 | 100 | Serine protease | H, W |
| Fibrinogen (Factor I) | 2500 | 120 | Clot structure | |
| Factor XIII (fibrin stabilizing factor) | 10 | 150 | Transglutamate | |

tional change in factor Xa that accelerates the enzymatic activity of Xa by some 300,000-fold in the presence of phospholipid![16]

The clotting cascade serves as a powerful biologic amplifier because each activated serine protease is able to activate many molecules of the next factor in the pathway; it is a biochemical "snowball." This ability to rapidly generate large quantities of fibrin necessitates mechanisms that localize clot formation to the specific site of vascular injury and maintain blood fluidity. Several such mechanisms have been identified. (1) Many of the reactions require activated platelets in order to proceed, thus localizing coagulation to the sites where platelets have become activated on the damaged endothelium. (2) The so-called vitamin K–dependent factors (II, VII, IX, X) (see Fig. 3–5) have a specialized "homing device" that is required for them to participate normally in coagulation reactions. Specialized gamma-carboxyglutamic acid (gla) residues are added to these proteins by a vitamin K–dependent reaction in the liver. These unique amino acids appear to be required to form a multimolecular complex with calcium ions and the altered endothelial or platelet surface (Fig. 3–6).[17] In the absence of these gamma-carboxyglutamate residues (vitamin K deficiency or warfarin administration), normal hemostasis is impaired. (3) The physiologic inhibitors, antithrombin-III and Protein C, act to neutralize specific activated coagulation factors and are discussed in a subsequent section.

## Coagulation: The Intrinsic and Extrinsic Pathways

Factor X activation, the initial step in the common pathway (see Fig. 3–5), can be accomplished by two interrelated, arbitrarily defined mechanisms, the intrinsic and extrinsic pathways. These have been reviewed elsewhere,[1, 18] but it is worthwhile to discuss the components of these pathways so that one may better understand how the normal physiology may go awry and how it may be modified pharmacologically. Both pathways are activated when normally hidden components of the vascular endothelium come into contact with blood. Blood drawn into a test tube will clot slowly over several minutes

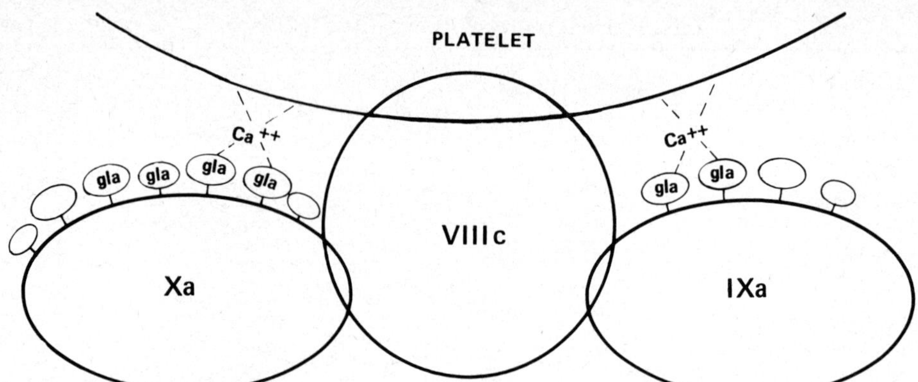


*Figure 3–6.* Vitamin K–dependent factors: role of γ-carboxyglutamic acid (gla) residues and calcium in localizing coagulation reactions to platelet or endothelial surface.

unless a blood-free tissue extract ("tissue factor" or tissue thromboplastin) is added. Tissue factor is the cofactor that catalyzes the activation of factor VII. Because tissue factor is not found in the blood (but is found in rather high concentration in brain and lung), it is said to be "extrinsic" to blood and therefore initiates the "extrinsic" clotting pathway. The prothrombin time (protime, PT) assay measures the function of extrinsic and final common pathways (VII, X, V, II, I) and generally is used to monitor warfarin therapy. Such an exogenous factor is not necessary to activate the so-called "intrinsic" cascade. All the factors are present in plasma and are activated by surface-mediated contact activation reactions (see Fig. 3–5). The partial thromboplastin time (PTT) is the most widely used assay of the intrinsic pathway and heparin therapy. It is clear that both pathways are essential for normal hemostasis from the clinical observation that congenital defects in either pathway are usually associated with bleeding disorders. It should be evident that the PT and PTT are both influenced to some extent by effects of warfarin and heparin on coagulation factors in the intrinsic, extrinsic, and common pathways (see Fig. 3–5 and Table 3–1).

## The Intrinsic Pathway

The intrinsic pathway is initiated by the contact activation phase when circulating factor XII comes into contact with subendothelial collagen or basement membrane (see Fig. 3–5). Other contact activation factors, high molecular weight kininogen (HMWK) and prekallikrein (PK) participate in the contact activation phase. In addition to its role in the intrinsic pathway, factor XII is important in initiating three other important biologic cascades: fibrinolysis, the complement cascade, and kinin generation (Fig. 3–7). Thus, it appears that factor XII, HMWK, and PK may exert effects on several key aspects of hemostasis. It is not certain that their role in initiating the intrinsic coagulation cascade is the most important.

Although patients with factor XII deficiency have a markedly prolonged PTT, they have no bleeding tendency. In fact, they may have a thrombotic tendency.[19] This suggests that some of factor XII's other actions, such as its stimulation of fibrinolysis, may be important in vivo; factor XII may play a key

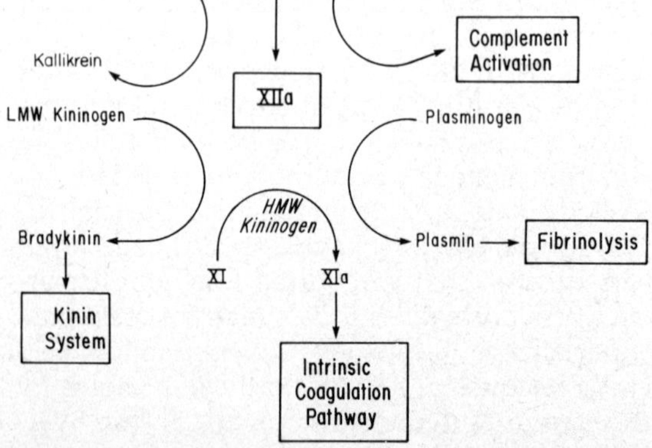


*Figure 3–7.* Roles of factor XII. In addition to its role in the intrinsic pathway, it exerts other important effects, including changes in vasomotor tone vis-à-vis the kinin system and in stimulating fibrinolysis.

role in the balance between coagulation and fibrinolysis. Factor XI–deficient patients, on the other hand, also have a markedly prolonged PTT and often do have a significant hemostatic defect. Taken together, these observations cast some doubt on the physiologic importance of factor XII in the intrinsic pathway and also raise the possibility of alternate mechanisms for the activation of factor XI in vivo.

Factor XI is activated by factor XIIa with high molecular weight kininogen participating as a cofactor (see Figs. 3–5 and 3–7). Once formed, factor XIa activates factor IX to factor IXa via a two-step protolytic cleavage (see Fig. 3–5). Alternatively, factor IX may be activated via the extrinsic pathway by the action of tissue factor and factor VIIa on factor IX (see Fig. 3–5),[20] although the physiologic importance of this mechanism is uncertain.

Factor X becomes bound to a multimolecular complex (see Fig. 3–6) by its gamma-carboxyglutamate residues and is activated by factor IXa in the presence of calcium and platelet phospholipid (Fig. 3–5). This proceeds via a two-step proteolytic cleavage (analogous to the activation of factor IX), producing factor Xa and a small activation fragment. Factor VIIIc (the antihemophilic factor) serves as an essential protein cofactor in the activation of factor X (see Fig. 3–5).

### Activation of Factor X by the Extrinsic Cascade

Tissue factor is normally "hidden" unless membrane damage or proteolysis exposes it. Factor VII is activated in the presence of tissue factor (see Fig. 3–5) in a poorly understood manner. It complexes via calcium to the phospholipid surface by its gamma-carboxyglutamate residues and can then activate factor X directly, by a proteolytic mechanism.

### Coagulation: The Common Pathway

The intrinsic and extrinsic pathways converge in the common pathway to generate thrombin (factor IIa), which in turn cleaves fibrinogen (factor I) to form a fibrin gel (see Fig. 3–8). The fibrin monomer can then be polymerized and stabilized into an insoluble clot (Fig. 3–9*B*).

Once Factor Xa is generated, by either the intrinsic or extrinsic pathway, it enzymatically cleaves prothrombin (II) into thrombin (IIa) and a small peptide "activation fragment" $F_{1+2}$.[16] (Fig. 3–8, [1]). This reaction is catalyzed by factor Va in the presence of platelet phospholipid and calcium. Factor V is released by activated platelets and may be activated to Va by thrombin. Va in turn binds to platelets, setting up high-affinity receptors for the activation of factor X. Thus, the production of thrombin has an autocatalytic effect because thrombin activates Factors VIII and V (Fig. 3–8, [4]), further increasing the rate of thrombin generation. Once generated, thrombin acts on fibrinogen (Fig. 3–8, [1]) to sequentially release two small peptide products, fibrinopeptide-A (FPA) and fibrinopeptide-B (FPB) and to expose specific sites necessary for fibrin polymerization (Fig. 3–9*A*). Fibrin initially forms a polymer stabilized by hydrophobic and electrostatic bonding between alpha and gamma chains in the D domain. The polymer is still somewhat soluble at this point. The activation fragments $F_{1+2}$ (thrombin) and FPA (fibrinogen) are indices of factor Xa and thrombin activity (Fig. 3–8), respectively, which may prove clinically useful in assessing anticoagulant therapy and in screening for the suspected hypercoagulable patient.[21, 22, 23]

### Fibrin Stabilization

In parallel with the formation of fibrin, thrombin also activates factor XIII (see Fig. 3–8, [2]), exposing a sulfhydryl active center of factor XIIIa. Factor XIIIa is able to form covalent cross linkages between the alpha and gamma chain of neighboring fibrin monomers (see Fig. 3–9*B*). The cross-linked clot is chemically and mechanically more stable, forming a structure resembling reinforced concrete, the insoluble fibrin clot.

## FIBRINOLYSIS

Whereas rapid, effective, and localized thrombosis is essential for survival, it is also apparent that recanalization and repair of the damaged endothelium are also important if flow is to be reestablished in the vessel and the organism is to recover from injury. The fibrinolytic system is a part of this "cleanup" or repair mechanism.

Once the fibrin polymer has been formed

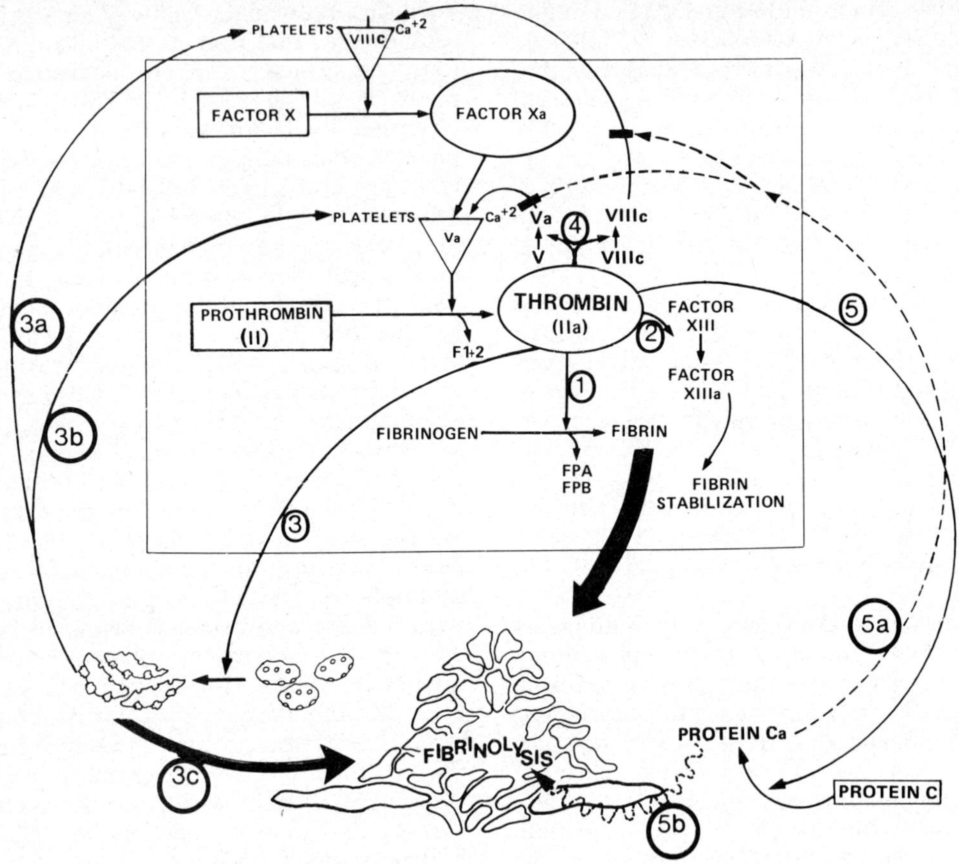


*Figure 3–8.* The common pathway and the central role of thrombin in the hemostatic system: [1] fibrin formation; [2] fibrin stabilization; [3] platelet aggregation; activated platelets adhere to factor VIIIc [3a], factor Va [3b], and form the initial platelet plug [3c]; [4] activation of factors V and VIIIc; and [5] activation of Protein C with its [5a] anticoagulant and [5b] fibrinolytic effects. Solid lines represent positive feedback loops. Hatched lines represent negative feedback loops. See text for details.

and cross-linked, it is very resistant to disruption and must be enzymatically "digested" by the serine protease *plasmin.* Plasminogen, the circulating precursor, is also trapped within the fibrin meshwork but can be converted to active plasmin by at least two types of physiologic *plasminogen activators* as well as fibrinolytic agents such as streptokinase and urokinase[24] (Fig. 3–10). The two physiologic plasminogen activators are: (1) *plasma* plasminogen activator,[25] which is activated by factor XIIa; and (2) *vascular* (tissue) plasminogen activators (tPA),[26] located in high concentrations in venous and capillary endothelial cells, which are released from the vessel walls in response to a number of stimuli, including exercise, hypotensive shock, pharmacologic agents, and Protein C.[27] Protein C is a vitamin K–dependent inhibitor of coagulation (anticoagulant), which also appears to activate fibrinolysis in vivo by the release of vascular (tissue) plasminogen activator (see Figs. 3–8, [5b] and 3–10). Protein C must first be activated by thrombin to form protein Ca (see Fig. 3–8, [5]).

Once formed, plasmin enzymatically digests fibrin (see Fig. 3–9*B*) to release a number of fibrin degradation products (also termed fibrin split products) (see Fig. 3–9C). These products are themselves potent anticoagulants that inhibit fibrin generation and polymerization. Plasmin is a serine protease with wide substrate specificity,[24] allowing it to cleave numerous biologically active proteins, including several activated clotting factors, low molecular weight kininogen, and several components of the complement cascade. The physiologic importance of these reactions remains to be determined.

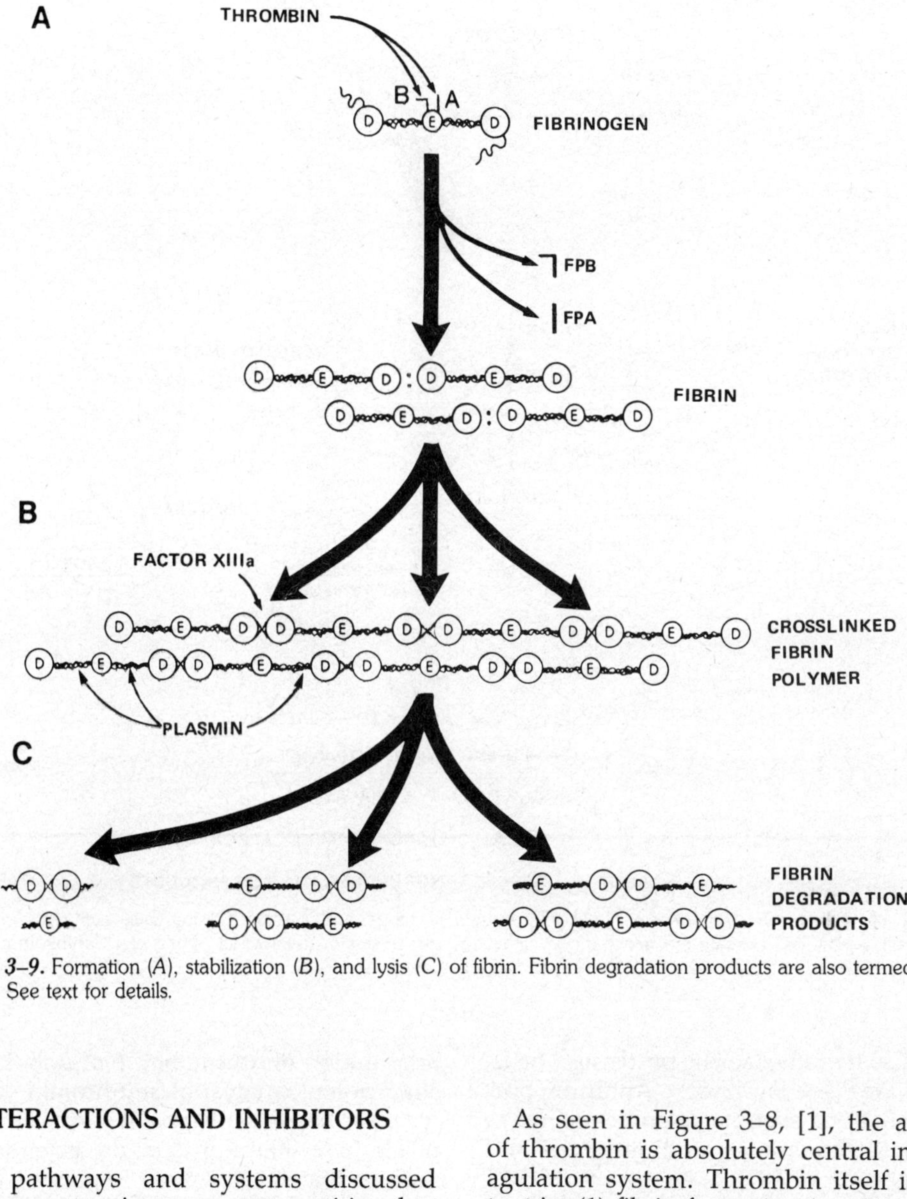


***Figure 3–9.*** Formation (*A*), stabilization (*B*), and lysis (*C*) of fibrin. Fibrin degradation products are also termed fibrin split products. See text for details.

## INTERACTIONS AND INHIBITORS

The pathways and systems discussed above are not unique, separate entities, but rather they interact and modulate one another by a complex set of positive and negative controls. The initial events in the physiology of clotting involve platelet–vessel wall interactions, including the release of metabolites, $TxA_2$ from platelets, and $PGI_2$ from the vessel wall, which have diametrically opposite effects on vessel wall tone and platelet aggregation (see Fig. 3–4). It seems likely that this difference in arachidonate metabolism plays an important role in the regulation of the delicate balance between blood fluidity and thrombosis, though this has recently been questioned.[37]

As seen in Figure 3–8, [1], the activation of thrombin is absolutely central in the coagulation system. Thrombin itself is important in: (1) fibrin formation (see Figs. 3–8, [1] and 3–9*A*); (2) fibrin stabilization (see Figs. 3–8, [2] and 3–9*B*); (3) induction of platelet aggregation (see Fig. 3–8, [3]); (4) activation of factors V and VIII (see Fig. 3–8, [4]); and (5) the activation of Protein C with its anticoagulant and profibrinolytic effects (see Fig. 3–8, [5]). Given this powerful and multifocal activation of the hemostatic system, it is not surprising that the generation of thrombin is the focus of important regulatory controls. Antithrombin III (AT III) is the major inhibitor of thrombin and is present in excess amounts in plasma. AT III not only complexes with and inactivates thrombin (factor

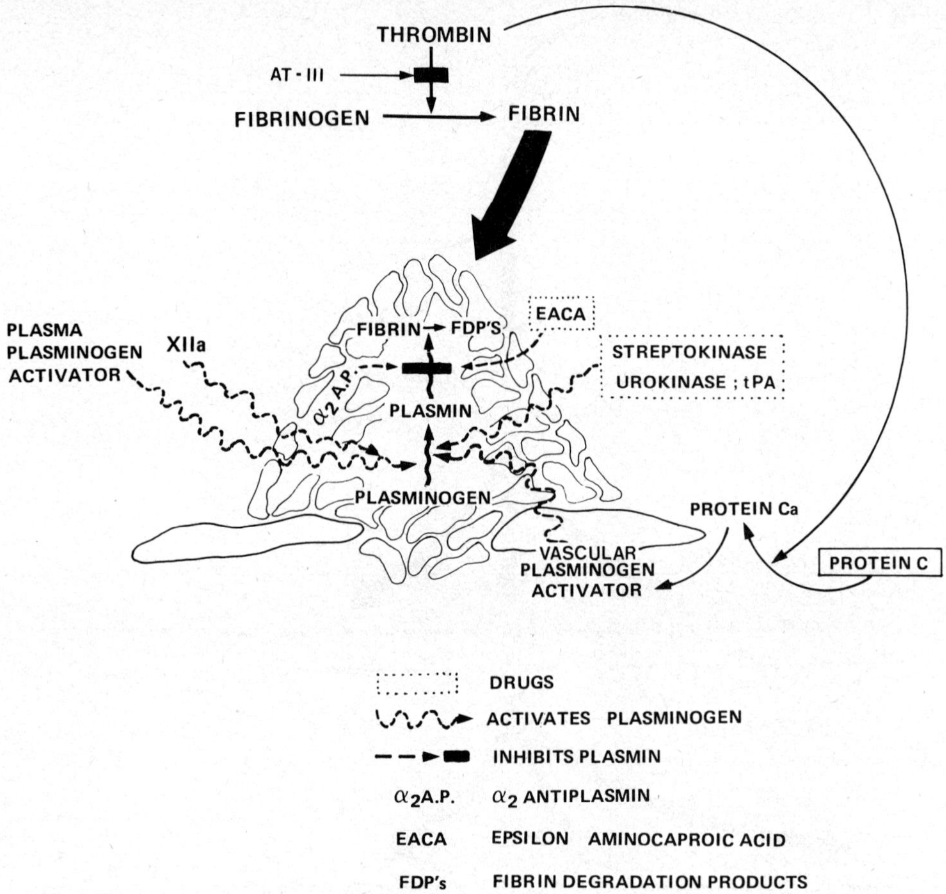


***Figure 3–10.*** Schematic view of the fibrinolytic system. Vascular and plasma plasminogen activators as well as pharmacologic agents can activate plasmin trapped within the clot. Plasmin dissolves the fibrin clot. Inhibitors of plasmin include $\alpha_2$ antiplasmin, also trapped within the clot, and pharmacologic agents.

IIa) but also the other serine proteases[28] (XIIa, XIa, IXa, Xa) (see Fig. 3–5). "Antithrombin" is somewhat of a misnomer, understating the physiologic importance and range of this inhibitor.

AT III slowly and progressively neutralizes thrombin in vitro. Heparin dramatically catalyzes the action of antithrombin III; the addition of small amounts of heparin causes nearly instantaneous, complete inactivation of thrombin. Heparin binds to a specific site on the antithrombin molecules, inducing a conformational change that results in a rapid neutralization of thrombin via formation of a stable, inactive thrombin:antithrombin (T:AT) complex (see Chapter 6, Fig. 6–4). Heparin can then dissociate from the T:AT complex and catalyze another round of thrombin:antithrombin interaction. The inactivation of the other serine proteases appears to proceed by an analogous mechanism with binding of the serine-active site to an arginine on antithrombin. Not only is heparin a potent catalyst of antithrombin activity in vitro, but there is recent in vivo evidence of a heparin-like substance on the endothelial surface that may play an important physiologic role in regulating thrombosis (see Chapter 9, Fig. 9–3).[29, 35] The physiologic importance of antithrombin is apparent from numerous reports of families in which heterozygous AT-deficient members have a high incidence of recurrent thromboembolic disease.[30]

Protein C, a vitamin K–dependent protein,[31–33] has recently been recognized as an important inhibitor of coagulation (anticoagulant) (see Fig. 3–8, [5a]) and stimulator of fibrinolysis (see Fig. 3–8, [5b]).[38] Several families have recently been described with Protein C deficiency associated with a high incidence of thromboembolic events (see Chapter 9). Protein C circulates as an inactive molecule that is activated by thrombin (see

Fig. 3–8, [5]) in the presence of a cofactor, thrombomodulin, on the endothelial surface. Activated Protein C has two important roles in limiting coagulation: it acts as an anticoagulant by inactivating Va and VIIIc to decrease thrombin production (see Fig. 3–8, [5a]),[32] and it appears to initiate fibrinolysis by releasing plasminogen activator from the vessel wall (see Fig. 3–8, [5b]).[27]

Thus, thrombin potentially may initiate both positive and negative feedback loops, which regulate further thrombin generation (see Fig. 3–8). On one hand, thrombin creates a positive feedback loop by activating V and VIIIc (see Fig. 3–8, [4]), which increases the rate of thrombin generation. On the other hand, thrombin participates in a negative feedback loop by its activation of Protein C (see Fig. 3–8, [5]), which in turn inactivates Va and VIIIc (see Fig. 3–8, [5a]) and stimulates fibrinolysis (see Fig. 3–8, [5b]). The factors that control this balance are not understood. Protein C and antithrombin III are inhibitors of the coagulation cascade (see Fig. 3–5) that operate by complementary mechanisms. Whereas antithrombin III specifically neutralizes the activated serine proteases (XIIa, XIa, IXa, IIa), Protein C inactivates two other cofactors in the coagulation cascade, Va and VIIIc (see Fig. 3–5).

Alpha-2 antiplasmin is a specific inhibitor of plasmin that appears to be active locally within the fibrin clot. (see Fig. 3–10).[24] It binds to fibrin and fibrinogen within the clot, as does plasminogen, and is the primary inhibitor of plasmin. The deficiency of this inhibitor of fibrinolysis is associated with a hemorrhagic disorder, as would be anticipated.

From the previous discussion and our knowledge of the variety of defects that may cause "primary hypercoagulable disorders," it seems likely that the regulation of fibrinolysis is as important as the regulation of the coagulation cascade in determining the overall balance of the hemostatic system. Indeed, these two systems are not discrete, isolated pathways, but are interrelated by at least two known systems. As noted above, the contact activation phase, involving XIIa, may be pivotal in this balance (see Fig. 3–7). Protein C, by its stimulation of fibrinolysis (see Fig. 3–8, [5b]) and inhibition of coagulation (see Fig. 3–8, [5a]), may also be important much later in the course of events, once thrombin is formed. The mechanisms that activate coagulation in vivo also appear to activate the fibrinolytic system in parallel, providing a mechanism to restore vascular patency. This delicate balance between clot formation and dissolution may be readily perturbed, in either direction, by a number of pharmacologic or pathologic mechanisms. Chapter 6 will review the drugs that shift the balance away from clot formation and Chapter 9 will discuss the primary and secondary disorders associated with the hypercoagulable state.

## REFERENCES

1. Thompson, A. R., and Harker, C. A.: Manual of Thrombosis and Hemostasis. F. A. Davis, Philadelphia, 1983, p. 5.
2. Berndt, M. C., and Phillips, D. R.: Platelet Membrane Proteins: Composition and Receptor Function. *In* Gordon, J. F. (Ed.): Platelets in Biology and Pathology, 2nd ed. New York, Elsevier, 1981, p. 43.
3. Nurden, A. T., and Caen, J. P.: The different glycoprotein abnormalities in thrombasthenic and Bernard-Solier platelets. Semin. Hematol., *16*:234, 1979.
4. Holmsen, H.: Platelet Secretion. *In* Colman, R. W., Hirsh, J., Marder, V. J., et al. (Eds.): Hemostasis and Thrombosis. J. B. Lippincott, Philadelphia, 1982, p. 392.
5. Files, J. C., et al.: Studies of human platelet alpha granule release in vivo. Blood, *58*:607, 1981.
6. Gerrard, J. M., and White, J. G.: Prostaglandins and thromboxanes: "Middlemen" modulating platelet function in hemostasis and thrombosis. Prog. Hemost. Thromb., *4*:87, 1978.
7. Hathaway, D. R., Eaton, C. R., and Adelstein, R. S.: Regulation of Human Platelet Myosin Kinase by Calcium-Calmodulin and Cyclic AMP. *In* Mann, K. G., and Taylor, F. B. (Eds.): The Regulation of Coagulation. Elsevier, New York, 1980, p. 271.
8. Vane, J. R.: Inhibition of prostaglandin synthesis as a mechanism of action of aspirin-like drugs. Nature, *231*:232, 1971.
9. Roth, G. J., and Majerius, P. W.: The mechanism of the effect of aspirin on human platelets. I. Activation of a particulate fraction protein. J. Clin. Invest., *56*:624, 1975.
10. Needleman, P., Minkes, M., and Raz, A.: Thromboxanes: Selected biosynthesis and distinct biologic properties. Science, *193*:163, 1976.
11. Moncada, S., Bunting, S., Mullane, K., et al.: Imidazole: A selective inhibitor of thromboxane synthetase. Prostaglandins, *13*:611, 1977.
12. Moncada, S., Gryglewski, R., Bunting, S.,et al.: An enzyme isolated from arteries transforms endoperoxides to an unstable substance that inhibits platelet aggregation. Nature, *263*:663, 1976.
13. Moncada, S., Higgs, E. A., and Vane, J. R.: Human arterial and venous tissues generate prostacyclin (prostaglandin X), a potent inhibitor of platelet aggregation. Lancet, *1*:18, 1977.
14. Preston, E. F., Whipps, S., Jackson, C. A., et al.: Inhibition of prostacyclin and platelet thromboxane $A_2$ after low-dose aspirin. New Engl. J. Med., *304*:76, 1981.
15. Fitzgerald, G. A., Oates, J. A., Hawiger, J., et al.: Endogenous biosynthesis of prostacycline and thromboxane and platelet function during chronic

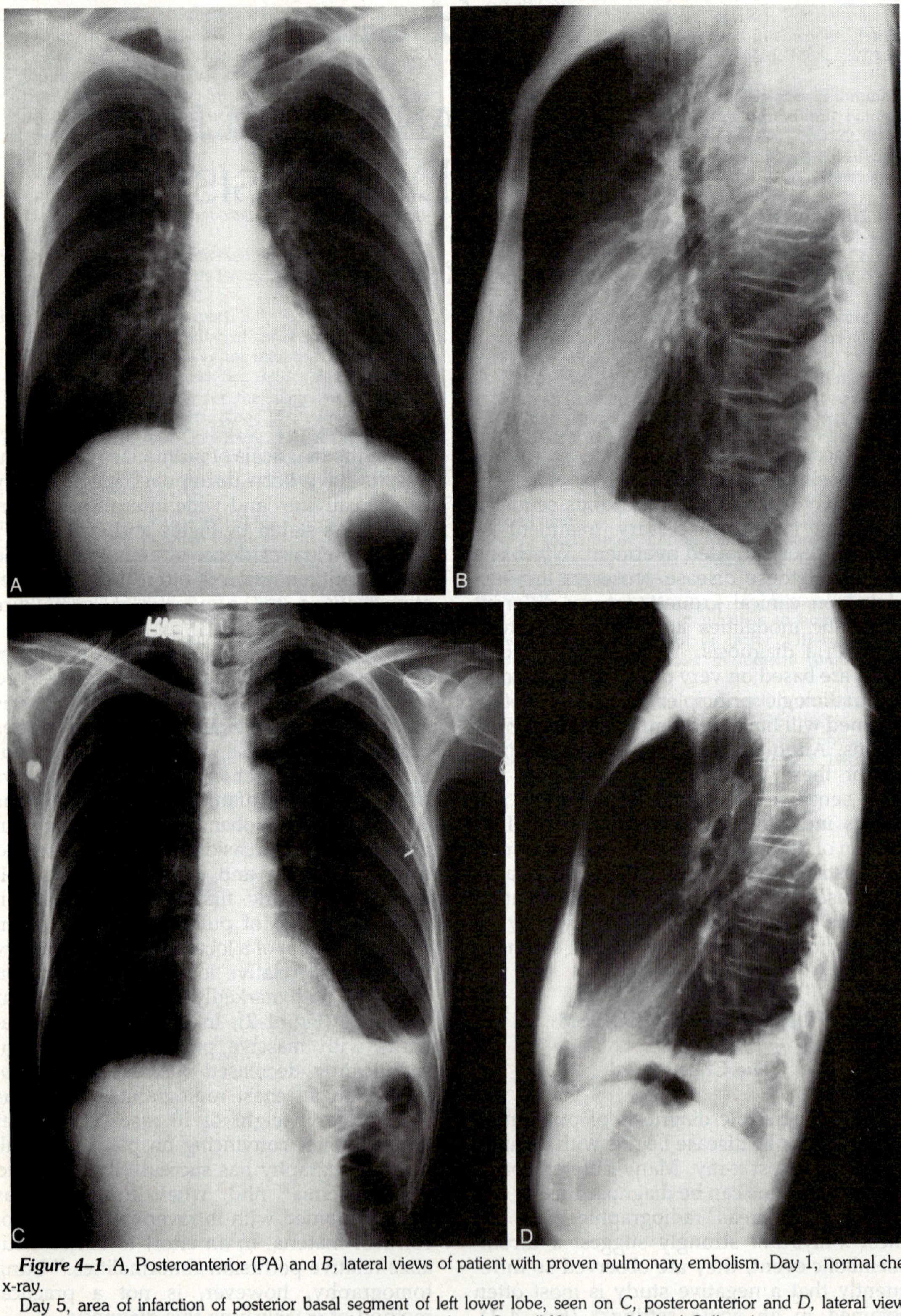


***Figure 4–1.*** *A*, Posteroanterior (PA) and *B*, lateral views of patient with proven pulmonary embolism. Day 1, normal chest x-ray.

Day 5, area of infarction of posterior basal segment of left lower lobe, seen on *C*, posteroanterior and *D*, lateral views. (Courtesy of Dr. Antonio F. Govoni, The New York Hospital and Cornell University Medical College.)

Fig. 3–8, [5]) in the presence of a cofactor, thrombomodulin, on the endothelial surface. Activated Protein C has two important roles in limiting coagulation: it acts as an anticoagulant by inactivating Va and VIIIc to decrease thrombin production (see Fig. 3–8, [5a]),[32] and it appears to initiate fibrinolysis by releasing plasminogen activator from the vessel wall (see Fig. 3–8, [5b]).[27]

Thus, thrombin potentially may initiate both positive and negative feedback loops, which regulate further thrombin generation (see Fig. 3–8). On one hand, thrombin creates a positive feedback loop by activating V and VIIIc (see Fig. 3–8, [4]), which increases the rate of thrombin generation. On the other hand, thrombin participates in a negative feedback loop by its activation of Protein C (see Fig. 3–8, [5]), which in turn inactivates Va and VIIIc (see Fig. 3–8, [5a]) and stimulates fibrinolysis (see Fig. 3–8, [5b]). The factors that control this balance are not understood. Protein C and antithrombin III are inhibitors of the coagulation cascade (see Fig. 3–5) that operate by complementary mechanisms. Whereas antithrombin III specifically neutralizes the activated serine proteases (XIIa, XIa, IXa, IIa), Protein C inactivates two other cofactors in the coagulation cascade, Va and VIIIc (see Fig. 3–5).

Alpha-2 antiplasmin is a specific inhibitor of plasmin that appears to be active locally within the fibrin clot. (see Fig. 3–10).[24] It binds to fibrin and fibrinogen within the clot, as does plasminogen, and is the primary inhibitor of plasmin. The deficiency of this inhibitor of fibrinolysis is associated with a hemorrhagic disorder, as would be anticipated.

From the previous discussion and our knowledge of the variety of defects that may cause "primary hypercoagulable disorders," it seems likely that the regulation of fibrinolysis is as important as the regulation of the coagulation cascade in determining the overall balance of the hemostatic system. Indeed, these two systems are not discrete, isolated pathways, but are interrelated by at least two known systems. As noted above, the contact activation phase, involving XIIa, may be pivotal in this balance (see Fig. 3–7). Protein C, by its stimulation of fibrinolysis (see Fig. 3–8, [5b]) and inhibition of coagulation (see Fig. 3–8, [5a]), may also be important much later in the course of events, once thrombin is formed. The mechanisms that activate coagulation in vivo also appear to activate the fibrinolytic system in parallel, providing a mechanism to restore vascular patency. This delicate balance between clot formation and dissolution may be readily perturbed, in either direction, by a number of pharmacologic or pathologic mechanisms. Chapter 6 will review the drugs that shift the balance away from clot formation and Chapter 9 will discuss the primary and secondary disorders associated with the hypercoagulable state.

## REFERENCES


1. Thompson, A. R., and Harker, C. A.: Manual of Thrombosis and Hemostasis. F. A. Davis, Philadelphia, 1983, p. 5.
2. Berndt, M. C., and Phillips, D. R.: Platelet Membrane Proteins: Composition and Receptor Function. *In* Gordon, J. F. (Ed.): Platelets in Biology and Pathology, 2nd ed. New York, Elsevier, 1981, p. 43.
3. Nurden, A. T., and Caen, J. P.: The different glycoprotein abnormalities in thrombasthenic and Bernard-Solier platelets. Semin. Hematol., *16*:234, 1979.
4. Holmsen, H.: Platelet Secretion. *In* Colman, R. W., Hirsh, J., Marder, V. J., et al. (Eds.): Hemostasis and Thrombosis. J. B. Lippincott, Philadelphia, 1982, p. 392.
5. Files, J. C., et al.: Studies of human platelet alpha granule release in vivo. Blood, *58*:607, 1981.
6. Gerrard, J. M., and White, J. G.: Prostaglandins and thromboxanes: "Middlemen" modulating platelet function in hemostasis and thrombosis. Prog. Hemost. Thromb., *4*:87, 1978.
7. Hathaway, D. R., Eaton, C. R., and Adelstein, R. S.: Regulation of Human Platelet Myosin Kinase by Calcium-Calmodulin and Cyclic AMP. *In* Mann, K. G., and Taylor, F. B. (Eds.): The Regulation of Coagulation. Elsevier, New York, 1980, p. 271.
8. Vane, J. R.: Inhibition of prostaglandin synthesis as a mechanism of action of aspirin-like drugs. Nature, *231*:232, 1971.
9. Roth, G. J., and Majerius, P. W.: The mechanism of the effect of aspirin on human platelets. I. Activation of a particulate fraction protein. J. Clin. Invest., *56*:624, 1975.
10. Needleman, P., Minkes, M., and Raz, A.: Thromboxanes: Selected biosynthesis and distinct biologic properties. Science, *193*:163, 1976.
11. Moncada, S., Bunting, S., Mullane, K., et al.: Imidazole: A selective inhibitor of thromboxane synthetase. Prostaglandins, *13*:611, 1977.
12. Moncada, S., Gryglewski, R., Bunting, S.,et al.: An enzyme isolated from arteries transforms endoperoxides to an unstable substance that inhibits platelet aggregation. Nature, *263*:663, 1976.
13. Moncada, S., Higgs, E. A., and Vane, J. R.: Human arterial and venous tissues generate prostacyclin (prostaglandin X), a potent inhibitor of platelet aggregation. Lancet, *1*:18, 1977.
14. Preston, E. F., Whipps, S., Jackson, C. A., et al.: Inhibition of prostacyclin and platelet thromboxane $A_2$ after low-dose aspirin. New Engl. J. Med., *304*:76, 1981.
15. Fitzgerald, G. A., Oates, J. A., Hawiger, J., et al.: Endogenous biosynthesis of prostacycline and thromboxane and platelet function during chronic

administration of aspirin in man. J. Clin. Invest., *71*:676, 1983.
16. Jackson, C. M.: Mechanisms of Prothrombin Activation. *In* Colman, R. W., Hirsh, J., Marder, V. J., et al. (Eds.): Hemostasis and Thrombosis. J. B. Lippincott, Philadelphia, 1982, p. 106.
17. Esmon, C. T., Suttie, J. W., and Jackson, C. M.: The functional significance of vitamin K action. Difference in phospholipid binding between normal and abnormal prothrombin. J. Biol. Chem., *250*:4095, 1975.
18. Colman, R. W., Hirsh, J., Marder, V. J., et al.: Hemostasis and Thrombosis. J. B. Lippincott, Philadelphia, 1982.
19. Dyerberg, J., and Stoffersen, E.: Recurrent thrombosis in a patient with Factor XII deficiency. Acta Hematol., *63*:278, 1980.
20. Osterud, B., and Rapaport, S. I.: Activation of Factor IX by the reaction product of tissue factor and Factor VII: Additional pathway for initiating blood coagulation. Proc. Natl. Acad. Sci. (USA), *74*:5260, 1977.
21. Hirsh, J.: Blood tests for the diagnosis of venous and arterial thrombosis. Blood, *57*:1, 1981.
22. Yudelman, I., and Greenberg, J.: Factors affecting fibrinopeptide-A levels in patients with venous thromboembolism during anticoagulant therapy. Blood, *59*:787, 1982.
23. Bauer, K. A., and Rosenberg, R. D.: Assays for thrombin generation in humans with prethrombotic states. Thromb. Haemost., *50*:159(a), 1983.
24. Robbins, K. C.: The Plasminogen-plasmin Enzyme System. *In* Colman, R. W., Hirsh, J., Marder, V. J., et al. (Eds.): Hemostasis and Thrombosis. J. B. Lippincott, Philadelphia, 1982, p. 623.
25. Goldsmith, G. H., Jr., Sacto, H., and Ratnoff, O. D.: The activation of plasminogen by Hageman factors (factor XII) and Hageman factor fragments. J. Clin. Invest., *62*:54, 1978.
26. Binder, B. R., Spragg, J., and Austen, K. F.: Purification and characterization of human vascular plasminogen activators derived from blood vessel perfusates. J. Biol. Chem., *244*:1998, 1979.
27. Comp, P. C., and Esmon, C. T.: Generation of fibrinolytic activity by infusion of activated protein C in dogs. J. Clin. Invest., *68*:1221, 1981.
28. Rosenberg, R. D.: Actions and interactions of antithrombin and heparin. N. Engl. J. Med., *292*:146, 1975.
29. Lollar, P., and Owen, W. G.: Clearance of thrombin from circulation in rabbits by high affinity binding sites on endothelium. J. Clin. Invest., *66*:1222, 1980.
30. Thaler, E., and Lechner, K.: Antithrombin-III deficiency and thromboembolism. Clin. Haematol., *10*:369, 1981.
31. Esmon, C. T., Stenflo, J., Suttie, J. W., et al.: A new vitamin K–dependent protein. A phospholipid-binding zymogen of a serine esterase. J. Biol. Chem., *251*:3052, 1976.
32. Kisiel, W., Canfield, W., Ericsson, L., et al.: Anticoagulant properties of bovine plasma protein C following activation by thrombin. Biochemistry, *16*:5824, 1977.
33. Morlar, R. A., Kleiss, A. J ., and Griffin, J. H.: Human protein C: Inactivation of factors V and VIII by the activated molecule. Ann. N.Y. Acad. Sci., *370*:303, 1981.
34. Hirsh, P. D., Campbell, W. B., Willerson, J. T., et al.: Prostaglandins and ischemic heart disease. Am. J. Med., *71*:1009, 1981.
35. Rosenberg, R. D., Marcum, J., and McKinney, J.: In vivo acceleration of antithrombin action by heparin-like molecules on the endothelium. Thromb. Haemost., *50*:90(a), 1983.
36. Sixma, J. J., Sakariassen, K. S., Beeser-Visser, N. H., et al.: Adhesion of platelets to human artery subendothelium: Effect of factor VIII–von Willebrand factor of various multimeric composition. Blood, *63*:128, 1984.
37. Marcus, A. J.: Aspirin as an antithrombotic medication. New Engl. J. Med., *309*:1515, 1983.
38. Esmon, C. T.: Protein C: Biochemistry, physiology, and clinical implications. Blood, *62*:1155, 1983.

CHAPTER 4

# RADIOLOGIC AND NUCLEAR MEDICINE DIAGNOSIS

JOHN A. MARKISZ, M.D., Ph.D.

An accurate diagnosis of deep venous thrombosis or pulmonary embolism is essential to avoid potentially hazardous sequelae stemming from unnecessary treatment or from a lack of indicated treatment. When one or both of these disease processes are suspected on clinical grounds, many different diagnostic modalities are available to help establish a diagnosis. These various procedures are based on very different physiologic and radiologic principles, and information obtained will have different diagnostic implications. Although sensitivities and specificities of these procedures vary greatly, the most sensitive or specific technique is not always indicated in a given situation. It is the aim of this chapter to discuss the different diagnostic tests available, their advantages and disadvantages, and the information available from them, so that they may be properly utilized in various clinical settings.

## PULMONARY EMBOLISM

### The Chest X-ray

The radiographic diagnosis of pulmonary thromboembolic disease begins with an analysis of the chest x-ray. Many different pathologic conditions can be diagnosed using this modality. Whereas radiographic signs on chest x-rays *can* strongly suggest a thromboembolic event, they are observed so infrequently that a negative study is most often obtained in an acute setting[1–6] (Fig. 4–1). Several studies[3–6] have been undertaken in an attempt to determine the role of the chest film in the diagnosis of pulmonary embolism. Results have been disappointing, with very low sensitivities and wide interobserver variability. As stated by Figley and coworkers[1]: "The principal evidence of embolism on the chest roentgenogram is often the paucity of abnormalities for a patient in such dire straits."

The "classic" signs of pulmonary embolism (emphasizing that these are rarely observed in an acute event, except when embolism is massive) can be divided into two categories radiologically—those with and those without evidence of infarction. Those chest x-rays without signs of infarction may exhibit signs of segmental or lobar oligemia, changes in vessel size and, occasionally, cardiac size and contour changes and diminished lung volume. Westermark[7] first described local oligemia as a sign of pulmonary embolism in 1938. Occlusion of a lobar or segmental artery will cause a relative local hyperlucency on plain film with markedly diminished vascular markings (Fig. 4–2). In one study of 25 patients with massive pulmonary embolism, significantly decreased vascularity was observed on all chest radiographs.[8] This was also found in eight of 10 cases in another study.[9] If not convincing on plain film, full lung tomography has successfully evaluated local oligemia[10] and, when equivocal, has been combined with intravenous infusion of contrast material in an effort to better visualize relative perfusion abnormalities.[11] Lung tomography, however, is not a practical method of establishing this diagnosis.

Engorgement of a major hilar artery becomes a significant diagnostic sign on plain

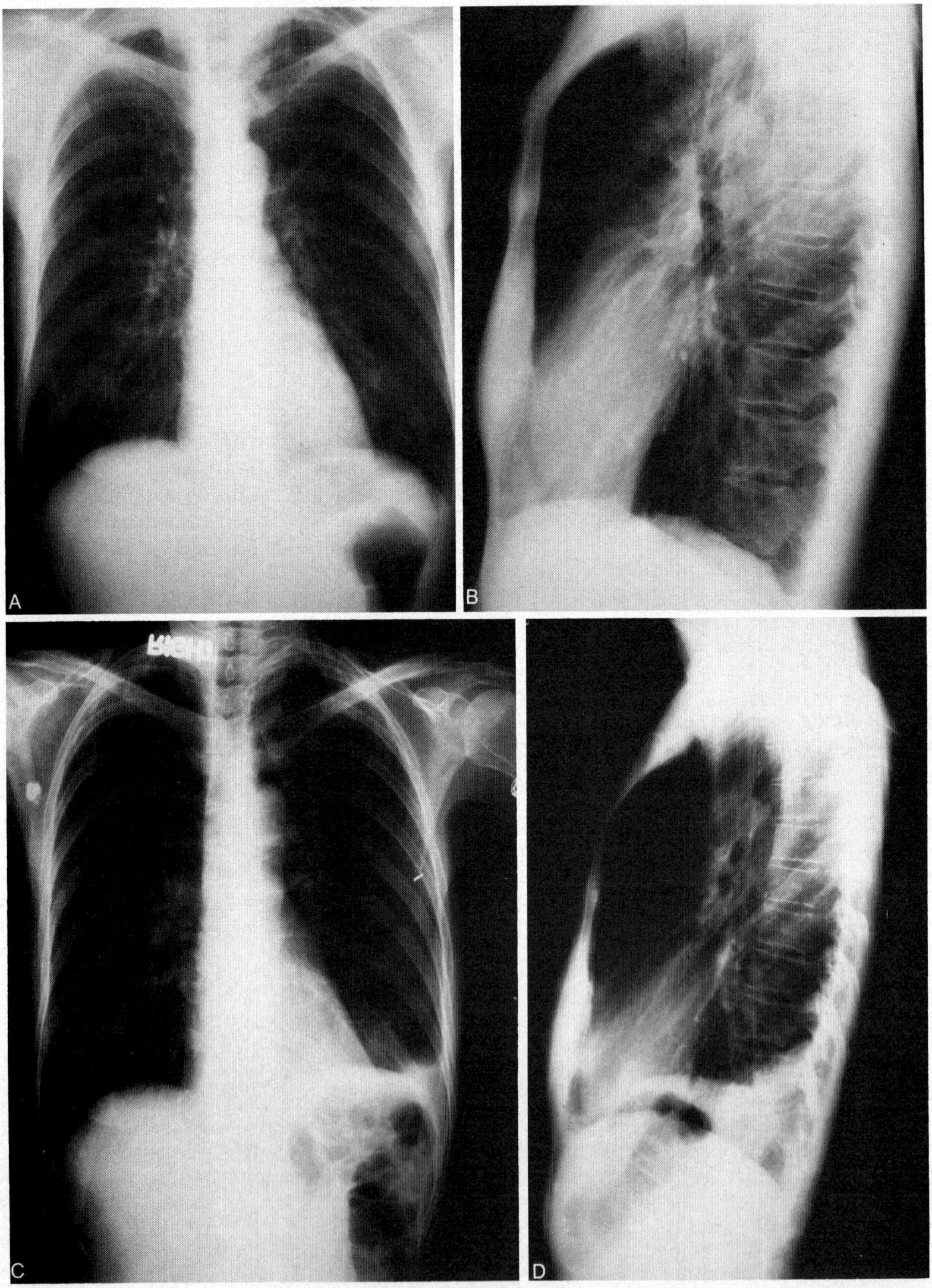


***Figure 4–1.*** *A,* Posteroanterior (PA) and *B,* lateral views of patient with proven pulmonary embolism. Day 1, normal chest x-ray.

Day 5, area of infarction of posterior basal segment of left lower lobe, seen on *C,* posteroanterior and *D,* lateral views. (Courtesy of Dr. Antonio F. Govoni, The New York Hospital and Cornell University Medical College.)

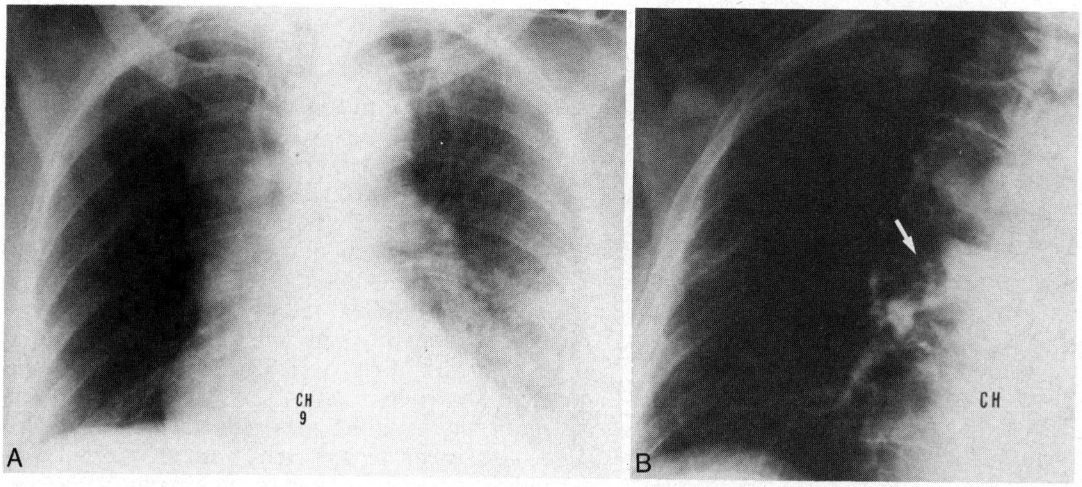


*Figure 4–2.* *A*, Chest x-ray of patient with clinical signs of pulmonary embolism demonstrating marked oligemia (Westermark's sign) in entire right lobe. *B*, Arteriogram of same patient demonstrating massive saddle embolus in right main pulmonary artery (arrow). (Courtesy of Dr. Jack L. Westcott, The New York Hospital and Cornell University Medical College.)

film for massive pulmonary embolism, especially when serial studies are available.[12, 13] Acutely appearing *plump* hilar arteries are strongly suggestive of embolic disease. In an examination of 25 arteriographically determined cases of massive pulmonary artery occlusion, 14 had such findings on chest x-ray.[8] That 13 of these 14 findings were on the right is not surprising because of the difficulty in appreciating left-sided hilar signs owing to cardiac and main pulmonary artery shadows. As pointed out by Fraser and Paré,[14] the increased size of the vessel is due to distention by bulk thrombus and not to increased vascular resistance of the lung. Increased vascular resistance secondary to arterial thrombus will increase flow to non-affected lung segments, causing an actual hyperemia through normal vasculature (observed in 10 of 25 cases by Kerr et al.[8]). The normal maximum diameter of the descending right pulmonary artery has been given as 16 mm in adult males and 15 mm in adult females.[15] The presence of massive thrombi can conceivably be determined by such measurement, but the most reliable utilization of this sign would be observation over recent sequential studies. Decreased pulsation under fluoroscopy in enlarged, thrombosed hilar arteries has been reported[16, 17]; however, the practicality of this observation appears questionable.

Abrupt tapering or termination of a vessel, the "knuckle sign," is very rarely noted, but can be diagnostic when present.[2, 9, 17] Non-specific signs that sometimes accompany thromboembolic disease are acute cor pulmonale (10 per cent) and diminished volume of a lower lobe (28 per cent) with displacement of a major fissure or elevation of a hemidiaphragm.[8, 18] These signs are obviously not diagnostic, but in the proper clinical setting may increase or even arouse suspicion.

Radiographic abnormalities in pulmonary embolism with infarction would essentially be the same as described previously, except that parenchymal consolidation is observed as an increased radiographic density rather than the hyperlucency of oligemia. Changes in arterial size may still be noted, and loss of lung volume has been reported in as high as 50 per cent of patients in this category.[14, 19] Parenchymal consolidation may be due to actual tissue necrosis or to so-called "reversible infarction" (i.e., hemorrhage and edema). In the latter case, the consolidation may clear within three to seven days,[20] but if infarction leads to necrosis, the average time of resolution is about three weeks, usually with permanent residual fibrotic changes.[1, 21]

The time of onset of increased radiographic density after the acute embolic event may vary from 10 hours to one week.[22–24] The "classic" configuration, first described by Hampton and Castleman,[25] is a homogeneous wedge-shaped density in the peripheral region of the lung with a rounded, convex apex pointing toward the hilum—commonly referred to as a "Hampton's hump" (Fig.

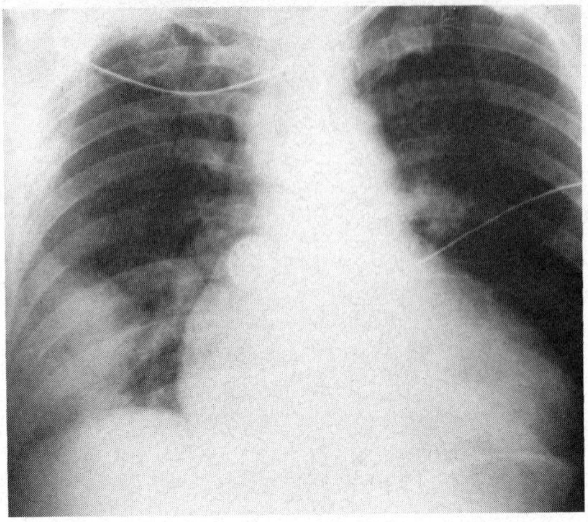

*Figure 4–3.* Posteroanterior chest x-ray of patient with pulmonary embolism, demonstrating "Hampton's hump." (Courtesy of Dr. Jack L. Westcott, The New York Hospital and Cornell University Medical College.)

4–3). The absence of an air bronchogram in a parenchymal consolidation is indicative of infarction[26] as opposed to a pneumonic process, but the presence of an air bronchogram is inconclusive because it can sometimes be observed in patients with pulmonary embolism.

Although not valuable as a diagnostic aid, the pattern of resolution described by Woesner and coworkers[27] may be useful during the latter stages of the disease process. Their "melting sign" (Fig. 4–4) refers to the relatively homogeneous manner in which parenchymal densities due to infarction diminish on serial radiographs. These shadows maintain their uniform consistency and shape as they gradually decrease in intensity. This is in sharp contrast to the clearing of a pneumonia, in which an originally homogeneous density becomes patchy with areas of lucency and significant changes in shape.

The chest x-ray, then, is the starting point in the diagnostic work-up for suspected pulmonary embolism. It will only rarely establish a diagnosis, may yield information directing suspicion elsewhere (pneumonia, tumor, and so forth), or may serve to increase the possibility that the patient has suffered a thromboembolic event and point to further testing. The next diagnostic step is almost always to obtain a lung scan.

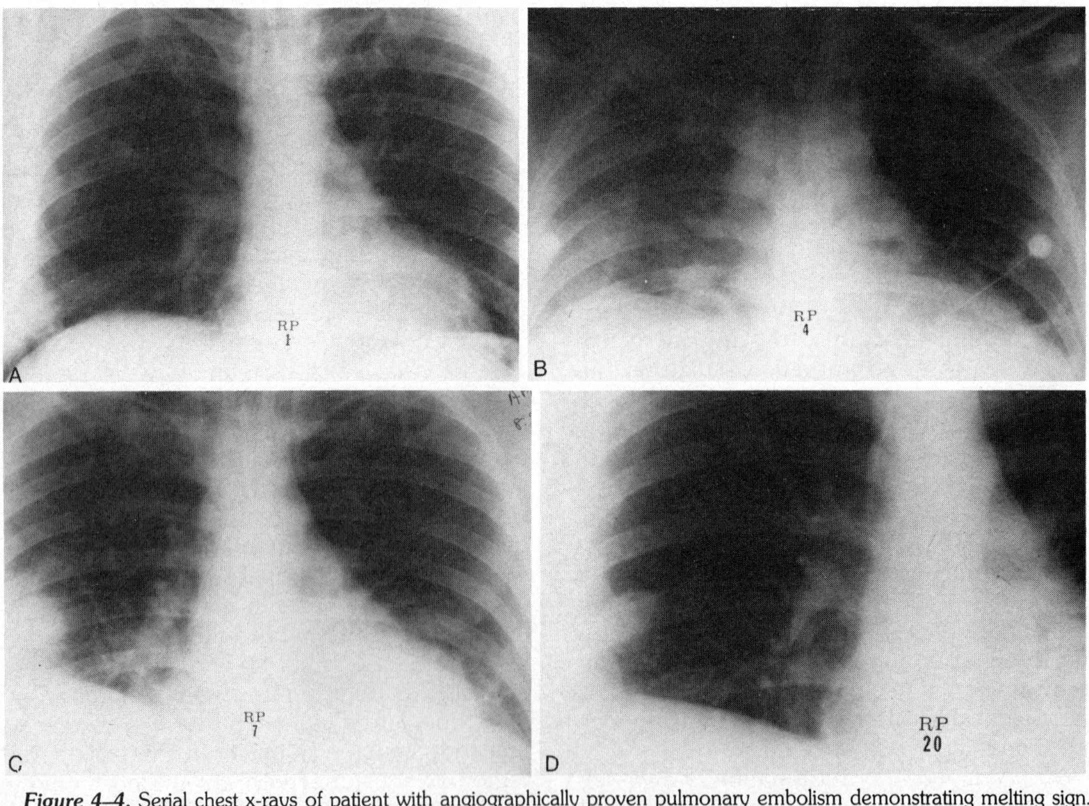


*Figure 4–4.* Serial chest x-rays of patient with angiographically proven pulmonary embolism demonstrating melting sign. *A,* Day 1, consolidation due to right lower lobe infarct; *B,* Day 4, increased density in right lower lobe due to edema and hemorrhage around infarcted parenchyma; *C,* Day 7, homogeneous clearing (melting); *D,* Day 20, further homogeneous resolution (melting). (Courtesy of Dr. Jack L. Westcott, The New York Hospital and Cornell University Medical College.)

### Radionuclide Studies

The lung scan is the diagnostic examination most often utilized for patients with suspected pulmonary embolism. The results of this study can also be misused by the clinician. An appreciation of the principles involved in the performance and interpretation of these studies may aid in the proper clinical management of these patients.

Radioisotopes have been used to study pulmonary physiology and pathology for 30 years.[28] Inhalation of radioactive gases was utilized as early as 1955 in an effort to quantitate pulmonary function and was later used together with perfusion scans to increase specificity with regard to the diagnosis of pulmonary embolism.[29, 30] Radionuclides were introduced for the study of lung perfusion in 1959.[31, 32] Radioactive gases were injected intravenously and would diffuse into the alveoli during the first transit through the lungs. Scintillation counters were then used to estimate regional blood flow. In 1964, radiolabeled particles were shown to accurately demonstrate the pattern of pulmonary blood flow, and clinical applications soon followed (Table 4–1).[33–35]

Because pulmonary emboli will diminish blood flow to regions of lung parenchyma, a radionuclide perfusion study is performed in patients suspected of an embolic event. In addition, a baseline perfusion scan should be obtained for patients with documented acute deep venous thrombosis. These patients are at high risk for developing pulmonary emboli and may have a chronically abnormal perfusion pattern on lung scan without acute pulmonary embolism. In any patient at high risk for PE, a baseline study becomes an invaluable aid to interpretation of later scans, should pulmonary embolism be suspected subsequently (Fig. 4–5).

Pulmonary perfusion scanning usually involves the use of $^{99m}$Tc-labeled particles of macroaggregated albumin (MAA) or albumin microspheres. Known hypersensitivity to albumin is a relative contraindication to this procedure. These perfusion techniques employ the lungs as a filter to remove intravenously injected particulate matter. With the pulmonary arteriolar capillary bed varying from 6 to 10 μ in diameter, particles entering the pulmonary circulation that are greater than 10 μ will be lodged within these vessels, effectively functioning as microemboli. Injected particles are thoroughly mixed within the right heart chambers so that distribution will be uniform and will remain trapped within the pulmonary vasculature; thus, gamma cameras can record areas of lung perfusion. Normal lungs contain about 280 million precapillary arterioles capable of trapping the administered particles.[36] The usual injection of albumin aggregates or microspheres is about 200,000 to 300,000 particles, up to a maximum of 500,000. Significantly less than 0.2 per cent of the precapillary vessels are occluded during the study, and no changes in pulmonary function have been noted.[37] Patients with severe pulmonary hypertension pose a special problem, because injection of a standard dose of particles can prove fatal.[38] Those patients with a significant right-to-left shunt will dispatch a proportionate fraction of these microembolic particles systemically. For patients with severe pulmonary hypertension or significant right-to-left shunt, the study can be safely performed if the number of injected particles is decreased to about 50,000. The biologic halftime for breakdown and clearance is 4 to 8 hours. The breakdown products will then be phagocytized by the reticuloendothelial system. The minimum toxic dose for MAA has been reported to be 20 mg/kg,[39] which exceeds the usual total imaging dose of 10 μg by a factor of about $10^3$. The primary difference between the two types of particles currently being used is one of size distribution. MAA injections contain about 90 per cent of the particles with diameters between 10 and 40 μ, whereas albumin microspheres contain a more uniform particle size, with a distribution between 20 and 40 μ. Because of the difficulty in preparing microspheres and the ready availability of MAA kits, the latter are employed in most clinical units.

A special problem arises regarding pregnant women presenting with symptoms of pulmonary embolism. Although no abnormalities of pregnancy due to a lung scan have been reported, minimizing radiation exposure to the fetus must be of prime concern. The estimated radiation dose to the unborn child has been approximated as 30 millirads/milliCurie,[40] which, while not excessive and significantly less than that received from pulmonary arteriography, should be avoided unless the clinical situation appears life-threatening.

Because pulmonary blood flow is influenced significantly by both gravity and ventilation,[41] the patient is placed in a supine position and asked to breathe deeply prior to injection. This will counteract the de-

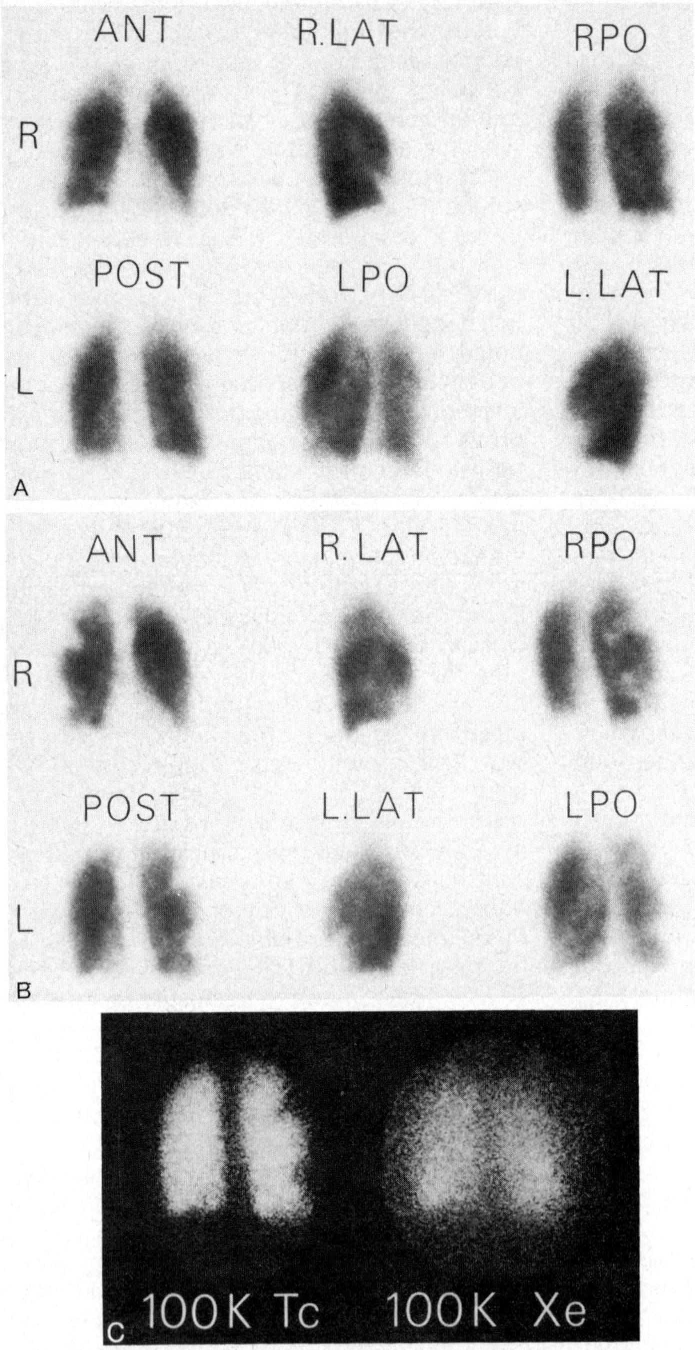


***Figure 4–5.*** *A*, Essentially normal $^{99m}$Tc macroaggregated albumin perfusion study done as part of a preoperative protocol. *B*, One week later, multiple right-sided perfusion defects are demonstrated in the postoperative perfusion scan, consistent with pulmonary embolism. *C*, Posterior ventilation with $^{133}$Xe (right panel) demonstrating normal ventilation—a V/Q mismatch consistent with a high probability of pulmonary embolism. A 100,000-count $^{99m}$Tc perfusion image (left panel) is shown for comparison. (Courtesy of Dr. Barbara J. McNeil, Brigham and Women's Hospital and Harvard Medical School.)

creased apical perfusion normally observed in the erect healthy patient. Care must be taken not to allow blood to clot within the syringe, because clots will absorb the particulate albumin, causing "hot spots" on the scan. Radioactive aggregates will also adhere to intravenous tubing, making injection through a central venous access line a potential source of artifact. Although imaging can be done immediately post injection, waiting 3 to 5 minutes permits the reticuloendothelial system to clear smaller particles, reducing background interference. Imaging is usually done in an upright position, if possible, to allow better visualization of the bases. In addition to anterior, posterior and both lateral views, both posterior oblique views should usually be obtained, because they have been shown to improve definition of perfusion defects, especially in the posterior and lateral basal segments.[42–44] Scanning in the anterior oblique positions has also been proposed,[45] but this is not routinely done in most centers unless additional views are necessary to clarify questionable perfusion defects.

A normal perfusion study will effectively eliminate a diagnosis of pulmonary embolism. Perfusion defects due to an embolism can begin to resolve within 24 to 48 hours after the acute event, especially in younger patients. Older patients, on the other hand, may never experience complete resolution. A lung scan should therefore be obtained as temporally close to the onset of clinical symptoms as possible. Although emboli will cause abnormalities, perfusion defects are not at all specific. In addition to pulmonary pathology causing infiltrative densities on chest x-rays, conditions such as asthma, chronic obstructive pulmonary disease (COPD), and bronchial mucus plugs, normally associated with a clear chest x-ray, produce regional hypoxia and a secondary decrease in perfusion. These airway abnormalities will not ventilate normally, whereas lung parenchyma affected by a primary reduction in blood flow, an embolic event, has been shown to exhibit a normal ventilation pattern.[46, 47] For these reasons, both Wagner[29] and DeNardo[30] suggested adding a radionuclide ventilation scan to the study to increase the specificity for the diagnosis of pulmonary thromboembolic disease.

That perfusion scans are not at all specific can be seen from the data in Table 4–2 (p. 50). Data obtained from several sources show that only 62 per cent of patients with at least one segmental perfusion defect had angio-

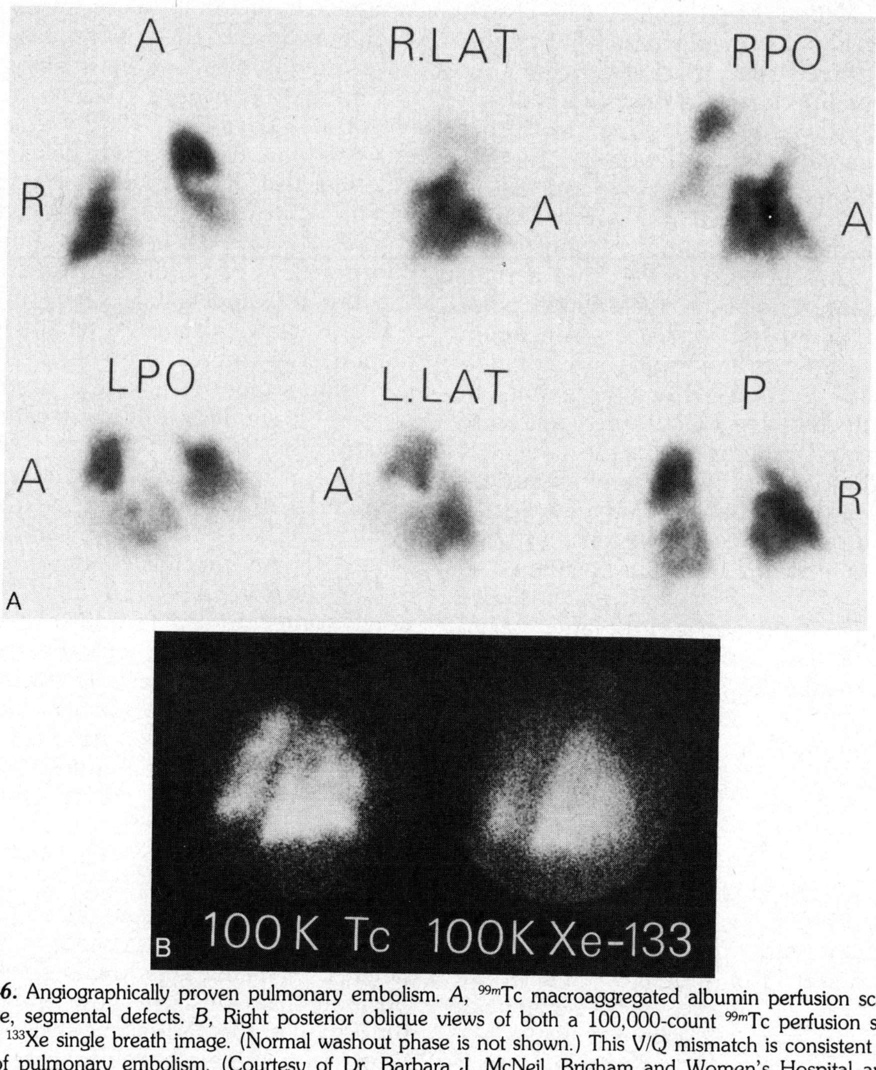


*Figure 4–6.* Angiographically proven pulmonary embolism. *A*, $^{99m}$Tc macroaggregated albumin perfusion scan showing multiple large, segmental defects. *B*, Right posterior oblique views of both a 100,000-count $^{99m}$Tc perfusion study and a mismatching $^{133}$Xe single breath image. (Normal washout phase is not shown.) This V/Q mismatch is consistent with a high probability of pulmonary embolism. (Courtesy of Dr. Barbara J. McNeil, Brigham and Women's Hospital and Harvard Medical School.)

graphically proven pulmonary embolism.[48–52] Studies by McNeil[48] and by Alderson et al.[49] have documented the significantly increased specificity for pulmonary embolism obtained by the use of combined ventilation-perfusion scintigraphy. This premise has been confirmed in several subsequent studies.[50–52] Perfusion defects that ventilate normally are called ventilation-perfusion (V/Q) mismatches and reflect a high probability of pulmonary embolism (Fig. 4–6). Regions of abnormal perfusion that do not ventilate (primary ventilatory pathology) or that retain significant activity during the washout phase (obstructive lung disease) are referred to as V/Q matches and have been shown clinically to represent a low probability of pulmonary embolism. McNeil[53] has further refined probabilities of disease by employing Bayes theorem using lung scan results along with posterior probabilities of pulmonary embolism.

Ventilation scans involve either inhalation of a radioactive gas or, much less frequently, intravenous injection of a diffusible radioactive gas dissolved in saline. The most usual type of ventilation study involves direct inhalation of a radioactive gas dissolved in oxygen. A closed system is used, which includes a mask or mouthpiece; intake, rebreathing, and exhaust valves; and a trap, usually charcoal, to absorb the exhaled radioactive gas. Ventilation studies are dependent on patient cooperation for proper inspiration and up to 30 seconds of breath-holding. In clinical units that use a mouthpiece and nose clips instead of a face mask, the patient is additionally required to maintain an airtight seal around the mouthpiece with his lips. If ventilation precedes the perfusion study, the study is done with the patient positioned so that the lungs are imaged in the posterior position. If ventilation is done after perfusion, the patient is positioned for the view that best delineates the perfusion defects. The face mask is securely fastened to form an airtight breathing system, and the radioactive gas, most commonly $^{133}$Xe, is injected into the system while the patient is instructed to inspire as deeply as possible. An initial "single-breath" view, usually 100,000 counts, is obtained. The patient then rebreathes in the closed system for 3 to 5 minutes to reach equilibration, with views taken for 300,000 to 500,000 counts. The system is adjusted so that room air is inhaled, with exhaled air going to the trap. "Washout" images are obtained sequentially every 30 to 45 seconds until no significant activity from inspired gas remains.

The radioactive gases currently being used for ventilation scanning include $^{133}$Xe, $^{127}$Xe, and $^{81m}$Kr (Table 4–1). Because $^{133}$Xe is a fission by-product, it is inexpensive. In addition, $^{133}$Xe is widely available and is transportable (half-life of 5 days). Its main drawback is that the imaging photon is only 81 keV, potentially allowing down scatter from $^{99m}$Tc (140 keV) to interfere with the study if it is administered after the perfusion examination. On the other hand, $^{81m}$Kr, with an imaging photon of 190 keV, has no such liability, and its half-life of 13 seconds eliminates the necessity of special collection and disposal devices. For clinical use, $^{81m}$Kr is obtained from $^{81}$Rb, which is cyclotron-produced and has a half-life of 4.6 hours. Therefore, $^{81m}$Kr can only be used at sites in relatively close proximity to cyclotron facilities. Radiation dose to the patient is significantly lowered with this isotope, making imaging in multiple projections possible. $^{127}$Xe (half-life of 36.4 days and 172 keV and 203 keV imaging photons) appears to be of significant potential use, but its availability is limited, and it is quite expensive. Several comparative studies[58–60] have shown little difference in interpretation of ventilation scans using the two xenon isotopes.

Controversy exists as to whether the ventilation scan should precede or follow the perfusion study when $^{133}$Xe is used.[61–65] This question is significant in many clinical units, because the use of $^{127}$Xe and $^{81m}$Kr is not practical in most areas, and the majority of ventilation examinations utilize the readily available $^{133}$Xe and its 81-keV imaging photon. With the imaging windows set for the 81-keV photon, it is feared by some that down scatter from $^{99m}$Tc (140 keV), if present from prior perfusion, will adversely affect the quality of the image and potentially obscure trapping during the washout phase. Postperfusion ventilation has been found to be less reliable than preperfusion ventilation by some investigators. Many others, however, feel that interpretation of ventilation images is unaffected by the relatively small amount of scatter and that this very slight disadvantage is more than offset by avoiding unnecessary ventilation and, when it is needed, by being able to choose the proper position that will best allow observation of the region of the perfusion defect. One study found that 48 per cent of lung scans would

***Table 4–1.*** Commonly Used Radionuclides

| Radionuclide | Half-life | Principal Photon Energies (keV) | Principal Photon Energies (% abundance) | Usual Dose (mCi) | Radiopharmaceutical | Radiation Dose (rads/mCi) | |
|---|---|---|---|---|---|---|---|
| $^{99m}Tc$ | 6.0 h | 140 | 90 | 3 | MAA | 0.002<br>0.26 | (whole body)<br>(lungs) |
| | | | | 10–15 | Red blood cells | 0.027 | (whole body) |
| | | | | 3 | Microspheres | 0.23 | (lungs) |
| $^{133}Xe$ | 5.27 d | 81 | 37 | 10–20 | Gas | 0.02<br>0.1 | (lungs)<br>(trachea) |
| | | | | | Intravenous solution | 0.018 | (lungs) |
| $^{127}Xe$ | 36.4 d | 172<br>203<br>375 | 22<br>66<br>20 | 5–10 | Gas | 0.0013<br>0.0047<br>0.0017 | (whole body)<br>(lungs)<br>(red marrow) |
| $^{81m}Kr$ | 13 s | 190 | 65 | 3–5 | Gas | 0.0047<br>0.019 | (lungs)<br>(trachea) |
| | | | | | Intravenous solution | 0.001 | (lungs) |
| $^{111}In$ | 2.8 d | 173<br>247 | 87<br>94 | 0.5 | Platelets | 0.6<br>33.5 | (whole body)<br>(spleen) |
| $^{131}I$ | 8.05 d | 284<br>364<br>637 | 4.8<br>83<br>6.9 | 0.3 | MAA | 0.008<br>2.0 | (whole body)<br>(lungs) |
| | | 723 | 1.6 | 0.3 | Fibrinogen | 0.3<br>1.0 | (whole body)<br>(liver) |
| $^{125}I$ | 60.2 d | 35 | 7 | 0.1–0.3 | Fibrinogen | 0.01<br>0.2 | (whole body)<br>(liver) |

d = days; h = hours; s = seconds; MAA = macroaggregated albumin.

not require ventilation, either because of a normal perfusion or a chest x-ray abnormality matching a perfusion defect.[65] Further, Alderson and coworkers[44] demonstrated experimentally that of 23 dogs studied, six had angiographically proven embolic defects that could only be visualized in oblique projections. It would appear, on balance, that a ventilatory study in the position that best shows the perfusion defect would be optimal for precise interpretation. Alderson[62] has proposed a compromise solution by suggesting a preperfusion posterior ventilation with a postperfusion study, if necessary, in the most advantageous position. Although a single posterior preperfusion ventilation scan has been traditional, the practice of obtaining a ventilation study solely after the perfusion scan has become widespread.

The radionuclide lung scan is the most frequently employed modality for the diagnosis of pulmonary embolism; therefore, accurate analysis of the scan results is most important. The diagnostic scheme will usually contain five categories: normal, indeterminate, high, moderate, or low probability of pulmonary embolism, based on prior clinical experience. Agreement is universal that a normal study, one without perfusion defects, will essentially exclude a clinical diagnosis of an embolic event. If the perfusion scan is normal, no ventilation study is needed. Experimental studies in animals have demonstrated that perfusion defects will be seen in 80 per cent of occluded vessels between 1.1 and 2.0 mm in size.[44] Embolic defects smaller than this are not usually clinically significant.

The indeterminate study shows perfusion defects in regions of abnormality on chest films. Severely diminished pulmonary blood flow is a nonspecific finding (Table 4–2) and can be caused by a large number of disease states that will demonstrate opacified irregularities on chest radiographs (e.g., pneumonia, tumor, edema, effusion, atelectasis, and so forth). Some of these nonembolic diseases *may*, early in their course, ventilate normally and could give the erroneous impression of pulmonary embolism if the chest x-ray is not taken into consideration. Therefore, no ventilation is performed, and

*Table 4–2.* Scintigraphic Results for Angiographically Proven Pulmonary Embolism*

| Scintigraphy | Perfusion Only PE+ (%) | Perfusion Only PE− | V/Q Mismatch PE+ (%) | V/Q Mismatch PE− | V/Q Match PE+ (%) | V/Q Match PE− |
|---|---|---|---|---|---|---|
| Indeterminate | 63 (35) | 116 | | | | |
| One or more segmental or larger defects | 141 (62) | 88 | 155 (86) | 25 | 8 (9) | 77 |
| Nothing more than subsegmental defects | 15 (9) | 162 | 7 (16) | 36 | 1 (3) | 28 |
| Multiple defects, the largest being: | | | | | | |
| Lung | 3 (60) | 2 | 2 (100) | 0 | | |
| Lobar | 56 (75) | 19 | 39 (95) | 2 | 2 (33) | 4 |
| Segmental | 40 (63) | 24 | 30 (91) | 3 | | |
| Subsegmental | 6 (7) | 85 | 4 (36) | 7 | 0 (0) | 17 |
| Single defect: | | | | | | |
| Lung | 1 | 2 | 1 | 0 | | |
| Lobar | 3 | 6 | 1 | 0 | | |
| Segmental | 2 | 6 | 0 | 4 | | |
| Subsegmental | 3 | 31 | 0 | 0 | | |

*A compilation of data from several major studies.

the study is considered nondiagnostic. If clinical suspicion is high, an arteriogram is usually required to establish a diagnosis. Attempts at lowering the number of indeterminate examinations by an analysis of both the scan and the chest x-ray have been made by Biello and coworkers.[66] A series of 111 indeterminate scans was studied by comparing the size of the perfusion defect with the size of the radiographic abnormality. Their criterion for size discrepancy was that the perfusion defect be *substantially* larger or smaller than the radiographic abnormality. Comparing the results with arteriograms obtained in each case, they found that if the radiographic abnormality was larger than the perfusion defect, one of 14 (7 per cent) had an embolism. If the relative abnormalities were of comparable size, 26 per cent (20 of 77) had positive angiograms. If the perfusion defect was significantly larger than the chest film irregularity, a ventilation scan was obtained. Arteriograms were positive in 89 per cent (16 of 18) with a V/Q mismatch and were negative in two additional patients with a V/Q match.

A correct understanding of the significance of interpretations attached to abnormal lung scintigraphy in the presence of a normal chest x-ray is essential for proper evaluation and treatment. The analysis of the lung scan and its usefulness in diagnosing pulmonary embolism have been a controversial subject in recent years because of questions raised by Robin.[67] This controversy has continued,[52, 68] even though the major portion of the data he quoted was based on antiquated procedures ($^{131}$I MAA, rectilinear scans, only anterior and posterior views), and the interpretive procedures employed were not consistent with current clinical practice.[62, 69] Recent clinical data have generally supported the concept that V/Q mismatches are highly specific for emboli, and V/Q matches minimize the probability of the disease.[50–53]

Various clinical studies have grouped data pertaining to perfusion defects in different ways, making direct and exact comparison difficult. Perfusion abnormalities will be listed as either lobar, segmental, or subsegmental by some authors[49, 51]; whereas others[50] will categorize them as up to 25 per cent of a segment, between 25 and 75 per cent of a segment, and greater than 75 per cent of a segment; and still others[52] will separate such defects into two classifications: (1) subsegmental and (2) segmental or larger. Table 4–2 is a compilation of perfusion and V/Q data extrapolated (when possible) from several major studies[48–52] of perfusion and ventilation scans for suspected pulmonary embolism, all using angiographic confirmation. Defects greater than half of a segment are treated as segmental in nature when appropriate, and anything smaller is considered subsegmental. From these data, several statements can be made about angiographically proven pulmonary embolism:

1. Isolated subsegmental defects rarely indicate disease.
2. Multiple defects predominate.
3. A V/Q mismatch is very strongly suggestive of PE.
4. A V/Q match is indicative of a low probability of PE.

These findings and clinical recommendations are summarized in Table 4–3.

Chronic obstructive pulmonary disease

***Table 4–3.*** Guidelines for Interpretation of Ventilation-Perfusion Scans

| Perfusion | Chest X-ray | Ventilation | Interpretation | Prob. PE† (%) | Recommendation |
|---|---|---|---|---|---|
| Normal | | Not indicated | Normal study | 0 | PE excluded |
| Single subsegmental defect | Normal | Not indicated | Low probability | 10 | No treatment indicated |
| Multiple subsegmental defects | Normal | Not done | Low probability* | 10* | No treatment indicated* |
| Multiple subsegmental defects | Normal | V/Q match | Low probability* | 5* | No treatment indicated* |
| Multiple subsegmental defects | Normal | V/Q mismatch | Intermediate (i.e., moderate) probability | 19 | Arteriography |
| Segmental or larger defects | Normal | V/Q match | Low probability* | 10* | No treatment indicated* |
| Segmental or larger defects | Normal | V/Q mismatch | High probability | 86 | Anticoagulate |
| Abnormal | Severe COPD | | Indeterminate | 19 | Arteriography |
| Abnormal | Abnormal in region of perfusion defect | Not indicated | Indeterminate | 35 | Arteriography |

*Currently the focus of an ongoing multicentered NIH-sponsored trial.
†An estimate based on data from several major studies.

(COPD) is the single most common cause of false-positive results in perfusion scintigraphy (Fig. 4–7). Defects observed represent both permanent pathologic changes and acute exacerbations of bronchitis. Ventilation studies will sometimes detect these primary airway abnormalities as matching defects on the single-breath image, but more often noted is retention of activity in diseased areas of lung with regionally delayed washout of radioactive gas.[70] COPD, especially when severe, has caused considerable difficulty in the interpretation of lung scans. With highly irregular perfusion and large areas of retention on ventilation, the appearance of underlying embolic disease can often be missed. Alderson and coworkers[71] have reported a significant number of false-negative studies (3 of 16) in patients with severe COPD that affected more than 50 per cent of the pulmonary parenchyma. These patients pose a significant diagnostic problem and, rather than be classified in the standard manner, they should be treated as indeterminate and should generally undergo arteriography.

Improved specificity in the diagnosis of pulmonary embolism has been reported with the use of positron-emitting $^{15}$O-labeled carbon dioxide.[72–74] $^{15}$O is a cyclotron-produced radionuclide with a very short half-life of 2.1 minutes. $C^{15}O_2$ is inhaled and very rapidly diffuses across alveolar membranes and into the pulmonary capillary beds. It is almost instantaneously hydrated and dissociated into bicarbonate ion, which undergoes rapid oxygen exchange, resulting in $^{15}$O-labeled water. This $H_2{}^{15}O$ is cleared by pulmonary blood flow. The rate of clearance is proportional to regional blood flow. In angiographically diagnosed pulmonary embolism, clearance of $^{15}$O-labeled water from embolized segments is markedly delayed, secondary to diminished or absent perfusion distal to the site of an embolus. Animal studies have demonstrated that abnormally decreased regions of perfusion are more easily observable as "hot spots" rather than the absence of activity noted on MAA scans.[72] A comparison study was undertaken in which 27 patients suspected of having pulmonary emboli had a conventional V/Q scan with $^{99m}$Tc MAA and $^{133}$Xe and a $C^{15}O_2$ inhalation study, in addition to a pulmonary arteriogram.[73] Combined perfusion-ventilation imaging had a sensitivity of 80 per cent and a specificity of 50 per cent, whereas the positron imaging showed a sensitivity of 87 per cent and a specificity of 92 per cent. This increased specificity was presumably due to the large number of patients with COPD or CHF. Inhaled $C^{15}O_2$ is not delivered to poorly ventilated regions of the lungs. False-negative studies will result from failure to ventilate areas of consolidation secondary to emboli. Repeated studies are quite feasible because of the low radiation dose to the patient (9 mR to the lungs and 4.5 mR whole body for a 70-kg adult). The major limitation of this technique is the necessity of a nearby cyclotron for the production of the short-lived $^{15}$O.

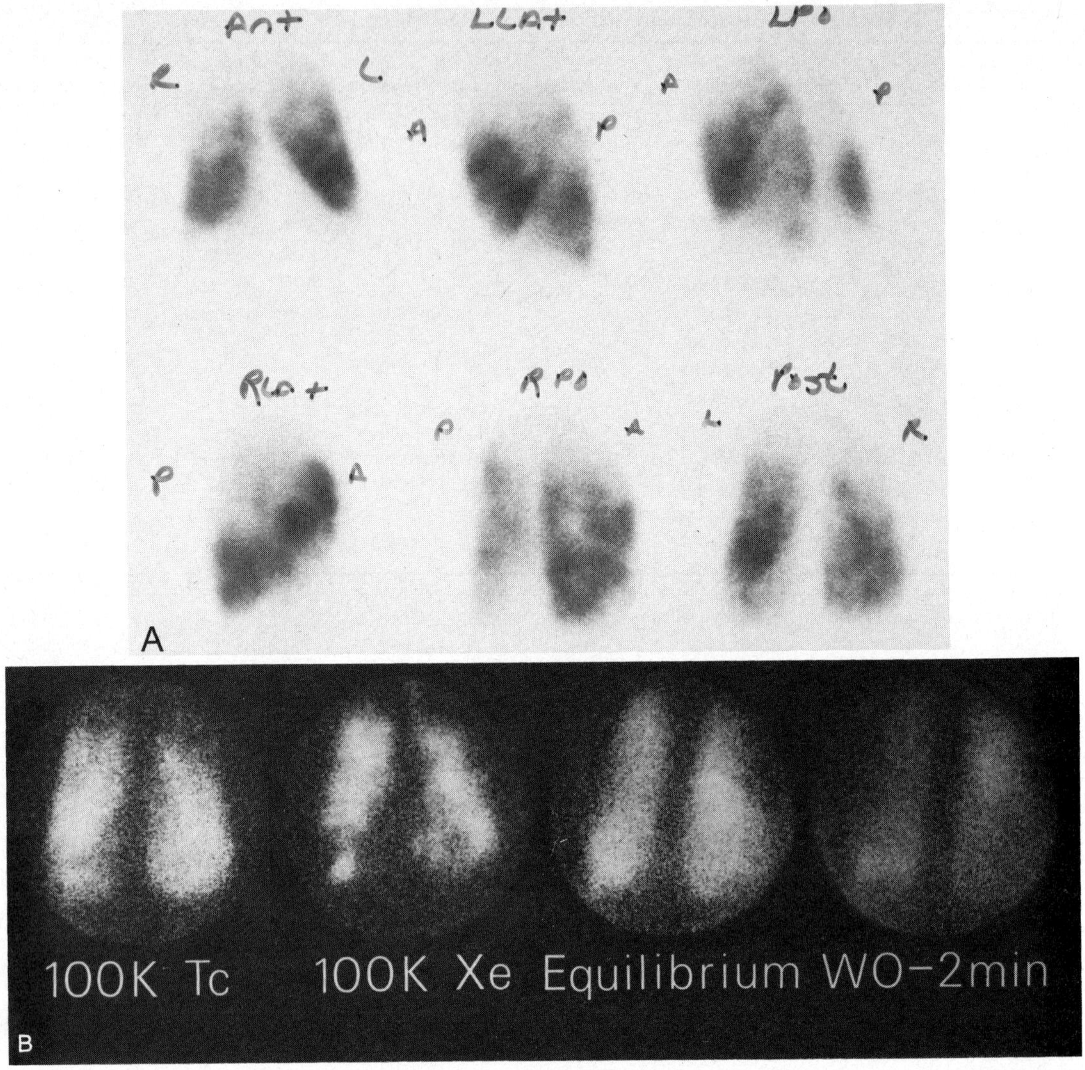


*Figure 4–7.* A, Highly abnormal perfusion study in patient with severe chronic obstructive pulmonary disease. B, Posterior views demonstrating: 100-K $^{99m}Tc$ perfusion; abnormal single breath image with matching defects; relative ventilation of both lungs during equilibrium; and areas of retention during washout, matching perfusion abnormalities. (Courtesy of Dr. Barbara J. McNeil, Brigham and Women's Hospital and Harvard Medical School.)

$^{111}In$-labeled platelets, in addition to their use in detecting deep venous thrombi, are also being used in an attempt to detect pulmonary emboli[75, 76] (see also Chapter 13). Experimental results appear promising, if imaging is accomplished prior to heparinization, but large-scale clinical trials have yet to be reported.

In summary, combined V/Q scintigraphy, although not a perfect diagnostic examination, offers a reasonable compromise between diagnostic accuracy and potential patient morbidity. A normal perfusion scan will definitely exclude pulmonary embolism. High- and low-probability studies are not absolutely diagnostic, and the decision to proceed with angiography will usually hinge on the overall clinical picture. Studies that are interpreted as moderate probability or indeterminate add little significant information to the diagnostic work-up. These patients should proceed to arteriography.

## Pulmonary Arteriography

Radiographic visualization of human vasculature was reported within two months of Roentgen's announcement of the discovery of x-rays, with the injection of radiopaque material into vessels in an amputated hand. Visualization of the human pulmonary vasculature following intravenous injection of contrast material was accomplished in 1923, and in 1928 Forssman, after practicing on a cadaver, was able to successfully introduce a catheter into his own heart, using an antecubital approach. The first attempt to diagnose pulmonary embolism arteriographically was reported by Jesser and deTakats in 1941.[77] Further advances continue to this day, including ongoing research in angiopharmaceuticals leading to less toxic contrast materials and the development and refinement of selective catheterization techniques, which are now very successfully employed and used almost exclusively for the visualization of the pulmonary circulation.

Pulmonary arteriography is accepted as the "gold standard" for the determination of pulmonary thromboembolic disease.[78–80] An invasive procedure, it affords direct, high-resolution radiographic visualization of contrast-filled arteries. Indications for an arteriogram are not universally established. However, it is generally agreed that a normal radioisotopic perfusion study excludes significant pulmonary emboli and the need for an arteriogram. An angiogram will usually be obtained prior to embolectomy, inferior vena caval interruption, and thrombolytic therapy. For patients who have had high-probability lung scans, the complications of anticoagulant therapy must be considered before treatment is begun. If there are relative contraindications to heparinization (e.g., gastrointestinal bleeding, immediate postoperative or postpartum period, and so forth), a definitive diagnosis is often desirable prior to anticoagulation. For those patients with a low-probability scan but with a high clinical suspicion of disease, a pulmonary angiogram may be warranted solely on the basis of strong clinical suspicion. Only a "normal" perfusion study (not a low-probability scan) excludes a diagnosis of pulmonary embolism. Some patients with high- or low-probability studies will be misdiagnosed by the lung scan alone. Those patients with an indeterminate or moderate-probability scan are no closer to a final diagnosis than before the lung scan. In these rather frequent situations, clinical judgment must be used. However, in general, clinical intuition should not be substituted for a definitive radiologic diagnosis. The risks inherent in angiography for most patients are considerably less than the potential complications of treating a disease-free patient or of nontreatment in the face of embolic disease.[79, 81] Marsh and coworkers[82] have urged a reanalysis of criteria used in analyzing lung scans, suggesting that the distribution of underlying disease states in patients currently undergoing pulmonary arteriography has significantly changed over the last 10 to 15 years, so that oncologic and postoperative patients now predominate. In their study, six of 18 patients with low-probability lung scans had positive arteriograms and six of 11 patients with high-probability studies had negative arteriograms. They concluded that in this new patient population, arteriography is becoming increasingly important in arriving at a correct diagnosis. The patient population in this study, however, is small compared with other recent series,[51, 52] the results of which continue to compare favorably with the older reports.

Arteriography is *the* definitive procedure for establishing a diagnosis of pulmonary embolism. Even so, it must be noted that arteriograms are not always diagnostic, with as many as 17 per cent of indeterminate examinations occurring in one early series.[81] There are probably no absolute contraindications to pulmonary arteriography. Known allergy to contrast material (which can be pretreated with steroids and diphenhydramine [Benadryl]), recent myocardial infarction, cardiac arrhythmias, renal failure, and pulmonary arterial hypertension have been considered relative contraindications to attempting the study.

The method employed for the arteriographic evaluation of pulmonary embolism usually involves selective catheterization techniques.[83] Injection of contrast material into a main pulmonary artery opacifies the entire arterial tree of the lung. Radiographs obtained with this nonselective technique will show significant overlap of opacified vessels and can be difficult to interpret. Selective angiography delivers contrast media through a catheter that has been advanced directly into the artery being investigated. This procedure allows unobscured, highly detailed visualization of the vascular anatomy in question (Fig. 4–8). A catheter is introduced into a peripheral access vein, usually the median basilic or the femoral vein. Although both are used, a brachial approach is preferred if there is any suspicion of potential dislodgement of clot. Introduction of a catheter into the internal jugular, axillary,

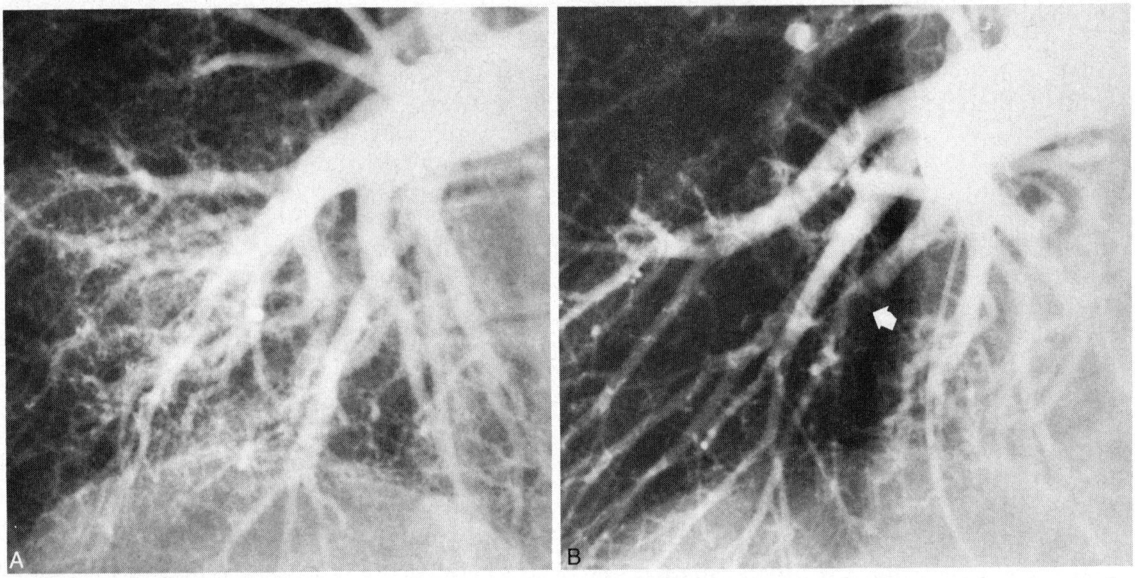


*Figure 4–8.* Selective right pulmonary arteriogram. *A*, Left posterior oblique projection of right lower lobe with normal appearing pulmonary arteriogram, due to overlap of vasculature. *B*, Right posterior oblique projection of the same area exhibiting an intravascular filling defect (arrow) in the artery to the lateral basal segment of the right lower lobe. (Courtesy of Dr. Thomas A. Sos, The New York Hospital and Cornell University Medical College.)

or subclavian veins has also been done when necessary. Catheters with side holes are employed to minimize potential complications of right ventricular perforation or other cardiac injury from whipping of the tip under power injection. The catheter is advanced into the right heart and main pulmonary artery under fluoroscopy, using small injections of contrast material as needed. As the catheter is advanced, hemodynamic measurements of right heart pressures should be obtained routinely. Radiographs can be obtained after injection of contrast material into the main pulmonary artery, and more selective views are obtained after advancing the catheter distally. These selective injections opacify only a small portion of the pulmonary vasculature and allow direct, detailed observation of structures, unhindered by overlying vessels from other segments. The volume of contrast agent is continually decreased as the examination becomes more peripheral, so that contrast reactions and toxic intimal damage to injected vessels can be minimized.

A definitive diagnosis of pulmonary embolism depends on visualization of a clot.[2, 80, 84] Primary arteriographic signs of emboli include persistent lucent defects without obstruction to flow or a trailing edge of an intraluminal lucency if there is complete obstruction to flow distally. If no abnormality is demonstrated, radiographs should be obtained in a second projection to exclude pulmonary embolism. As shown by Bossart and coworkers[85] in a study of 127 consecutive patients referred for arteriography because of suspected pulmonary emboli, in four of 47 positive arteriograms the abnormality was not viewed in the initial projection (see Fig. 4–8*A*), but was seen only in a different obliquity (see Fig. 4–8*B*). A fifth lesion was detected on the first selective study but not in a second view, which was attempted to better view the abnormality. Secondary signs, not in themselves diagnostic but simply indicators of decreased pulmonary perfusion, include areas of avascularity or oligemia, a prolonged arterial phase, tortuosity of peripheral vessels, and delayed visualization of pulmonary venous circulation. Secondary signs are often associated with pulmonary embolism but can occur in other conditions (e.g., bronchial asthma, severe mitral stenosis with associated pulmonary hypertension, or left ventricular failure) and thus are not specific.[86] Adherence to observation of a primary sign for diagnosing an embolus is necessary to prevent false-positive diagnoses.[86, 87] There should be no hesitation to read an equivocal study as indeterminate.

Pulmonary arteriography is an invasive procedure and, as such, does carry the risk of morbidity and mortality, due both to catheterization and contrast reactions.[81, 88–90]

Complications include severe bronchospasm, pulmonary edema, hypotension, anaphylaxis, cardiogenic shock, cardiac perforation, major arrhythmias, endocardial or myocardial injury, pyrogen reactions, and cardiac arrest. In two large reported series involving a total of 1894 patients who underwent pulmonary angiography,[89, 90] the combined morbidity was 4.5 per cent, and a total of five deaths were reported (0.26 per cent). At least four of those deaths involved patients with severe pulmonary hypertension, consistent with earlier reports of increased frequency of deaths during angiocardiography in this subgroup of patients. Hypertonic solutions and ionic contrast agents have been shown experimentally to increase right ventricular and pulmonary artery pressures. Severe hypotensive episodes following the administration of a bolus of contrast material may be due to a severely compromised right ventricle, indicated by an elevated right ventricular end-diastolic pressure (RVEDP), which is incapable of tolerating further increases in pulmonary artery resistance and pressure. All three deaths in one of these series involved patients with an elevated RVEDP of 20 mm Hg or higher.[89] RVEDP can easily be measured during catheterization and should be done routinely. Mills and coworkers[89] have chosen a RVEDP of 20 mm Hg as the safe upper limit for using contrast material and are reluctant to complete studies for patients with more elevated values.

Pulmonary angiography is the most definitive diagnostic modality available. However, it is too invasive to use as a screening or routine diagnostic measure and should be obtained only after performing a lung scan according to the criteria in Table 9–3. The lung scan will help guide the angiographer in choosing appropriate selective and subselective views.[91] Although pulmonary embolism is being diagnosed with increasing frequency,[92] the ability to diagnose this condition accurately remains a major clinical challenge.[93]

### Digital Subtraction Pulmonary Arteriography

Probably the most promising new radiographic modality for diagnosing pulmonary embolism is digital subtraction angiography (DSA). This technique can provide visualization of the pulmonary arterial circulation with peripheral intravenous injection of contrast material. Therefore, there is much potential for reducing the time, expense, morbidity, and mortality usually associated with pulmonary arteriography.[94, 159]

Intravenous arteriography was advocated by Robb and Steinberg[95] in 1939, predating conventional arteriography. Large volumes of contrast material were injected into an extremity and delayed x-rays were taken of the vasculature. The quality of films obtained was not sufficiently detailed, and the procedure became impractical after the advent of arteriographic catheterization procedures. Photographic film subtraction techniques were introduced by Des Plantes[96] in 1935. An initial x-ray is taken without contrast material, and a second film is obtained after the intravenous injection of contrast agent. Initial images are photographically subtracted from the image with contrast in the arterial tree. All extraneous information is thereby removed, enhancing contrast-containing structures. In principle, this procedure should provide maximum enhancement of contrast agent, but in practice, films obtained are suboptimal. Images obtained are diagnostically useful, especially for extracranial arteries, but techniques are cumbersome, motion artifacts abound, and iodinated contrast material is nonuniform.

Recent advances in computer technology have allowed the digitization of images[97–100] (Fig. 4–9). Conventional radiographic or fluoroscopic images are referred to as analog images. Analog images have a continuous gray scale at any and every point. In digital processing of these images, a video camera will record the image by scanning it as a series of lines and outputting a voltage wave that varies at each point along the line in direct proportion to the brightness of the image (Fig. 4–10). This signal is then transmitted to an analog-to-digital converter. A digital image has a discrete number of well-defined shades of gray. Each successive shade of gray is designated by a successive integer. The image matrix is broken up into a defined number of small squares, called pixels, and the analog information for each pixel is converted into a number corresponding to the closest of the defined gray shades available that will match the analog information. The smaller the pixels and the larger the gray scale, the better the resolution of the image (Fig. 4–11). This information is stored in a computer to be retrieved when necessary.

For procedures involving the introduction

to determine the region of maximum concern and to allow imaging efforts to be concentrated there. Coupled closely to the size of the image intensifier is the somewhat inferior resolution obtained, when compared with conventional arteriography. However, larger field of view intensifiers with an increased matrix size may eliminate this shortcoming. An additional problem involves the overlap of contrast-containing vessels on radiographs because of the nonselective nature of intravenous injections. Anteroposterior and oblique projections will eliminate most, but not all, overlap.

Although most digital subtraction pulmonary arteriography has been performed on experimental animals, several clinical trials have been reported, with very encouraging results.[101–104] Twenty to forty ml of contrast material is power injected into a catheter placed in the superior vena cava (SCV) or right atrium, or directly into an antecubital vein. Goodman and Brant-Zawadzki[102] studied 14 patients suspected of having pulmonary emboli using digital subtraction methods. Injection was done through a catheter placed in the right atrium or through an indwelling Swan-Ganz catheter already in place in the main pulmonary artery. Thirteen studies were felt to be of diagnostic quality; the single inadequate examination was due to patient motion. Nine studies were confirmed by conventional arteriography (four positive, five negative) and four patients (all negative studies) were not candidates for arteriography because of their "precarious clinical situation."

A larger series of 57 patients suspected of having pulmonary emboli was studied by Pond and coworkers[101] using a 14.5-inch image intensifier. Thirty-three of these patients had agreed to participate in a protocol comparing digital subtraction pulmonary arteriography with conventional pulmonary arteriography. Catheters were inserted into the SVC or right atrium, and diagnostic examinations were obtained in 31 of the 33 patients, with two patients unable to control respiratory movements for the required 15 seconds. Thirteen patients were diagnosed as having pulmonary emboli; 12 of these were confirmed by arteriography (one was false-positive), and all 18 negative studies were confirmed by arteriograms (specificity 96 per cent, sensitivity 100 per cent). Emboli as small as 2 mm were detected. Of the 24 patients who did not undergo arteriography, 10 had a diagnosis of pulmonary embolism based on the digital study alone. Ludwig and coworkers[103] reported on a comparative study examining the relative merits of digital subtraction techniques with ventilation-perfusion scanning, employing antecubital injection techniques. In 11 patients without preexisting lung disease, five of whom had pulmonary emboli, V/Q scanning had a sensitivity of 100 per cent and a specificity of 63 per cent, compared with a sensitivity of 83 per cent and a specificity of 100 per cent for digital methods. In seven patients with COPD, four of whom had pulmonary emboli, most scans were reported as being too irregular for interpretation. The digital studies in these cases had both a sensitivity and specificity of 100 per cent.

The current state of imaging, utilizing digital subtraction methods as applied to the detection of pulmonary emboli, still appears to be somewhat experimental. Although this method appears to have the potential to offer an acceptable alternative to the morbidity and mortality inherent in conventional pulmonary arteriography, especially in the high-risk patient population (e.g., possible recent myocardial infarction, pulmonary hypertension, cardiac arrhythmias), techniques and diagnostic criteria are not yet standardized or accepted. Because of motion artifacts, overlap of contrast-containing vessels, and decreased resolution (compared with arteriography), emboli smaller than 2 mm will be missed. With further technologic advances aimed at increasing resolution and the field of view, utilization of these techniques should be of ever-increasing clinical value, and routine diagnostic studies should be obtained in a rapid, inexpensive manner that will entail significantly reduced rates of complications. Gating of images to the cardiac cycles is quite promising; there is a well-established precedent in cardiac nuclear medicine. The technology of gating is well refined, available, and essentially "waiting" to be applied to cardiopulmonary DSA.[159]

## DEEP VENOUS THROMBOSIS

### Contrast Venography

The most accurate method of determining the presence of venous thrombosis is contrast venography.[105–107] This is an invasive procedure that, when done properly, allows direct radiographic visualization of the patency of the venous system and the existence of thrombi. Interpretation of the roentgenographic findings is based on the anatomy of the venous system, properties of the contrast agent, and hemodynamics of flow within the veins of the lower extremities.

The normal venous anatomy of the lower extremity (Fig. 4–13) can be divided into four categories:

1. The deep veins
2. The deep muscle veins
3. The superficial veins
4. The communicating or perforating veins

The deep veins are embedded within muscle except at the ankle, where they are surrounded by fat. The most distal part of the system is the plantar arch of the foot, which continues as the lateral plantar veins. When joined by the medial plantar veins, they become the posterior tibial veins—one of three main trunks of paired vessels comprising the deep calf veins. The anterior tibial veins (continuations of the dorsal foot veins) and the peroneal veins (arising from small vessels around the ankle) complete the triad within the calf. These all merge in the upper calf to form the popliteal vein (paired in 20 per cent of normal subjects), which becomes the superficial femoral vein at the proximal popliteal fossa. It is joined by the deep femoral vein in the proximal thigh, forming the common femoral vein, which becomes the external iliac vein at the level of the inguinal ligament.

The deep muscle veins are the gastrocnemius and soleus veins, which are embedded within the corresponding muscles. The gastrocnemius veins, which are variable but usually include two pairs each of lateral and medial veins, drain into the proximal popliteal veins (usual) or the peroneal veins (variant). Multiple pairs of soleus veins drain into the posterior tibial and peroneal veins, and the soleus arch vein connects to the posterior tibial vein at both its proximal and distal ends.

The superficial veins are found in the subcutaneous fascia, beginning with the dorsal metatarsal veins, which form the superficial dorsal arch, branching laterally as the lesser saphenous vein and medially as the greater saphenous vein. The lesser saphenous empties into the popliteal vein and the greater saphenous joins the common femoral vein in the groin. Variable accessory saphenous veins are common.

The communicating or perforating veins are short vessels that connect the superficial system to the deep system. They are present from the foot to the groin and are thought to number at least 90 in each extremity. They contain valves that direct flow only from the superficial to the deep system. Valves directing flow centrally are found in all veins of the lower extremity except within the foot.

Blood flow through the lower extremity is very dependent on position and degree of muscle activity. The veins of the deep system contain little smooth muscle within their walls and can act as distensible reservoirs, with an estimated capacity of 250 to 300 ml when in an upright position. When supine, pressures in the venous system are primarily hydraulic, slightly higher than those in the right atrium, 7 to 16 mm Hg; when standing, they are essentially hydrostatic, being measured as 78 to 92 mm Hg at the ankle.[108–109] If the legs are elevated to a level above the right heart, there is a passive gravitational drainage centrally. Large volumes of blood are expelled from the deep venous system of the legs with each contraction of the muscles of the calf and thigh.[110] Pressure within a maximally contracted calf muscle can reach 250 mm Hg and cause a transient venous pressure of up to 100 mm Hg.[111, 112] A single contraction of a calf muscle can eject 50 to 85 ml of blood from the leg in an upright position.

The specific gravity and viscosity of radiopaque contrast material is significantly higher than that of blood; therefore, mixing is incomplete when injected into a peripheral foot vein. If the patient is injected while supine, there is considerable layering of contrast material under blood, with resultant incomplete filling of veins. This layering and incomplete mixing can be erroneously interpreted as filling defects. Kjellberg showed that complete filling could not be attained until positioning was vertical.[112]

For these reasons, venographic methods utilizing supine injections have generally been abandoned in favor of ascending phlebography. This method, as outlined by Rabinov and Paulin,[105] involves positioning the patient in a semierect manner, about 40° above horizontal, on a tilting fluoroscopic table. Elevations of less than 30° result in layering and poor venous distention. The patient supports himself on a box on his unaffected leg, and the leg to be injected is left completely free of weightbearing. The patient is told to keep it relaxed and not to tense his muscles at any time during the procedure, to insure adequate filling and distention of the deep venous system. Injection is made through a small-caliber needle into a distal superficial dorsal vein, which will communicate with both the superficial and deep venous systems. The dorsal metatarsal vein of the great toe is preferred. Injec-

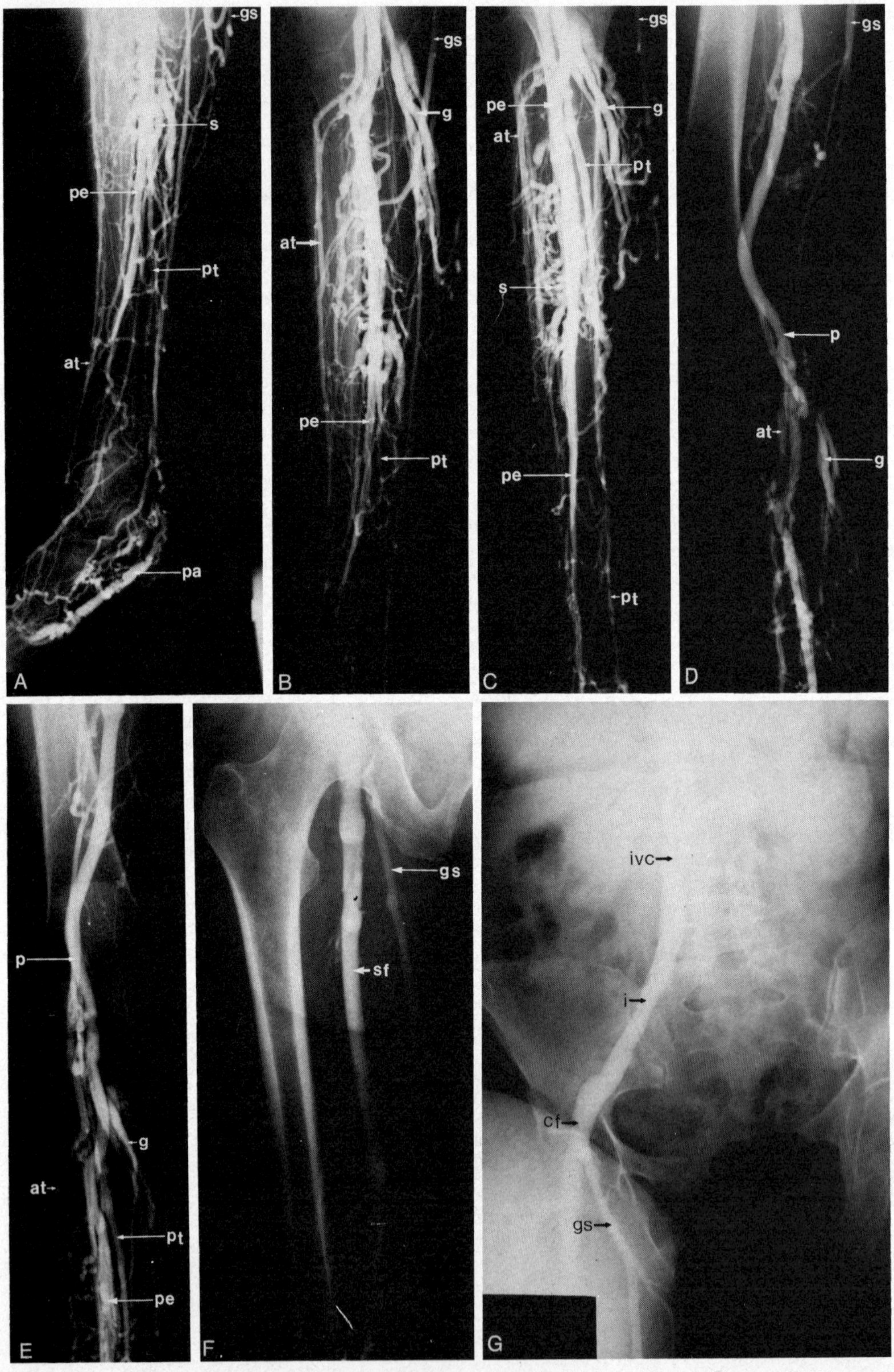


***Figure 4–13.*** A normal venogram demonstrating normal venous anatomy. *A,* lateral foot and lower calf; *B,* lateral calf; *C,* anteroposterior calf; *D,* lateral knee; *E,* anteroposterior knee; *F,* anteroposterior thigh; *G,* anteroposterior pelvis.

at, anterior tibial; cf, common femoral; g, gastrocnemius; gs, greater saphenous; i, iliac; ivc, inferior vena cava; p, popliteal; pa, palmer arch; pe, peroneal; pt, posterior tibial; s, soleus; sf, superficial femoral. (Courtesy of Dr. Souheil Saddekni, The New York Hospital and Cornell University Medical College.)

tions can be monitored fluoroscopically, with multiple spot films and overhead radiographs taken over the entire leg. Contrast material should enter the deep veins freely, and the use of a tourniquet during injection may prevent their filling. To minimize complications due to contrast material, after all radiographs have been taken, the entire venous system should be flushed with 100 ml of heparinized saline.

In a normal study, all deep and superficial veins will be opacified, with the possible exception of the deep femoral vein, which is only observed in about half of all venograms. The most reliable, direct sign of venous thrombosis is a constant, sharply delineated filling defect seen on all films, in different projections (Figs. 4–14 and 4–15). Other indirect signs, suggestive of but not diagnostic of deep venous thrombosis, are abrupt termination of opacification of a vein, either proximally or distally; nonopacification of a vein or veins; or abnormal diversion of contrast material, representing collateral flow. These indirect signs are only suggestive of disease, because they can also be caused by edema, cellulitis, muscle rupture, hematoma, or periarticular cysts. Thin intraluminal streaky defects, irregular venous margins, the absence of venous valves, and occluded veins with large collaterals are indicative of chronic disease.

There are several common causes of false-positive results. Weightbearing or tensing of muscles during injection may cause incomplete filling of the deep veins. Tourniquets, once proposed as an aid in filling the deep system, can actually prevent their filling. If the vein chosen for injection is too proximal, this may cause contrast material to bypass distal deep veins, giving an impression of thrombophlebitis. Defects due to improper mixing will simulate clots, but these will usually have changes in contour or position on different views. The use of small volumes of contrast material will increase the frequency of spurious defects due to improper

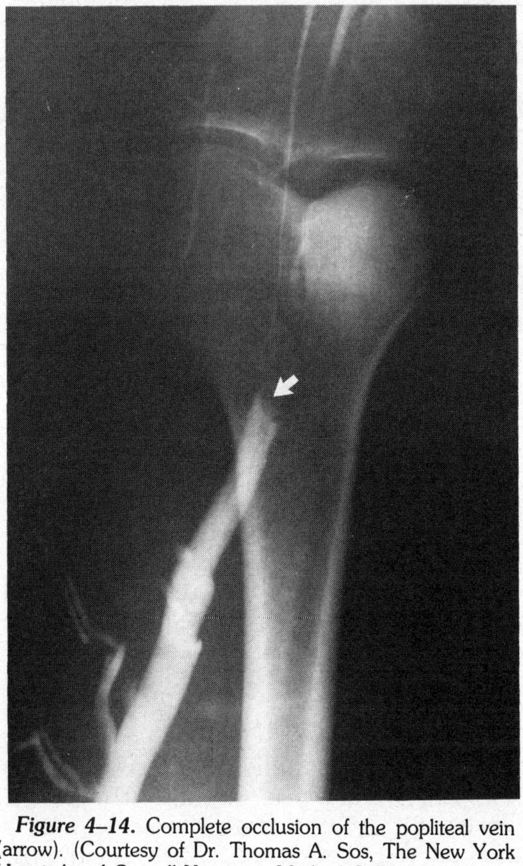

*Figure 4–14.* Complete occlusion of the popliteal vein (arrow). (Courtesy of Dr. Thomas A. Sos, The New York Hospital and Cornell University Medical College.)

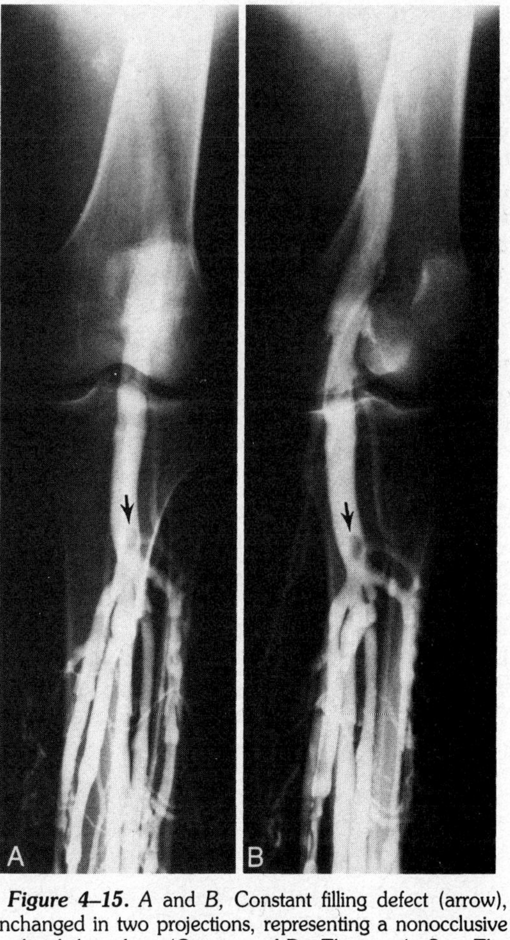


*Figure 4–15.* *A* and *B*, Constant filling defect (arrow), unchanged in two projections, representing a nonocclusive popliteal thrombus. (Courtesy of Dr. Thomas A. Sos, The New York Hospital and Cornell University Medical College.)

mixing. Usual volumes of contrast material employed are between 100 and 150 ml.

A wide variety of complications, both in type and severity, have been reported in patients after contrast venography.[113–115] Severe systemic reactions are uncommon and similar to other contrast studies. Warm flushing sensations, nausea, vomiting, metallic taste, and urticaria are common immediately postinjection. Muscle pain during the examination is thought to be secondary to the hyperosmolarity of the contrast material. The postphlebographic syndrome—pain, swelling, tenderness, and erythema up to 36 hours after administration of contrast material—has been reported in as many as 24 per cent of venograms performed.[113] Decreasing the concentration of contrast material from 60 to 45 per cent reduced the frequency of these effects to 7.5 per cent. The use of nonionic, low-osmolarity contrast materials has also been reported to decrease patient pain and discomfort. Pulmonary embolism secondary to phlebography, although reported,[116] is rare. Extravasation of contrast material has led to tissue necrosis at the injection site.[114] Gangrene of the toes has been reported, due to trapping of contrast material within foot veins.[117] To minimize patient discomfort and the possibility of thrombosis subsequent to the procedure, it has been suggested that the venous system be flushed well with heparinized saline once the examination is completed, but this is somewhat controversial.[112, 118]

Contrast venography that is properly performed is the most accurate diagnostic test available for the detection of deep venous thrombosis. The examination is invasive and not without serious side effects. The frequency and severity of these complications can be diminished by decreasing the concentration of contrast material. Venography is not readily repeatable and is not suitable as a screening modality. Radionuclide studies, impedance plethysmography (IPG), and Doppler ultrasound studies are noninvasive and, when used in combination, quite sensitive and applicable for screening high-risk patients.

### Doppler Ultrasound Flow Detection

The Doppler shift is a well-known physical phenomenon that refers to the change in frequency detected by a stationary observer when a sound wave is emitted from a moving source. This principle can be applied to ultrasonic techniques to detect dynamics of blood flow.[119–121] The ultrasonic probe employed in these studies uses two piezoelectric crystals. One is electrically stimulated and produces a constant ultrasonic beam at a given frequency. The probe is coupled to the skin by a gel and the beam is directed toward the blood vessel being examined. The beam is reflected by blood cells within the vein back to the probe, where it is detected by the second crystal. If the blood cells are moving, the frequency of the reflected beam is different from the initial, incident frequency (Doppler shift), and it is this difference in frequencies that is amplified and recorded. This alteration in the reflected wave is proportional to the velocity of flow. If there is no blood flow (secondary to thrombosis), there will be no Doppler shift and no detectable frequency difference.

Normal venous blood flow varies with respiration. Flow ceases during breath-holding or a Valsalva maneuver and becomes rapid with the sudden release of intrathoracic pressure. Flow distal to total venous occlusion is unchanged by respiration or a Valsalva maneuver. Sudden increases in blood flow can be caused by squeezing the muscles or by sudden release of pressure over a compressed vein. During the examination, the patient is supine, with his legs in external rotation. The pulsatile femoral artery is easily identified and the probe positioned medially over the common femoral vein. A low-pitched phasic sound, changing with respiration, is normally heard. If the external iliac vein is compressed, no respiratory variation is noted. When compression is released, an augmented sound is heard, due to a sudden increase in blood flow. Further augmentation can be detected if the calf or thigh is compressed. The superficial femoral, popliteal (performed with the patient in the prone position), and posterior tibial veins are sequentially examined, and the respiratory influences and the changes due to proximal and distal compression of veins and muscle groups are noted (Table 4–4).

The diagnosis of venous outflow obstruction by Doppler ultrasound is based on a lack of normal response within the vein being examined to respiration and compression (Fig. 4–16). Table 4–4 outlines changes observed with thrombosis. The sensitivity of the method, compared with venography,

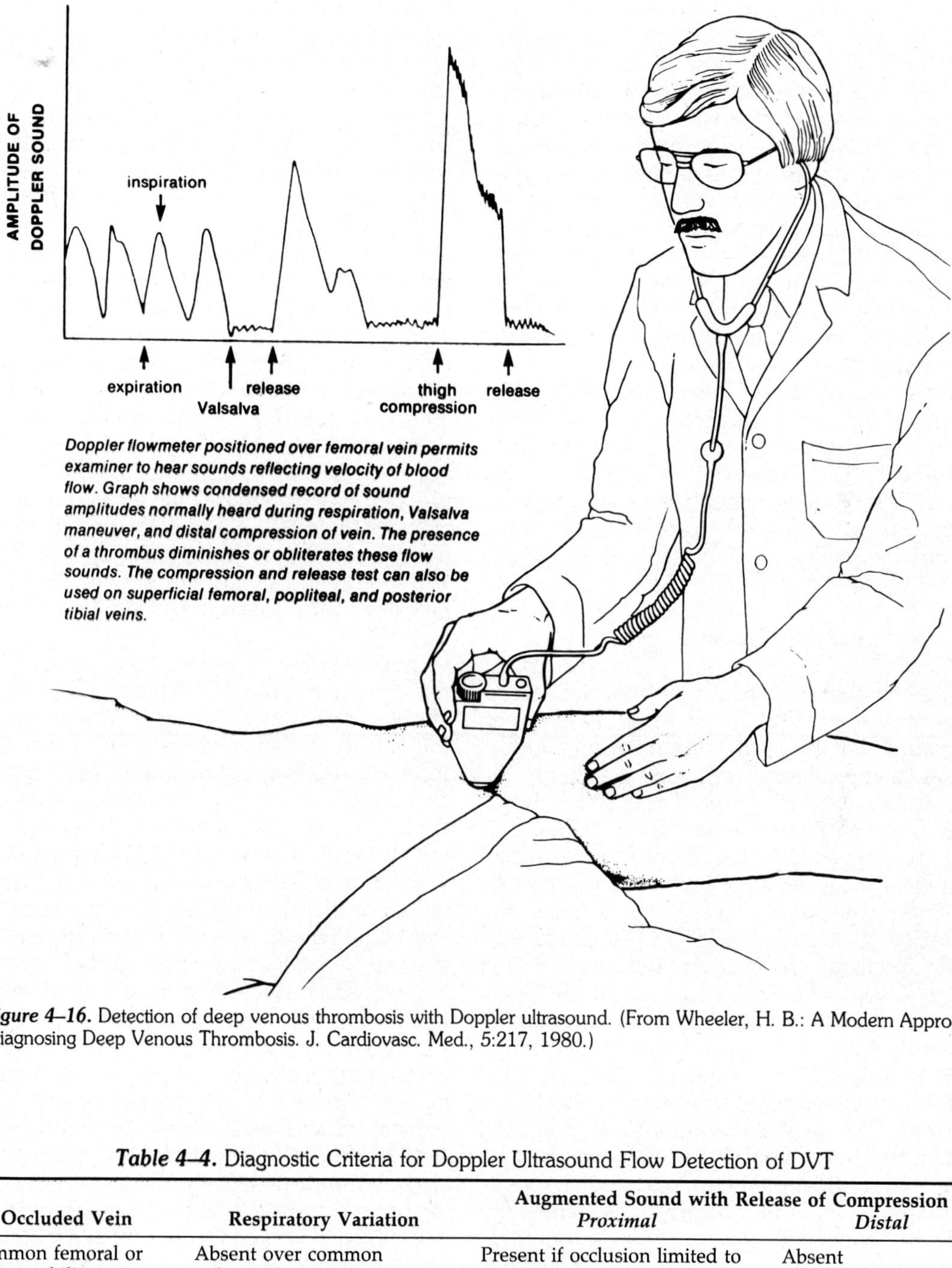


***Figure 4–16.*** Detection of deep venous thrombosis with Doppler ultrasound. (From Wheeler, H. B.: A Modern Approach to Diagnosing Deep Venous Thrombosis. J. Cardiovasc. Med., 5:217, 1980.)

***Table 4–4.*** Diagnostic Criteria for Doppler Ultrasound Flow Detection of DVT

| Occluded Vein | Respiratory Variation | Augmented Sound with Release of Compression *Proximal* | *Distal* |
|---|---|---|---|
| Common femoral or external iliac | Absent over common femoral | Present if occlusion limited to external iliac | Absent |
| Superficial femoral | Phasic over common femoral | Present with abdominal compression | Absent or impaired |
| Popliteal | Phasic over common femoral | Present over common femoral | Absent or impaired |
| | Absent over posterior tibial and popliteal | Absent or impaired over posterior tibial and popliteal | Absent or impaired |
| Calf | Absent over posterior tibial | Absent or impaired with calf compression | Present with foot compression |

varies according to the position of the thrombus. Proximal vein thrombosis (popliteal, femoral, or iliac) is readily detected by this method, with reported diagnostic accuracies of over 90 per cent in most studies, whereas calf vein thrombosis is only occasionally detected, with reported sensitivities of less than 50 per cent.[119–123] False-negative studies in proximal veins are due to nonocclusive proximal thrombi, which are not large enough to significantly alter blood flow. False-positive studies have been attributed to external venous compression, e.g., by the transducer or by constricting garments, to poor patient positioning, and to the examination of veins drained of blood.[65]

Detection of deep venous thrombosis by Doppler ultrasound techniques is a noninvasive, inexpensive, versatile method that requires no preparation and little patient cooperation. It does depend a great deal on technical expertise, and results are not uniformly favorable.

### Impedance Plethysmography

Plethysmographic techniques for the detection of deep venous thrombosis involve the measurement of blood volume within a limb. Impedance plethysmography (IPG),[124–126] measuring changes in electrical resistance,* has been employed most often; however, strain-gauge plethysmography,[127] measuring changes in limb circumference, and air-cuff plethysmography,[128] measuring changes in resistive pressure, have also been used. For IPG, electrical changes are detected. From Ohm's law, voltage is equal to the product of current and resistance; thus, for a constant current, changes in resistance (or impedance) will be reflected by voltage changes.

Blood is an excellent conductor of electrical current. The greater the amount of blood in a region, the lower the impedance (resistance) to conducting the current. If electrodes are applied to the calf, the resistance to current flow will vary according to the amount of blood within the tissues.[129] The lower the blood volume, the higher the resistance. In practice, an imperceptible small current is applied to the electrodes attached to the calf, and a blood pressure cuff is inflated around the mid-thigh, just sufficient to occlude venous return but not enough to disrupt arterial supply. Voltage changes are continuously recorded and, after a predetermined interval, the cuff is rapidly deflated and the pattern of voltage changes noted. In a normal leg, one without occlusive thrombi, blood volume will increase on inflation of the cuff, more rapidly at first, then more slowly as pressures increase. When the cuff is deflated, there will be a sudden surge of blood out of the limb, producing a sharp change in voltage. If occlusive venous thrombi are present, extensive blood pooling has already occurred; thus, the venous capacitance is minimal, which is reflected by a minimal voltage change and minimal change in blood outflow after deflation (Fig. 4–17). To minimize temporary occlusion due to improper positioning, the hip and knee are flexed 30°, the hip is externally rotated, and the entire leg is elevated 20 to 30°. A series of three 45-second occlusions and two 120-second occlusions, with 30-second deflation intervals, has been proposed for maximum sensitivity and specificity.[65]

Interpretation of the results is obtained by use of a nomogram,[125, 130] plotting the rise of venous capacitance during occlusion against the fall in venous outflow during the first three seconds after deflation, with normal and abnormal regions well established (see Fig. 4–17). The sensitivity of IPG is dependent on location of the thrombus. For proximal vein thrombi, IPG approaches a sensitivity of 95 per cent and specificity of 98 per cent. For calf vein thrombi, however, the sensitivity is extremely poor (<30 per cent).[124–126, 130–132] False-positive studies can be caused by external constriction due to clothing, electrodes, the thigh cuff, a pelvic mass, or faulty leg positioning. Muscle tension, arterial insufficiency, increased venous pressure secondary to congestive heart failure, or venoconstriction due to shock will also yield abnormal tests without evidence of thrombi by venography. A normal study in the presence of thrombi can occur in nonocclusive thrombosis, significant collateral circulation (caused by previous thrombosis), and artifact caused by skin stretching when the thigh cuff is inflated.[132]

IPG studies can be used as screening tests for proximal vein thrombosis. They can be done quickly, are highly sensitive, are repeatable, and require little patient cooperation. Although not sensitive to calf vein

*Although impedance and resistance are not identical, they are equivalent in direct circuits and can be used interchangeably in this application.

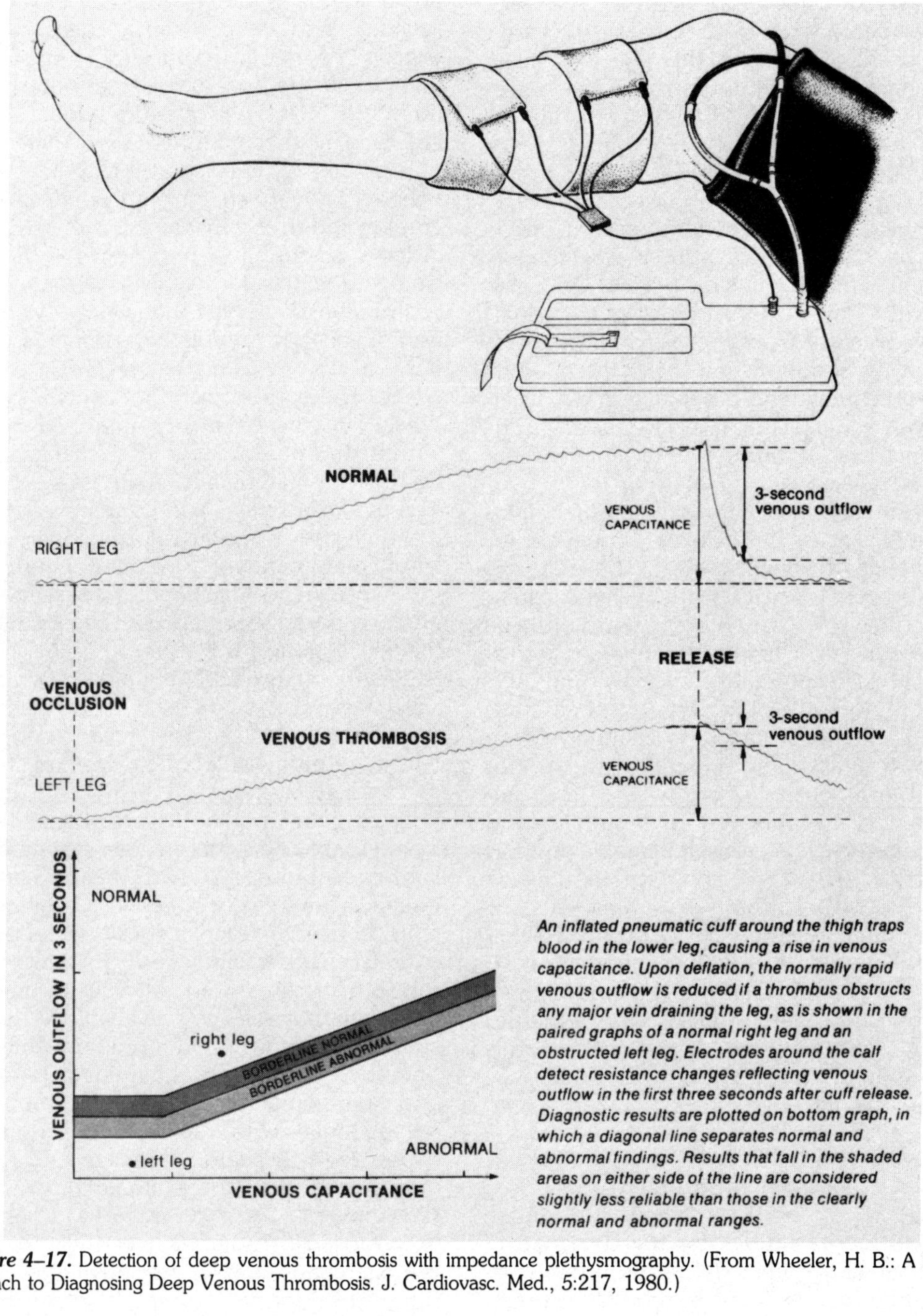


***Figure 4–17.*** Detection of deep venous thrombosis with impedance plethysmography. (From Wheeler, H. B.: A Modern Approach to Diagnosing Deep Venous Thrombosis. J. Cardiovasc. Med., 5:217, 1980.)

thrombosis, the test can be repeated at frequent intervals to detect calf vein thrombosis extending into the thigh. The combination of IPG and $^{125}$I fibrinogen leg scanning increases the diagnostic accuracy of both proximal and calf vein thrombosis.[133, 134] However, technical skill and experience are crucial in obtaining accurate results.

### Thermography

In the presence of deep venous thrombosis, there is a significant diversion of blood flow from the obstructed or partially occluded deep system to the superficial system and the skin. There is also an inflammatory reaction in the surrounding tissue. Both of these events result in an increased skin surface temperature, which leads to increased infrared radiation from the affected areas. Thermographic techniques have been applied in an effort to utilize this radiation to detect thrombosis of the deep veins.[135–137]

Detection of this infrared radiation necessitates a special thermographic scanning camera, which can resolve temperature differences of 0.2°C at 30°C, much less than is apparent clinically.[138] The normal temperature in the lower extremity shows a gradual, 2 to 6° decrease from the proximal thigh to the foot, with diminished thermal emissions in the prepatellar and pretibial regions. Deep venous thrombosis is associated with a diffuse increase in infrared emissions in the affected areas.

Several early thermographic studies demonstrated sensitivities of over 90 per cent for deep venous thrombosis.[136, 137] These appear to have been based on patients with extensive occlusive disease. More recently, Ritchie and coworkers[138, 139] found diagnostic agreement between contrast venography and thermography of only 79 per cent. In their studies, thermography failed to diagnose deep venous thrombosis in patients with early or limited thrombosis. Nevertheless, the examination can be done rapidly, simply, and noninvasively. It is easily repeatable and has a high diagnostic accuracy for established and extensive thrombosis. False-positive studies can be caused by a ruptured Baker cyst, inflammation, inflamed synovial cyst, and venous insufficiency. If equipment is available and causes of false-positive studies can be eliminated, positive results in this simple, noninvasive study will usually be clinically useful.

### Radionuclide Studies

Radioisotopic studies for the detection of deep venous thrombosis can be broadly divided into two categories—those that examine the patency of the deep venous system (radionuclide venography) and those that attempt to incorporate or entrap radiopharmaceuticals within a thrombus.

Radionuclide venography became practicable with the routine availability of gamma camera systems capable of dynamic studies—rapid sequence imaging. In these studies, radioactive materials are injected into a pedal vein, and images are obtained. Diagnostic accuracy above the knee is excellent (greater than 90 per cent), comparable to contrast venography, but can be unsatisfactory below the knee because of poor resolution.[140–146] Two types of radiopharmaceuticals are used in these studies. Particulate materials ($^{99m}$Tc human serum albumin microspheres or $^{99m}$Tc macroaggregated albumin) employ multiple bipedal injections with sequential scanning of both lower extremities from the ankles to the pelvis.[143] Absence or obstruction of deep venous flow, visualization of collateral circulation, or increased superficial flow is taken as a sign of a positive study. The presence of "hot spots" is sometimes due to the incorporation of activity within thrombi but is a less reliable sign.[146] Both of the materials used are lung scanning agents and as such, will be removed during the first pass through the pulmonary circulation, eliminating background interference for subsequent injections. A baseline pulmonary perfusion scan can be obtained at the conclusion of the study.

Continuously circulating radiopharmaceuticals have also been used for radionuclide venography. $^{99m}$Tc-labeled red blood cells, labeled either in vivo or in vitro, are allowed to circulate systemically. Any vein can be injected, not only or necessarily in the affected limb. The entire venous system can be continuously imaged, with repeated and angulated views easily obtained. Combined results from two recent series[144, 145] show that overall sensitivity and specificity are excellent for both proximal and calf vein thrombosis. Although not routinely available, $^{81m}$Kr infusion has been proposed for radionuclide venography.[147] With a short half-life (13 seconds) and high count rate, high-resolution images are obtained with relatively little radiation exposure to the patient. Background rapidly disappears; thus, the examination is readily repeatable.

A forming thrombus will incorporate fibrinogen, and this is the physiologic basis for $^{125}$I fibrinogen scanning.[148, 149] Fibrinogen is labeled with $^{125}$I (which has replaced $^{131}$I because of its longer half-life and lower radiation dose [see Table 4–1]). Experimental studies have demonstrated that, when properly labeled, this compound, in vivo, behaves like normal fibrinogen.[150] Twenty-four hours prior to intravenous injection, at least 100 mg of oral nonradioactive iodide should be administered to block the thyroid from taking up any free $^{125}$I and to eliminate any unnecessary radiation dose to the gland. For at least two weeks after injection, one should continue to administer daily nonradioactive iodide. After injection, the radioactive fibrinogen will circulate within the intravascular space, and activity can be detected with a hand-held scintillation counter along a predetermined and precisely marked map. Marks are made and numbered on the patient's legs with an indelible marker at approximately two-inch intervals, so that precisely the same spot can be counted at each session (Fig. 4–18). Counting can be started as early as four hours but is more usually done at 24, 48, and 72 hours post injection. Activity is sufficient to continue scanning for seven days if warranted. Because of changing backgrounds, ratios of leg to precordial activity rather than absolute counts are recorded for each location. An increase of 15 to 50 per cent between any two points that is consistent for 24 hours is considered a positive study. The diagnostic accuracy of the test distal to the mid-thigh is reported to be as high as 92 per cent.[148] Increased false-negative results are found along the common femoral and iliac veins. High proximal vein thrombi are difficult to detect because the photon emitted is of such low energy that it is attenuated by the large overlying muscle mass. Other reasons for false-negative studies throughout the leg include thrombus formation being completed when $^{125}$I fibrinogen is low (either early or late thrombus formation) and very small thrombi. Additionally, metabolism of the radiopharmaceutical yields free $^{125}$I, which eventually is excreted into the bladder, producing an obscuring background in the pelvic region. False-positive studies can occur because of cellulitis, skin ulcers, surgical incisions, hematoma, inflammation, or varicose veins. Fibrinogen tests also become positive in approximately 50 per cent of patients who have recently undergone contrast venography.[151] On occasion, this is due to thrombus formation; however, animal experiments have demonstrated that there is a transient deposition of fibrin on venous

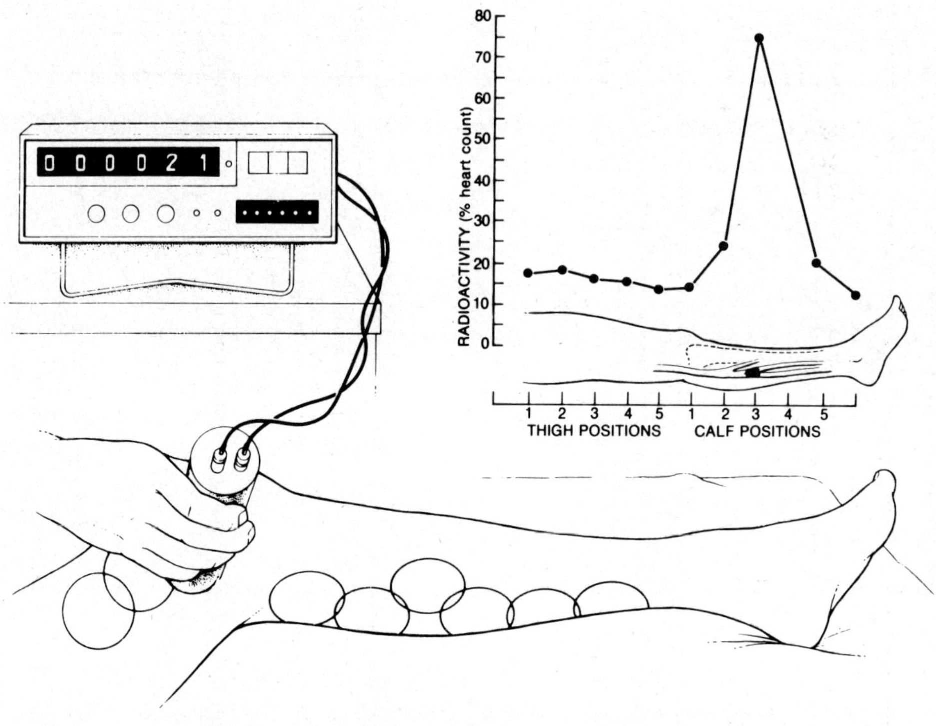


*After IV administration of $^{125}$I fibrinogen and a waiting period to allow it to concentrate in any thrombi, a scintillation counter is used to measure radioactivity levels at circled sites on calf and thigh. In graph, a calf thrombus is indicated by a "hot spot" of radioactivity plotted in relation to maximum count detected over the heart. The test is sensitive and accurate in detecting calf thrombi but not those in the groin or pelvis.*

***Figure 4–18.*** Detection of deep venous thrombosis with $^{125}$I fibrinogen. (From Wheeler, H. B.: A Modern Approach to Diagnosing Deep Venous Thrombosis. J. Cardiovasc. Med., 5:217, 1980.)

***Table 4–5.*** Characteristics of Diagnostic Examinations Available for Evaluation of Suspected Pulmonary Embolism (PE) and Deep Venous Thrombosis (DVT)

| Modality | Indications | Contraindications (* = relative contraindication) | Advantages | Disadvantages | False-Positives | False-Negatives | Comments |
|---|---|---|---|---|---|---|---|
| Chest x-ray (CXR) | Pulmonary symptoms | None | Can narrow differential<br>Occasionally strongly suggestive of PE | Rarely, if ever, diagnostic for PE | Consolidation may be due to infarction secondary to PE or to many other disease states | Normal study does not rule out PE | Necessary for evaluation of pulmonary pathology and further workup of PE |
| Perfusion scan | Suspicion of PE | Known albumin hypersensitivity* (can be pretreated)<br>Pulmonary hypertension*<br>Right-to-left shunt* (exam can be done if particles decreased to 50,000) | High sensitivity<br>Physiologic perfusion demonstrated | Low specificity<br>Indeterminate study if matching CXR abnormality | COPD<br>Pneumonia<br>Tumor<br>Atelectasis<br>Congenital abnormalities | None | Except for a normal study that effectively excludes PE, results are reported in terms of probabilities. Treatment can and should be based on V/Q interpretation; however, low probability does not completely exclude, nor high probability completely confirm the presence of PE |
| Ventilation scan | Abnormal perfusion scan | Normal perfusion scan<br>Small subsegmental perfusion defects<br>CXR abnormality in region of perfusion defect | Increases specificity of perfusion scan for PE | Patient cooperation required | | Severe COPD | |
| Arteriography | Indeterminate lung scan<br>Moderate probability lung scan<br>High probability scan with contraindication to anticoagulation<br>Prior to IVC interruption, embolectomy, or thrombolytic therapy | Normal perfusion scan<br>Pulmonary hypertension with RVEDP $\geq$ 20 mm Hg<br>Contrast allergy* can be pretreated<br>Recent myocardial infarction*<br>Cardiac arrhythmia*<br>Renal failure* | Most specific and sensitive diagnostic study<br>Allows direct radiographic visualization of thrombi | Significant morbidity and mortality due to both invasive procedure and contrast reactions | None, if primary diagnostic criteria adhered to | Possible if multiple projections not obtained | "Gold standard" for PE, but indeterminate studies do occur |

| | | | | | | | |
|---|---|---|---|---|---|---|---|
| Digital subtraction pulmonary arteriography | Not definitely established, but high-risk patient may be better served than with angiogram, in departments experienced in this procedure | Contrast allergy* | Minimally invasive<br>Direct radiographic visualization of thrombi<br>Increased sensitivity for severe COPD patients compared with V/Q scans | Resolution less than arteriogram<br>Motion artifacts<br>Nonselective injections | Similar to arteriography | Similar to arteriography | Standards and diagnostic criteria not yet established, but method holds great potential as a highly sensitive, minimally invasive test for PE |
| Contrast venography | Unavailable or inconclusive noninvasive studies<br>Negative noninvasive studies with a high clinical suspicion of DVT<br>Inexperience with noninvasive studies | Hypersensitivity to contrast*<br>Renal failure* | Highly specific<br>Allows direct radiographic visualizatiion of thrombi | Contrast reactions including postvenogram thrombo-phlebitis<br>Extravasation of contrast<br>Not readily repeatable | Improper procedure (poor injection, inadequate volume, faulty positioning)<br>Muscle tensing<br>Weight bearing<br>Tourniquet<br>Proximal injection | Rare, with multiple projections and adherence to direct signs | "Gold standard" for DVT |
| Doppler ultrasound | Suspected proximal DVT<br>Screening high-risk patient populations | None | Rapid<br>Minimal patient cooperation required<br>Noninvasive<br>Repeatable<br>High sensitivity for proximal thrombi<br>Inexpensive<br>Portable<br>Useful in amputees and patients in traction | Relatively insensitive for calf vein thrombi<br>Subjective interpretation—accuracy varies with expertise of observer<br>Risk of dislodgement of thrombus during compression | External compression<br>Poor patient positioning<br>Examining gravity-drained venous system | Nonocclusive thrombi<br>Calf vein thrombi<br>Patent collateral circulation<br>Improper probe positioning | Good screening test for proximal thrombi |
| Impedance plethysmog-raphy (IPG) | Suspected proximal DVT<br>Screening high-risk patient populations | None | Rapid<br>Noninvasive<br>Repeatable<br>High sensitivity for proximal thrombi<br>Portable | Relatively insensitive for calf vein thrombi<br>Technique-dependent | External compression<br>Poor patient positioning<br>Venous compression by pelvic mass<br>Muscle tensing<br>Arterial insufficiency<br>Increased venous pressure due to CHF<br>Venoconstriction secondary to shock | Nonocclusive thrombi<br>Patent collateral circulation<br>Skin stretching artifact | Excellent screening test for DVT when combined with $^{125}I$ fibrinogen scanning |

*Table continued on the following page*

***Table 4–5.*** Characteristics of Diagnostic Examinations Available for Evaluation of Suspected Pulmonary Embolism (PE) and Deep Venous Thrombosis (DVT) (*Continued*)

| Modality | Indications | Contraindications (* = relative contraindication) | Advantages | Disadvantages | False-Positives | False-Negatives | Comments |
|---|---|---|---|---|---|---|---|
| Thermography | Suspected DVT | None | Rapid<br>Noninvasive<br>Repeatable<br>High sensitivity to extensive thrombosis<br>High sensitivity to small calf vein thrombi<br>Portable | Decreased sensitivity for early or limited thrombosis | Inflammation<br>Ruptured Baker's cyst<br>Inflamed synovial cyst<br>Superficial thrombophlebitis<br>Infected hematoma | Early or limited thrombosis | Positive test is highly significant if causes of false-positive studies can be ruled out |
| $^{125}I$ fibrinogen scanning | Suspected calf vein thrombosis<br>Screening high-risk patient populations | None | Minimally invasive<br>No patient cooperation required<br>High sensitivity for early calf vein thrombi<br>Permits daily scanning<br>Portable | Low sensitivity for proximal thrombi<br>Positive results not available for at least 12–24 hours<br>Patient cannot be anticoagulated until examination is complete† | Cellulitis<br>Ulcerations<br>Surgical incisions<br>Hematoma<br>Inflammation<br>Varicose veins<br>Recent contrast venography | Proximal thrombi<br>Small thrombi<br>Thrombi completely formed prior to injection | Sensitive screening procedure for calf vein thrombosis<br>Increased sensitivity when combined with IPG or Doppler ultrasound<br>Extension of calf vein thrombi can be monitored |
| Radionuclide venography with MAA or $^{99m}Tc$ red blood cells (RBC) | Suspected DVT | MAA: as with perfusion scanning<br>RBC: none | Minimally invasive<br>High sensitivity<br>Rapid<br>Baseline lung perfusion scan obtained (MAA)<br>Little or no morbidity<br>Easily repeatable (RBC) | Diminished resolution compared with contrast venography | Varicose veins<br>Extrinsic compression (e.g., by Baker's cyst)<br>Old collateral circulation<br>Poor peripheral circulation | Small thrombi<br>Nonocclusive thrombi | Although a positive study is significant, poor resolution may allow smaller thrombi to escape detection<br>More extensive studies are needed to establish guidelines |

†Anticoagulation interferes with deposition of fibrin and will increase the rate of false-negative studies.

endothelium following intravenous contrast injection.[152] To avoid false-positive studies on this basis, scanning should always be completed prior to contrast venography.

Because platelets and leukocytes will localize within thrombi, $^{111}$In-labeled platelets and white blood cells have been successfully used for the detection of deep venous thrombosis, with sensitivities of over 90 per cent reported for the platelet studies[75, 76, 153, 154] (see also Chapter 13). Fibrinolytic agents have been labeled as potential detectors of thrombi.[155–158] Streptokinase has proved unsatisfactory, probably because the labeling procedure destroyed its enzymatic activity.[40] Urokinase has been shown to produce results within one hour, but labeling has been heterogeneous and not reproducible.[40] $^{99m}$Tc-labeled plasmin,[158] injected intravenously, has recently shown considerable promise.

As has been described, many different examinations are available for the detection of thromboembolic disease. Each has its own particular advantages and disadvantages. In forging a diagnostic strategy, the clinician and radiologist should work as a team to plan an appropriate series of tests tailored to a particular patient's needs. Table 4–5 summarizes the various procedures that are available.

## REFERENCES

1. Figley, M. M., Gerdes, A. J., and Ricketts, H. S.: Radiographic aspects of pulmonary embolism. Semin. Roentgenol., *2*:389, 1967.
2. Williams, J. R., and Wilcox, W. C.: Pulmonary embolism: Roentgenographic and angiographic considerations. AJR, *89*:333, 1963.
3. Maddison, F. E., Wright, R. R., and Tooley, W. H.: Chest radiography following unilateral pulmonary artery occlusion. An experimental study. Radiology, *88*:435, 1967.
4. Szucs, M. M., Jr., Brooks, H. L., Grossman, W., et al.: Diagnostic sensitivity of laboratory findings in acute pulmonary embolism. Ann. Intern. Med., *74*:161, 1971.
5. Wolfe, W. G., and Sabiston, D. C., Jr.: A study of changes in the roentgenogram of the chest in experimental pulmonary embolism. Surg. Gynecol. Obstet., *127*:492, 1968.
6. Greenspan, R. H., Ravin, C. E., Polansky, S., et al.: Accuracy of chest radiographs in diagnosis of pulmonary embolism. Invest. Radiol., *17*:539, 1982.
7. Westermark, N.: On the roentgen diagnosis of lung embolism. Acta Radiol. (Stockh.), *19*:357, 1938.
8. Kerr, I. H., Simon, G., and Sutton, G. C.: The value of the plain radiograph in acute massive pulmonary embolism. Br. J. Radiol., *44*:751, 1971.
9. Llamas, R., and Swenson, E. W.: Diagnostic clues in pulmonary thromboembolism evaluated by angiographic and ventilation–blood flow studies. Thorax, *20*:327, 1965.
10. Fletcher, B. D., and Donner, M. W.: The use of full-chest tomography in the roentgenographic evaluation of pulmonary embolism. Dis. Chest, *54*:13, 1968.
11. Beamish, W. E.: Radiologic diagnosis of pulmonary embolism including the application of full chest tomography. J. Can. Assoc. Radiol., *21*:217, 1970.
12. Fleischner, F. G.: Pulmonary embolism. Clin. Radiol., *13*:169, 1962.
13. Teplick, J. G., Haskin, M. E., and Steinberg, S. B.: Changes in the main pulmonary artery segment following pulmonary embolism. AJR, *92*:557, 1964.
14. Fraser, R. G., and Paré, J. A. P.: Embolic and Thrombotic Diseases of the Lung. *In* Fraser, R. G., and Paré, J. A. P. (Eds.): Diagnosis of Diseases of the Chest. W. B. Saunders, Philadelphia, 1977.
15. Chang, C. H., and Davis, W. C.: A roentgen sign of pulmonary infarction. Clin. Radiol., *16*:141, 1965.
16. Ring, A., and Bakke, J. R.: Chronic massive pulmonary artery thrombosis. Ann. Intern. Med., *43*:781, 1955.
17. Ball, K. P., Goodwin, J. F., and Harrison, C. V.: Massive thrombotic occlusion of the large pulmonary arteries. Circulation, *14*:766, 1956.
18. Laur, A.: Roentgen diagnosis of pulmonary embolism and its differentiation from myocardial infarction. AJR, *90*:632, 1963.
19. Talbot, S., Worthington, B. S., and Roebuck, E. J.: Radiographic signs of pulmonary embolism and infarction. Thorax, *28*:198, 1973.
20. Castleman, B.: Pathologic Observations on Pulmonary Infarction in Man. *In* Sasahara, A. A., and Stein, M. (Eds.): Pulmonary Embolic Disease. Grune and Stratton, New York, 1965.
21. Fleischner, F. G.: Observations on the Radiologic Changes in Pulmonary Embolism. *In* Sasahara, A. A., and Stein, M. (Eds.): Pulmonary Embolic Disease. Grune and Stratton, New York, 1965.
22. Beilin, D. S., Fink, J. P., and Leslie, L. W.: Correlation of postmortem pathological observations with chest roentgenograms. Radiology, *57*:361, 1951.
23. Fleischner, F. G.: Roentgenology of the pulmonary infarct. Semin. Roentgenol., *2*:61, 1967.
24. Stein, G. N., Chen, J. T., Goldstein, F., et al.: The importance of the chest roentgenograph in the diagnosis of pulmonary embolism. AJR, *81*:255, 1959.
25. Hampton, A. O., and Castleman, B.: Correlation of postmortem chest teleroentgenograms with autopsy findings with special reference to pulmonary embolism and infarction. AJR, *43*:305, 1940.
26. Bachynski, J. E.: Absence of the air bronchogram sign: a reliable finding in pulmonary embolism with infarction or hemorrhage. Radiology, *100*:547, 1971.
27. Woesner, M. E., Sanders, I., and White, G. W.: The melting sign in resolving transient pulmonary infarction. AJR, *111*:782, 1971.
28. Albert, R. B., and Arnett, L. C.: Clearance of radioactive dust from the human lung. Arch. Indust. Health, *12*:99, 1955.
29. Wagner, H. N., Jr., Lopez-Majano, V., Langan, J. K., et al.: Radioactive xenon in the differential diagnosis of pulmonary embolism. Radiology, *91*:1168, 1968.
30. DeNardo, G. L., Goodwin, D. A., Ravasini, R., et al.: The ventilation lung scan in the diagnosis of pulmonary embolism. N. Engl. J. Med., *282*:1334, 1970.

31. West, J. B., and Dollery, C. T.: Distribution of blood flow and ventilation-perfusion ratio in the lung, measured with radioactive $CO_2$. J. Appl. Physiol., *15*:405, 1960.
32. Dyson, N. A., Hugh-Hones, P., Newberry, G. R., et al.: Studies of regional lung function using radioactive oxygen. Br. Med. J., *1*:231, 1960.
33. Quinn, J. L. III, Whitley, J. E., Hudspeth, A. S., et al.: Early clinical applications of lung scintiscanning. Radiology, *82*:315, 1964.
34. Wagner, H. N., Jr., Sabiston, D. C., Iio, M., et al.: Regional pulmonary blood flow in man by radioisotope scanning. JAMA, *187*:601, 1964.
35. Wagner, H. N., Jr., Sabiston, D. C., Jr., McAfee, J. G., et al.: Diagnosis of massive pulmonary embolism in man by radioisotope scanning. N. Engl. J. Med., *271*:377, 1964.
36. Weibel, E. R.: Morphometry of the Human Lung. Academic Press, New York, 1963.
37. Gold, W. M., and McCormack, K. R.: Pulmonary function response to radioisotope scanning of the lungs. JAMA, *197*:146, 1966.
38. Vincent, W. R., Goldberg, S. J., and Desilets, D.: Fatality immediately following rapid infusion of macroaggregates of 99m-Tc albumin (MAA) for lung scan. Radiology, *91*:1181, 1968.
39. Taplin, G. V., and McDonald, N. S.: Radiochemistry of macroaggregated albumin and newer lung scanning agents. Semin. Nucl. Med., *1*:132, 1971.
40. Henkin, R. E.: Radionuclide Detection of Thromboembolic Diseases. *In* Kwaan, H. C., and Bowie, E. J. W. (Eds.): Thrombosis. W. B. Saunders, Philadelphia, 1982.
41. West, J. B.: Regional differences in gas exchange in the lung of erect man. J. Appl. Physiol., *17*:893, 1962.
42. Wellman, H. N., Mack, J. F., Saenger, E. L., et al.: Clinical experiences with oblique views in pulmonary perfusion scintiphotography in normal and pathologic anatomy. J. Nucl. Med., *9*:374, 1968 (Abstr.).
43. Caride, V. J., Puri, S., Slavin, J. D., et al.: The usefulness of posterior oblique views in perfusion lung imaging. Radiology, *121*:669, 1976.
44. Alderson, P. O., Doppman, J. L., Diamond, S. S., et al.: Ventilation-perfusion lung imaging and selective pulmonary angiography in dogs with experimental pulmonary embolism. J. Nucl. Med., *19*:164, 1978.
45. Nielson, P. E., Kirchner, P. T., and Gerber, F. H.: Oblique views in perfusion lung scanning: Clinical utility and limitations. J. Nucl. Med., *18*:967, 1977.
46. Bryan, A. C., Bentivoglio, L. C., Beerel, F., et al.: Factors affecting regional distribution of ventilation and perfusion in the lung. J. Appl. Physiol., *19*:395, 1964.
47. Quinn, J. I. III: The lung: The challenge of nuclear medicine. AJR, *105*:251, 1969.
48. McNeil, B. J.: Diagnostic strategy using ventilation-perfusion studies in patients suspect for pulmonary embolism. J. Nucl. Med., *17*:613, 1976.
49. Alderson, P. O., Rujanavech, N., Secker-Walker, R. H., et al.: The role of $^{133}$Xe ventilation studies in the scintigraphic detection of pulmonary embolism. Radiology, *120*:633, 1976.
50. Biello, D. R., Mattar, A. G., McKnight, R. C., et al.: Ventilation-perfusion studies in suspected pulmonary embolism. AJR, *133*:1033, 1979.
51. Cheely, R., McCartney, W. H., Perry, J. R., et al.: The role of noninvasive tests versus pulmonary angiography in the diagnosis of pulmonary embolism. Am. J. Med., *70*:17, 1981.
52. Hull, R. D., Hirsh, J., Carter, C. J., et al.: Pulmonary angiography, ventilation lung scanning, and venography for clinically suspected pulmonary embolism with abnormal perfusion lung scan. Ann. Intern. Med., *98*:891, 1983.
53. McNeil, P. J.: Ventilation-perfusion studies and the diagnosis of pulmonary embolism: Concise communication. J. Nucl. Med., *21*:319, 1980.
54. Yano, Y., McRae, J., and Anger, H. O.: Lung function studies using short-lived 81m-Kr and the scintillation camera. J. Nuc. Med., *11*:674, 1970.
55. Fazio, F., and Jones, T.: Assessment of regional ventilation by continuous inhalation of radioactive krypton 81-m. Br. Med. J., *1*:673, 1975.
56. Li, D. K., Treves, S., Heyman, S., et al.: Krypton-81m: A better radiopharmaceutical for assessment of regional lung function in children. Radiology, *130*:741, 1979.
57. Clarke, J. C., Finn, R. D., Bolomey, L., et al.: Krypton-81m generators. Radiochem. Radioanal. Lett., *25*:245, 1976.
58. Atkins, H. L., Susskind, H., Klopper, J. F., et al.: A clinical comparison of Xe-127 and Xe-133 for ventilation studies. J. Nucl. Med., *18*:653, 1977.
59. Coates, G., and Nahmia, C.: Xenon-127, a comparison with xenon-133 for ventilation studies. J. Nucl. Med., *18*:21, 1977.
60. McCartney, W. H., Perry, R. J., Cheely, R., et al.: Comparison of Xe-127 and Xe-133 for ventilation-perfusion imaging in the diagnosis of pulmonary embolism. Proc. RSNA, *65*:374, 1979 (Abstr.).
61. Neumann, R. D., Sostman, H. D., and Gottschalk, A.: Current status of ventilation-perfusion imaging. Semin. Nucl. Med., *10*:198, 1980.
62. Alderson, P. O.: Pulmonary Nuclear Medicine. *In* Freeman, L. M., and Weissman, H. S. (Eds.): Nuclear Medicine Annual 1980. Raven Press, New York, 1980.
63. Ryo, U. Y., Bilow, P. A., and Pinsky, S.: Lateral view ventilation images with $^{133}$Xe. Clin. Nucl. Med., *4*:47, 1979.
64. Alderson, P. O., and Line, B. R.: Scintigraphic regional pulmonary ventilation. Semin. Nucl. Med., *10*:218, 1980.
65. Hirsh, J., Genton, E., and Hull, R.: Venous Thromboembolism. Grune and Stratton, New York, 1981.
66. Biello, D. R., Matlar, A. G., Osel-Wusu, A., et al.: Interpretation of indeterminate lung scintigrams. Radiology, *133*:189, 1979.
67. Robin, E. D.: Overdiagnosis and overtreatment of pulmonary embolism: The emperor may have no clothes. Ann. Intern. Med., *87*:775, 1977.
68. Seckler-Walker, R. H.: On purple emperors, pulmonary embolism, and venous thrombosis. Ann. Intern. Med., *98*:1006, 1983.
69. Alderson, P. O., and Gottschalk, A.: Ventilation-perfusion studies for pulmonary embolism: A rebuttal to Dr. Eugene Robin. Semin. Nucl. Med., *9*:145, 1979.
70. Alderson, P. O., Biello, D. R., Khan, A. R., et al.: Comparison of Xe-133 single breath and washout images in the scintigraphic diagnosis of pulmonary embolism. Radiology, *137*:481, 1980.
71. Alderson, P. O., Biello, D. R., Sachariah, K. G., et al.: Scintigraphic detection of pulmonary embolism in patients with obstructive pulmonary disease. Radiology, *138*:661, 1981.
72. Nichols, A. B., Cochavi, S., Moore, R. H., et al.:

Detection of experimental pulmonary emboli in dogs by sequential positron imaging after inhalation of 15-O carbon dioxide. Circ. Res., *42*:53, 1978.

73. Nichols, A. B., Cochavi, S., Hales, C. A., et al.: Scintigraphic detection of pulmonary embolism by serial positron imaging of inhaled 15-O–labeled carbon dioxide. N. Engl. J. Med., *299*:279, 1978.
74. Nichols, A. B., Beller, G. A., Cochavi, S., et al.: Detection of pulmonary embolism by positron imaging of inhaled 15-O–labeled carbon dioxide. Semin. Nucl. Med., *10*:252, 1980.
75. McIlmoyle, G., Davis, H. H., Welch, M. J., et al.: Scintigraphic diagnosis of experimental pulmonary embolism with In-111 labeled platelets. J. Nucl. Med., *18*:910, 1977.
76. Moser, K. M., Spragg, R. G., Bender, F., et al.: Study of factors that may condition scintigraphic detection of venous thrombi and pulmonary emboli with indium-111 labeled platelets. J. Nucl. Med., *21*:1051, 1980.
77. Abrams, H. L.: Introduction and Historical Notes. *In* Abrams, H. L. (Ed.): Abrams Angiography: Vascular and Interventional Radiology, 3rd ed. Little, Brown and Co., Boston, 1983.
78. Menzoian, J. O., and Williams, F. L.: Is pulmonary angiography essential for the diagnosis of acute pulmonary embolism? Am. J. Surg., *137*:543, 1979.
79. Sasahara, A. A., Stein, M., Simon, M., et al.: Pulmonary angiography in the diagnosis of thromboembolic disease. N. Engl. J. Med., *270*:1075, 1964.
80. Greenspan, R. H.: Angiography in Pulmonary Embolism. *In* Abrams, H. L.: Abrams Angiography: Vascular and Interventional Radiology, 3rd ed. Little, Brown and Co., Boston, 1983.
81. Dalen, J. E., Brooks, H. L., Johnson, L. W., et al.: Pulmonary angiography in acute pulmonary embolism: Indications, techinques and results in 367 patients. Am. Heart J., *81*:175, 1971.
82. Marsh, J. D., Glynn, M. A., and Torman, H. A.: Pulmonary angiography: Application in a new spectrum of patients. Am. J. Med., *75*:763, 1983.
83. Johnson, B. A., James, A. E., Jr., and White, R. I., Jr.: Oblique and selective pulmonary angiography in diagnosis of pulmonary embolism. AJR, *118*:801, 1977.
84. Williams, J. R., Wilcos, W. C., Andrews, G. J., et al.: Angiography in pulmonary embolism. JAMA, *184*:473, 1968.
85. Bossart, P. J., Sniderman, K. W., Beinart, C., et al.: Pulmonary arteriography: The importance of multiple projections. Cardiovasc. Intervent. Radiol., *5*:105, 1982.
86. Greenspan, R. H., and Capps, J. H.: Pulmonary angiography: Its use in diagnosis and as a guide to therapy in lesions of the chest. Radiol. Clin. North Am., *1*:315, 1963.
87. Stein, P. D., O'Connor, J. F., Dalen, J. E., et al.: The angiographic diagnosis of acute pulmonary embolism: Evaluation of criteria. Am. Heart J., *73*:730, 1967.
88. Wennevold, A., Christiansen, I., and Lindeney, O.: Complications in 4,413 catheterizations of the right side of the heart. Am. Heart J., *69*:173, 1965.
89. Mills, S. R., Jackson, D. C., Older, R. A., et al.: The incidence, etiologies and avoidance of complications of pulmonary angiography in a large series. Radiology, *136*:295, 1980.
90. Grossman, W.: Pulmonary Angiography. *In* Grossman, W. (Ed.): Cardiac Catheterization and Angiography, 2nd ed. Lea and Febiger, Philadelphia, 1980.
91. Bookstein, J. J., Feigin, D. S., Seo, K. W., et al.: Diagnosis of pulmonary embolism: Experimental evaluation of the accuracy of scintigraphically guided pulmonary arteriography. Radiology, *136*:15, 1980.
92. Goldhaber, S. Z., and Hennekens, C. H.: Time trends in hospital mortality and diagnosis of pulmonary embolism. Am. Heart J., *104*:305, 1982.
93. Goldhaber, S. Z., Hennenkens, C. H., Evans, D. A., et al.: Factors associated with the correct antemortem diagnosis of pulmonary embolus. Am. J. Med., *73*:822, 1982.
94. Jolles, H., Reilley, R., Price, R. R., et al.: Pulmonary Applications of Digital Radiography. *In* Price, R. R., Rollo, F. D., Monahan, W. G., et al. (Eds.): Digital Radiography: A Focus on Clinical Utility. Grune and Stratton, New York, 1982.
95. Robb, G. P., and Steinberg, I.: Visualization of the chambers of the heart, the pulmonary circulation and the great blood vessels in man. AJR, *41*:1, 1939.
96. Des Plantes, B.G.Z.: Subtraction: cine roentgograhische methode zur sepuraten. Abbildung bestimmater teile des objekts. ROFEO, *52*:69, 1935.
97. Mistretta, C. A., Ort, M. G., Cameron, J. R., et al.: Multiple images subtraction technique for enhancing low contrast periodic objects. Invest. Radiol., *8*:43, 1973.
98. Kruger, R. A., Mistretta, C. A., Houk, T. L., et al.: Computerized fluoroscopy in real-time for noninvasive evaluation of the cardiovascular system. Radiology, *130*:49, 1979.
99. Ergun, D. L., Mistretta, C. A., Kruger, R. A., et al.: A hybrid computerized fluoroscopy technique for non-invasive cardiovascular imaging. Radiology, *132*:739, 1979.
100. Crummy, A. B., Strother, C. M., Sackett, J. F., et al.: Computerized fluoroscopy: Digital subtraction for intravenous angiocardiography and arteriography. AJR, *135*:1131, 1980.
101. Pond, G. D., Ovitt, T. W., and Capp, M. P.: Comparison of conventional pulmonary angiography with intravenous digital subtraction angiography for pulmonary embolic disease. Radiology, *147*:345, 1983.
102. Goodman, P. C., and Brant-Zawadzki, M.: Digital subtraction pulmonary angiography. AJR, *139*:305, 1982.
103. Ludwig, J. W., Verhoeven, L. A. J., Kersbergen, J. J., et al.: Digital subtraction of the pulmonary arteries for the diagnosis of pulmonary embolism. Radiology, *147*:639, 1983.
104. Kollath, J., and Riemann, H.: Pulmonary digital subtraction angiography. Cardiovasc. Intervent. Radiol., *6*:233, 1983.
105. Rabinov, K., and Paulin, S.: Roentgen diagnosis of venous thrombosis of the leg. Arch. Surg., *104*:134, 1972.
106. Hull, R., Hirsh, J., Sackett, D. L., et al.: Cost effectiveness of clinical diagnosis venography and non-invasive testing in patients with symptomatic deep-vein thrombosis. N. Engl. J. Med., *304*:1561, 1981.
107. Hull, R.: Current approach to diagnosis of deep vein thrombosis. Mod. Con. Cardiovasc. Dis., *51*:129, 1982.
108. Sumner, D. S.: The Hemodynamics and Pathophysiology of Venous Disease. *In* Rutherford, R. B. (Ed.): Vascular Surgery. W. B. Saunders, Philadelphia, 1977.
109. Pollack, A. A., and Wood, E. H.: Venous pressure in the saphenous vein at the ankle in man during

exercise and changes in posture. J. Appl. Physiol., *1*:649, 1949.
110. Arnoldi, C. C.: On the conditions for the venous return from the lower leg in healthy subjects and in patients with chronic venous insufficiency. Angiology, *17*:153, 1966.
111. Ludbrook, J.: Applied Physiology of the Veins. *In* Dodd, H., and Crockett, F. B. (Eds.): The Pathology and Surgery of the Veins of the Lower Limb, 2nd ed. Churchill Livingstone, New York, 1976.
112. Rabinov, K., and Paulin, S.: Venography of the Lower Extremities. *In* Abrams, H. (Ed.): Abrams Angiography: Vascular and Interventional Radiology, 3rd ed. Little, Brown and Co., Boston, 1983.
113. Bettmann, M. A., and Paulin, S.: Leg phlebography: The incidence, nature and modification of undesirable side effects. Radiology, *122*:101, 1977.
114. Coel, M. N., and Dodge, W.: Complication rate with supine phlebography. AJR, *131*:821, 1978.
115. Thomas, M. L., McAllister, V., and Tonge, K.: Simplified phlebography in deep venous thrombosis. Clin. Radiol., *22*:490, 1971.
116. Albrechtsson, U., and Olsson, C. G.: Thrombotic side-effects of lower limb phlebography. Lancet, *1*:723, 1976.
117. Thomas, M. L.: Gangrene following peripheral phlebography of the legs. Br. J. Radiol., *43*:528, 1970.
118. Arndt, R. D., Grollman, J. H., Gomes, A. S., et al.: The heparin flush: An aid in preventing post-venography thrombophlebitis. Radiology, *130*:249, 1979.
119. Evans, D. S.: The early diagnosis of deep-vein thrombosis by ultrasound. Br. J. Surg., *57*:726, 1970.
120. Strandness, D. E., and Sumner, D. S.: Ultrasonic velocity detector in the diagnosis of thrombophlebitis. Arch. Surg., *104*:180, 1972.
121. Sigel, B., Feliz, W. R., Propky, G. L., et al.: Diagnosis of lower limb venous thrombosis by Doppler ultrasound technique. Arch. Surg., *104*:172, 1972.
122. Sumner, D. S., and Lambwith, A.: Reliability of Doppler ultrasound in the diagnosis of acute venous thrombosis both above and below the knee. Am. J. Surg., *138*:205, 1979.
123. Barnes, R. W., Russell, H. E., Wu, K. K., et al.: Accuracy of Doppler ultrasound in clinically suspected venous thrombosis of the calf. Surg. Gynecol. Obstet., *143*:425, 1976.
124. Wheeler, H. B., Pearson, D., O'Connell, D., et al.: Impedance phlebography. Technique, interpretation and results. Arch. Surg., *104*:164, 1972.
125. Hull, R., van Aken, W. G., Hirsh, J., et al.: Impedance plethysmography using the occlusive cuff technique in the diagnosis of venous thrombosis. Circulation, *53*:696, 1976.
126. Hull, R., Taylor, D. W., and Hirsh, J.: Impedance plethysmography: The relationship between venous filling and sensitivity and specificity for proximal vein thrombosis. Circulation, *58*:898, 1978.
127. Barnes, R. W., Hokanson, D. W., Wu, K. K., et al.: Detection of deep vein thrombosis with an automatic electrically calibrated strain-gauge plethysmography. Surgery, *82*:219, 1977.
128. Bynum, L. J., Wilson, J. E. III, Crotty, C. M., et al.: Noninvasive diagnosis of deep venous thrombosis by phleborheography. Ann. Int. Med., *89*:162, 1978.
129. Mullick, S. C., Wheeler, H. B., and Songster, G. P.: Diagnosis of deep venous thrombosis by measurement of electrical impedance. Am. J. Surg., *119*:417, 1970.
130. Wheeler, H. B., O'Donnell, J. A., Anderson, F. A., et al.: Occlusive impedance plethysmography: A diagnostic procedure for venous thrombosis and pulmonary embolism. Prog. Cardiovasc. Dis., *17*:199, 1974.
131. Young, A. E., Henderson, B. A., Phillips, D. A., et al.: Impedance plethysmography: Its limitations as a substitute for phlebography. Cardiovasc. Radiol., *1*:233, 1978.
132. Benedict, K. T., Wheeler, H. B., and Patwardham, N. A.: Impedance plethysmography: Correlation with contrast venography. Radiology, *125*:695, 1977.
133. Hume, M., Kuriakose, T. X., Jamieson, J., et al.: Extent of leg vein thrombosis determined by impedance and 125-I-fibrinogen. Am. J. Surg., *129*:455, 1975.
134. Hull, R., Hirsh, J., Sackett, D. L., et al.: The value of adding impedance plethysmography to 125-I-fibrinogen leg scanning for the detection of deep vein thrombosis in high risk surgical patients: A comparative study between patients undergoing general surgery and hip surgery. Thromb. Res., *15*:227, 1979.
135. Soulen, R. L., Lapayowker, M. S., Tyson R. R., et al.: Angiography, ultrasound and thermography in the study of peripheral vascular disease. Radiology, *105*:115, 1972.
136. Cooke, E. D., and Pilcher, M. F.: Thermography in diagnosis of deep venous thrombosis. Br. Med. J., *2*:523, 1973.
137. Berqvist, D., Efsing, H. O., and Hallbook, T.: Thermography. Arch. Surg., *112*:600, 1977.
138. Ritchie, W. G. M., Soulen, R. L., and Lapayowker, M. S.: Thermographic diagnosis of deep venous thrombosis. Radiology, *131*:341, 1979.
139. Ritchie, W. G. M., Lapayowker, M. S., and Soulen, R. L.: Thermographic diagnosis of deep venous thrombosis: Anatomically based diagnostic criteria. Radiology, *132*:321, 1979.
140. Ryo, U. Y., Qazi, M., Srikantaswamy, S., et al.: Radionuclide venography: Correlation with contrast venography. J. Nucl. Med., *18*:11, 1977.
141. Henkin, R. E., Yao, J. S. T., Quinn, J. L., et al.: Radionuclide venography (RVN) in lower extremity venous disease. J. Nucl. Med., *15*:171, 1974.
142. Hayt, D. B., Blatt, C. J., and Freeman, L. M.: Radionuclide venography: Its place as a modality for the investigation of thromboembolic phenomena. Semin. Nucl. Med., *7*:263, 1977.
143. Rosenthall, L.: Combined inferior vena cavography, iliac venography, and lung imaging with 99m-Tc albumin macroaggregates. Radiology, *98*:623, 1971.
144. Beswick, W., Chmiel, R., Booth, R., et al.: Detection of deep venous thrombosis by scanning of 99m-technetium-labelled red-cell venous pool. Br. Med. J., *1*:82, 1979.
145. Lisbona, R., Stern, J., and Derbekyan, V.: $^{99m}$Tc red blood cell venography in deep vein thrombosis of the leg: A correlation with contrast venography. Radiology, *143*:771, 1982.
146. Gomes, A., Webber, M. M., and Buffkin, D.: Contrast venography vs. radionuclide venography: A study of discrepancies and their possible significance. Radiology, *142*:719, 1982.
147. Ham, H. R., Vandevivere, J., Guillaume, M., et al.: Radionuclide venography using continuous Kr-81m

infusion: Preliminary note. Clin. Nucl. Med., *6*:461, 1981.
148. Kakkar, V.: The diagnosis of deep vein thrombosis using the $^{125}I$ fibrinogen test. Arch. Surg., *104*:152, 1972.
149. Kakkar, V.: Fibrinogen uptake test for detection of deep vein thrombosis—a review of current practice. Semin. Nucl. Med., *7*:229, 1977.
150. McFarlane, A. S.: Method of iodinating human fibrinogen. J. Clin. Invest., *42*:346, 1963.
151. Ritchie, W. G. M., Soulen, R. L., and Rogers, P.: The effect of ascending venography on the fibrinogen uptake test. Invest. Radiol., *12*:416, 1977 (Abstr.).
152. Ritchie, W. G. M., Stewart, G. J., and Lynch, P. R.: The effects of simulated phlebography on the venous endothelium: A scanning electron microscopy study. Invest. Radiol., *4*:279, 1973 (Abstr.).
153. Davis, H. H., Siegel, B. A., Sherman, L. A., et al.: Scintigraphy with $^{111}In$-labeled autologous platelets in venous thromboembolism. Radiology, *136*:203, 1980.
154. Fenech, A., Hussey, J. K., Smith, F. W., et al.: Diagnosis of deep vein thrombosis using autologous indium-111-labelled platelets. Br. Med. J., *282*:1020, 1981.
155. Siegel, B. A., Malmud, L. S., Rhodes, B. A., et al.: Scanning of thromboemboli with iodine-131 streptokinase. Radiology, *103*:695, 1972.
156. Kempi, V., Vander Linden, W., and Von Scheele, C.: Diagnosis of deep vein thrombosis with $^{99m}Tc$-streptokinase: A clinical comparison with phlebography. Br. Med. J., *4*:748, 1974.
157. Millar, W. T., and Smith, J. F. B.: Localization of deep venous thrombosis using technetium-99m labeled urokinase. Lancet, *2*:695, 1974.
158. Deacon, J. M., Anderson, P., and Khan, O.: Technetium 99m-plasmin: A new test for the detection of deep vein thrombosis. Br. J. Radiol., *53*:673, 1980.
159. Goldhaber, S. Z., and Markisz, J.: Digital subtraction pulmonary angiography: An internist's and radiologist's view. Cardiovasc. Intervent. Radiol., *6*:239, 1983.

# PART II

# CLINICAL CONSIDERATIONS

CHAPTER 5

# STRATEGIES FOR DIAGNOSIS

SAMUEL Z. GOLDHABER, M.D.

An accurate diagnosis of PE or DVT is often difficult to establish. Because they are usually nonspecific, symptoms and signs of venous thromboembolism can be misleading. Furthermore, in the hospital setting, PE often occurs concomitantly with other major illnesses such as pneumonia or congestive heart failure. These latter conditions are relatively easily diagnosed, and even the most vigilant physician may overlook the possibility of coexistent PE.

## DIAGNOSIS OF PE

### Sources of Data

#### AUTOPSY STUDIES

From autopsy studies, one may determine the frequency of PE among hospitalized patients (Table 5–1) and the proportion of major PEs diagnosed ante mortem (Table 5–2). A problem in interpreting the results of autopsy series is in distinguishing between clinically significant and clinically incidental PE. Although most series attempt to differentiate between *major* pulmonary emboli that caused or significantly contributed to the patient's death and *minor* PEs that were clinically incidental, this distinction is somewhat subjective, even when stringent anatomic criteria are applied.

Table 5–1 lists 15 autopsy series published from 1934 to 1982.[1–15] The percentage of patients autopsied ranged from 34 to 76 per cent, and the proportion of patients with pulmonary emboli *(minor plus major)* varied from 8 to 52 per cent. It is evident that the more meticulous the dissection of the lungs, the higher the rate of PE.[16] Table 5–1 also shows that *major* PE occurred in 2 to 14 per cent of autopsied patients. These figures vary greatly from study to study because of differences in patient populations and in criteria for anatomically and clinically major PE.

When autopsy findings are correlated with clinical chart review, one can determine the proportion of patients suspected of having major PE prior to death (Table 5–2). This proportion varied from 16 to 38 per cent. Factors that have helped to establish the correct diagnosis of PE are DVT[11, 13, 14] and the postoperative state.[11, 14]

Few studies have examined factors associated with failure to establish the diagnosis of PE.[11–14] It does appear, however, that the presence of pneumonia greatly misleads clinicians. Although pneumonia can occur concomitantly with pulmonary embolism, sometimes *only* the pneumonia may be recognized clinically. In one series, physicians concluded that their antibiotic treatment of pneumonia was failing when, in fact, the patients were deteriorating because of concomitant PE.[14] Other medical conditions hindering the diagnosis of PE include congestive heart failure[14] and cancer.[11] Increasing age has also been associated with less frequent clinical detection of PE (Fig. 5–1).[14]

Besides *underdiagnosis* of PE, *overdiagnosis* of PE also occurs[17] but has been less well studied. In patients with clinically diagnosed PE who were subsequently autopsied, the proportion of diagnoses of PE that can be confirmed at autopsy ranges from 38 to 68 per cent (Table 5–3).

Autopsy series have also been used to investigate embolic sources and clinical settings for PE. In 1846, the German pathologist Virchow published the first examples of PE in which leg and pelvic veins were implicated

***Table 5–1.*** Prevalence of PE at Autopsy

| Reference | Study Period | Per Cent of Patients Autopsied | Number of Autopsies | Number of Minor and Major PE (%) | Number of Major PE (%) |
|---|---|---|---|---|---|
| Belt[1] | — | — | 567 | 56 (10) | 37 (6.5) |
| Collins[2] | 1928–1935 | — | 10,940 | — | 226 (2.1) |
| McCartney[3] | 1919–1938 | — | 25,771 | 2603 (10.1) | 689 (2.7) |
| Roe[4] | 1930–1947 | — | 5906 | 464 (7.9) | 211 (3.6) |
| Ochsner[5] | 1938–1950 | 34 | 10,947 | — | 383 (3.5) |
| Fowler[6] | 1930–1953 | 37 | 2457 | — | 97 (3.9) |
| Towbin[7] | 1949–1954 | 58 | 512 | 132 (25.7) | 73 (14.2) |
| Coon[8] | 1945–1954 | 69 | 4391 | 606 (13.8) | 388 (8.8) |
| Uhland[9] | 1956–1960 | — | 981 | 118 (12.0) | 70 (7.1) |
| Morrell[10]* | 1964–1965 | 76 | 263 | 136 (51.7) | 37 (14) |
| Modan[11] | 1961–1964 | 66 | 2107 | 353 (16.8) | 223 (10.6) |
| MacIntyre[12] | 1967–1971 | 46 | 2291 | 303 (13.2) | 204 (8.9) |
| Coon[13] | 1964–1974 | 70 | 4600 | 567 (12.3) | 325 (7.1) |
| Goldhaber[14] | 1973–1977 | 61 | 1455 | 216 (14.8) | 54 (3.7) |
| Mossey[15] | 1969–1981 | — | 2255 | 731 (32.3) | 224 (9.9) |
| | | | 95† | 9 (9.5) | 0 (0) |

*Every fourth autopsy was included in this series.
†Subset of patients with chronic renal failure.

as the source of the thrombus. These early cases occurred in the settings of childbirth, trauma, and medical illness. Subsequently, the association of pulmonary embolism with deep leg vein thrombosis has been emphasized repeatedly.[2, 4, 5, 8] Nevertheless, it is difficult to determine the frequency of DVT in autopsied cases of PE because even in the 1980s, some states have implicit agreements with pathologists that discourage extensive dissection of the deep leg veins and pelvic veins.

Many autopsied patients with pulmonary embolism died after surgical procedures.[2–5, 8–10, 13, 18–21] Concomitant heart disease, advanced age, cancer, and obesity were additional common associated findings.[6, 22, 23] On the other hand, Mossey and coworkers have reported an *inverse* relationship between pulmonary embolism found at autopsy and chronic renal failure.[15]

Several autopsy studies have compared the frequency of PE in vastly different populations.[24, 25] Thomas and coworkers studied patients autopsied in Uganda and St. Louis.[24] Deep venous thrombosis and pulmonary embolism were found at autopsy in 24 per cent of St. Louis whites and 22 per cent of St. Louis blacks but in only 2 per cent of Ugandan blacks. In another study comparing findings in Boston and Kyushu, Japan, both minor and major PE occurred in 24 per cent of the Boston patients but in only 1 per cent of the Japanese patients.[25] These descriptive studies may prove useful in generating additional hypotheses about genetic versus environmental influences on the frequency of PE and DVT.

## DEATH CERTIFICATES

Studies that rely solely upon coding from death certificates may be inaccurate owing to both the difficulty in clinically diagnosing

***Table 5–2.*** Proportion of Major PE Found at Autopsy That Were Clinically Diagnosed Ante Mortem

| Reference | Number of Autopsies Showing Major PE | Number of Major PE Diagnosed Ante Mortem (%) | Factors Aiding Diagnosis | Factors Hindering Diagnosis |
|---|---|---|---|---|
| Uhland[9] | 70 | 11 (16) | — | — |
| Modan[11] | 223 | 85 (38) | Postoperative state<br>Thrombophlebitis<br>Chest x-ray | Cancer<br>Pneumonia |
| Coon[13] | 325 | 53 (16) | Venous thrombosis | — |
| Goldhaber[14] | 54 | 16 (30) | Postoperative state<br>Deep venous thrombosis<br>Lung scans<br>Pulmonary angiograms | Pneumonia<br>Increasing age<br>Congestive heart failure |

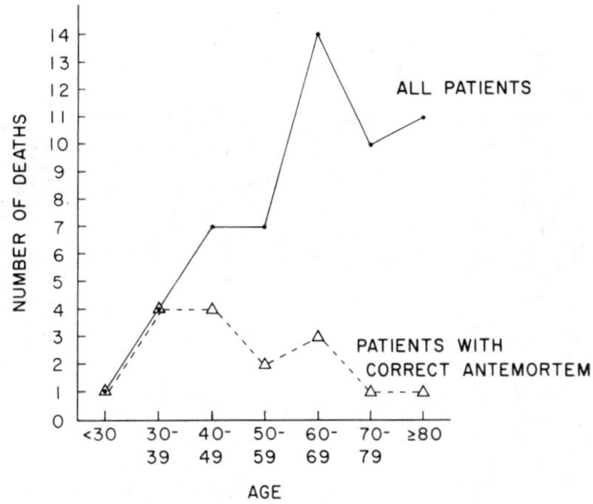


***Figure 5–1.*** Increase in proportion of undiagnosed PE deaths with increasing age. (From Goldhaber, S. Z., Hennekens, C. H., Evans, D. A., et al.: Factors associated with correct antemortem diagnosis of major pulmonary embolism. Am. J. Med., *73*:822, 1982.)

pulmonary embolism and the problems related to proper coding of death certificates. Rossman reviewed 6385 death certificates filed in New York City during a single month and found that 207 listed pulmonary embolism as the major cause or a contributory cause of death.[26] However, improper coding methods reduced this figure to 31, so that the clinical impression of pulmonary embolism at the time of death was being grossly underreported. In any study that relies on coding for PE on death certificates, researchers should acknowledge the inherent limitations in terms of ascertaining the true frequency of PE.[27]

### National Hospital Discharge Survey

Another source of descriptive survey information is the United States National Hospital Discharge Survey conducted by the National Center for Health Statistics (NCHS).[28] From 1971 to 1978, the NCHS selected approximately 400 hospitals to be surveyed from among 7903 acute care hospitals in which the average length of stay was less than 30 days. Approximately 216,000 acute care charts were reviewed annually. From 1971 to 1978, the number of patients whose deaths were certified primarily due to PE decreased (Fig. 5–2*A*); in contrast, the overall number of patients with PE as a primary or secondary discharge diagnosis increased (Fig. 5–2*B*). The case fatality rate (mortality divided by incidence) decreased significantly during the study period—from 20 per cent in 1971 to 13 per cent in 1978 (Fig. 5–2*C*). The greatest decrease in the proportion of fatal PEs occurred in patients 65 years and over. This survey was limited in that it (1) relied on a sampling of hospital charts rather than ascertaining diagnoses in all patients admitted to all acute care hospitals; (2) included few autopsies, with most PE deaths diagnosed based on the attending physician's clinical impression; (3) lacked diagnostic confirmation by lung scanning or pulmonary angiography (so that both underdiagnosis and overdiagnosis were possible shortcomings); and (4) did not determine the number of hospitalizations per patient per year. Nevertheless, this study suggests that PE is being diagnosed with increasing frequency and that the case fatality rate is decreasing. One cannot surmise from these data, however, whether the decreasing case fatality rate is due to a decline in frequency of massive PE, increased diagnosis of minor PE, improved treatment of PE, or a combination of these factors.

***Table 5–3.*** Proportion of PE Diagnosed Clinically That Were Not Present at Autopsy

| Reference | Number of PE Diagnosed Clinically in Patients Subsequently Autopsied | Number of Clinical Diagnoses Confirmed at Autopsy (%) |
|---|---|---|
| Modan[11] | 310 | 118 (38) |
| Smith[17] | — | — (60) |
| Goldhaber[46] | 25 | 17 (68) |

## Assessment of Long-term Risk Factors for PE

Although the Framingham Heart Study did not ascertain information prospectively on PE or DVT, a cohort of Framingham patients with autopsy-confirmed PE was identified

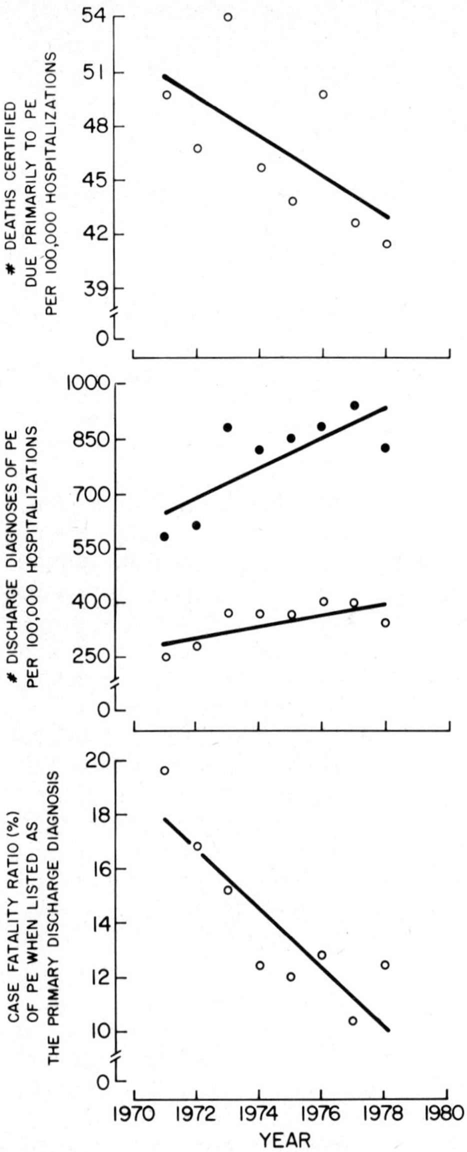


***Figure 5–2.*** *A,* Number of patients whose death was certified as primarily due to PE per 100,000 hospitalizations is shown from 1971 through 1978. For the annual decrease in patient deaths, 95% confidence limits are +0.2% to −2.5%. *B,* Number of patients with discharge diagnoses of PE per 100,000 hospitalizations is shown from 1971 through 1978. Open circles = patients with PE as the primary discharge diagnosis; closed circles = patients with PE listed as either a primary or secondary discharge diagnosis. For the annual increase in primary discharge diagnoses, 95% confidence limits are 0.0 to +3.1%. For PE listed as either a primary or a secondary discharge diagnosis, 95% confidence limits for the annual increase are +0.6% to +7.6%. *C,* Case fatality ratio (%) of PE listed as the primary discharge diagnosis is shown from 1971 through 1978. For the annual decrease in case fatality ratio, 95% confidence limits are −0.4% to −1.7%. (From Goldhaber, S. Z., and Hennekens, C. H.: Time trends in hospital mortality and diagnosis of pulmonary embolism. Am. Heart J., *104*:305, 1982.)

retrospectively, and potential long-term risk factors for PE were examined. These patients were then compared with all Framingham Heart Study patients who died.[29] Potential risk factors at entry into the study included age, systolic blood pressure, cholesterol level, cigarette use, blood glucose level, Metropolitan Relative Weight (based on normal weight-for-height data generated by the Metropolitan Life Insurance Company), and varicose veins (Table 5–4). When patients found to have major PE at autopsy were compared with all those who died within 26 years of follow-up, multiple logistic regression analysis showed that only Metropolitan Relative Weight among women was a significantly associated long-term risk factor for PE ($p<0.001$).

### Symptoms and Signs Suggestive of PE

Despite the difficulties in diagnosing pulmonary embolism clinically, suspicion of PE is of paramount importance. Without a high index of suspicion, clinicians may not perform the proper diagnostic tests to confirm or exclude this condition.

In the Urokinase-Streptokinase Pulmonary Embolism Trial, clinical symptoms and signs were observed in 327 patients with angiographically documented PE.[33] The most common symptoms were chest pain (88 per cent), which was usually pleuritic (74 per cent), and dyspnea (84 per cent). Apprehension (59 per cent) and cough (53 per cent) occurred often, whereas hemoptysis (30 per cent), diaphoresis (27 per cent), and syncope (13 per cent) were uncommon.

The most common sign in these patients was tachypnea (92 per cent), defined as more than 16 respirations per minute. Also observed were rales (58 per cent); an accentuated second heart sound (53 per cent); tachycardia (44 per cent), defined as a heart rate greater than 100 beats per minute; and fever (43 per cent), defined as temperature above 37.8°C. Phlebitis occurred in only 32 per cent of the patients. Other less common signs included diaphoresis (36 per cent), cardiac gallop (34 per cent), edema (24 per cent), heart murmur (23 per cent), and cyanosis (19 per cent).

It is interesting that certain "classic" triads of symptoms and signs were virtually absent, such as hemoptysis, cough, and sweating;

***Table 5–4.*** Potential Long-term Risk Factors for Major PE in the Framingham Heart Study

| Parameter | Entered Into Study | | Death During 26 Years of Follow-up | | Major PE at Autopsy | |
|---|---|---|---|---|---|---|
| | *Men (n = 1619)* | *Women (n = 1851)* | *Men (n = 567)* | *Women (n = 431)* | *Men (n = 27)* | *Women (n = 19)* |
| Mean age (years) | 43.7 | 43.9 | 49.1 | 49.5 | 48.9 | 47.6 |
| Mean systolic blood pressure (mm Hg) | 137 | 136 | 145 | 150 | 144 | 156 |
| Mean blood cholesterol (mg/100 ml) | 227 | 227 | 233 | 244 | 229 | 255 |
| Cigarette use (%) | 66 | 43 | 68 | 43 | 78 | 42 |
| Mean blood glucose (mg/100 ml) | 82 | 82 | 87 | 86 | 83 | 101 |
| Metropolitan Relative Weight (%) | 119 | 120 | 121 | 125 | 124 | 149* |
| Varicose veins (% present) | 11 | 28 | 15 | 37 | 11 | 42 |

From Goldhaber, S. Z., Savage, D. D., Garrison, R. J., et al.: Risk factors for pulmonary embolism: The Framingham study. Am. J. Med., *74*:1023, 1983.

*$p < 0.001$.

hemoptysis, chest pain, and dyspnea; or dyspnea, chest pain, and apprehension. Allen's sign (the triad of fever, tachypnea, and tachycardia) was present in only 23 per cent of patients. When the 65 per cent of patients in this study without preexisting cardiac or pulmonary disease were analyzed separately, the frequency of presenting symptoms and signs was virtually identical.[34]

Coexisting conditions included venous disease (49 per cent), immobilization (55 per cent), and congestive heart failure or chronic lung disease (38 per cent). However, almost half the patients in this trial had no apparent predisposing conditions. This reflects selection bias in favor of patients sufficiently healthy to withstand required angiography and potential thrombolytic therapy.

The trial described previously examined clinical presentation only among patients with angiographically proven PE and did not compare their symptoms and signs with those of patients suspected of having PE who were subsequently found to have normal pulmonary angiograms. In contrast, a case series from the Medical College of Virginia reviewed clinical presentations in 73 patients examined angiographically for PE over a one-year period (1976 to 1977).[35] In only 29 per cent of those suspected of having PE was the condition confirmed at angiography. Symptoms did *not* help to discriminate between patients with true PE and those with no evidence of PE on arteriograms. Ironically, chest pain (77 per cent versus 57 per cent) and hemoptysis (23 per cent versus 10 per cent) occurred more often in those without PE. Dyspnea and sweating occurred with virtually identical frequency in both groups. Signs on physical examination were *not* useful in discriminating between those with PE and those without. Of those with PE, 21 per cent had heart rates less than 100 beats per minute. All patients in both groups had respiratory rates greater than 16 per minute. This latter study supports the concept that symptoms and signs of PE are so nonspecific that it behooves the physician to pursue radiologic diagnosis (Chapter 4) in virtually all patients with suspected PE.

## Less Common Clinical Presentations

Small case series have helped to elucidate certain unusual symptoms and signs of PE. In 1935, Sylvester McGinn and Paul Dudley White published a report of nine patients with *acute cor pulmonale* due to pulmonary embolism.[36] Six of these patients were postoperative. The authors described a right ventricular gallop, best heard at the second and third intercostal spaces at the left sternal border, which they suggested might be due to right ventricular dilatation.

Other signs of PE include fever, syncope, paradoxical arterial embolization, and wheezing. Murray and coworkers reviewed 35 consecutive patients with angiographically documented pulmonary embolism and found that 24 had *fever* (rectal temperature ≥38°C); in 20, fever was attributed solely to PE.[37] In five of these 20 patients, the peak temperature was 39°C or above.

Thames and coworkers reviewed 132 consecutive cases of angiographically documented pulmonary embolism and found that *syncope* was the initial or predominant clinical feature in 13 per cent of the patients.[38] The syncope associated with PE may be vagal in origin and has been observed with simultaneous slowing of the sinus rate and atrioventricular block.[41]

In another case series, each of five patients presented with a syndrome of (1) DVT and/or PE, (2) arterial embolism, (3) a right-to-left intracardiac shunt, and (4) no evidence for a source of embolism in the left side of the heart.[39] These five patients met criteria for *paradoxical arterial embolism* from a venous site to an arterial site, either through a patent foramen ovale or an atrial septal defect.

Three patients with *wheezing* who had pulmonary embolism that masqueraded as asthma were described by Olazábai and coworkers.[40] These diverse case series suggest that we should maintain vigilance for unusual manifestations of PE as well as for the more classic presentations. In another case series of six patients, unrecognized pulmonary embolism presented as *disseminated intravascular coagulation*.[122]

## Diagnostic Tests

### Electrocardiogram

The electrocardiogram tends to have characteristic abnormalities only in patients with massive PE (see Fig. 10–1). Traditional manifestations of acute cor pulmonale such as $S_1Q_3T_3$, right bundle branch block, P pulmonale, or right axis deviation occurred in only 26 per cent of the patients evaluated in the Urokinase Pulmonary Embolism Trial.[42] Usually, when the electrocardiogram suggests PE, the diagnosis tends to be apparent for other reasons, such as the clinical presentation.

### Chest Roentgenogram and Pleural Effusion

The chest x-ray can be a valuable diagnostic aid, especially in massive PE (see Figure 4–2). Virtually all patients with massive PE will demonstrate zones of oligemia and a widened right pulmonary artery.[43] Pleural effusions are frequent, occurring in approximately half of 155 patients with PE in one prospective series.[44] However, pleural effusions are nonspecific and also occur commonly in patients with congestive heart failure, pneumonia, and cancer. Thus, the diagnostic value of this finding is low. Furthermore, the results of pleural fluid analysis are so variable[45] that thoracentesis in patients with suspected PE is generally not worthwhile unless a concomitant infectious process is considered likely. One should keep in mind that after thoracentesis has been performed, thrombolytic agents should not be administered for 10 days (see pages 110 to 113 and 123 to 125).

### Arterial Blood Gas

Hypoxia, as detected by measurement of arterial blood gases, has generally been considered an important screening test for pulmonary embolism. Yet patients suspected of PE who are then found to have negative lung scans or pulmonary angiograms may be as hypoxic as or more hypoxic than those with documented PE. For example, on evaluation of arterial blood gases in 97 patients between ages 18 and 40 years who underwent lung scanning for pleuritic chest pain, the average $PO_2$ for those *with* PE was 81 torr, compared with 77 torr for those *without* PE.[47, 48] In the personal experience of Dr. Eugene Robin, 14 per cent of 43 patients with an arterial $PO_2$ of 85 or greater had angiographically documented PE.[49] One of these six patients had an arterial $PO_2$ of 108 torr (with the measurement repeated twice) yet demonstrated multiple bilateral PE at angiography. While a high $PO_2$ can mistakenly dissuade the physician from pursuing the diagnosis of PE, a low $PO_2$ is nonspecific and consistent with a variety of illnesses that may mimic PE. Although a high $PO_2$ militates against PE, we believe lung scanning should be obtained in virtually all patients suspected of PE, regardless of the blood gas result.

### Lung Scanning

McNeil and colleagues have described a diagnostic strategy for assessing the probability of PE with lung scanning[50–52] (see Chapter 4, pages 45 to 52). Generally, perfusion lung scans are interpreted as indicating a high, moderate, or low probability of PE or as being indeterminate (see Table 4–2). In patients who undergo ventilation-perfusion lung scanning, the correlation between a scan showing a high probability of PE (segmental or greater perfusion defects with normal ventilation [i.e., ventilation-perfusion scan mismatch]) and the presence of PE on angiography is greater than 90%.[51, 53] Conversely, a normal lung scan, with few exceptions,[54, 55] will exclude the possibility of clinically significant PE. This latter tenet has been confirmed on long-term follow-up of patients with normal lung scans.[56]

### Pulmonary Angiography

Pulmonary angiography is the most specific examination available to establish the clinical diagnosis of PE (see Chapter 4, pages 52 to 55, and Figure 5–3). Much of the pioneering work in this area was undertaken by Dexter and colleagues at the Peter Bent Brigham Hospital.[57, 58] In 1971, they reported a 4 per cent morbidity rate and 0.3 per cent mortality rate in a series of 367 patients.[58] Even with their extensive experience using pulmonary angiography, they classified 17 per cent of the pulmonary angiograms as diagnostically equivocal for the presence of PE. In 1980, Mills and coworkers from Duke reviewed their experience with 1350 pulmonary angiograms during the previous 11 years.[59] Their morbidity rate (5 per cent) and their mortality rate (0.2 per cent) were similar to those reported by Dexter and coworkers. The three patients of Mills and coworkers who died all had severe pulmonary hypertension and experienced irreversible systemic hypotension after injection of radiographic contrast material. It is likely that in patients with pulmonary hypertension, the high osmolality of standard contrast agents is responsible for increases in pulmonary artery and right ventricular pressures, which further depress an already compromised right ventricle and decrease cardiac output. In view of this potential hazard, the Duke group generally will not perform pulmonary angiography if the right ventricular end diastolic pressure exceeds 20 mm Hg. In the future, however, newer contrast agents of lower osmolality will probably be utilized in patients with pulmonary hypertension.[60]

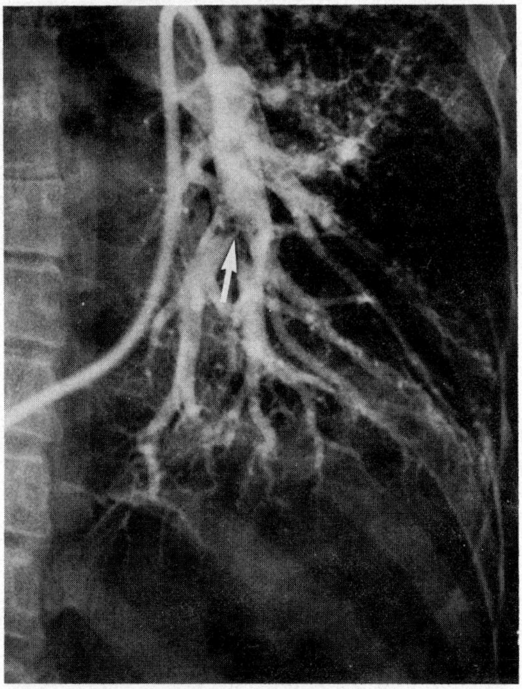

***Figure 5–3.*** Angiographically demonstrated pulmonary embolism. There is a saddle-shaped filling defect (white arrow) at the origin of the left lateral and left posterior medial basilar pulmonary arteries. (Courtesy of Dr. John A. Markisz, The New York Hospital and Cornell University Medical College.)

A normal pulmonary angiogram in patients with suspected PE almost always excludes clinically significant PE. At Massachusetts General Hospital, the clinical course of 180 patients suspected of having PE prior to negative pulmonary angiography was followed for at least six months after the procedure.[61] Ten of the 20 patients who died were autopsied, and none was found to have major PE. Of those who survived, none showed evidence of recurrent venous thromboembolism.

**Indications for Pulmonary Angiography.** The most controversial issue concerning diagnostic strategy for PE centers on the indications for pulmonary angiography. Unless the physician is confronted with a patient with life-threatening massive PE (see Chapter 10), lung scanning will routinely precede pulmonary angiography. Even if the odds of obtaining a diagnostic lung scan are low, such as in a patient with chronic obstructive pulmonary disease, lung scanning will usually aid the angiographer in catheter placement for optimal selective and subselective pulmonary angiography.

When a lung scan is normal, there is generally no reason to pursue the diagnosis of PE (Fig. 5–4). Instead, other diagnostic possibilities should be considered, such as pleuritis, pleurodynia, or costochondritis. Conversely, when ventilation-perfusion lung scanning indicates a high probability of PE and clinical suspicion is high prior to scanning, it is generally not necessary to proceed with pulmonary angiography when standard therapy is contemplated. However, if thrombolytic therapy or inferior vena caval inter-

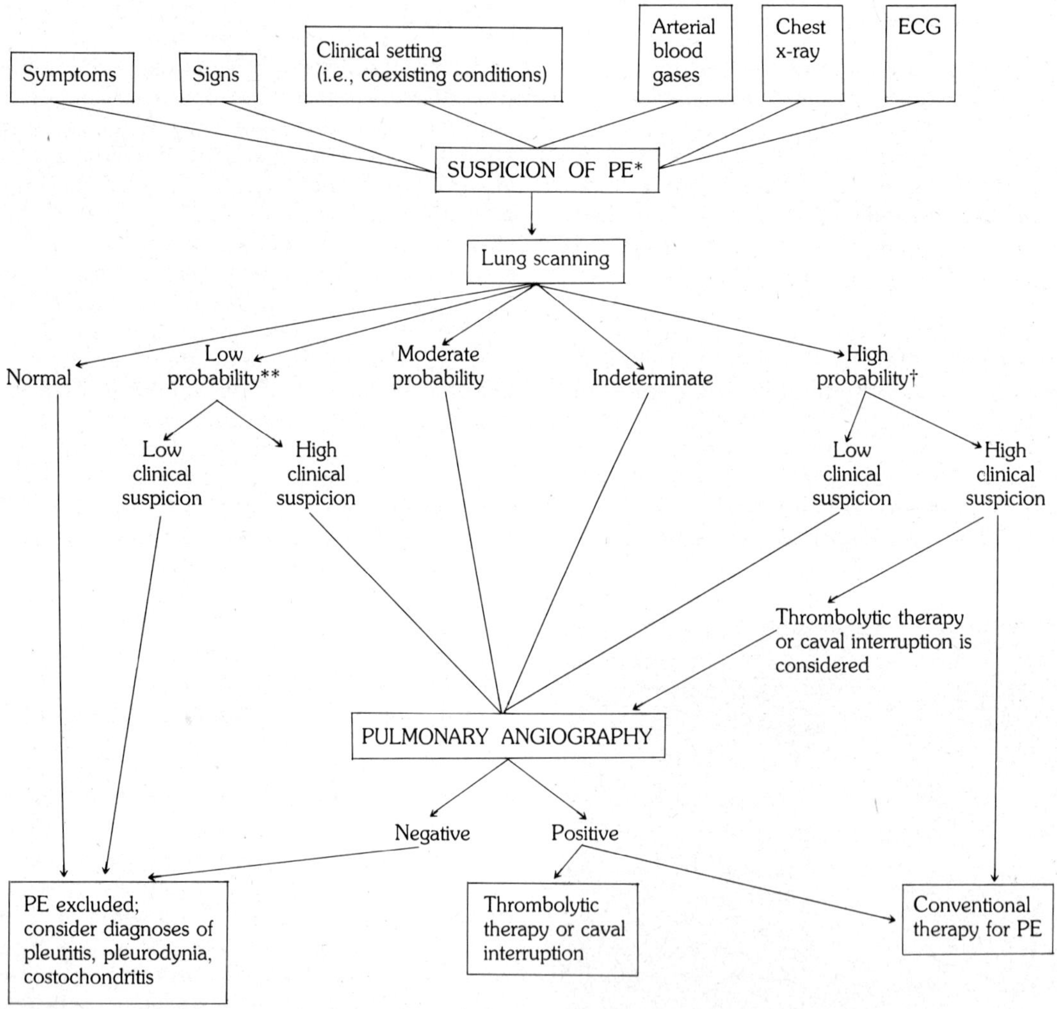


*Patients suspected of having PE should generally undergo lung scanning, regardless of blood gas results.
**Subsegmental perfusion defects with matching ventilation defects (i.e., a ventilation-perfusion scan match).
†Segmental or greater perfusion defects with normal ventilation (i.e., a ventilation-perfusion scan mismatch).

***Figure 5–4.*** Strategy for clinical use of lung scanning and pulmonary angiography in patients with suspected PE.

ruption is being considered, one may wish to eliminate even the slightest diagnostic uncertainty by obtaining a pulmonary angiogram.

To further clarify indications for pulmonary angiography, Hull and colleagues performed a prospective study in which patients with suspected PE and abnormal lung scans underwent routine pulmonary angiography and routine ascending leg venography.[62] Not surprisingly, they found that 86 per cent of patients with one or more segmental or greater perfusion defects coupled with normal ventilation scans (i.e., a ventilation-perfusion mismatch) had PE at angiography. However, the predictive value of ventilation-perfusion scanning was low for other categories of patients—i.e., one or more segmental or greater perfusion defects coupled with a ventilation scan that had matching defects (i.e., a ventilation-perfusion match), or one or more subsegmental perfusion defects regardless of the ventilation results, or an indeterminate perfusion scan in which the perfusion defect matched a radiologic abnormality.

The association between angiographically demonstrated PE and venographically demonstrated DVT was also examined. Of 41 patients with positive pulmonary angiograms, 12 (29 per cent) had negative venograms. Thus, substitution of venography for pulmonary angiography can be misleading, and this strategy is not recommended.

A study by Marsh and coworkers[63] has suggested that in the rare instances when lung scan results differ markedly from the clinical impression, a diagnostic pulmonary angiogram should be obtained. Of 30 patients who underwent angiography despite low probability scans, 10 had positive pulmonary angiograms. Of 18 patients who underwent pulmonary angiography despite high probability scans, 10 had negative pulmonary angiograms. These patients were distinctly unusual and underwent angiography because their clinical status was particularly perplexing. In most situations, however, multiple segmental or lobar perfusion defects in areas of normal ventilation will correspond with angiographically documented PE; conversely, many subsegmental and nonsegmental perfusion defects that match ventilation defects will correspond with normal angiographic findings.[64]

Despite studies to date, controversy persists regarding indications for pulmonary angiography among patients with lung scans that are neither normal nor markedly positive for PE.[65] Therefore, the National Institutes of Health is currently sponsoring a prospective multihospital study in which all patients suspected of PE with abnormal lung scans are undergoing routine pulmonary angiography. The results of this study are awaited with interest. In the meantime, we have outlined a strategy based on currently available information to guide our clinical use of pulmonary angiography in patients with suspected PE (see Figure 5–4). We generally reserve pulmonary angiography for patients with moderate probability or indeterminate lung scans. In unusual situations, in which our level of clinical suspicion for PE differs markedly from scan results, or when we are considering thrombolytic therapy or caval interruption, we tend to obtain pulmonary angiograms. We do not substitute venography or impedance plethysmography for pulmonary angiography. As technology for digital subtraction pulmonary angiography improves (see Chapter 4, pages 55 to 58), we anticipate that the threshold for obtaining angiographic assessment will be lowered.

### Echocardiogram

The diagnosis of massive PE can sometimes be established by means of two-dimensional echocardiography.[66–68] In addition to imaging the echo-dense clot, this technique also allows one to visualize right atrial and right ventricular dilatation and hypokinesis (see Figures 10–3 and 10–4).

### Computed Tomography

Computed tomography has been used to demonstrate chronic PE in patients with pulmonary hypertension.[68, 69] Because of the risks associated with conventional pulmonary angiography in these patients, CT should be considered as a possible alternative diagnostic modality. It can also be used to evaluate noninvasively the results of medical thrombolysis or surgical embolectomy.

### Blood Tests

The concept of a rapid, inexpensive, and accurate blood test to screen for PE or DVT is very appealing. Such a test would be analogous to the CK-MB assay used to diagnose acute myocardial infarction. To date, however, no diagnostic blood test of equal utility has been found for venous thromboembolism despite transient enthusiasm for a variety of assays. We shall briefly review the difficulties associated with the use of several of these blood tests as screening maneuvers.

In 1961, Wacker and colleagues proposed a new method of diagnosing PE based on serial measurements of lactic dehydrogenase (LDH), serum glutamic oxaloacetic transaminase (SGOT), and serum bilirubin concentration.[70] In 17 patients with PE, they found that the LDH was consistently elevated and that SGOT was consistently normal. In 12 of these 17 patients, the bilirubin level was significantly increased. They believed that this triad of blood tests would permit the differentiation of PE from acute myocardial infarction (in which SGOT would be elevated as well as LDH) and from pneumonia (in which LDH and SGOT levels would both be normal). Five of the 17 patients had massive PE proved at autopsy. Of the remaining 12 patients, most had massive PE, manifested by electrocardiographic signs of right heart strain. Ten years later, the diagnostic utility of serial LDH, SGOT, and bilirubin levels could not be confirmed in 50 more recent PE patients from the same institution,[71] probably because most patients in the latter study did not have massive PE. Of the 50 patients with angiographically documented PE, only nine had electrocardiographic evidence of right heart strain. The triad of increased LDH, normal SGOT, and increased bilirubin was present in only 12 per cent of patients. Therefore, we do not recommend the serial measurement of these three blood tests to diagnose PE.

For the past 15 years, there has been clinical interest in using tests of fibrin metabolism to help screen for venous thromboembolism.[72–78] The most frequently studied of these potential screening tests is fibrin split products (FSP), also known as fibrinogen/fibrin degradation products (FDP/fdp). Less frequently used tests of fibrin metabolism have included fibrinopeptide A (FPA), which is a peptide cleaved from fibrinogen by thrombin, and soluble fibrin complexes (SFC), which are circulating fibrin monomer complexes (see Figure 3–9). Most reports of FSP measurement in PE patients note a marked elevation in FSPs compared with normal levels.[74–78] Unfortunately, FSPs also tend to be elevated in many ill patients who do not have PE. One report suggested that *simultaneous* elevation of FDP/fdp and of SFC could accurately differentiate PE from nonthromboembolic lung disease.[76] However, simultaneous elevations of these two parameters were found in only 55 per cent of PE patients—a rate far too insensitive for a reliable screening test. Similar problems exist when FPA measurements are used in an attempt to screen for PE or DVT.[79, 80]

Transient enthusiasm also existed for elevations in plasma DNA as a rapid, accurate, inexpensive, and noninvasive screening test for PE.[81, 82] In a report published by Sipes and coworkers,[81] plasma DNA was elevated in 19 of 23 patients with PE but in none of 49 patients with pneumonia, myocardial infarction, DVT, or normal lung scans. Unfortunately, these promising results could not be confirmed by other research groups.[83, 84]

## Differential Diagnosis of PE

### In Patients Without Pulmonary Hypertension

*Pneumonia, congestive heart failure,* and *myocardial infarction* may have clinical presentations that obscure or simulate the diagnosis of PE. Patients with pneumonia and congestive heart failure generally have chest x-ray and lung scan abnormalities that make noninvasive diagnosis of PE more difficult. Use of the MB fraction of creatine phosphokinase has proved to be very accurate in diagnosing myocardial infarction.[87] Nevertheless, PE is a frequent concomitant illness in these three settings. For patients who fail to respond to appropriate therapy for these three conditions, it may be prudent to consider the possibility of coexisting PE.

### In Patients with Pulmonary Hypertension

Manifestations of pulmonary hypertension can vary from obvious (e.g., cor pulmonale) to subtle. When physical findings are present, such as a right ventricular heave, right ventricular third heart sound, and loud, single second heart sound, establishing the presence of pulmonary hypertension is relatively straightforward. In these circumstances, the chest x-ray often demonstrates an enlarged pulmonary artery.

***Recurrent PE Versus Primary Pulmonary Hypertension.*** Recurrent PE can cause pulmonary hypertension and can be mistaken for primary pulmonary hypertension, which should be considered a diagnosis of exclusion. The symptoms, clinical course, and

***Table 5–5.*** Common Features of Primary Pulmonary Hypertension and Recurrent PE

| | |
|---|---|
| Symptoms | Fatigue, dyspnea on exertion—most common<br>Chest pain, syncope, hemoptysis, cyanosis—also common |
| Clinical course | Progressive dyspnea<br>Right heart failure |
| Hemodynamics | Elevated right heart pressures<br>Normal pulmonary capillary wedge pressure |

hemodynamics of recurrent PE and primary pulmonary hypertension share many common features (Table 5–5). Variables that may help differentiate these entities are listed in Table 5–6.[88–97]

***Chronic Obstructive Pulmonary Disease (COPD).*** Patients with PE or COPD may also have similar clinical presentations and similar abnormalities on chest x-ray and lung scanning. Sharma and Sasahara found that lung scanning reliably established or excluded the diagnosis of PE in fewer than 20 per cent of their COPD patients.[98] Even pulmonary angiography at times yielded equivocal results, because nondiagnostic findings in PE patients, such as retarded blood flow and blood vessel pruning, are also common in COPD patients. Definitive diagnosis of PE in COPD patients thus requires observation of a vessel cut-off and an intravascular filling defect. Nevertheless, microemboli in vessels 2 mm or less in diameter can be present despite an apparently normal angiogram.[99]

***Other Conditions.*** In patients with pulmonary hypertension and possible PE, other illnesses that may coexist with or mimic PE include *sarcoidosis, sickle cell disease,*[100] *pulmonary veno-occlusive disease,*[101] *pulmonary arteriovenous fistula,*[102] *schistosomiasis, vasculitis, chronic interstitial lung disease, left-to-right shunting,* and *increased left heart filling pressure. Nonthrombotic PE* (e.g., tumor embolism[103]) is discussed in Chapter 11. When any of these conditions occur chronically, patients with these disorders may benefit from baseline lung scanning so that if new symptoms or signs suggest PE acutely, an emergent lung scan can be obtained and compared with a previous scan.

## DIAGNOSIS OF PULMONARY INFARCTION

The clinical diagnosis of pulmonary infarction due to PE cannot be established unless an infiltrate is present on chest x-ray (see Figure 4–4), and the usual criteria for PE on lung scan or pulmonary angiography are met. Patients with PE and pulmonary infarction are likely to experience intense pleuritic pain and tend to have a unilateral, distal, and less extensive embolism on angiography than do PE patients *without* pulmonary infarction, who are more likely to suffer massive bilateral proximal embolism.[85, 86] Thus, pulmonary infarction, although often characterized by intense pleuritic pain, may signify an anatomically small, peripheral PE.

***Table 5–6.*** Differentiation Between Primary Pulmonary Hypertension (PPH) and Recurrent PE

| Variable | PPH | Recurrent PE |
|---|---|---|
| Age (years) | 20 to 40 | >50 |
| Female:male ratio | 4:1 | 1:1 |
| Clinical course | Continued downhill | Downhill, with stabilization between episodes |
| Lung scan | No segmental perfusion defects | Segmental or larger perfusion defects |
| Pulmonary artery systolic pressure (mm Hg) | >60 | <60 |
| Pulmonary arteriogram | "Pruning" | Intraluminal filling defects |
| Confounding problems with arteriogram | Thrombi may occur on or distal to PPH lesion | "Pruning," a common angiographic finding in PPH, can also be an angiographic sign of PE. Furthermore, late in the clinical course, arteriogram may not show emboli. |
| Diagnostic alternatives | Open lung biopsy | Pulmonary angioscopy (see Chapter 14) |
| Therapy | Isoproterenol[123]<br>Hydralazine<br>Nifedipine<br><br>Anticoagulation | Anticoagulation (see Chapter 7)<br>IVC interruption (see Chapter 10)<br>Thromboendarterectomy (see Chapter 15)<br>? Ketanserin (see Chapter 16) |

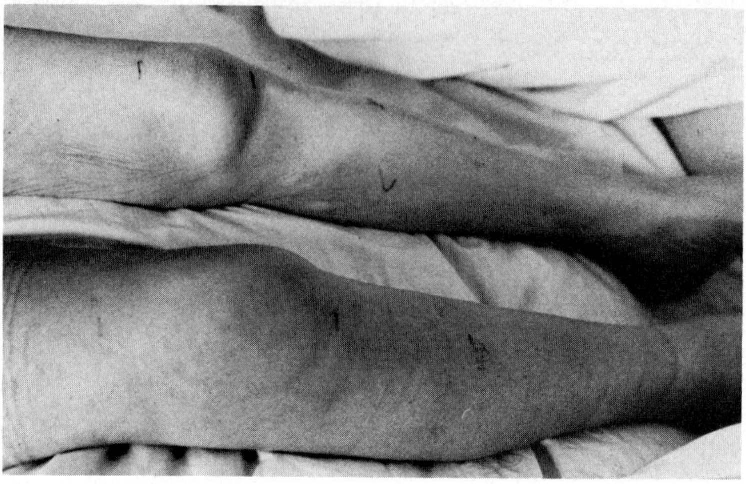

***Figure 5–5.*** Right leg iliofemoral venous thrombosis causing leg swelling and leg discoloration. (Figure kindly contributed by Dr. Nathan P. Couch, Brigham and Women's Hospital and Harvard Medical School.)

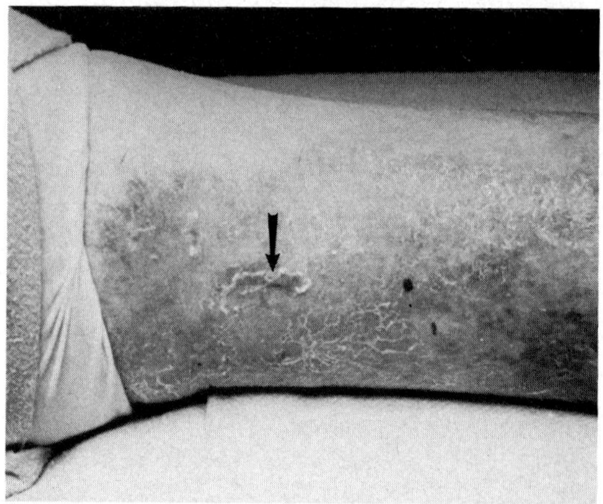

***Figure 5–6.*** Mild postphlebitic syndrome, manifested as stasis dermatitis with scaling of skin and brawny pigmentation in a patient who suffered a prior episode of DVT. A well-healing stasis ulcer can be seen (arrow). (Figure kindly contributed by Dr. Nathan P. Couch, Brigham and Women's Hospital and Harvard Medical School.)

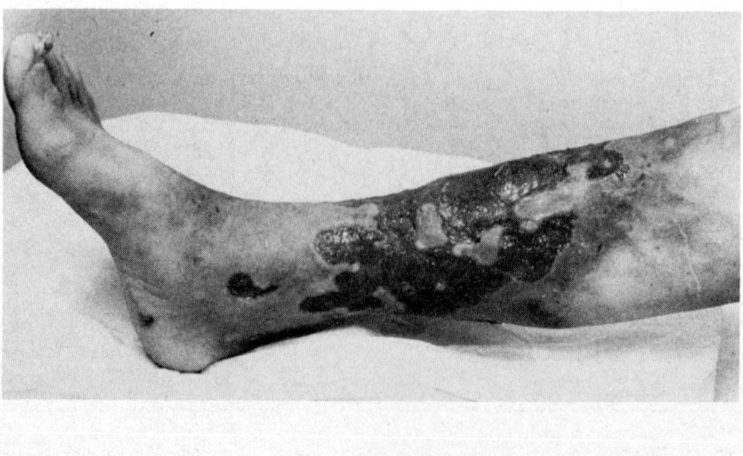

***Figure 5–7.*** Severe postphlebitic syndrome, manifested as deep leg ulceration in a patient with prior DVT. These extensive ulcers required skin grafting. (Figure kindly contributed by Dr. Nathan P. Couch, Brigham and Women's Hospital and Harvard Medical School.)

## DIAGNOSIS OF DVT

### Symptoms and Signs Suggestive of DVT

DVT often occurs without any symptoms or signs. When present, however, the major symptoms are leg pain, tenderness, and swelling, and the major signs are leg edema, discomfort in the calf upon forced dorsiflexion of the foot (Homans' sign), venous distention of subcutaneous vessels, discoloration (Fig. 5–5), and a palpable cord (i.e., thrombus). Unfortunately, these symptoms and signs are not specific for DVT, so that diagnoses based on clinical findings are often incorrect. For example, when Hull and coworkers evaluated 478 symptomatic patients who were referred for treatment after clinically diagnosed DVT, the venograms were found to be normal in 277 (58 per cent).[104] Therefore, clinical suspicion of DVT should be supplemented by definitive radiologic evaluation (see Chapter 4).

Obstructive iliofemoral vein thrombosis, which is rare, causes marked leg swelling and cyanosis and is termed *phlegmasia cerulea dolens.* Venous occlusion obstructs blood flow and causes severe leg edema, which in turn can impair arterial inflow and cause marked tissue ischemia.

When iliofemoral vein thrombosis is associated with arterial spasm, leg pulses may be weak or absent and the extremity will be cold and pale. This condition is known as *phlegmasia alba dolens.*[116]

*Postphlebitic syndrome* can develop weeks to years after an episode of DVT. Its manifestations can range from mild stasis dermatitis with brawny pigmentation (Fig. 5–6) to severe ulceration requiring skin grafting (Fig. 5–7).

### Association Between PE and DVT

PE is associated with clinically silent DVT and, conversely, DVT is associated with clinically silent PE. For example, of 86 patients with clinical syndromes and lung scans diagnostic of PE, none had symptoms or signs of DVT. In search of a source for PE, the investigators carried out bilateral leg phlebography in all 86 patients; in 34, the venograms demonstrated nonocclusive thrombus.[32] Conversely, Kistner and coworkers reported a series of 46 patients with phlebographically confirmed DVT who initially had no symptoms of PE.[30] Serial perfusion lung scans were obtained in all patients, and 24 (52 per cent) developed lung scans positive for PE, although only four developed clinical syndromes suggestive of PE. More recently, Moser and LeMoine performed contrast venography to document DVT in 36 patients, 21 with thrombosis limited to the calf veins and 15 with thrombosis involving both thigh and calf veins.[31] All 36 patients underwent ventilation and perfusion lung scanning. The 21 patients with only calf vein thromboses had normal lung scans. However, of the 15 patients with proximal DVT, eight had evidence of embolism on the scan, yet only one patient was symptomatic. Thus, embolic risk appears to depend on the location of the leg vein thrombosis. In patients with proximal thrombosis in thigh veins, a lack of symptoms of PE does not exclude the presence of PE, and therefore routine baseline and predischarge lung scanning may be warranted.

### Radiographic Assessment

*Leg phlebography* remains the most accurate modality to establish or exclude DVT. It is the standard by which noninvasive techniques for examining leg veins are judged. Despite the fairly high cost, relatively invasive nature, and occasional complications of venography, we find that this technique is generally safe, rapid, and reliable, and we use it routinely to diagnose DVT at our institution.[105] Three-month follow-up of patients with clinically suspected DVT but negative venograms has confirmed that it is safe to withhold anticoagulant therapy in this group of patients.[115]

The utility of venography in relation to noninvasive tests for DVT (e.g., radionuclide phlebography, Doppler ultrasound, fibrinogen leg scanning, or impedance plethysmography) is discussed in detail in the previous chapter. *Fibrinogen leg scanning,* although potentially useful in patients with equivocal venograms,[114] cannot distinguish superficial from deep venous thrombi. In addition, it is unreliable for detecting DVT proximal to the calves and may yield false-positive results in the presence of hemorrhagic or inflammatory exudates.[106, 107] *Impedance plethysmography* (IPG) is not a reliable means of detecting calf vein thrombi,[108, 109] but if operators are sufficiently experienced, it can be used to diagnose most cases of proximal DVT.[110, 111] IPG is particularly useful for serial screening of

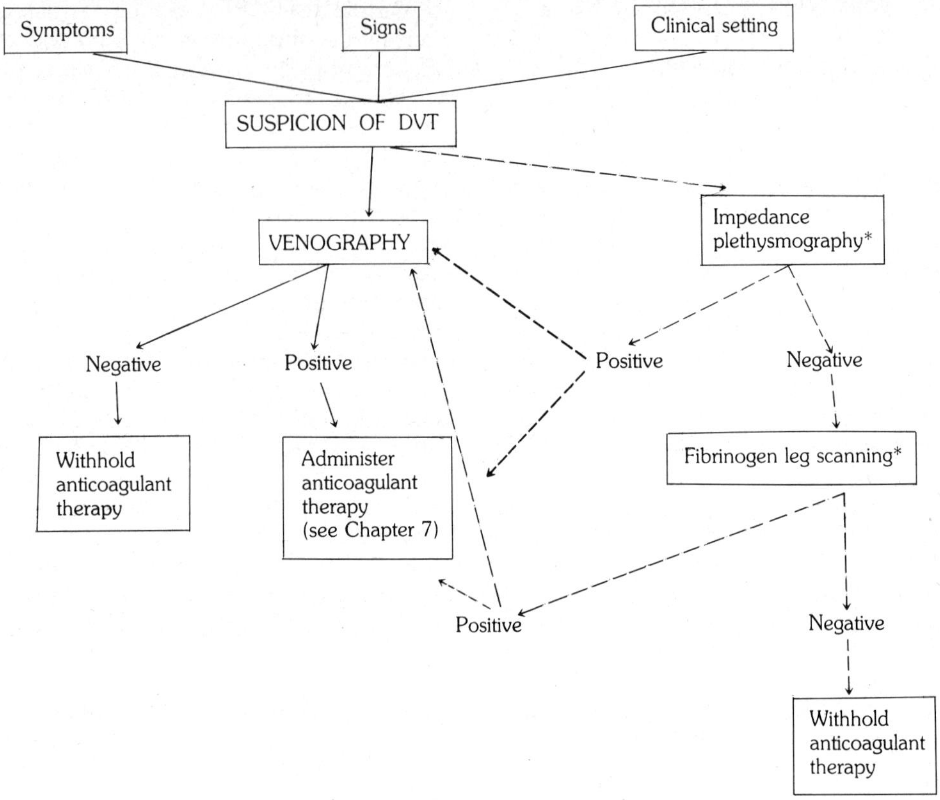


Solid lines indicate our preferred strategy.
Dashed lines indicate alternative approaches.
*Other noninvasive tests to detect DVT are discussed in Chapter 4.

***Figure 5–8.*** Strategy for diagnosing DVT.

patients at high risk for developing DVT. The combined use of these two complementary procedures—fibrinogen leg scanning and IPG—has been advocated as an alternative to leg phlebography.[112, 113] In institutions where the accuracy of these noninvasive techniques has been confirmed by comparison with venography, such an alternative approach is reasonable. However, it should be noted that leg phlebography can provide information about venous valve morphology that cannot be obtained using noninvasive tests.

In summary, the clinician's strategy for diagnosing DVT should be to maintain a high level of suspicion for this condition and a low threshold for proceeding with radiologic imaging. Approaches to diagnosing DVT are outlined in Figure 5–8.

## Differential Diagnosis of DVT

In patients with leg pain, tenderness, or swelling who are suspected clinically of having DVT, a negative venogram is frequently obtained,[113] and an alternative explanation for the clinical presentation is often not established. The frequent exclusion of DVT based on venographic findings despite a strong clinical suspicion reinforces the concept that laboratory confirmation of the presence of DVT is essential. When alternative diagnoses have been established after venography is negative (Table 5–7), the most frequent explanation has been *muscle strain* associated with unaccustomed exercise.[115]

*Varicose veins* are abnormally dilated vessels with incompetent valves that permit venous reflux. They can be classified as primary, in the absence of prior deep venous disease, or secondary, occurring subsequent to deep venous disease. Symptoms may include leg fatigue, ankle swelling, calf muscle cramping, and itching or burning.[116] Diagnosis is readily established by visual inspection of the legs with the patient in the upright position. Initial management involves elastic compression stockings and leg elevation.

***Table 5–7.*** Alternative Diagnoses When Venograms Are Normal in Patients Suspected of Having DVT*

| |
|---|
| Muscle strain or tear |
| Venous reflux due to varicose veins |
| Stasis dermatitis due to postphlebitic syndrome |
| Cellulitis |
| Superficial thrombophlebitis |
| Ruptured popliteal (Baker's) cyst |
| Spontaneous muscle hematoma |
| Swelling in a paralyzed leg |
| Lymphatic obstruction |
| Arterial insufficiency |
| Neurogenic pain |

*Often, no definitive alternative diagnosis is established.

When these simple measures fail, the postphlebitic syndrome (PPS) may result, manifested by stasis dermatitis, ulceration, and superficial thrombophlebitis. The reader is referred to Chapter 7 for a discussion of the management of PPS (page 129).

Although leg *cellulitis* may be misdiagnosed as stasis dermatitis, the converse is more likely. Leg cellulitis can also mimic DVT because both conditions cause leg inflammation, swelling, and tenderness. However, fever and leukocytosis occur more often with cellulitis than with DVT.

*Superficial thrombophlebitis*[117–119] may present as a tender, reddened superficial vein with a palpable thrombus. Rarely, extensive superficial thrombophlebitis may be associated with propagation of clot to the deep venous system (Table 5–8). While saphenous vein stripping used to be commonly employed to manage this condition, enthusiasm for this approach has waned with the advent of saphenous vein aortocoronary bypass grafting. Consequently, superficial thrombophlebitis is usually managed conservatively, with heat, leg elevation, and anti-inflammatory agents.

A *ruptured popliteal (Baker's) cyst* should be considered in any patient suspected of DVT who has knee arthritis in the ipsilateral leg.

***Table 5–8.*** Association of Superficial Thrombophlebitis with PE and DVT

| Reference | Number of Patients with Superficial Thrombophlebitis | Number of Patients with Associated DVT | Number of Patients with Associated PE |
|---|---|---|---|
| Hafner and coworkers[117] | 324 | 23 | 3 |
| Muller and coworkers[118] | 344 | 1 | 3 |
| Husni and Williams[119] | 221 | 10 | 10 |

Symptoms and signs may be identical in the two conditions, and to complicate matters further, DVT and ruptured Baker's cyst may occur simultaneously in the same patient. Swelling due to ruptured Baker's cyst may occur higher and more medially than with DVT,[120] but these subtle distinctions are not reliable for clinical differentiation. A definitive diagnosis of ruptured Baker's cyst may be made with ultrasound or arthrography. Leg phlebography shows stretching and compression of the popliteal vein around the cyst, at times with coexisting thrombus.

*Leg swelling in a paralyzed leg* and *lymphatic obstruction* may also mimic DVT. *Arterial insufficiency*, however, can usually be differentiated by sudden onset of pain; coolness and pallor of the leg; a nonpalpable pulse; and the absence of leg swelling.[121] *Neurogenic pain* from sciatic or lateral cutaneous nerve compression is generally sudden in onset and is exacerbated by maneuvers that stretch the nerve.

## SUMMARY

A high level of suspicion should be maintained for the presence of PE and DVT, especially in patients with other illnesses that can mimic venous thromboembolic disease. Frequently, two clinically similar conditions can coexist in the same patient, such as pneumonia *and* PE, or ruptured Baker's cyst *and* DVT. Because both overdiagnosis and underdiagnosis of PE and DVT are notoriously common problems, clinical suspicion should be accompanied by definitive radiologic evaluation. To date, nonradiologic methods of diagnosing venous thromboembolism, such as blood tests to assess fibrin metabolism, have not proved sufficiently accurate to be considered reliable. Furthermore, we believe that the extent to which PE occurs *without* DVT and *without* hypoxia indicates that the evaluation of leg veins or arterial blood gases to detect PE can be misleading in situations in which clinical suspicion is high.

Although the indications for pulmonary angiography remain somewhat controversial, we believe that our investigative strategy (as outlined in Figure 5–4) is reasonable and will provide an accurate diagnosis without overutilization of this invasive procedure. In the future, digital subtraction pulmonary angiography (see Figure 4–12) may require only the injection of contrast agent into a peripheral vein and may obviate right heart catheterization for pulmonary angiographic evaluation. Development of a rapid and reliable blood test to screen for PE and DVT, analogous to the MB band of creatine phosphokinase for myocardial infarction, would greatly facilitate the clinician's diagnostic strategy.

ACKNOWLEDGMENT: I wish to thank Ms. Nancy Orendain for her research assistance in the differential diagnosis section of this chapter.

## REFERENCES


1. Belt, T. H.: Thrombosis and pulmonary embolism. Am. J. Path., *10*:129, 1934.
2. Collins, D. C.: Pulmonary embolism, based on a study of 271 instances. Am. J. Surg., *33*:210, 1936.
3. McCartney, J. S.: Postoperative pulmonary embolism. Surgery, *17*:191, 1945.
4. Roe, B. B., and Goldthwait, J. C.: Pulmonary embolism: A statistical study of post-mortem material at the Massachusetts General Hospital. New Engl. J. Med., *241*:679, 1949.
5. Ochsner, A., DeBakey, M. E., DeCamp, P. T., et al.: Thromboembolism: An analysis of cases at the Charity Hospital in New Orleans over a 12-year period. Ann. Surg., *134*:405, 1951.
6. Fowler, E. F., and Bollinger, J. A.: Pulmonary embolism: A clinical study of ninety-seven fatal cases. Surgery, *36*:650, 1954.
7. Towbin, A.: Pulmonary embolism: Incidence and significance. JAMA, *156*:209, 1954.
8. Coon, W. W., and Coller, F. A.: Clinicopathologic correlation in thromboembolism. Surg. Gynecol. Obstet., *109*:259, 1959.
9. Uhland, H., and Goldberg, L. M.: Pulmonary embolism: A commonly missed clinical entity. Dis. Chest, *45*:533, 1964.
10. Morrell, M. T., and Dunnill, M. S.: The postmortem incidence of pulmonary embolism in a hospital population. Br. Med. J., *55*:347, 1968.
11. Modan, B., Sharon, E., and Jelin, N.: Factors contributing to the incorrect diagnosis of pulmonary embolic disease. Chest, *62*:388, 1972.
12. MacIntyre, I. M. C., and Ruckley, C. V.: Pulmonary embolism: A clinical and autopsy study. Scott. Med. J., *19*:20, 1974.
13. Coon, W. W.: Risk factors in pulmonary embolism. Surg. Gynecol. Obstet., *143*:385, 1976.
14. Goldhaber, S. Z., Hennekens, C. H., Evans, D. A., et al.: Factors associated with correct antemortem diagnosis of major pulmonary embolism. Am. J. Med., *73*:822, 1982.
15. Mossey, R. T., Kasabian, A. A., Wilkes, B. M., et al.: Pulmonary embolism: Low incidence in chronic renal failure. Arch. Intern. Med., *142*:1646, 1982.
16. Freiman, D. G., Suyemoto, J., and Wessler, S.: Frequency of pulmonary thromboembolism in man. New Engl. J. Med., *272*:1278, 1965.
17. Smith, G. T., Dexter, L., and Dammin, G. J.: Postmortem quantitative studies in pulmonary embolism. *In* Sasahara, A. A., and Stein, M. (Eds.): Pulmonary Embolic Disease. Grune and Stratton, New York, 1965, p. 120.
18. Henderson, E. F.: Fatal pulmonary embolism: A statistical review. Arch. Surg., *15*:231, 1927.
19. Barker, N. W., Nygaard, K. K., Walters, W., et al.: A statistical study of postoperative venous thrombosis and pulmonary embolism: I. Incidence in various types of operations. Mayo Clin., *15*:769, 1940.
20. Hermann, R. E., Davis, J. H., and Holden, W. D.: Pulmonary embolism: A clinical and pathologic study with emphasis on the effect of prophylactic therapy with anticoagulants. Am. J. Surg., *102*:19, 1961.
21. Morrell, M. T., Truelove, S. C., and Barr, A.: Pulmonary embolism. Br. Med. J., *2*:830, 1963.
22. Carlotti, J., Hardy, I. B., Jr., Linton, R. R., et al.: Pulmonary embolism in medical patients. JAMA, *134*:1447, 1947.
23. Kucera, M.: Some problems of venous thromboembolism in patients with heart disease. Rev. Czech. Med., *14*:50, 1968.
24. Thomas, W. A., Davies, J. N. P., O'Neal, R. M., et al.: Incidence of myocardial infarction correlated with venous and pulmonary thrombosis and embolism. Am. J. Cardiol., *5*:41, 1960.
25. Gore, I., Hirst, A. E., and Tanaka, E.: Myocardial infarction and thromboembolism: A comparative study in Boston and in Kyushu, Japan. Arch. Intern. Med., *113*:323, 1964.
26. Rossman, I.: True incidence of pulmonary embolization and vital statistics. JAMA, *230*:1677, 1974.
27. Samkoff, J. S., and Comstock, G. W.: Epidemiology of pulmonary embolism: Mortality in a general population. Am. J. Epidemiol., *114*:488, 1981.
28. Goldhaber, S. Z., and Hennekens, C. H.: Time trends in hospital mortality and diagnosis of pulmonary embolism. Am. Heart J., *104*:305, 1982.
29. Goldhaber, S. Z., Savage, D. D., Garrison, R. J., et al.: Risk factors for pulmonary embolism: the Framingham Study. Am. J. Med., *74*:1023, 1983.
30. Kistner, R. L., Ball, J. J., Nordyke, R. A., et al.: Incidence of pulmonary embolism in the course of thrombophlebitis of the lower extremities. Am. J. Surg., *124*:169, 1972.
31. Moser, K. M., and LeMoine, J. R.: Is embolic risk conditioned by location of deep venous thrombosis? Ann. Intern. Med., *94*:439, 1981.
32. Walker, M. G.: The natural history of venous thrombo-embolism. Br. J. Surg., *59*:753, 1972.
33. Bell, W. R., Simon, T. L., and DeMets, D. L.: The clinical features of submassive and massive pulmonary emboli. Am. J. Med., *62*:355, 1977.
34. Stein, P. D., Willis, P. W. III, and DeMets, D. L.: History and physical examination in acute pulmonary embolism in patients without preexisting cardiac or pulmonary disease. Am. J. Cardiol., *47*:218, 1981.
35. Goodall, R. J. R., and Greenfield, L. J.: Clinical correlations in the diagnosis of pulmonary embolism. Ann. Surg., *191*:219, 1980.
36. McGinn, S., and White, P. D.: Acute cor pulmonale resulting from pulmonary embolism: Its clinical recognition. JAMA, *104*:1473, 1935.
37. Murray, H. W., Ellis, G. C., Blumenthal, D. S., et al.: Fever and pulmonary thromboembolism. Am. J. Med., *67*:232, 1979.
38. Thames, M. D., Alpert, J. S., and Dalen, J. E.: Syncope in patients with pulmonary embolism. JAMA, *238*:2509, 1977.
39. Meister, S. G., Grossman, W., Dexter, L., et al.: Paradoxical embolism: Diagnosis during life. Am. J. Med., *53*:292, 1972.
40. Olazábai, F., Jr., Román-Irizarry, L. A., Oms, J.

D., et al.: Pulmonary emboli masquerading as asthma. New Engl. J. Med., *278*:999, 1968.
41. Simpson, R. J., Jr., Podolak, R., Mangano, C. A., Jr., et al.: Vagal syncope during recurrent pulmonary embolism. JAMA, *249*:390, 1983.
42. Stein, P. D., Dalen, J. E., McIntyre, K. M., et al.: The electrocardiogram in acute pulmonary embolism. Prog. Cardiovasc. Dis., *17*:247, 1975.
43. Kerr, I. H., Simon, G., and Sutton, G. C.: The value of the plain radiograph in acute massive pulmonary embolism. Br. J. Radiol., *44*:751, 1971.
44. Bynum, L. J., and Wilson, J. E. III: Radiographic features of pleural effusions in pulmonary embolism. Am. Rev. Respir. Dis., *117*:829, 1978.
45. Bynum, L. J., and Wilson, J. E. III: Characteristics of pleural effusions associated with pulmonary embolism. Arch. Intern. Med., *136*:159, 1976.
46. Goldhaber, S. Z., Buring, J. E., Godleski, J. J., et al.: The predictive value of the antemortem diagnosis of pulmonary embolism. Unpublished observations.
47. McNeil, B. J., Hessel, S. J., Branch, W. T., et al.: Measures of clinical efficacy. III. The value of the lung scan in the evaluation of young patients with pleuritic chest pain. J. Nucl. Med., *17*:163, 1976.
48. Branch, W. T., Jr., and McNeil, B. J.: Analysis of the differential diagnosis and assessment of pleuritic chest pain in young adults. Am. J. Med., *75*:671, 1983.
49. Robin, E. D.: Overdiagnosis and overtreatment of pulmonary embolism: the emperor may have no clothes. Ann. Intern. Med., *87*:775, 1977.
50. McNeil, B. J., Holman, B. L., and Adelstein, S. J.: The scintigraphic definition of pulmonary embolism. JAMA, *277*:753, 1974.
51. McNeil, B. J.: A diagnostic strategy using ventilation-perfusion studies in patients suspect for pulmonary embolism. J. Nucl. Med., *17*:613, 1976.
52. McNeil, B. J.: Ventilation-perfusion studies and the diagnosis of pulmonary embolism: Concise communication. J. Nucl. Med., *21*:319, 1980.
53. Biello, D. R., Mattar, A. G., McKnight, R. C., et al.: Ventilation-perfusion studies in suspected pulmonary embolism. AJR, *133*:1033, 1979.
54. McDougall, I. R., Goris, M. L., and Kriss, J. P.: Pulmonary embolism (Letter). Ann. Intern. Med., *88*:711, 1978.
55. Robin, E. D.: Pulmonary embolism (Letter). Ann. Intern. Med., *88*:713, 1978.
56. Kipper, M. S., Moser, K. M., Kortman, K. E., et al.: Longterm follow-up of patients with suspected pulmonary embolism and a normal lung scan. Perfusion scans in embolic subjects. Chest, *82*:411, 1982.
57. Stein, P. D., O'Connor, J. F., Dalen, J. E., et al.: The angiographic diagnosis of acute pulmonary embolism: Evaluation of criteria. Am. Heart J., *73*:730, 1967.
58. Dalen, J. E., Brooks, H. L., Johnson, L. W., et al.: Pulmonary angiography in acute pulmonary embolism: Indications, techniques, and results in 367 patients. Am. Heart J., *81*:175, 1971.
59. Mills, S. R., Jackson, D. C., Older, R. A., et al.: The incidence, etiologies, and avoidance of complications of pulmonary angiography in a large series. Radiology, *136*:295, 1980.
60. McCracken, S., and Bettmann, M.: Current status of ionic and non-ionic intravascular contrast media. Postgrad. Radiol., *3*:345, 1983.
61. Novelline, R. A., Baltarowich, O. H., Athanasoulis, C. A., et al.: The clinical course of patients with suspected pulmonary embolism and a negative pulmonary arteriogram. Radiology, *126*:561, 1978.
62. Hull, R. D., Hirsh, J., Carter, C. J., et al.: Pulmonary angiography, ventilation lung scanning, and venography for clinically suspected pulmonary embolism with abnormal perfusion lung scan. Ann. Intern. Med., *98*:891, 1983.
63. Marsh, J. D., Glynn, M. A., and Torman, H. A.: Pulmonary angiography: Application in a new spectrum of patients. Am. J. Med., *75*:763, 1983.
64. Cheely, R., McCartney, W. H., Perry, J. R., et al.: The role of noninvasive tests versus pulmonary angiography in the diagnosis of pulmonary embolism. Am. J. Med., *70*:17, 1981.
65. Secker-Walker, R. H.: On purple emperors, pulmonary embolism, and venous thrombosis. Ann. Intern. Med., *98*:1006, 1983.
66. Starkey, I. R., and de Bono, D. P.: Echocardiographic identification of right-sided cardiac intracavitary thromboembolus in massive pulmonary embolism. Circulation, *66*:1322, 1982.
67. Woolridge, J. D., and Healey, J.: Echocardiographic diagnosis of right ventricular thromboembolism. Am. Heart J., *106*:590, 1983.
68. DiCarlo, L. A., Jr., Schiller, N. B., Herfkens, R. L., et al.: Noninvasive detection of proximal pulmonary artery thrombosis by two-dimensional echocardiography and computerized tomography. Am. Heart J., *104*:879, 1982.
69. Kereiakes, D. J., Herfkens, R. J., Brundage, B. H., et al.: Computerized tomography in chronic thromboembolic pulmonary hypertension. Am. Heart J., *106*:1432, 1983.
70. Wacker, W. E. C., Rosenthal, M., Snodgrass, P. J., et al.: A triad for the diagnosis of pulmonary embolism and infarction. JAMA, *178*:108, 1961.
71. Szucs, M. M., Jr., Brooks, H. L., Grossman, W., et al.: Diagnostic sensitivity of laboratory findings in acute pulmonary embolism. Ann. Intern. Med., *74*:161, 1971.
72. Hirsh, J.: Laboratory diagnosis of thrombosis. *In*: Colman, R. W., Hirsh, J., Marder, V. J., et al. (Eds.): Hemostasis and Thrombosis: Basic Principles and Clinical Practice. J. B. Lippincott Co., Philadelphia, 1982, p. 789.
73. Yudelman, I. M., Nossel, H. L., Kaplan, K. L., et al.: Plasma fibrinopeptide A levels in symptomatic venous thromboembolism. Blood, *51*:1189, 1978.
74. Wilson, J. E. III, Frenkel, E. P., Pierce, A. K., et al.: Spontaneous fibrinolysis in pulmonary embolism. J. Clin. Invest., *50*:474, 1971.
75. Rickman, F. D., Handin, R., Howe, J. P., et al.: Fibrin split products in acute pulmonary embolism. Ann. Intern. Med., *79*:664, 1973.
76. Bynum, L. J., Crotty, C., and Wilson, J. E. III: Use of fibrinogen/fibrin degradation products and soluble fibrin complexes for differentiating pulmonary embolism from nonthromboembolic lung disease. Am. Rev. Respir. Dis., *114*:285, 1976.
77. Bynum, L. J., Parkey, R. W., and Wilson, J. E. III: Tests of fibrin metabolism in recurrent venous thromboembolism. Arch. Intern. Med., *137*:1385, 1977.
78. Bynum, L. J., Crotty, C. M., and Wilson, J. E. III: Diagnostic value of tests of fibrin metabolism in patients predisposed to pulmonary embolism. Arch. Intern. Med., *139*:283, 1979.
79. Nossel, H. L., Yudelman, I., Canfield, R. E., et al.: Measurement of fibrinopeptide A in human blood. J. Clin. Invest., *54*:43, 1974.
80. Nossel, H. L., Ti, M., Kaplan, K. L., et al..: The

generation of fibrinopeptide A in clinical blood samples: Evidence for thrombin activity. J. Clin. Invest., *58*:1136, 1976.
81. Sipes, J. N., Suratt, P. M., Teates, C. D., et al.: A prospective study of plasma DNA in the diagnosis of pulmonary embolism. Am. Rev. Respir. Dis., *118*:475, 1978.
82. Barada, F. A., Jr., Suratt, P. M., Davis, J. S. IV, et al.: Free plasma DNA in patients with pulmonary embolism. South. Med. J., *73*:345, 1980.
83. Lippmann, M. L., Morgan, L., Fein, A., et al.: Plasma and serum concentrations of DNA in pulmonary thromboembolism. Am. Rev. Respir. Dis., *125*:416, 1982.
84. Goldhaber, S. Z., Hennekens, C. E., Markisz, J. A., et al.: Low sensitivity of plasma DNA in screening for pulmonary embolism. Am. Rev. Respir. Dis., *126*:360, 1982.
85. Dalen, J. E., Haffajee, C. I., Alpert, J. S., et al.: Pulmonary embolism, pulmonary hemorrhage and pulmonary infarction. New Engl. J. Med., *296*:1431, 1977.
86. Tsao, M.-S., Schraufnagel, D., and Wang, N.-S.: Pathogenesis of pulmonary infarction. Am. J. Med., *72*:599, 1982.
87. Goldhaber, S. Z., and Smith, T. W.: Blood tests. *In*: Cohn, P. F., and Wynne, J. (Eds.): Diagnostic Methods in Clinical Cardiology. Little, Brown and Co., Boston, 1982, p. 333.
88. Sleeper, J. C., Orgain, E. S., and McIntosh, H. D.: Primary pulmonary hypertension: Review of clinical features and pathologic physiology with a report of pulmonary hemodynamics derived from repeated catheterization. Circulation, *26*:1358, 1962.
89. Wagenvoort, C. A., and Wagenvoort, N.: Primary pulmonary hypertension: A pathologic study of lung vessels in 156 clinically diagnosed cases. Circulation, *42*:1163, 1970.
90. Walcott, G., Burchell, H. B., and Brown, A. L., Jr.: Primary pulmonary hypertension. Am. J. Med., *49*:70, 1970.
91. Case Records of the Massachusetts General Hospital: Case 8-1976. New Engl. J. Med., *294*:433, 1976.
92. Edwards, W. D., and Edwards, J. E.: Clinical primary pulmonary hypertension: Three pathologic types. Circulation, *56*:884, 1977.
93. Daoud, F. S., Reeves, J. T., and Kelly, D. B.: Isoproterenol as a potential pulmonary vasodilator in primary pulmonary hypertension. Am. J. Cardiol., *42*:817, 1978.
94. Camerini, F., Alberti, E., Klugmann, S., et al.: Primary pulmonary hypertension: Effects of nifedipine. Br. Heart J., *44*:352, 1980.
95. Fishman, A. P., and Pietra, G. G.: Primary pulmonary hypertension. Ann. Rev. Med., *31*:421, 1980.
96. Rubin, L. J., and Peter, R. H.: Oral hydralazine therapy for primary pulmonary hypertension. New Engl. J. Med., *302*:69, 1980.
97. Case Records of the Massachusetts General Hospital: Case 38-1981. New Engl. J. Med., *305*:685, 1981.
98. Sharma, G. V. R. K., and Sasahara, A. A.: Diagnosis of pulmonary embolism in patients with chronic obstructive pulmonary disease. J. Chron. Dis., *28*:253, 1975.
99. Fanta, C. H., Wright, T. C., and McFadden, E. R., Jr.: Differentiation of recurrent pulmonary emboli from chronic obstructive lung disease as a cause of cor pulmonale. Chest, *79*:92, 1981.
100. Walker, B. K., Ballas, S. K., and Burka, E. R.: The diagnosis of pulmonary thromboembolism in sickle cell disease. Am. J. Hematol., *7*:219, 1979.
101. Case Records of the Massachusetts General Hospital: Case 14-1983. New Engl. J. Med., *308*:823, 1983.
102. Sperling, D. C., Cheitlin, M., Sullivan, R. W., et al.: Pulmonary arteriovenous fistulas with pulmonary hypertension. Chest, *71*:753, 1977.
103. Case Records of the Massachusetts General Hospital: Case 43-1980. New Engl. J. Med., *303*:1049, 1980.
104. Hull, R., Hirsh, J., Sackett, D. L., et al.: Cost effectiveness of clinical diagnosis, venography, and noninvasive testing in patients with symptomatic deep-vein thrombosis. New Engl. J. Med., *304*:1561, 1981.
105. Bettmann, M. A.: Leg phlebography. Postgrad. Radiol., *1*:127, 1981.
106. Hirsh, J., and Gallus, A. S.: I-125–labeled fibrinogen scanning. Use in the diagnosis of venous thrombosis. JAMA, *233*:970, 1975.
107. Harris, W. H., Salzman, E. W., Athanasoulis, C., et al.: Comparison of I-125–fibrinogen count scanning with phlebography for detection of venous thrombi after elective hip surgery. New Engl. J. Med., *299*:665, 1975.
108. Harris, W., Athanasoulis, C., Waltman, A. C., et al.: Cuff-impedance phlebography and I-125–fibrinogen scanning versus roentgenographic phlebography for diagnosis of thrombophlebitis following hip surgery. A preliminary report. J. Bone Joint Surg., *58A*:939, 1976.
109. Young, A. E., Henderson, B. A., Phillips, D. A., et al.: Impedance plethysmography: Its limitations as a substitute for phlebography. Cardiovasc. Radiol. *1*:233, 1978.
110. Wheeler, H. B.: A modern approach to diagnosing deep venous thrombosis. J. Cardiovasc. Med., *5*:217, 1980.
111. Sasahara, A. A., Sharma, G. V. R. K., and Parisi, A. F.: New developments in the detection and prevention of venous thromboembolism. Am. J. Cardiol., *43*:1214, 1979.
112. Hull, R., Hirsh, J., Sackett, D. L., et al.: Combined use of leg scanning and impedance plethysmography in suspected venous thrombosis. An alternative to venography. New Engl. J. Med., *296*:1497, 1977.
113. Hull, R., Hirsh, J., Sackett, D. L., et al.: Replacement of venography in suspected venous thrombosis by impedance plethysmography and I-125–fibrinogen leg scanning. Ann. Intern. Med., *94*:12, 1981.
114. Hull, R. D., Carter, C. J., Jay, R. M., et al.: The diagnosis of acute, recurrent, deep-vein thrombosis: A diagnostic challenge. Circulation, *67*:901, 1983.
115. Hull, R., Hirsh, J., Sackett, D. L., et al.: Clinical validity of a negative venogram in patients with clinically suspected venous thrombosis. Circulation, *64*:622, 1981.
116. Lofgren, K. A.: Varicose veins. Their symptoms, complications, and management. Postgrad. Med., *65*:131, 1979.

117. Hafner, C. D., Cranley, J. J., Krause, R. J., et al.: A method of managing superficial thrombophlebitis. Surgery, *55*:201, 1964.
118. Muller, M., and Rosenberg, H.: Thrombosis of varicose veins in lower extremities: Experiences with 334 patients. Rev. Med. Chile, *104*:718, 1976.
119. Husni, E. A., and Williams, W. A.: Superficial thrombophlebitis of lower limbs. Surgery, *91*:70, 1982.
120. Pitney, W. R.: Venous and Arterial Thrombosis: Evaluation, Prevention and Management. Churchill Livingstone, Edinburgh, 1981, p. 123.
121. Hirsh, J., and Hull, R.: Natural history and clinical features of venous thrombosis. *In* Colman, R. W., Hirsh, J., Marder, V. J., et al. (Eds.): Hemostasis and Thrombosis: Basic Principles and Clinical Practice. J. B. Lippincott Co., Philadelphia, 1982, p. 831.
122. Stahl, R. L., Javid, J. P., and Lackner, H.: Unrecognized pulmonary embolism presenting as disseminated intravascular coagulation. Am. J. Med., *76*:772, 1984.
123. Pietro, D. A., LaBresh, K. A., Shulman, R. M., et al: Sustained improvement in primary pulmonary hypertension during six years of treatment with sublingual isoproterenol. New Engl. J. Med., *310*:1032, 1984.

CHAPTER 6

# CLINICAL PHARMACOLOGY

RICHARD B. STEAD, M.D.

The agents considered here are those that have some clinical utility in the management of thromboembolic disease. They range from the relatively innocuous antiplatelet agents to extremely potent inhibitors of coagulation and stimulators of fibrinolysis that have narrow therapeutic/toxic ratios. Each of these agents affects a specific mechanism of the hemostatic system; interference with more than one arm of the hemostatic system, either intentionally or inadvertently, may cause a potentially serious bleeding diathesis.

## HEPARIN

Heparin has been the drug of choice in the prevention and management of thromboembolic disease because of its immediate, potent, multifocal inhibition of several steps of the coagulation cascade vis-à-vis its interaction with antithrombin[1–4] (Fig. 6–1).

Heparin is a sulfated, acidic mucopolysaccharide, composed of alternating hexosamines and hexuronic acids, attached to a protein backbone (Fig. 6–2). The hexuronic acid residues as well as side chains of the sugar moiety may vary, giving a wide variety of structural sequences. A unique tetrasaccharide sequence appears to interact with antithrombin. Rosenberg[5] has recently reviewed heparin biosynthesis and structure-function relationships.

### Mechanism of Action

Heparin exerts its anticoagulant action by binding to antithrombin; the anticoagulant effect of a given heparin sequence is proportional to its antithrombin affinity.[6] The anticoagulant activity (and direct effects on platelets) may vary according to the source of the heparin. Commercially available heparin is a heterogeneous mixture of molecules ranging in molecular weight from 4000 to 40,000 with varying antithrombin affinity. Less than one-third of the heparin in commercial preparations actually has significant anticoagulant activity; the other two thirds, with low antithrombin affinity, has little anticoagulant activity.[7] Thus, only a small portion of heparin, containing a short, highly active sequence, appears to account for the major anticoagulant effects.

Heparin acts to catalyze the interaction of antithrombin III, the heparin cofactor, with the activated coagulation factors (serine proteases), including XIIa, XIa, IXa, Xa, and thrombin (IIa) (see Fig. 6–1). The heparin:antithrombin III complex is an immediate, potent inhibitor of all of these activated clotting factors.[6] Heparin increases the rate of neutralization of thrombin by antithrombin III approximately 1000-fold in an in vitro system. As can be seen in Figure 6–3, antithrombin III alone slowly neutralizes thrombin over the course of 20 minutes; the addition of heparin dramatically accelerates this reaction, completely neutralizing thrombin in a matter of seconds. Figure 6–4 shows a schematic diagram of the mechanism of action of the heparin:antithrombin III system in neutralizing thrombin. Heparin is shown to greatly increase the affinity of antithrombin III for thrombin by binding to a remote site on antithrombin III (Fig. 6–4*A* and *B*). The enzymatic active center of thrombin containing a negatively charged serine residue is specifically bound by positively charged

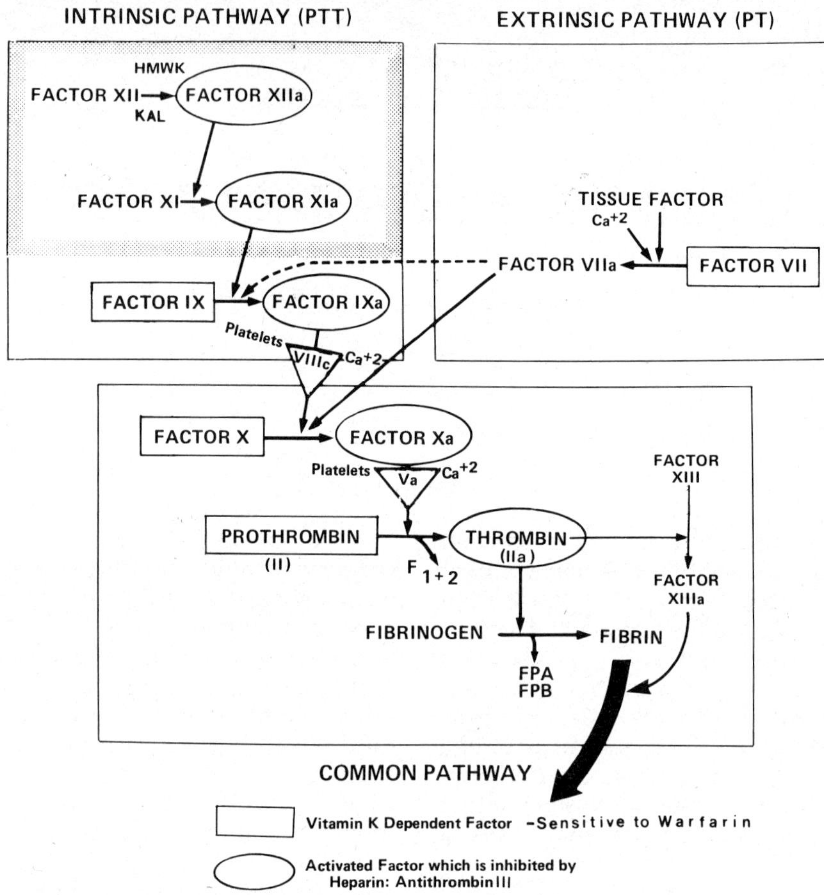


***Figure 6–1.*** Coagulation pathways: actions of warfarin and heparin. Vitamin K–dependent factors (in boxes) are affected by warfarin; activated serine proteases (in ovals) are neutralized by heparin:antithrombin. The partial thromboplastin time (PTT) measures the overall function of the intrinsic and common pathways and is primarily sensitive to heparin. The prothrombin time (PT) measures the overall function of the extrinsic and common pathways and is primarily sensitive to warfarin.

arginine on antithrombin (Fig. 6–4C), forming a stable thrombin:antithrombin (T:AT) complex. Heparin is released from the complex to catalyze further interactions of antithrombin with thrombin (or other proteases) (Fig. 6–4*D* and *E*).

The coagulation system serves as a biologic amplifier with small numbers of molecules of the early clotting factors generating a progressively larger number of molecules of the later clotting factors. Thus, it may require less heparin to prevent thrombosis by neutralizing small amounts of early factors in the cascade such as XIIa and XIa than it does to neutralize factors Xa and thrombin (IIa), which are present in much greater concentrations, once thrombosis has been initiated (see Fig. 6–1). Thus, small doses of subcutaneous

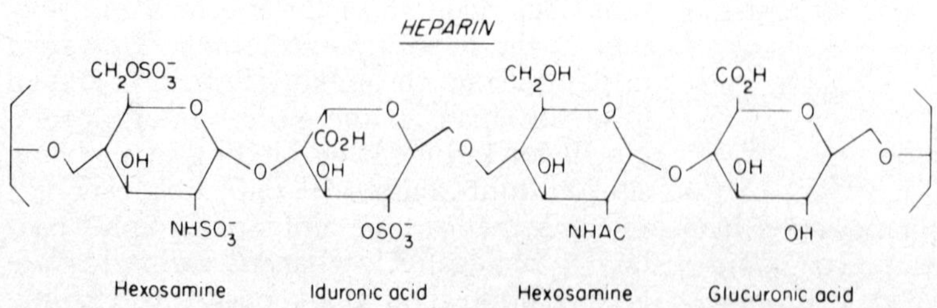


***Figure 6–2.*** One of the many possible arrangements of heparin's hexosamine and uronic acid residues. (From Rosenberg, R. D.: Heparin, antithrombin, and abnormal clotting. Ann. Rev. Med., *29*:367, 1978.)

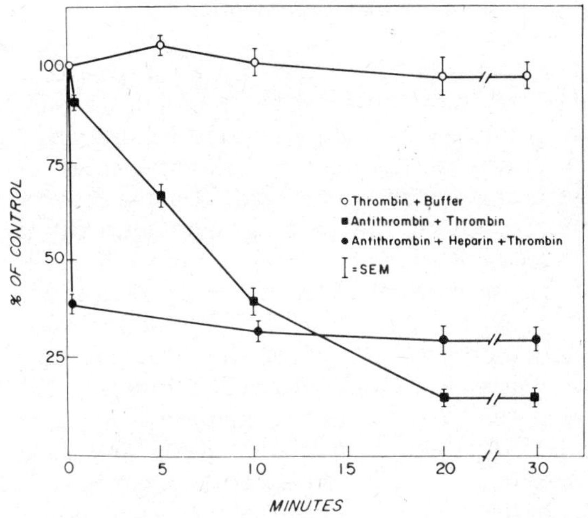


***Figure 6–3.*** Inhibition of thrombin by antithrombin-heparin cofactor in the presence and absence of heparin. Antithrombin neutralizes thrombin slowly (squares). The addition of heparin increases the rate of neutralization over 1000-fold (solid circles). (From Rosenberg, R. D.: Heparin, antithrombin, and abnormal clotting. Ann. Rev. Med., *29*:367, 1978.)

heparin may be effective prophylactically, whereas they would not be effective in the treatment of overt thrombosis. A similar mechanism may be important physiologically, because it has been recently shown that heparin-like material exists on endothelial cells and can interact with antithrombin (see Fig. 9–3).

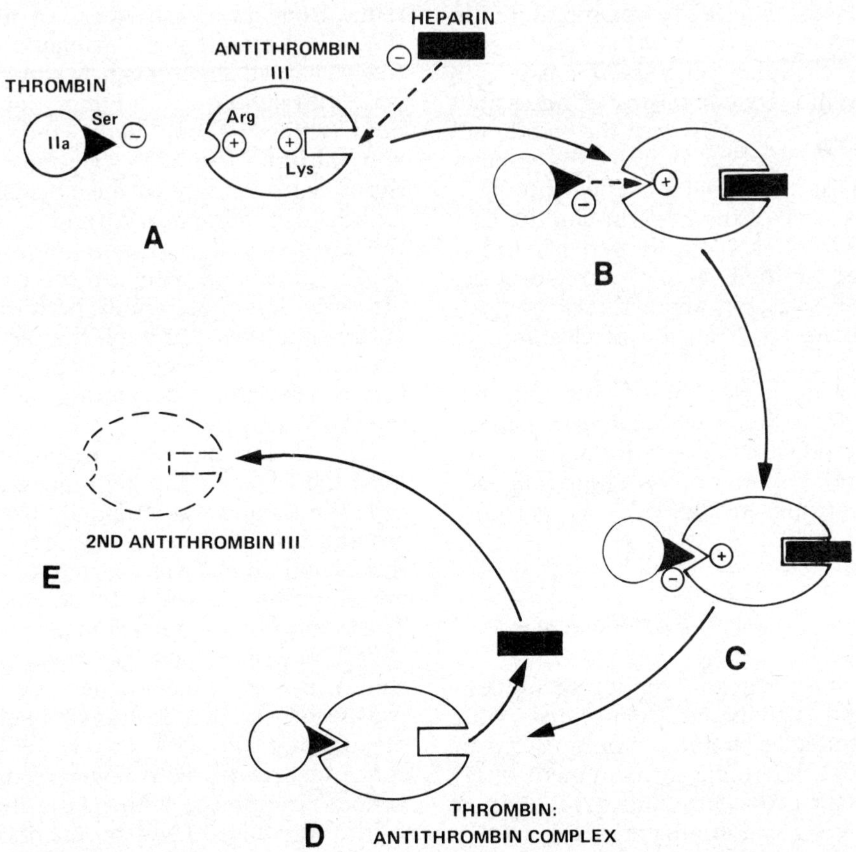


***Figure 6–4.*** Mechanism of action of heparin. Heparin interacts with antithrombin III, which catalyzes the formation of thrombin:antithrombin complexes. Heparin and antithrombin also inactivate factors XIIa, XIa, and Xa by a similar mechanism. (See text for details.)

### Pharmacokinetics

Heparin is not absorbed by the gastrointestinal tract and must be given parenterally by intravenous bolus, continuous infusion, or subcutaneous injection. Intramuscular injection is not recommended, because absorption is erratic and is associated with intramuscular hematomas. The half-life of heparin is highly variable, fitting neither zero order nor first order kinetics.[2, 8, 9] With higher intravenous doses of heparin, the apparent half-life increases, ranging from 56 minutes to 152 minutes.[9] At low doses, heparin levels rise very slowly, but at higher doses, the dose response curve is very steep and can lead to extremely high heparin levels. Thus, when high doses are administered by intravenous bolus, not only is the coagulation system essentially paralyzed, but the duration of action is more prolonged, in proportion to the dose. This may account for evidence that major bleeding complications were more frequent when heparin was administered in large doses by intermittent injection than by continuous infusion, even though the partial thromboplastin time (PTT) was monitored in both groups.[10]

Heparin clearance may be increased in massive pulmonary embolism,[11, 12] necessitating higher doses early in the treatment course. This may be due to the greater amount of thrombin that must be neutralized or to the release of the heparin-binding protein platelet factor 4.[13] Although heparin is metabolized by the liver and excreted in the urine, little is known about the exact clearance mechanisms. The rate of clearance of heparin appears to be unchanged in renal failure and decreased in hepatic failure.[11] However, in patients with renal or hepatic failure, the effects on clearance are not predictable and heparin doses should be adjusted according to the PTT, as in other patients.

### Monitoring and Dose Adjustment

Current methods for monitoring heparin therapy and activity are suboptimal. Four general strategies for monitoring heparin therapy exist, including measurement of (1) plasma heparin concentrations, (2) inhibition of specific coagulation enzymes, e.g., Xa or thrombin (IIa), (3) inhibition of overall coagulation activity, e.g., activated partial thromboplastin time (aPTT, also termed PTT), and (4) thrombin generation or activity.

All four strategies suffer from limitations. Plasma heparin concentrations can be measured by assays utilizing chromogenic substrates, but because of the heterogeneity of anticoagulant activity among heparin preparations, heparin concentrations often do not correlate with the anticoagulant effects. Such assays are not clinically useful. The inhibition of specific coagulation reactions by heparin can be measured, e.g., Xa inhibition or the thrombin time. Each of these assays measures a specific reaction in the coagulation cascade but is more technically demanding than other assays. Furthermore, it is not clear that they correlate with the clinical outcome any better than simpler tests that measure the overall in vitro effects of heparin on the coagulation system. The latter tests include the activated whole blood clotting time (WBCT), the whole blood recalcification time, the Lee-White clotting time, and the activated partial thromboplastin time.

Of these, none is more widely used or advantageous than the aPTT. It derives its name from its measurement of the clotting time of plasma that is "activated" by negatively charged agents such as kaolin or ellagic acid with subsequent additions of phospholipid (without tissue factor, thus "partial") and calcium. The aPTT therefore measures the in vitro activity of the intrinsic cascade and the common pathway and is sensitive to the effects of the heparin-antithrombin III system at several points in the cascade (see Fig. 6–1). It can be rapidly performed on an automated basis, although the precise measurement may vary significantly from laboratory to laboratory, depending on the equipment and reagents used.

The therapeutic recommendation[1, 6] to keep the PTT at 1½ to 2½ times the baseline or control value was originally based on the amount of heparin needed to prevent clotting in isolated animal vein segments in vitro as measured by the whole blood clotting time. These and other animal studies[15, 16] using the WBCT and PTT have been extrapolated to clinical use in humans using the PTT. Two prospective studies in humans suggest that maintaining the PTT at 1½ to 2½ times control correlates with fewer recurrences of venous thrombosis both in the initial treatment, with high doses by continuous infusion,[17] and in the long-term treatment with intermittent doses of subcutaneous heparin.[18]

Others suggest that the PTT may serve better as an indicator of potential heparin toxicity (when the PTT is greater than 2½ to 3 times control) than as a biologic measure of efficacy.[4]

In the future, newly developed assays that measure thrombin generation or activity may prove useful in monitoring heparin therapy. For example, fibrinopeptide A (FPA) is a peptide fragment released when thrombin cleaves fibrinogen to form fibrin (see Fig. 3–8). Yudelman[19] has shown a prompt drop in concentrations of FPA immediately upon initiation of heparin therapy in those patients responding to heparin, indicating that fibrin formation has ceased. Tests that reflect thrombin generation (or Xa activity) such as assays for the activation fragment of prothrombin ($F_{1+2}$) and the thrombin:antithrombin (T:AT) complex will also be evaluated for their role in assessing anticoagulant therapy.

The required duration of therapy has not been adequately studied, but the common clinical practice is for 7 to 10 days of intravenous heparin. Recently, Teitel and Rosenberg[20] have described a possible physiologic basis for this clinical maxim. Activated platelets retain Xa activity on their surface, which is apparently protected from inactivation by heparin and antithrombin. Thus, therapy may have to be continued until this platelet:Xa complex is cleared or inactivated and is no longer a potential source of ongoing thrombin generation.

## Heparin Preparations

As noted earlier, commercially available heparin preparations are heterogeneous; anticoagulant activity may vary from lot to lot. Furthermore, heparin is available from different animal sources and as either a sodium or calcium salt.

Although there is no evidence to suggest that there is a difference in the anticoagulant activity between bovine lung and porcine intestinal mucosal heparin, there is evidence[21, 22] that the use of beef lung heparin is associated with substantially higher risk of heparin-associated thrombocytopenia and thrombosis.

Some investigators have reported that calcium heparin is absorbed more slowly than sodium heparin when administered subcutaneously and that calcium heparin is associated with slightly fewer and milder bleeding complications. However, at this time, it does not appear that calcium heparin is superior to sodium heparin.[23]

Finally, new, more highly purified heparin preparations are now becoming available. As noted previously, heparin anticoagulant activity is proportional to antithrombin affinity. This forms the basis for fractionating or purifying heparin by its ability to bind antithrombin to make heparin preparations with greater purity and anticoagulant activity. There is evidence that low molecular weight, high antithrombin–affinity heparin has a less pronounced effect on platelet aggregation than do other fractions of heparin.[24] Clinical trials are in progress to determine whether the use of these new heparin fractions will translate into a better therapeutic index with a lower incidence of heparin-associated thrombocytopenia and thrombosis.

## Toxicity

The most obvious and important toxic effect of heparin is hemorrhage. In fact, heparin therapy is a leading cause of drug-related deaths in medical inpatients.[25]

The risk of bleeding with prophylactic subcutaneous heparin is quite low.[26] At least four double-blind randomized prospective trials have failed to show an excess of bleeding complications in patients receiving prophylactic heparin who underwent general surgery or lower limb orthopedic procedures.[27–29, 112] There are, however, other nonblinded studies that suggest an increase in transfusion requirements and a greater drop in the postoperative hematocrit.[30, 31] Overall, prophylactic low dose heparin is not associated with an increase of major hemorrhage.

In contrast, the risk of major bleeding with full therapeutic doses of heparin for the treatment of thromboembolic disease has been reported to range from 1 per cent to 33 per cent,[26] although most studies have found a frequency between 5 per cent and 10 per cent.[10, 26, 32, 33] Variables that correlate with the risk of bleeding in patients treated with full doses of heparin are summarized in Table 6–1.

There have been no optimally designed studies to test the relationship of bleeding to dose adjustment using different monitoring assays. One study[34] found a lower incidence of bleeding when 40,000 compared with

***Table 6–1.*** Factors Associated with an Increased Risk of Bleeding During Heparin Therapy[26, 33]

1. Dose of heparin
2. Anticoagulant response to a given dose of heparin (indicated by the PTT > 3× control)
3. Method of administration—intermittent vs. continuous; subcutaneous vs. intravenous
4. Specific patient risk factors
   a. Other coagulopathy, including thrombocytopenia, vitamin K deficiency
   b. Age
   c. Underlying disease—recent surgery, trauma, history of gastrointestinal bleeding, severe hypertension, malignancy, alcoholism, uremia
   d. Drugs—aspirin, nonsteroidal anti-inflammatory drugs, streptokinase

60,000 units of heparin were administered over 24 hours by intermittent intravenous infusion. Several other studies have found that the risk of major bleeding significantly increases when the PTT (or WBCT or Lee-White clotting time) was prolonged to greater than 2½ to 3 times the control value. The risk increased the longer the PTT remained above the therapeutic range.[26]

At least five[10, 35–38] controlled randomized studies have compared continuous infusion with intermittent injection. Four of the five studies have shown that continuous infusion is associated with a lower frequency of bleeding than intermittent injection. Although these studies are not absolutely conclusive because the total daily dose of heparin was higher in the group treated with the intermittent injection, we recommend administration by continuous infusion.[26]

Other features that may predispose to clinical bleeding are an associated coagulopathy such as thrombocytopenia (idiopathic or drug-related) or the concurrent use of other hemostatically active drugs such as streptokinase, aspirin,[33] or nonsteroidal anti-inflammatory agents. Advanced age and underlying disease, including alcoholism, may also be risk factors.[33] In addition to avoidance of other drugs that affect the hemostatic system, several other precautions should be taken.[26] Invasive procedures such as lumbar puncture or pericardiocentesis should be performed only if absolutely necessary and at least two to three hours after cessation of heparin therapy.[1] Platelet counts and prothrombin time should be performed at least every other day to detect a coagulopathy such as heparin-associated thrombocytopenia or vitamin K deficiency.

The therapeutic approach to the heparinized patient who is bleeding will depend on the severity of bleeding and the extent to which the PTT is elevated above the therapeutic range. For most cases of moderate bleeding, cessation of heparin therapy will suffice; the PTT will usually return to normal within two to three hours. Resumption of heparin at a lower dose or alternate means of therapy will depend on consideration of the severity of the bleeding, the risk of recurrent thromboembolism, and the extent to which bleeding may have resulted from excessive anticoagulation, i.e., a PTT greater than three times the baseline value. In the event of life-threatening or intracranial hemorrhage, protamine sulfate should be administered at the same time that heparin is discontinued. Protamine is a strongly basic protein that will immediately reverse the anticoagulant activity of heparin by forming a stable complex with the acidic heparin. For life-threatening hemorrhage, the usual dose is approximately 1 mg per 100 units of heparin, administered slowly (less than 50 mg over 10 minutes).[39] It should be noted that protamine sulfate is not necessarily innocuous; it can cause allergic reactions that vary from mild to life-threatening.

Heparin has been advocated over warfarin in pregnancy. Heparin does not cross the placenta nor is it found in human milk.[8] Although there are no teratogenic or hemorrhagic effects on the newborn, there is a higher incidence of prematurity and stillbirths in pregnant women treated with heparin, such that a "normal" outcome of pregnancy occurs only two-thirds of the time. Although the overall fetal mortality is approximately 20 per cent in both groups, warfarin is associated with a tenfold higher in-

***Table 6–2.*** Fetal and Neonatal Outcome After Anticoagulant Use During Pregnancy

| | Per Cent of Pregnancies | |
|---|---|---|
| | *Warfarin* | *Heparin* |
| Mortality | | |
| Spontaneous abortions | 8.6 | 1.5 |
| Stillbirths | 7.7 | 12.6 |
| Subsequent infant death | 2.4 | 7.4 |
| TOTAL | 18.7 | 21.5 |
| Complications | | |
| Premature, otherwise normal | 1.9 | 14.1 |
| Congenital anomalies | 10.4 | 0.7 |

From Hall, J. G., Pauli, R. M., and Wilson, K. M.: Maternal and fetal sequelae of anticoagulation during pregnancy. Am. J. Med., *68*:122, 1980.

***Table 6–3.*** Other Toxic Effects of Heparin Therapy

| Side Effect | Dose | Onset | Risk Factor |
|---|---|---|---|
| Heparin-associated thrombocytopenia-thrombosis (HAT) | Low or high IV or SQ | 5–7 days | Previous history of HAT<br>Use of beef lung heparin |
| Osteopenia/pathologic bone fractures | High dose 15–30,000 IU/day IV or SQ | 4–6 mo. | Preexisting osteopenia |
| Hypoaldosteronism | 5,000–10,000 IU/day IV or SQ | 4–8 days | Mineralocorticoid deficiency<br>Diabetes<br>Renal disease(?) |

crease of congenital anomalies (Table 6–2).[14] For this reason, heparin is the anticoagulant of choice in pregnancy.

In addition to predictable side effects of bleeding, three other less common toxic effects should be noted. These are summarized in Table 6–3.

## THROMBOCYTOPENIA

Heparin-associated thrombocytopenia appears in some cases to be an immune-related process that occurs more frequently with beef lung heparin than with pork gut heparin[21] and that may be associated with clinically significant, even life-threatening, thrombosis.[21, 22, 26, 118] It is believed that the pathogenesis of both the thrombocytopenia and thrombosis involves in vivo heparin-induced platelet aggregation. This apparent paradox results because the systemic platelet aggregation not only lowers the platelet count and predisposes to bleeding but may also trigger coagulation reactions and initiate thrombosis. The sera of these patients contain a factor that induces in vitro aggregation of normal platelets only in the presence of heparin (Fig. 6–5). Multiple studies have indicated that this factor is an antibody[43–47] (usually IgG), involves complement fixation,[43] and is probably directed at heparin itself [42] rather than a protein contaminant.

The thrombotic events are often of distinctly unusual character[40] and clearly not related to the initial thrombotic event for which the heparin was initiated. For instance, thrombosis involving skin[40] or major arteries,[41] including the femoral or radial arteries, may develop. Heparin may be associated with an increased frequency of pulmonary emboli following coronary artery bypass surgery, an otherwise rare event.[42] The syndrome usually occurs five to seven days after the initiation of therapy but may occur more rapidly if the patient has been treated with heparin previously. The potential for bleeding or thrombosis is heightened by the continuation of heparin or by rechallenge at a later time.

It is important that the diagnosis of heparin-dependent platelet aggregation be confirmed with in vitro tests (see Fig. 6–5); the diagnosis has profound therapeutic implications for the immediate discontinuation of heparin and its avoidance in the future. It is not known whether switching to different preparations, particularly purified heparin fractions, will reduce the risk of further heparin therapy. The treatment is to stop the heparin[26] and to use alternative modes of therapy. Protamine has no role in reversing this indirect effect of heparin. More commonly, mild thrombocytopenia may develop with heparin therapy; this may be a direct, nonimmune-mediated effect of heparin and

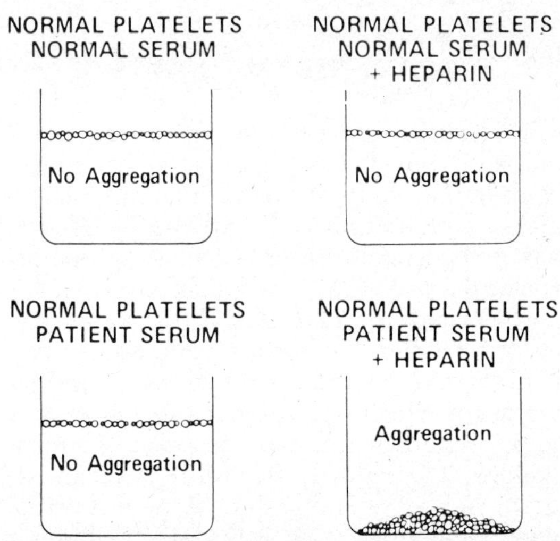


***Figure 6–5.*** Schematic drawing showing how platelet antibodies (in patient's serum) plus heparin can cause aggregation of platelets (thrombosis and/or hemorrhage). This is the basis of the in vitro diagnostic test for heparin-dependent platelet aggregation. (From Rice, L., and Jackson, D.: Can heparin cause clotting? Heart and Lung, *10*:331, 1981.)

is not associated with serious clinical consequences. Whether the mild and severe forms are related is not known.

#### OSTEOPENIA

Heparin has also been associated with osteopenia and pathologic bone fractures in a number of patients undergoing prolonged heparin therapy at relatively high doses. In one series it was found that 6 of 10 patients receiving 15,000 to 30,000 units of heparin for six months or longer developed spontaneous bone fractures.[48] The use of prolonged therapy with adjusted-dose subcutaneous heparin instead of warfarin has recently been advocated;[18] however, potential complications of long-term heparin administration should be considered and evaluated in future trials. The use of baseline skeletal surveys or of vitamin D and calcium to prevent osteopenia remains to be assessed.

#### HYPOALDOSTERONISM

Heparin predictably depresses aldosterone by an unknown mechanism within four to eight days of initiation of therapy.[49] In patients with a normally functioning renin-angiotensin-aldosterone axis, this is probably of no clinical significance, although the serum sodium may drop slightly. However, it may cause clinically important hyperkalemia in certain patients such as those with diabetes[50] or renal failure.[51]

## ORAL ANTICOAGULANTS

Oral anticoagulants are derivatives of dicumarol, which was discovered serendipitously to be a potent anticoagulant in the late 1930s. Link and his colleagues at the University of Wisconsin traced a menacing hemorrhagic disease of cattle to spoiled sweet clover and isolated and identified dicumarol as the culprit.[52] Over the next several years they synthesized multiple congeners including warfarin, which had the most favorable biologic properties and had been used the most widely. It is named after the Wisconsin Alumni Research Foundation, where most of this pioneering work was done. Although the chemistry and mechanism of action of these drugs are well understood and they have been in use clinically for over 40 years, there is still considerable controversy regarding their optimal use. In the United States, warfarin sodium (Coumadin®) is the most widely prescribed oral anticoagulant. This discussion focuses on the clinical use of warfarin; the clinical pharmacology of other oral anticoagulants has been reviewed elsewhere.[8]

### Mechanism of Action

The oral anticoagulants are similar in structure to vitamin K and competitively inhibit a crucial enzyme in vitamin K metabolism,[53] vitamin K epoxide reductase (Fig. 6–6*A*). Factors II, VII, IX, and X as well as Protein C are synthesized in hepatocytes but must undergo a vitamin K–dependent addition of carboxyl groups onto glutamic acid (glu) residues before they become biologically active.[54] The gamma-carboxyglutamic acid (gla) residues so formed are important for the participation of these factors in coagulation reactions vis-à-vis calcium bridging (Fig. 6–6*B*). The principal effect of warfarin is to competitively inhibit the vitamin K epoxide reductase. This prevents the regeneration of the active vitamin $K_1H_2$ so that carboxylation of the vitamin K–dependent clotting factors is reduced. The unmodified clotting factors are released and circulate in the blood where they can be measured immunologically but are functionally inactive.[54] As can be seen from Figure 6–1, warfarin acts on vitamin K–dependent clotting factors and reduces the functional levels of key components of the extrinsic (factor VII), intrinsic (factor IX), and common pathways (factor X and prothrombin [II]).

### Pharmacokinetics

Warfarin is absorbed completely from the gastrointestinal tract within two to four hours and is over 90 per cent bound to albumin. Its half-life varies widely between 15 and 44 hours with a mean of approximately 35 hours.[55] This wide variation in metabolism may account for some of the variations in dosage requirements seen clinically. Because warfarin acts to prevent modification of newly synthesized clotting factors, its biologic effects are not apparent until the previously synthesized normal factors become depleted and new factors without the vitamin K–dependent modification have accumulated. This depletion takes place according to the biologic half-life (see Table 3–1) of the clotting factors (factor VII—four to six hours, factors IX and X—20 to 65 hours, and prothrombin [factor II]—over 100 hours). Thus, the initial prolongation of the PT into the "therapeutic range" principally reflects depletion of factor VII, but this has only minimal therapeutic impact,[55] because normal, functional prothrombin (factor II), IX, and X are still present in adequate amounts to generate thrombin. In practice, this means that when patients are initiating oral coagulation there should be an overlap of three to four days with the prothrombin time (PT)[54, 55] in the therapeutic range before full-dose heparin is discontinued. The long half-life of the drug (approximately 35 hours) and the delayed action mean that the effects of a dose adjustment will not be reflected in the PT for approximately 36 to 48 hours.

The dosage of warfarin required to prolong the PT into the therapeutic range is extremely variable,[55] ranging from 2 to 12 mg per day. In addition to the two different monitoring assays, many other factors influence the patient's response to warfarin. As noted previously, there is a threefold range of normal

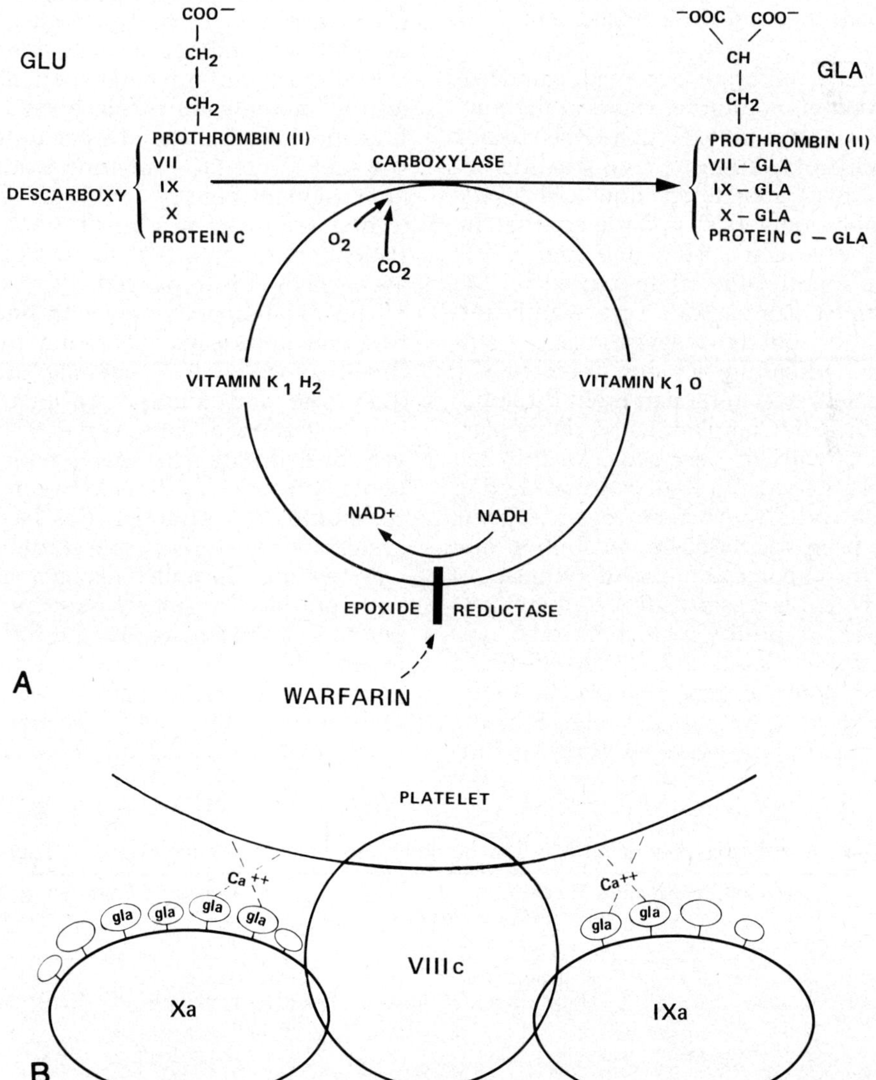


***Figure 6–6.*** *A,* The mechanism of action of warfarin: Warfarin inhibits an important step in vitamin K metabolism, decreasing vitamin $K_1H_2$–dependent carboxylation of factor II, VII, IX, X, and protein C. *B,* The gamma-carboxyglutamic acid (GLA) residues on the vitamin K–dependent factors are essential for participation of these factors in coagulation reactions. (GLU, glutamic acid).

for the rate of metabolism of warfarin. In addition, there are a large number of drug interactions[53] as well as disease states that alter the response to warfarin (see Table 6–4). Important drug interactions have been described that affect absorption, protein binding, metabolism, and excretion. Furthermore, as with heparin, any drug that interferes with the hemostatic system may increase the risk of bleeding.[54] *It should be emphasized that warfarin therapy must be individualized; the PT should be followed closely and the patient should be examined frequently for evidence of bleeding.*

### Monitoring and Dose Adjustment

There is no uniformly accepted, standardized method of monitoring warfarin therapy. This makes it difficult to compare the efficacy and toxicity of warfarin found in different studies. Most laboratories now utilize the prothrombin time (PT) and determine the ratio of the patient's PT to the control PT. Most importantly, the PT measured on the same plasma sample can vary significantly depending on the reagents used.[26, 54] In the United Kingdom, PT measurement has been standardized to human brain thromboplastin (British Comparative Thromboplastin—BCT), which is very sensitive to small changes in the vitamin K–dependent clotting factors. In North America, however, reagents have not been standardized; most often rabbit brain thromboplastin reagent (Simplastin) is used, which is less sensitive to the effects of warfarin. A prothrombin time ratio (patient:control) of 1.3 to 1.7, measured using the rabbit brain reagent (Simplastin time), corresponds to a ratio of 2.0 to 2.75 in the same plasma samples assayed using the British Comparative Thromboplastin (BCT) reagent.[26] Thus, the British reagent is more sensitive and would suggest that a patient is at the upper end of the therapeutic range (2 to 2½ times control), whereas the same patient monitored by the Simplastin reagent would be judged to be only marginally anticoagulated (approximately 1½ times control).

Recently, these two assays have been compared prospectively in a series of almost 100 patients with DVT.[111] Patients had their therapy monitored and adjusted to either the Simplastin time at 1½ to 2 times control (18 to 22 seconds) or the BCT-measured protime at 2 times control (26 to 30 seconds). There was no difference in the recurrence rate of DVT—about 2 per cent in each group. The Simplastin-monitored group, however, received more warfarin and experienced significantly more hemorrhagic events than the BCT-monitored group, 22 per cent versus 4 per cent. Thus, in comparing studies of oral anticoagulant efficacy and toxicity or in selecting a dose of warfarin for an individual patient, it is important to recognize which assay method is employed.

The initiation of therapy with small loading doses of approximately 10 mg per day for three to four days is generally agreed to be less toxic and more efficacious than the administration of large doses.[53–55] The conventional duration of therapy for most patients with DVT or PE is between three and six months.[53–55] Although this has not been systematically studied, one study of patients with venous thromboembolism not treated with oral anticoagulants sustained over 90 per cent of recurrences within the first three months, and the recurrence rate for both treated and untreated patients was negligible after four months.[57] Other patients at particularly high risk, such as those with docu-

***Table 6–4.*** Factors Associated with Changes in Prothrombin Time During Warfarin Therapy

| **Increased Prothrombin Time** | | **Decreased Prothrombin Time** | |
|---|---|---|---|
| *Drugs* | *Specific Patient Factors* | *Drugs* | *Specific Patient Factors* |
| Phenylbutazone | Hepatic disease | Barbiturates | Uremia |
| Sulfinpyrazone | Hypermetabolic states | Cholestyramine | Hereditary resistance |
| Clofibrate | | Rifampin | |
| Heparin | | Diuretics | |
| Acetylsalicylic acid | | | |
| Disulfiram | | | |
| Metronidazole | | | |
| Trimethoprim-sulfamethoxazole | | | |

From O'Reilly, R. A.: Vitamin K antagonists. *In* Colman, R. W., Hirsh, J., Marder, V. J., et al. (Eds.): Hemostasis and Thrombosis. J. B. Lippincott, Philadelphia, 1982, p. 955.

mented hypercoagulable disorders, may have to be treated with oral anticoagulants indefinitely (see Chapters 7 and 9).

### Toxicity

As with heparin, the major toxicity of warfarin is bleeding, an extension of its therapeutic effect. The overall frequency of hemorrhagic complications in many studies has ranged widely from 2.5 to 27 per cent.[26] Bleeding complications are proportional to the intensity of anticoagulation and are increased by the presence of risk factors such as underlying coagulopathy, severe hepatic or renal disease, alcoholism, drug interactions, trauma, malignancy, and known bleeding sites in the gastrointestinal tract.[26, 53–55] In two studies performed by Hull and coworkers,[56, 111] the frequency of all bleeding complications was approximately 20 per cent, but the frequency of major bleeding complications was less than 5 per cent. Furthermore, the overall frequency of bleeding was reduced to less than 5 per cent when oral anticoagulant therapy was adjusted based on the more sensitive BCT reagent test, resulting in less intense anticoagulation.[111]

Treatment of bleeding in patients on warfarin will depend on several factors:[26, 55] (1) the clinical severity of bleeding, including the rate of hemorrhage and the location (e.g., intracranial versus superficial skin); (2) the extent to which the PT is prolonged; (3) the expected duration of anticoagulation therapy; and (4) the initial indication for anticoagulation. Such factors will influence decisions regarding the use of vitamin K and the utility of diagnostic studies to search for an underlying bleeding lesion.

Major life-threatening bleeding requires immediate treatment with enough fresh frozen plasma (usually two units) to correct the PT to normal. The PT should be repeated 30 minutes after the completion of the infusion and periodically thereafter. Because the half-life of factor VII is only four to six hours, fresh frozen plasma (FFP) may have to be given every six to eight hours for several days if no other measures are taken, especially if the PT is prolonged to greater than 3 times control. If the risk of hemorrhage outweighs the need for long-term anticoagulation with warfarin, vitamin K may be administered parenterally. A dose of 10 mg subcutaneously or intramuscularly will usually reverse the effects of warfarin in six to 12 hours.[26] Administration of vitamin K at this dose or higher will make the patient relatively refractory to warfarin for variable periods of time, up to two weeks, making reinstitution of warfarin more difficult.[26, 55] There is no convincing evidence of a rebound hypercoagulable state following discontinuation of warfarin or the administration of vitamin K.[58, 59]

Minor bleeding with a prolonged PT may merely require interruption of warfarin therapy, with or without administration of fresh frozen plasma, until the PT has returned to the therapeutic range.

The decision of how extensively to evaluate the patient for an anatomic cause of bleeding will be influenced by the prolongation of the PT at the time of bleeding and by one's index of suspicion. Bleeding that occurs when the PT is within the therapeutic range should be evaluated as rigorously as in other patients;[55] a substantial number of patients have identifiable anatomic lesions, such as occult malignancies. The evaluation of patients with a PT above the therapeutic range is less productive. Such a prolongation of PT, unless otherwise explained, should raise the suspicion of a drug interaction or intercurrent illness.

Warfarin-induced skin necrosis is a rare but important complication that usually begins acutely within 10 days of the initiation of therapy and is more common in females. It is heralded by painful, discrete erythematous lesions on the lower extremities or trunk that rapidly progress to hemorrhagic bullae or infarction.[55] The pathogenesis is uncertain; warfarin should be discontinued. Recently, it has been suggested that this syndrome may be related to a reduction of Protein C.[116] This observation and its possible therapeutic implications deserve further study.

The use of warfarin during pregnancy is contraindicated.[14] During the first trimester of pregnancy, it has been associated with a specific "warfarin embryopathy" leading to skeletal anomalies including nasal hypoplasia. Even more alarming are multiple central nervous system abnormalities attributable to warfarin therapy in the second or third trimester. Because warfarin crosses the placenta, it also increases the risk of fetal intracranial hemorrhage at the time of delivery. Although heparin is associated with other complications (noted previously), it is the anticoagulant of choice during pregnancy (see Table 6–2).

## WARFARIN VS. SUBCUTANEOUS HEPARIN FOR DVT TREATMENT FOLLOWING INITIAL THERAPY WITH HEPARIN

Only a few studies have compared subcutaneous heparin and warfarin in the long-term treatment of DVT following initial heparin therapy. In comparing these studies, attention must be paid to the dose of heparin used and the methods used to monitor heparin or warfarin therapy. Initially, Hull and coworkers[56] found that at a fixed dose of 5000 units twice a day, subcutaneous heparin was not as effective as conventional warfarin therapy. Bynum and Wilson[60] found the same dose of heparin to be more efficacious and less toxic than warfarin, although the recurrence rates on both warfarin (38 per cent) and heparin (29 per cent) were unusually high. Hull[18] subsequently adjusted the dose of subcutaneous heparin to prolong the PTT to 1½ times control at six hours after an injection; the average dose was 10,000 units twice a day. In this study, the warfarin dose was adjusted to 1½ to 2 times the control value, according to the conventional North American Simplastin time assay. This prospective randomized study showed that dose-adjusted heparin administration was as effective as warfarin (4 per cent recurrence) but associated with a much lower rate of hemorrhage than warfarin (2 per cent versus 18 per cent). Further studies comparing these two regimens will be necessary to verify this.

Factors such as pregnancy, a history of warfarin-induced skin necrosis, or a hypercoagulable state induced by malignancy, which may be refractory to warfarin (see Chapter 9), may favor the use of subcutaneous heparin. On the other hand, a history of heparin-induced thrombocytopenia-thrombosis or concern over osteoporosis may favor the use of warfarin.

## FIBRINOLYTIC THERAPY

Fibrinolytic agents offer the promise of rapid and complete clot lysis, although the risk of bleeding is somewhat higher than with anticoagulant therapy.[26] At present, there are two fibrinolytic agents available for the treatment of established thrombosis:[62] streptokinase (SK) and urokinase (UK). In the future, availability of human tissue plasminogen activator (tPA),[63, 64] produced by recombinant DNA technology,[65] may overcome some of the disadvantages of currently available agents.

### Comparison of Fibrinolytic Agents

All of these agents are proteins with enzymatic activity that directly (UK, tPA) or indirectly (SK) activate endogenous plasminogen to form plasmin, *which actually lyses the clot* (Fig. 6–7). SK and UK cause generalized systemic activation of plasminogen circulating in whole blood.[62, 66, 67] Tissue plasminogen activator requires fibrin for the activation of plasminogen and should allow for better controlled, localized activation of fibrinolysis preferentially at the site of the actual clot, without depletion of fibrinogen. No systemic activation of plasminogen has been seen with the use of tPA in animal or human studies.[63, 64, 68, 69] UK and tPA are derived from human sources and, therefore, are nonantigenic compared with SK. The principal ad-

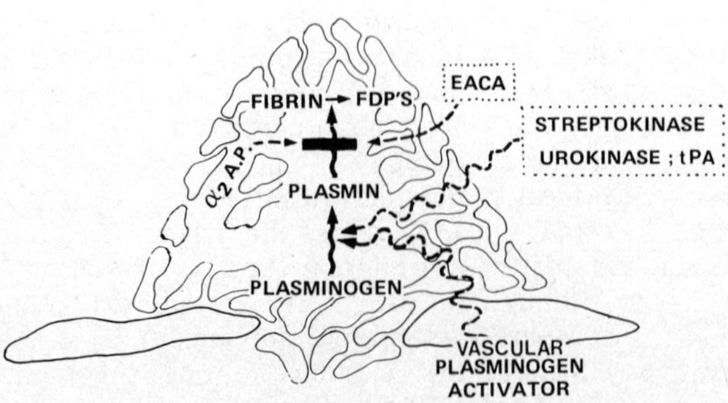


*Figure 6–7.* Mechanism of action of fibrinolytic agents. Urokinase and tissue plasminogen activator (tPA) directly activate plasminogen to form plasmin. Streptokinase activates plasminogen by an indirect mechanism. Plasmin enzymatically digests fibrin to smaller fibrin degradation products (FDPs). Epsilon-aminocaproic acid (EACA) can antagonize the action of fibrinolytic agents by inhibiting plasmin.

vantage of UK over SK is that approximately 5 per cent of the patients who have had recent streptococcal infection or SK therapy may develop allergic reactions or resistance to SK due to circulating antistreptococcal antibodies.[70] However, UK is currently 10 times more expensive than SK. tPA has theoretic advantages, noted previously, over both SK and UK, but the actual magnitude of these advantages and the cost of this agent remain to be determined. These three agents are compared in Table 6–5.

### Laboratory Monitoring

The onset of action of SK and UK is immediate and the duration of action is relatively short—several hours after therapy is discontinued. Almost all patients will rapidly develop a lytic state with the standard regimen, once naturally occurring and acquired inhibitors are overcome. Monitoring is directed at verifying that the "lytic state" has been achieved and sustained;[62, 119] there is no need to titrate the dose once the lytic state has been achieved.[71, 72] The lytic state can be verified by measuring a number of laboratory tests, including fibrin degradation products (FDPs) (also termed fibrin split products [FSPs]), thrombin time, whole blood euglobulin lysis time, PT, or PTT. The rationale and limitations of the available laboratory tests useful in monitoring the lytic state are listed in Table 6–6. The most sensitive, widely available test is the thrombin time, which reflects hypofibrinogenemia and elevated fibrin degradation products; however, this test is also extremely sensitive to heparin. Fibrin degradation products are also a sensitive and readily available indicator of the lytic state but may be elevated by the thromboembolic process itself or by other underlying diseases. The most specific test available is the whole blood euglobulin lysis time, but this is not generally available. The PT and PTT are useful, readily available indicators of the lytic state. In short, any *one* of these tests will suffice if the pretreatment value is normal

***Table 6–5.*** Comparison of Streptokinase, Urokinase, and Tissue Plasminogen Activator

| | SK | UK | tPA |
|---|---|---|---|
| ***Source*** | Streptococci bacteria | Human | Human |
| ***Purification Procedure*** | Cell culture | Fetal kidney-cell culture or urine extract | Recombinant DNA |
| ***Mechanism of Action*** | Plasminogen activation (indirect) | Plasminogen activation (direct) | Plasminogen activation (direct) in presence of fibrin |
| ***Clinical Changes*** | | | |
| Benefit | Rapid lysis of thrombi | Rapid lysis of thrombi | Rapid, specific lysis of thrombi |
| Side effects | | | |
| Biochemical | "Lytic state" | "Lytic state" | "Localized lytic state" |
| Time-related | Fever | Fever | ? |
| Dose-related | Nausea, headache, flushing, cramps, hypotension (rarely) | None | ? |
| Allergic | Pruritus, urticaria, anaphylaxis (rarely) | Pruritus (rarely) | ? (unlikely) |
| Complications | Bleeding | Bleeding | Bleeding (? less) |
| ***Cost (12-hour Infusion)*** | $150 | $1550 | ? |
| ***Advantages*** | Relatively low cost | Nonantigenic | Does not deplete fibrinogen; "localized" lytic state |
| ***Disadvantages*** | Antigenic, dose adjustment or change to UK with high titer anti-SK antibodies, generalized lytic state due to depletion of fibrinogen | Cost, generalized lytic state due to depletion of fibrinogen | Investigational agent with very limited availability |

*Table 6–6.* Laboratory Tests That Can Be Applied for Monitoring Fibrinolytic Therapy

| Test | Rationale | Disadvantage |
|---|---|---|
| Thrombin time | Sensitive screening for hypofibrinogenemia and circulating degradation products | Extremely sensitive to heparin |
| Plasma fibrinogen | Major plasma substrate of plasmin | Direct assay for clottable protein required |
| Fibrin(ogen) degradation products (FDPs); also termed fibrin split products (FSPs) | Specific for plasmin lysis of fibrinogen and/or fibrin | Pretreatment value may be abnormal |
| Lysis time (plasma or whole blood) | Direct measure of the lytic state | Specialized study that may not be readily available |
| PT, PTT | Will detect increased fibrin split products, hypofibrinogenemia; most widely available | Less sensitive and specific than thrombin time |

and a value obtained two to four hours after the initiation of fibrinolytic therapy is "abnormal." The *risk of bleeding does not correlate with any specific laboratory abnormality*[26] nor with the dose of the lytic agent,[26, 62] as long as contraindications to streptokinase and urokinase are heeded (Table 6–7).

## Dosage and Administration

The presently recommended loading dose of 250,000 units of streptokinase is sufficient to establish a lytic state in at least 90 per cent of the population.[62, 70, 71] If a lytic state is not established as judged by the assays previously noted, the loading dose may be empirically increased or adjusted by the in vitro SK resistance test.[67] Alternatively, UK may be used. Repeat administration of SK within six to 12 months will, in general, be limited by high antibody titers. In this situation, the use of UK is indicated. The current recommended regimens for the administration of SK and UK are given in Table 6–8.

*Table 6–7.* Contraindications to Streptokinase and Urokinase

I. Absolute contraindications
- A. Risk of CNS hemorrhage
  1. History of cerebrovascular accident
  2. Intracranial neoplasm
  3. Cranial surgery or head trauma within 10–14 days
- B. Risk of massive hemorrhage (Within 10 days)
  1. Major thoracic or abdominal surgery
  2. Cardiopulmonary resuscitation
  3. Biopsy in a location inaccessible to external compression
  4. Parturition

II. Relative contraindications
1. Coagulation defects (thrombocytopenia, coagulation factor deficiency)
2. Uncontrolled severe hypertension
3. Recent invasive procedures (lumbar puncture, thoracentesis, paracentesis, organ biopsy, or puncture of noncompressible blood vessel)
4. Other system diseases, including visceral carcinoma, endocarditis, and active tuberculosis

The duration of therapy depends on the agent used and the size of the clot. Generally, for PE, 12 hours of urokinase or 24 hours of streptokinase has been found to be optimal, whereas for DVT, the optimal duration is more variable—from 24 to 72 hours of streptokinase.[70] (Urokinase has not been approved for treatment of DVT.) The role of laboratory tests to monitor the adequacy of therapy remains to be determined. In the past, it has been recommended that heparin should not follow streptokinase or urokinase until the thrombin time or PTT has returned to less than twice the control value,[62] usually two to four hours following the cessation of fibrinolytic therapy. However, with renewed interest in intravenous streptokinase to treat acute myocardial infarction, some investigators, for example, Ganz,[113] have resumed heparin immediately after streptokinase administration. Ganz believes that the risk of delaying heparin therapy while awaiting the results of a laboratory assay outweighs the benefit of insuring that the PTT remains in the therapeutic range. In his patients, the rate of major bleeding complications has been 12 per cent.

## Contraindications and Toxicity

Contraindications to the use of streptokinase and urokinase include recent stroke, invasive procedures, surgery, or trauma (Table 6–7). Streptokinase and urokinase cannot

*Table 6–8.* Recommended Regimens for Administration of Streptokinase and Urokinase

| | Loading Dose | Hourly Dose | Duration | Indications |
|---|---|---|---|---|
| *Streptokinase* | 250,000 IU* over 30 min | 100,000 IU/hr** | PE: 24 hr<br>DVT: 48–72 hr | 1. Acute pulmonary embolism (within 7 days)<br>2. Deep vein thrombosis (within 7 days)<br>3. Arterial thrombosis†<br>4. Acute myocardial infarction††<br>5. Occlusion of vascular shunts and catheters† |
| *Urokinase* | 4400 IU/kg over 10 min | 4400 IU/kg/hr** | PE: 12 hr<br>DVT: not approved for use | 1. Acute pulmonary embolism (within 7 days)<br>2. Occlusion of vascular shunts and catheters† |

*If resistant, increase or change to UK.
**By continuous infusion pump.
†Lower doses, selective infusion.
††Intracoronary infusion at lower doses was approved by the FDA in 1982. Intravenous administration has not yet been approved by the FDA for acute myocardial infarction.

discriminately lyse pathologic clot while sparing thrombi required for normal hemostasis. Furthermore, replacement of the fibrin plug and healing generally requires at least seven to 10 days. Because the lysis of any hemostatic plug may lead to significant hemorrhage, all invasive procedures, including arterial punctures and venous cut-downs, should be minimized before or during lytic therapy. Arterial blood gases, if necessary, should be obtained from the radial artery with a 22-gauge needle followed by 20 minutes of manual compression.

Hemorrhage is obviously the major risk of fibrinolytic therapy. The risks of bleeding are not precisely known but are probably somewhat greater than conventional anticoagulant therapy.[26, 114] The overall frequency of bleeding in the urokinase trial was particularly high for both UK- (45 per cent) and heparin-treated (27 per cent) patients, largely as a result of invasive diagnostic procedures required by the study protocol.[32, 62, 70] Of the patients with bleeding complications, less than 10 per cent on UK and 4 per cent on heparin had bleeding of sufficient magnitude to require cessation of therapy or transfusion. In other studies, patients treated with SK had an overall frequency of bleeding between 10 and 20 per cent, with serious bleeding between 1 and 4 per cent.[26, 62] The risk of major hemorrhage can be reduced by careful patient selection and by minimizing invasive procedures.[62, 73]

The treatment of bleeding in patients undergoing fibrinolytic therapy depends on the location and magnitude of the bleeding. Bleeding from superficial sites such as cut-downs or arterial punctures may be controlled by local tamponade; rarely will the topical application of epsilon-aminocaproic acid (EACA) be necessary. Severe or life-threatening hemorrhage requires immediate discontinuation of the fibrinolytic agents; the lytic state will be promptly reversed, because the half-life of these agents is quite short. Replacement with fresh frozen plasma or whole blood will reverse the depletion of fibrinogen, factor V, and factor VIII that accompanies fibrinolytic therapy with SK or UK. In life-threatening circumstances, intravenous infusion of EACA may be used to reverse the lytic state immediately. One recommended regimen is a 5-gr loading dose administered over 30 minutes and followed by 1 gr per hour until hemostasis is achieved.[26]

A common but minor complication of SK is the acute febrile and vasomotor reaction that can occur after administration of the loading dose. This can usually be prevented by the intravenous administration of 100 mg of hydrocortisone immediately before therapy.[62]

## PLATELET-ACTIVE DRUGS

Antiplatelet agents may act by preventing platelet adhesion, aggregation, or release or by other less well-defined mechanisms. Most of the available agents, including aspirin, nonsteroidal anti-inflammatory drugs, and sulfinpyrazone, act by inhibiting cyclooxygenase.[74, 75] Dipyridamole, as well as other, newer agents, acts via different mechanisms

***Table 6–9.*** Pharmacology of Antiplatelet Agents

| | Aspirin | Sulfinpyrazone | Dipyridamole | Ticlopidine | $PGI_2$ |
|---|---|---|---|---|---|
| ***Mode of Action*** | Irreversible acetylation of cyclooxygenase | Competitive (reversible) inhibition of cyclooxygenase | Inhibitor of phosphodiesterase | ?Alters platelet membrane binding sites | Stimulates adenyl cyclase |
| ***Platelet Aggregation*** | Blocks except with thrombin | Inhibits dilute collagen | Weak Effect | Blocks | Blocks |
| ***Platelet Adhesion*** | No effect | No effect | Decreases | ? | Blocks |
| ***Platelet Survival*** | No effect | Improves | Improves | ? | Improves |
| ***Bleeding Time*** | Prolongs | No effect | No effect | Prolongs | Prolongs |
| ***Duration of Action*** | Days | Hours | Hours | ? | < 5 min. |
| ***Side Effects*** | Gastrointestinal bleeding and discomfort* | Minimal | Minimal | ? | Hypotension, headache |
| ***Dose*** | 150–325 mg PO once weekly to QID | 200 mg PO QID | 25–75 mg PO TID | 250 mg PO QID | 1–6 mg/kg/min IV (as limited by hypotension) |

*Minimal with low doses of buffered or enteric coated preparations.
Adapted from Thompson, A. R., and Harker, L. A.: Manual of Thrombosis and Hemostasis. F. A. Davis, Philadelphia, 1983.
TID = three times daily; QID = four times daily; IV = intravenously

(Table 6–9). Virtually all of the agents are available in oral form and are relatively safe. They have mild to moderate activity in certain clinical and laboratory models of thrombosis, most often when they are used prophylactically. Their role seems to be limited primarily to the prevention of microthrombi or embolism arising in the *arterial* circulation or from artificial surfaces.[74, 117]

*Aspirin* is an irreversible inhibitor of the enzyme cyclooxygenase, blocking platelet production of thromboxane $A_2$[76, 77] (Fig. 6–8), the potent platelet aggregrating agent and vasoconstrictor. (In larger doses, it also inhibits endothelial production of prostacyclin, a powerful vasodilator with antiaggregatory effects[78, 79] [see Fig. 3–4].) Ingestion of doses as small as 2 mg per kg of aspirin will cause a 80 to 90 per cent irreversible inhibition of platelet cyclooxygenase and cause prolongation of the bleeding time.[80, 81] The inability of platelets to synthesize new proteins means that this inhibition lasts for the life span of the platelet, from four to seven days after the ingestion of a single dose of aspirin. Endothelial production of $PGI_2$ seems to be relatively protected not only by the ability to overcome the blockade by the de novo synthesis of cyclooxygenase but probably also by virtue of the lower sensitivity of the endothelial enzyme to aspirin.[80, 81] Virtually all the initial clinical studies of aspirin for the prevention of coronary[82–86] or cerebrovascular[87, 88] thromboembolic events have employed aspirin at frequent (up to 4 times a day) high doses (up to 3000 mg per day). Such dosing schedules of aspirin may not have exploited the subtle pharmacologic differences between platelets and the endothelium. Careful clinical trials employing less frequent, lower doses of aspirin will be necessary to see whether these modifications of dose will result in improvement of clinical efficacy. A recent study of patients with unstable angina showed a significant reduction in myocardial infarction and death with 324 mg of buffered aspirin daily.[89] The ongoing Physicians Health Study, which uses 325 mg of buffered aspirin on alternate days in a primary prevention study of ischemic heart disease, should provide further useful information in this regard. Other nonsteroidal anti-inflammatory agents, including indomethacin, ibuprofen, naproxen, and zomepirac, reversibly block cyclooxygenase and have a shorter duration of action commensurate with the half-life of the drug.

*Sulfinpyrazone* is a uricosuric agent that has been used in the management of gout. It appears to act like other nonsteroidal anti-inflammatory drugs (NSAIDs) as a competitive, reversible inhibitor of cyclooxygenase[75, 90] (see Fig. 6–8), and as such it is effective only for the half-life of the drug. It has been shown to increase shortened platelet survival time in patients with artificial valves[91] or shunts or with other thrombotic tendencies such as cerebral vascular dis-

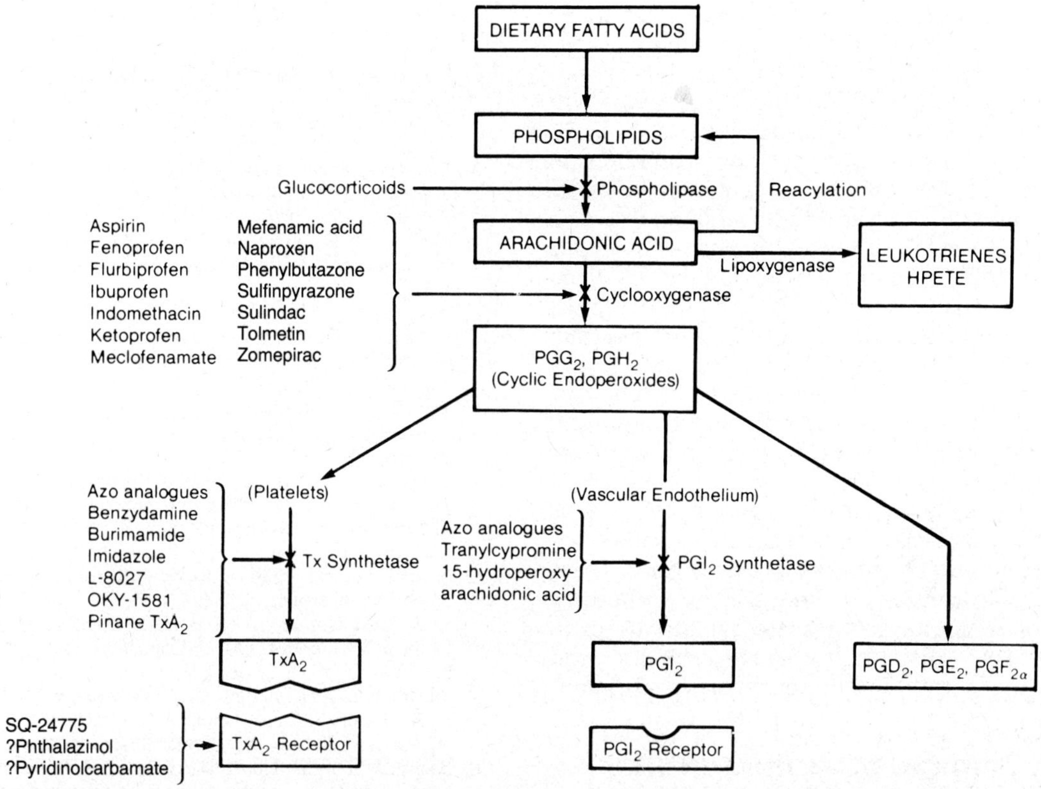


***Figure 6–8.*** Mechanism of action of certain antiplatelet agents—the pathway of arachidonic acid metabolism and the pharmacologic agents that block it. Arachidonic acid is enzymatically released from cell membrane phospholipids by a series of phospholipases, after which it enters one of three pathways: (1) reacylation into the phospholipid storage pool, (2) metabolism by the lipoxygenase enzymes to the leukotrienes and hydroperoxy-eicosatetraenoic acid (HPETE), and (3) conversion by cyclooxygenase to the prostaglandins ($PGD_2$, $PGE_2$, $PGF_{2\alpha}$) as well as to prostacyclin ($PGI_2$) and thromboxane $A_2$ ($TxA_2$). Glucocorticoids interfere with the phospholipases. The nonsteroidal anti-inflammatory drugs, including aspirin, inhibit cyclooxygenase activity, thereby preventing the synthesis of all prostaglandins and thromboxanes. Prostacyclin synthetase is found principally in vascular endothelial cells; there are several inhibitors of this enzyme that prevent the formation of $PGI_2$. Thromboxane synthetase is concentrated within platelets; inhibitors of this enzyme prevent $TxA_2$ formation. Finally, there are several compounds that inhibit $TxA_2$ activity by blocking the $TxA_2$ receptor. (From Hirsh, P. D., et al.: Prostaglandins and ischemic heart disease. Am. J. Med., *71*:1009, 1981.)

ease.[92] It does not prolong the bleeding time but weakly inhibits platelet aggregation in vitro; the exact mechanism and significance of improved platelet survival is uncertain. A controversial study[93] reported that sulfinpyrazone decreased the number of deaths following myocardial infarction. Because of flaws in clinical trial methodology, the conclusions of this study have generally not been accepted. The Food and Drug Administration has not approved sulfinpyrazone for post–myocardial infarction prophylaxis.

*Dipyridamole* is classified as a vasodilator but appears to have important antiplatelet activity.[74] Unlike the agents described previously, it does not inhibit cyclooxygenase.[75] At high levels it inhibits platelet phosphodiesterase (see Fig. 3–4), the enzyme that degrades cAMP, and results in increased platelet cAMP levels; high cAMP levels inhibit platelet aggregation. It has been suggested that dipyridamole may act,[94, 95] in vivo, by potentiating the effects of prostacyclin, inasmuch as prostacyclin stimulates cAMP production and dipyridamole inhibits its breakdown. However, dipyridamole may not inhibit phosphodiesterase at pharmacologic concentrations. Alone, dipyridamole is a weak antithrombotic agent that increases shortened platelet survival without prolonging the bleeding time. Its clinical utility appears to be in combination with warfarin[96] (in patients with prosthetic heart valves) or aspirin[97] (in patients with a tendency toward arterial thrombosis and a shortened platelet survival).

*Ticlopidine* is a new antiplatelet agent undergoing initial clinical trials that prolongs the bleeding time and is a potent inhibitor of aggregation induced by virtually all agonists.[99–102] It appears to affect platelet membrane glycoprotein binding sites for von Willebrand's factor and fibrinogen.

Other studies are currently ongoing to evaluate the efficacy of selective platelet thromboxane synthetase inhibitors[103] (see Fig. 6–8); none of these drugs is yet available for clinical use. Prostacyclin itself ($PGI_2$) is now available for a few investigational trials, but its use is limited by a half-life of less than 5 minutes[104] in vivo and its profound hypotensive effects.[105] It is the most potent, naturally occurring antiaggregatory compound; it prolongs the bleeding time and improves shortened platelet survival. Its most promising use so far appears to be in extracorporeal circuits such as hemodialysis[106, 107] and cardiopulmonary bypass. In this setting, it appears to reduce or eliminate the amount of heparin required for anticoagulation and to decrease platelet hyperaggregability and platelet thrombi in the extracorporeal circuit.

## FUTURE DIRECTIONS IN THE THERAPY OF THROMBOEMBOLIC DISEASE

Current therapy is imperfect, but recent developments are encouraging. Prevention of thrombin generation and fibrin formation is the target of anticoagulant therapy. New sensitive measurements of thrombin generation and activity may prove to be useful not only in screening but in monitoring the efficacy of therapy. Standardization of the PT with the BCT reagent may improve the therapeutic/toxic index of warfarin. Radioimmunoassays that measure noncarboxylated vitamin K–dependent factors are under development and appear promising for future monitoring of warfarin therapy. Purified heparin fractions may reduce the complications of thrombocytopenia and thrombosis. New, more potent antiplatelet agents are becoming available that selectively interfere with platelet aggregation and/or thromboxane production without inhibiting endothelial prostacyclin production. Finally, the availability of recombinant DNA human tissue plasminogen activator that is active preferentially at the site of fibrin clot may significantly increase the safety and efficacy and may reduce the expense of fibrinolytic therapy.

## REFERENCES


1. Thomas, D. P.: Heparin. Clin. Haematol., *10*:443, 1981.
2. Wessler, S., and Gitel, S. N.: Heparin: New concepts relevant to clinical use. Blood, *53*: 525, 1979.
3. Thomas, D. P.: Heparin in the prophylaxis and treatment of venous thromboembolism. Semin. Hematol., *15*:1, 1978.
4. Ryback, M. E., and Handin, R. I.: The science and art of using heparin. J. Cardiovasc. Med., *6*:265, 1981.
5. Rosenberg, R. D.: Heparin-antithrombin system. *In* Colman, R. W., Hirsh, J., Marder, V. J., et al. (Eds.): Hemostasis and Thrombosis. J. B. Lippincott, Philadelphia, 1982, p. 962.
6. Rosenberg, R. D.: Actions and interactions of antithrombin and heparin. New Engl. J. Med., *292*:146, 1975.
7. Lam, L. H., Silbert, J. E., and Rosenberg, R. D.: The separation of active and inactive forms of heparin. Biochem. Biophys. Res. Comm., *69*:570, 1976.
8. O'Reilly, R. A.: Anticoagulant, antithrombotic and thrombolytic drugs. *In* Gilman, G. G., Goodman, L. S., and Gilman, A. (Eds.): The Pharmacologic Basis of Therapeutics. Macmillan, New York, 1980, p. 1350.
9. deSwart, C. A. M., Nijmeter, B., Roelofs, J. M. M., et al.: Kinetics of intravenously administered heparin in normal humans. Blood, *60*:125, 1981.
10. Salzman, E. W., Degkin, D., Shapiro, R. M., et al.: Management of heparin therapy. Controlled prospective trial. New Engl. J. Med., *292*:1046, 1975.
11. Simon, T. L., Hyers, T. M., Gaston, J. P., et al.: Heparin pharmacokinetics: Increased requirements in pulmonary embolism. Br. J. Haematol., *39*:111, 1978.
12. Elliott, C. G. Michocki, R. J., Brown, R., et al.: Heparin requirements in pulmonary embolism and venous thrombosis: A prospective study. J. Clin. Pharm., *22*:102, 1982.
13. Thomas, D. P., Niewiarowski, S., and Ream, V. J.: Release of adenine nucleotides and platelet factor 4 from platelets of man and four other species. J. Lab. Clin. Med., *75*:607, 1970.
14. Hall, J. G., Pauli, R. M., and Wilson, K. M.: Maternal and fetal sequelae of anticoagulation during pregnancy. Am. J. Med., *68*:122, 1980.
15. Wessler, S., and Morris, L. E.: Studies in intravascular coagulation. IV. The effect of heparin and dicumarol on serum-induced venous thrombosis. Circulation, *12*:553, 1955.
16. Zucker, S., and Cathey, M. H.: Control of heparin therapy: Sensitivity of the activated partial thromboplastin time for monitoring the antithrombotic effects of heparin. J. Lab. Clin. Med., *73*:320, 1969.
17. Basura, D., Gallus, A., Hirsh, J., et al.: A prospective study of the value of monitoring heparin treatment with the activated partial thromboplastin time. New Engl. J. Med., *287*:372, 1972.
18. Hull, R., Delmore, T., Carter, C., et al.: Adjusted subcutaneous heparin versus warfarin sodium in the long-term treatment of venous thrombosis. New Engl. J. Med., *306*:189, 1982.
19. Yudelman, I., and Greenberg, A.: Factors affecting fibrinopeptide-A levels in patients with venous thromboembolism during anticoagulant therapy. Blood, *59*:787, 1982.

20. Teitel, J. M., and Rosenberg, R. D.: Protection of factor $X_a$ from neutralization by the heparin-antithrombin complex. J. Clin. Invest., *71*:1383, 1983.
21. Bell, W. R., and Royall, R. M.: Heparin associated thrombocytopenia: A comparison of three heparin preparations. New Engl. J. Med., *303*:902, 1980.
22. Ansell, J., Stepchuk, N., Kumas, R., et al.: Heparin induced thrombocytopenia: A prospective study. Thromb. Haemost., *43*:61, 1980.
23. Bergquist, D., and Hallböök, T.: A comparison between subcutaneous low-dose sodium and calcium heparin. Acta Chir. Scand., *144*:339, 1978.
24. Salzman, E. W., Rosenberg, R. D., Smith, M. H., et al.: Effect of heparin and heparin fractions on platelet aggregation. J. Clin. Invest., *65*:64, 1980.
25. Porter, J., and Jick, H.: Drug related deaths among medical inpatients. JAMA, *237*:879, 1977.
26. Kelton, J. G., and Hirsh, J.: Bleeding associated with antithrombotic therapy. Semin. Hematol., *17*:259, 1980.
27. Hampson, W. G. J., Harris., F. C., Lucas, H. K., et al.: Failure of low-dose heparin to prevent deep-vein thrombosis after hip replacement arthroplasty. Lancet, *2*:795, 1974.
28. Kiil, J., Kiil, J., Axelsen, F., et al.: Prophylaxis against postoperative pulmonary embolism and deep-vein thrombosis by low-dose heparin. Lancet, *1*:1115, 1978.
29. William, J. W., Eikman, E. A., Greenberg, S. H., et al.: Failure of low-dose heparin to prevent pulmonary embolism after hip surgery or above the knee amputation. Ann. Surg., *188*:468, 1978.
30. Gallus, A. S., Hirsh, J., O'Brien, S. E., et al: Prevention of venous thrombosis with small subcutaneous doses of heparin. JAMA, *235*:1980, 1976.
31. Gallus, A. S., Hirsh, J., Tuttle, R. J., et al.: Small subcutaneous doses of heparin in prevention of venous thrombosis. New Engl. J. Med., *288*:545, 1973.
32. Urokinase Pulmonary Embolism Trial: Morbidity and mortality. Circulation, *57*(Suppl. II):66, 1973.
33. Walker, A. M., and Jick, H.: Predictors of bleeding during heparin therapy. JAMA, *244*:1209, 1980.
34. Kernohan, R. J., and Todd, C.: Heparin therapy in thromboembolic disease. Lancet, *1*:621, 1966.
35. Glazier, R. I., and Crowell, E. B.: Randomized prospective trial of continuous versus intermittent heparin therapy. JAMA, *236*:1365, 1976.
36. Mant, M. J., O'Brien, B. D., Thong, K. L., et al.: Haemorrhagic complications of heparin therapy. Lancet, *1*:1133, 1977.
37. Wilson, J. R., and Lampman, J.: Heparin therapy: a randomized prospective study. Am. Heart J., *97*:155, 1979.
38. Wilson, J. E., Bynum, L. J., and Parkey, R. W.: Heparin therapy in venous thromboembolism. Am. J. Med., *70*:808, 1981.
39. O'Reilly, R. A.: Anticoagulant, antithrombotic and thrombolytic drugs. *In* Gilman, G. G., Goodman, L. S., and Gilman, A. (Eds.): The Pharmacologic Basis of Therapeutics. Macmillan, New York, 1980, p. 1352.
40. Weisman, R. E., and Tobin, R. W.: Arterial embolism occurring during systemic heparin therapy. AMA Arch. Surg., *76*:220, 1958.
41. White, P. W., Sodd, J. R., and Nensel, R. E.: Thrombotic complications of heparin therapy, including six cases of heparin-induced skin necrosis. Ann. Surg., *190*:595, 1979.
42. Stead, R. B., Schafer, A. I., Rosenberg, R. D., et al.: Heterogeneity of heparin lots associated with thrombocytopenia and thromboembolism. Am. J. Med., *77*:185, 1984.
43. Ames, D. V., Kaywin, P., Bina, M., et al.: Heparin-associated thrombocytopenia studies of antibody-heparin specificity. New Engl. J. Med., *303*:788, 1980.
44. Trowbridge, A. A., Caraveo, J., Green, B., et al.: Heparin-related immune thrombocytopenia studies of antibody-heparin specificity. Am. J. Med., *65*:278, 1978.
45. Cimo, P. L., Moake, J. L., Weinger, R. S., et al.: Heparin-induced thrombocytopenia aggregating factor and arterial thrombosis. Am. J. Hematol., *6*:125, 1979.
46. Green, D., Harris, K., Reynolds, N., et al.: Heparin immune thrombocytopenia: Evidence for a heparin-platelet complex as the antigenic determinant. J. Lab. Clin. Med., *91*:167, 1978.
47. Chong, B. H., Grace, C. S., and Rosenberg, M. C.: Heparin-induced thrombocytopenia: Effect of heparin platelet antibody on platelets. Br. J. Haematol., *49*:531, 1981.
48. Jaffe, M. D., and Willis, P. W. III: Multiple fractures associated with long term heparin therapy. JAMA *193*:158, 1965.
49. O'Kelly, R., Magee, F., and McKenna, T. J.: Routine heparin therapy inhibits adrenal aldosterone production. J. Clin. Endocrinol. Metab., *56*:108, 1983.
50. Phelps, K. R., Oh, M. S., and Caroll, H. J.: Heparin-induced hyperkalemia: Report of a case. Nephron, *25*:254, 1980.
51. Leekey, D., Gantt, C., and Lim, V.: Heparin-induced hypoaldosteronism—report of a case. JAMA, *246*:2189, 1981.
52. Campbell, H. A., and Link, K. P.: Studies on the hemorrhagic sweet clover disease. IV. The isolation and crystallization of the hemorrhagic agent. J. Biol. Chem., *138*:21, 1941.
53. O'Reilly, R. A.: Vitamin K antagonists. *In* Colman, R. W., Hirsh, J., Marder, V. J., et al. (Eds.): Hemostasis and Thrombosis. J. B. Lippincott, Philadelphia, 1982, p. 955.
54. Winter, J. H., and Douglas, A. S.: Oral anticoagulants. Clin. Haematol., *10*:549, 1981.
55. Deykin, D.: Anticoagulant therapy. *In* Colman, R. W., Hirsh, J., Marder, V. J., et al. (Eds.): Hemostasis and Thrombosis. J. B. Lippincott, Philadelphia, 1982, p. 1005.
56. Hull, R., Delmore, T., Genton, E., et al.: Warfarin sodium versus low-dose heparin in the long term treatment of venous thrombosis. New Engl. J. Med., *301*:855, 1979.
57. Conn, W. W., and Willis, P. W.: Recurrence of venous thromboembolism. Surgery, *73*:823, 1973.
58. Michaels, L.: Incidence of thromboembolism after stopping anticoagulant therapy. JAMA, *215*:595, 1971.
59. Kazmir, F. J.: Anticoagulation. *In* Kwaan, H. C., and Bowie, E. J. W. (Eds.): Thrombosis. W. B. Saunders, Philadelphia, 1982, p. 269.
60. Bynum, L. J., and Wilson, J. E.: Low dose heparin in the long-term management of venous thromboembolism. Am. J. Med., *67*:553, 1979.
61. Verstraete, M.: Biochemical and clinical aspects of thrombosis. Semin. Hematol., *15*:35, 1978.
62. Sharma, G. V. R. K., Cella, G., Parisi, A. F., et al.:

Thrombolytic therapy. New Engl. J. Med., *306*:1268, 1982.
63. Winman, B., and Collen, D.: Molecular mechanisms of physiological fibrinolysis. Nature, *272*:549, 1978.
64. Bergmann, S. R., Fox, K. A. A., Ter Pogossian, M. M., et al.: Clot selective thrombolysis with tissue type plasminogen activator. Science, *220*:1181, 1983.
65. Pennica, D., Holmes, W. E., Kohr, W. J., et al.: Cloning and expression of human tissue type plasminogen activator cDNA in *E. coli.* Nature, *301*:214, 1983.
66. Bell, W. R., and Meek, A. G.: Guidelines for the use of thrombolytic agents. New Engl. J. Med., *301*:1266, 1979.
67. Marder, V. J.: The use of thrombolytic agents: Choice of patient, drug administration, laboratory monitoring. Ann. Intern. Med., *90*:802, 1979.
68. Hoylaerts, M., Rijken, D. C., Lijen, H. R., et al.: Kinetics of the activation of plasminogen by human tissue plasminogen activator. Role of fibrin. J. Biol. Chem., *257*:2912, 1982.
69. Weiman, W., Stibbe, J., and van Seyen, A. J.: Specific lysis of an iliofemoral thrombus by administration of extrinsic (tissue-type) plasminogen activator. Lancet, *2*:1018, 1981.
70. Urokinase-Streptokinase Embolism Trial: Phase 2 results: A comparative study. JAMA, *229*:1606, 1974.
71. Olow, B., Johanson, C., Andersson, I., et al.: Deep venous thrombosis treated with a standard dosage of streptokinase. Acta Chir. Scand., *136*:181, 1970.
72. Hirsh, J., O'Sullivan, E. F., and Martin, M.: Evaluation of a standard dosage schedule with streptokinase. Bood, *35*:341, 1970.
73. Kwaan, H. C.: Thrombolytic therapy. *In* Kwaan, J. S., and Bowie, E. J. W. (Eds.): Thrombosis. W. B. Saunders, Philadelphia, 1982, p. 314.
74. Weiss, H. J.: Antiplatelet therapy (parts 1 and 2). New Engl. J. Med., *298*:1344 and 1403, 1978.
75. Packham, M. A., and Mustard, J. F.: Pharmacology of platelet-affecting drugs. Circulation *62*(Supp. V):V26, 1980.
76. Vane, J. R.: Inhibition of prostaglandin synthesis as a mechanism of action of aspirin-like drugs. Nature, *231*:232, 1971.
77. Roth, G. J., and Majerus, P. W.: The mechanism of the effect of aspirin on human platelets. I: Activation of a particulate fraction protein. J. Clin. Invest., *56*:624, 1975.
78. Moncada, S., Higgs, E. A., and Vane, J. R.: Human arterial and venous tissues generate prostacyclin (prostaglandin I), a potent inhibitor of platelet aggregation. Lancet, *1*:18, 1977.
79. Preston, E. F., Whipps, S., Jackson, C. A., et al.: Inhibition of prostacyclin and platelet thromboxane $A_2$ after low dose aspirin. New Engl. J. Med., *304*:76, 1981.
80. Burch, J. W., Baenziger, N. L., Stanford, N., et al.: Sensitivity of fatty acid cyclooxygenase from human aorta to acetylation by aspirin. Proc. Natl. Acad. Sci. USA, *75*:5181, 1978.
81. Burch, J. W., Stanford, N., and Majerus, P. W.: Inhibition of platelet prostaglandin synthesis by oral aspirin. J. Clin. Invest., *61*:314, 1978.
82. Aspirin Myocardial Infarction Study Research Group: A randomized, controlled trial of aspirin in persons recovered from myocardial infarction. JAMA, *243*:661, 1980.
83. Elwood, P. C., and Sweetnam, P. M.: Aspirin and secondary mortality. Lancet, *2*:314, 1979.
84. The Persantine-Aspirin Reinfarction Study Research Group: Persantine and aspirin in coronary heart disease. Circulation, *62*:449, 1980.
85. Coronary Drug Project Research Group: Aspirin in coronary heart disease. J. Chronic Dis., *29*:625, 1976.
86. Breddin, K., Loew, D., Lechner, K., et al.: Secondary prevention of myocardial infarction; comparison of acetylsalicylic acid, phenprocoumon and placebo: A multicenter two year prospective study. Thromb. Haemost., *41*:225, 1979.
87. Fields, W. S., Lemak, N. A., Frankowski, R. F., et al.: Controlled trial of aspirin in cerebral ischemia. Stroke, *8*:301, 1977.
88. Canadian Cooperative Study Group: A randomized trial of aspirin and sulfinpyrazone in threatened stroke. New Engl. J. Med., *299*:53, 1978.
89. Lewis, H. D., Davis, J. W., Archibald, D. G., et al.: Protective effects of aspirin against acute myocardial infarction and death in men with unstable angina. New Engl. J. Med. *309*:396, 1983.
90. Ali, N., and McDonald, J. W. D.: Effects of sulfinpyrazone on platelet prostaglandin synthesis and platelet release of serotonin. J. Lab. Clin. Med., *89*:868, 1977.
91. Steele, P., Rainwater, J., and Vogel, R.: Platelet suppressant therapy in patients with prosthetic cardiac valves: Relationship of clinical effectiveness to alteration of platelet survival time. Circulation, *60*:910, 1979.
92. Steele, P., Carroll, J., Overfield, D., et al.: Effect of sulfinpyrazone on platelet survival time in patients with transient cerebral ischemic attacks. Stroke, *8*:396, 1977.
93. Anturane Reinfarction Trial Research Group: Sulfinpyrazone in the prevention of cardiac death after myocardial infarction. New Engl. J. Med., *298*:289, 1977.
94. Moncada, S., and Vane, J. R.: Arachidonic acid metabolites and the interactions between platelets and blood-vessel walls. New Engl. J. Med., *300*:1142, 1979.
95. Smith, J. B.: Dipyridamole may be more effective with sodium salicylate than aspirin. Am. Heart J., *101*:686, 1981.
96. Sullivan, J. M., Harken, D. E., and Gorlin, R.: Pharmacologic control of thromboembolic complications of cardiac-valve replacement. New Engl. J. Med., *284*:1392, 1971.
97. Ritchie, J. L., and Harker, L. A.: Platelet and fibrinogen survival in coronary atherosclerosis: Response to medical and surgical therapy. Am. J. Cardiol, *39*:595, 1977.
98. Chesebro, J. H., Clements, I. P., Fuster, V., et al.: A platelet-inhibitor-drug trial in coronary-artery bypass operations: Benefit of perioperative dipyridamole and aspirin therapy on early postoperative vein-graft patency. New Engl. J. Med., *307*:73, 1982.
99. O'Brien, J. R., Etherington, M. D., and Shuttleworth, R. D.: Ticlopidine—an antiplatelet drug: Effects in human volunteers. Thromb. Res., *13*:245, 1978.

100. Ashida, S.-I., and Abiko, Y.: Inhibition of platelet aggregation by a new agent: ticlopidine. Thromb. Haemost., *40*:542, 1978.
101. Knudsen, J. B., and Gormsen, J.: The effects of ticlopidine on platelet function in normal volunteers and in patients with hyperaggregability *in vitro*. Thromb. Res., *16*:663, 1979.
102. Lee, H., Paton, R. C., Ruan, C., et al.: The in vitro effect of ticlopidine on fibrinogen and Factor VIII binding to human platelets. Thromb. Haemost., *46*:590, 1981.
103. Gorman, R. R., Shebuski, R. J., Aiken, J. W., et al.: Analysis of the biologic activity of azoprostanoids in human platelets. Fed. Proc., *40*:1997, 1981.
104. Dusting, G. J., Moncada, S., and Vane, J. R.: Disappearance of prostacyclin ($PGI_2$) in the circulation of the dog. Br. J. Pharmacol., *62*:414p, 1978.
105. Feigen, L. P.: Actions of prostaglandins in peripheral vascular beds. Fed. Proc., *40*:1987, 1981.
106. Zusman, R. M., Rubin, R. H., and Cato, A. E.: Hemodialysis using prostacyclin instead of heparin as the sole antithrombic agent. New Engl. J. Med., *304*:934, 1981.
107. Smith, M. C., Danviriyasup, K., Crow, J. W., et al.: Prostacyclin substitution for heparin in long term hemodialysis. Am. J. Med., *73*:669, 1982.
108. Thompson, A. R., and Harker, L. A.: Manual of Thrombosis and Hemostasis. F. A. Davis, Philadelphia, 1983, p. 160.
109. Rosenberg, R. D.: Heparin, antithrombin, and abnormal clotting. Ann. Rev. Med., *29*:367, 1978.
110. Rice, L., and Jackson, D.: Can heparin cause clotting? Heart and Lung, *10*:331, 1981.
111. Hull, R., Hirsh, J., Jay, R., et al.: Different intensities of oral anticoagulant therapy in the treatment of proximal-vein thrombosis. New Engl. J. Med., *307*:1676, 1982.
112. Leyvarz, P. F., Richard, J., Bachmann, F., et al.: Adjusted versus fixed-dose subcutaneous heparin in the prevention of deep-vein thrombosis after total hip replacement. New Engl. J. Med., *309*:954, 1983.
113. Ganz, W., Geft, I., Shah, P. K., et al.: Intravenous streptokinase in evolving acute myocardial infarction. Am. J. Cardiol., *53*:1209, 1984.
114. Goldhaber, S. Z., Buring, J. E., Lipnick, R. J., et al.: Pooled analyses of randomized trials of streptokinase and heparin in phlebographically documented acute deep venous thrombosis. Am. J. Med., *76*:393, 1984.
115. Hirsh, P. D., Campbell, W. B., Willerson, J. T., et al.: Prostaglandins and ischemic heart disease. Am. J. Med., *71*:1009, 1981.
116. Broekmans, A. W., Bertina, R. M., Loeliger, E. A., et al.: Protein C and the development of skin necrosis during anticoagulant therapy. Thromb. Haemost., *49*:251, 1983.
117. Marcus, A. J.: Aspirin as an antithrombotic medication. New Engl. J. Med., *309*:1515, 1983.
118. King, D. J., and Kelton, J. G.: Heparin-associated thrombocytopenia. Ann. Intern. Med., *100*:535, 1984.
119. Shafer, K. E., Santoro, S. A., Sobel, B. E., et al.: Monitoring activity of fibrinolytic agents: A therapeutic challenge. Am. J. Med., *76*:879, 1984.

CHAPTER 7

# STRATEGIES FOR MANAGEMENT

SAMUEL Z. GOLDHABER, M.D.

Whereas the previous chapter presented an overview of the clinical pharmacology of various antithrombotic agents, here we will concentrate on the selection of agents for treating PE or DVT. Patients with major (but not massive) PE are discussed here; Chapter 10 is devoted entirely to patients with massive PE.

Once the diagnosis of PE or DVT is established, a new set of problems emerges and revolves around the optimal strategy for managing these patients. One concern of the clinician is whether to institute conventional anticoagulant therapy using heparin or to take a more aggressive approach and employ thrombolytic therapy. To date, no study has adequately addressed this problem. Another question centers on duration of anticoagulant therapy. Traditionally, patients with PE or DVT have been treated for three to six months; however, one cannot be certain about the optimal duration of treatment on the basis of available data. In addition, strategies for managing DVT are in flux. For example, the optimal intensity of an oral anticoagulant regimen to treat DVT is now being reappraised. Although the usual recommendation has been to maintain the prothrombin level at twice the control value, such intense anticoagulation may be excessive for some patients with DVT. One recent and promising approach is the use of adjusted doses of subcutaneous heparin, which may prove safer than traditional treatment with warfarin.

## ANTICOAGULATION VS. THROMBOLYSIS

### Heparin Anticoagulation

**Rationale for Therapy.** The rationale for heparin therapy is to prevent recurrent PE or DVT. Unless PE patients have an underlying disease such as cancer, those who receive treatment with heparin anticoagulation usually improve. At the Peter Bent Brigham Hospital, Alpert and coworkers[1] reported on 144 consecutive patients with angiographically documented PE. Twelve died of PE and eight died of causes other than PE; 86% survived. The most important factor affecting mortality was shock due to acute right ventricular failure from massive PE. All patients in this series received heparin, and none was treated with thrombolytic agents. Thus heparin, used to avert recurrent PE, was associated with a low mortality from PE.

When heparin anticoagulation succeeds, it allows the body's natural lytic mechanisms to dissolve the previously formed clot and prevents these lytic mechanisms from being overwhelmed by recurrent venous thromboembolism. Even weeks after PE has occurred and has been treated with heparin, the clot usually persists to some extent on the angiogram, showing minimal to moderate resolution.[2] However, the degree of lysis is usually sufficient to restore right heart pressures to normal or near normal within the first week after embolization.

Although heparin has been accepted as the traditional therapy for PE, only one randomized trial has been published comparing heparin with no anticoagulation.[3] After 35 patients had been randomized, this trial was discontinued on ethical grounds because the mortality rate among the control subjects became unacceptably high. Trials using historical controls have also attested to heparin's efficacy.[4] However, one recent case series suggested that in patients with cancer, heparin therapy may be associated with surprisingly high rates of venous thromboembolic and hemorrhagic complications.[5] The authors hypothesized that in cancer patients, inter-

***Table 7–1.*** Procedures Prior to Initiating Heparin Therapy

1. Obtain a careful history directed toward:
   A. History of prior blood disease
   B. Prior response to anticoagulation
   C. Underlying diseases that might affect heparinization (e.g., recent surgery or trauma)
   D. Concomitant drug therapy
   E. Symptoms suggestive of active bleeding disorder
2. Physical examination to detect potential risk of bleeding:
   A. Blood pressure
   B. Skin examination to exclude petechiae and ecchymoses
   C. Rectal examination, with stool analysis for occult blood
3. Baseline laboratory evaluation:
   A. Complete blood count
   B. Platelet count (qualitative assessment on blood smear will suffice)
   C. Partial thromboplastin time
   D. Urine analysis (to detect hematuria)

ruption of the inferior vena cava might be more effective than heparin therapy. Nevertheless, heparin anticoagulation remains the foundation for treatment of PE.

Among 12 patients treated with therapeutic doses of heparin for DVT, quantitative venography after five days indicated minor extension of thrombus in three patients despite adequate anticoagulation.[6] In five of the 12 patients, no change occurred in the extent of leg vein thrombus; four showed improvement. These results indicate that heparin's utility in venous thromboembolism is primarily to halt major extension of previously formed thrombi. Analogous angiographic findings have been reported for PE patients treated with heparin.[7]

**Strategies for Initiating Heparin Therapy.** Obtaining a careful history is the most important first step to ensure safe initiation of heparin therapy. Factors associated with an increased risk of bleeding during heparin therapy were outlined in Table 6–1. In particular, one should consider risk factors such as a history of coagulopathy, thrombocytopenia, vitamin K deficiency, older age, underlying diseases, and concomitant drug therapy.

Before initiating heparin therapy, we follow the procedures listed in Table 7–1. If results of the screening evaluation are benign, we proceed with heparinization prior to lung scanning, pulmonary angiography, or venography (Table 7–2). If a potentially severe bleeding problem is detected, such as active gastrointestinal bleeding, we withhold heparin therapy until more definitive evaluation with angiography can be undertaken. If angiography or venography proves positive for PE or proximal DVT, we seriously consider and usually opt in favor of inferior vena caval (IVC) interruption for patients at high risk for bleeding with heparin, especially if such patients have had a prior episode of PE or DVT. When there is an intermediate risk of bleeding, we usually proceed cautiously with heparin but prepare for the possible need to switch strategies from heparinization to inferior vena caval interruption. For each patient we develop a stratifi-

***Table 7–2.*** Risk Profile for Bleeding Due to Heparin Therapy

| Risk Level | Examples | Treatment Modality for PE or Proximal DVT |
|---|---|---|
| 1. No increased risk | History, physical examination, and laboratory evaluation as outlined in Table 7–1 are negative | Heparinize before confirmation of diagnosis. |
| 2. Slightly increased risk | A. Has been taking aspirin for headaches within the week prior to hospitalization<br>*or* B. BP = 180/110<br>*or* C. Patient's PTT = 30 seconds and prolongation is unexplained (control value = 25 seconds) | Heparinize before confirmation of diagnosis. Increase nursing and laboratory surveillance for potential bleeding. |
| 3. Moderately increased risk | A. Cholecystectomy (or car accident) 1 week earlier<br>*and/or* B. Ecchymoses on skin<br>*and/or* C. HCT = 34 | Heparinize after confirmation of diagnosis. Notify patient, angiographer, and vascular surgeon of potential for IVC interruption. |
| 4. Markedly increased risk | A. Active gastrointestinal bleeding<br>*or* B. Has developed thrombocytopenia in the past from porcine and beef heparin preparations | Defer heparin. Confirm diagnosis with angiography or venography. If angiogram or venogram is positive, interrupt IVC. |

cation of potential risk for bleeding (see Table 7–2). Unless the risk for bleeding is markedly increased, we proceed with heparin therapy.

The dosage regimen for optimal heparinization is rather arbitrary. Usually we attempt to maintain heparin anticoagulation so that the partial thromboplastin time (PTT) remains two to three times greater than the control level. A PTT greater than 1.5 times control prevents the recurrence of venous thromboembolism in most cases.[8, 9] Interestingly, bleeding complications during heparin therapy do not correlate closely with elevated PTT levels.[8, 9] Thus, we are much more concerned about underheparinization for established PE than about a PTT that is four times the control value in a patient who is not at particularly increased risk for bleeding with heparin therapy.

We also favor continuous infusion of heparin rather than intermittent intravenous or subcutaneous administration. In our judgment, continuous intravenous heparinization is safer, despite several reports to the contrary,[10, 11] because wide fluctuations in the PTT level are avoided.[12–15] To achieve adequate heparinization, we employ dosing and laboratory monitoring as outlined in Table 7–3. These guidelines should, of course, be modified according to the individual patient's particular clinical history and evaluation.

Although complications of heparin therapy were covered in detail in the previous chapter, we should point out here that *heparin-associated thrombocytopenia* is more common than is generally recognized. Therefore, patients receiving heparin should be examined routinely for the development of petechiae, and serial qualitative or quantitative platelet counts should be determined during heparin administration.

## Thrombolytic Therapy

**Rationale for Therapy.** Whereas heparin acts primarily to prevent thrombus extension, streptokinase and urokinase are thrombolytic agents that promote dissolution of clots that have recently formed (i.e., within seven days). Although these thrombolytic agents were approved for treatment of PE in 1977, their use has not become as widespread as was initially predicted. Only three randomized trials of PE therapy have compared thrombolytic agents with heparin[16–18] (see Ta-

***Table 7–3.*** Guide to Dosing and Laboratory Monitoring of Heparin Therapy

I. Initial intravenous heparin dose and infusion rate as a function of body weight (assuming baseline laboratory evaluation in Table 7–1 reveals no abnormality).
Unless the patient is at markedly increased risk for bleeding (see Table 7–2), we initiate heparin therapy prior to lung scanning and pulmonary angiography.

| Body Weight (kg) | Initial Heparin Dose (units)* | Initial Heparin Infusion Rate (units/hour) |
|---|---|---|
| 40 | 3500 | 700 |
| 50 | 4000 | 800 |
| 60 | 4500 | 900 |
| 70 | 5000 | 1000 |
| 80 | 5500 | 1100 |
| 90 | 6000 | 1200 |
| 100 | 6500 | 1300 |

II. Determine PTT at 2 hours and 6 hours after initiation of continuous intravenous heparin infusion. Heparin infusion should be optimized according to PTT and patient's weight.

| PTT Less Than Twice or Greater Than Three Times Control Value and Body Weight (kg) is: | Incremental Adjustment of Heparin Infusion (units/hr) | |
|---|---|---|
| 40 | 100 | *Increase* heparin infusion when PTT less than twice control; *decrease* heparin infusion when PTT greater than 3 times control value |
| 50 | 100 | |
| 60 | 100 | |
| 70 | 100 | |
| 80 | 200 | |
| 90 | 200 | |
| 100 | 200 | |

III. Continue to adjust heparin dose every 4 hours until PTT is in the optimal therapeutic range of 2–3 times the control value.

IV. After PTT is in the therapeutic range, determine daily PTT and qod (alternate day) CBC and platelet count.

*If *massive* PE is suspected, we ordinarily administer much larger initial boluses of intravenous heparin (see Chapter 10).

ble 10–10). In these trials, no reduction in mortality from PE was apparent with streptokinase or urokinase, even though clots lysed more quickly when these agents were used. In two of the three studies, bleeding complications occurred more often after thrombolysis.[16, 18] Follow-up of patients treated with streptokinase or urokinase for PE has demonstrated increases in pulmonary capillary blood volume and pulmonary diffusing capacity compared with heparin-treated patients.[19] However, the clinical significance of these improvements in pulmonary parameters is uncertain.

**Strategies for Initiating Thrombolytic Therapy.** The clinical pharmacology of streptokinase and urokinase (i.e., contraindications, clinical effects, mode of action, dosing, and monitoring regimens) were discussed in Chapter 6. Many patients suspected of PE or DVT will be receiving heparin by continuous infusion while undergoing diagnostic evaluation. After a definitive diagnosis of venous thromboembolism is established, the physician must decide whether to continue heparin anticoagulation or to interrupt heparin treatment for a course of thrombolytic therapy. Immediately prior to initiation of thrombolytic therapy, heparin is discontinued. For PE, we administer a loading dose of 250,000 IU of *streptokinase* over 20 to 30 minutes, after pretreatment with 100 mg of intravenous hydrocortisone. We then administer a continuous infusion of streptokinase at 100,000 IU per hour for 24 hours in PE and for 48 to 72 hours in DVT. The lytic state can be confirmed by measuring any *one* of the following parameters: PTT, prothrombin time, thrombin time, fibrin split products, or whole blood euglobulin lysis time. Generally we use the PTT for the sake of convenience and familiarity. If a lytic state has not been achieved, we administer additional streptokinase. During the infusion period, we attempt to minimize physical handling of the patient and invasive procedures. Whenever possible, we avoid simultaneous administration of platelet-active drugs and we never employ simultaneous heparin anticoagulation. Upon discontinuing streptokinase, we administer heparin by continuous infusion without a loading dose when the PTT is approximately twice the control value.[23]

Phase I of the Urokinase Pulmonary Embolism Trial demonstrated that PEs were lysed more quickly with *urokinase* than with heparin.[16] Heparin was not studied in phase II of the trial, which showed that clot resolution after 24 hours of urokinase infusion was equal to that achieved after 12 hours of urokinase and after 24 hours of streptokinase.[67]

Our experience with urokinase is more limited than with streptokinase. Because urokinase is more expensive than streptokinase, we generally reserve urokinase for PE patients who have had a major adverse allergic reaction to streptokinase or for patients in whom we cannot readily attain a systemic lytic state with streptokinase. (Prior exposure to streptokinase, which is antigenic, can cause formation of antistreptokinase antibodies that prevent streptokinase from inducing a systemic lytic state.) The recommended dosage for urokinase is a loading dose of 4400 IU/kg over 10 minutes, followed by a continuous infusion of 4400 IU/kg/hour for 12 to 24 hours. After cessation of urokinase therapy, heparin is administered when the PTT decreases to approximately twice the control value. Urokinase has not been approved by the Food and Drug Administration for treatment of DVT.

In the event of excessive bleeding, we discontinue the thrombolytic agent. If necessary, we then administer fresh frozen plasma to restore the depleted plasma fibrinogen. Rarely, if hemorrhage persists, it may be necessary to administer epsilon aminocaproic acid (EACA). The recommended intravenous loading dose for adult patients with normal renal function is 0.1 g/kg over 20 to 30 minutes, followed by a continuous intravenous infusion of 0.5 to 1 g/hour.[75] However, most bleeding complications can be managed by applying local pressure.

In general, we feel that for patients with venous thromboembolism, thrombolytic agents have the highest benefit-to-risk ratio in patients with massive PE (see Chapter 10). For more detailed information on streptokinase and urokinase, the reader is referred to Chapters 3 and 6 and to several excellent reviews.[20–23]

### Benefits and Risks of Thrombolysis

Controversy persists regarding the roles of thrombolytic agents and anticoagulation in the treatment of PE and DVT. In 1980, an NIH Consensus Development Conference suggested that thrombolytic therapy was not being used often enough.[24] This view was echoed in an accompanying editorial,[25] which predicted that thrombolytic therapy would "slowly but progressively be incorporated into the routine management of patients with venous thrombotic and embolic disease." Several months later, a more skeptical view was expressed by Schrier, who urged prospective clinical studies to define subgroups for whom thrombolytic agents would be most beneficial.[26] The controversy regarding thrombolytic agents for PE has also been debated by Sasahara,[27] a proponent, and by Dalen,[28] an opponent. At present, we utilize streptokinase or urokinase primarily to treat massive PE (Fig. 7–1).

In the treatment of acute DVT, streptokinase has the potential to prevent venous valve damage and subsequent venous stasis disease in the legs. However, this possible benefit must be weighed against the potential risk of increased bleeding compared with standard heparin anticoagulation. Although streptokinase has been compared with heparin in several randomized trials of phlebographically documented DVT,[29–34] no individual study has included a sample of sufficient size to determine both the efficacy and the safety of this agent. When we pooled the results of the randomized trials, we found that although thrombolysis is achieved more often with streptokinase (see Figure 1–1), major bleeding complications are more frequent with streptokinase than with heparin.[35] Future trials involving larger numbers of patients should therefore be undertaken to evaluate streptokinase compared with heparin for treatment of DVT. At present, we do not advocate the routine use of streptokinase for DVT.

## TISSUE PLASMINOGEN ACTIVATOR

In the future, tissue plasminogen activator (tPA) may become an attractive alternative to heparin, streptokinase, and/or urokinase. tPA can lyse thrombus by activating plasminogen without depleting fibrinogen. Thus, it offers the potential of thrombolytic efficacy with fewer bleeding complications than are seen with streptokinase or urokinase.

When fibrin is formed, a small amount of plasminogen is specifically bound to it. tPA is adsorbed on the fibrin surface and efficiently activates the bound plasminogen (see Figure 6–7). The formed plasmin remains bound to the fibrin clot and degrades the fibrin to which it is attached. Therefore, because the plasmin is bound to the fibrin locally, the small amount of plasmin released from digested fibrin into the general circulation is rapidly and irreversibly neutralized by circulating antiplasmin.[36,37]

tPA has been isolated from human melanoma cells[38, 39] and has been synthesized using recombinant DNA techniques.[40] It is metabolized by the liver[41] and has a half-life of approximately 15 minutes.[36] To date, tPA has been used in dogs to lyse experimental coronary occlusions.[42–45, 72, 74] Recently, tPA was reported to lyse coronary thromboses in six of seven patients with evolving myocardial infarction.[73] If success in humans is confirmed, tPA may usher in a new era of safer, more widespread thrombolytic therapy for both arterial and venous clots.

## ADJUNCTIVE THERAPY FOR PE

While the cornerstone of PE treatment involves anticoagulation or thrombolysis, adjunctive measures are also useful. Hypoxia, as assessed by arterial blood gases, should be treated with supplemental oxygen. In most patients, 2 to 4 liters of oxygen via nasal prongs will suffice. In those patients prone to carbon dioxide narcosis, oxygen concentrations should be controlled by means of a Venturi mask, and arterial blood gas measurements should be repeated after oxygen therapy has begun.

Discomfort due to PE can be intense and can cause chest wall splinting, making the patient susceptible to pneumonia and increased hypoxia owing to poor ventilation. Therefore, pain should be aggressively controlled. Although the pleuritic pain of PE often has an inflammatory component, most patients can be managed satisfactorily with narcotics (e.g., codeine, morphine, or meperidine) rather than with anti-inflammatory agents, all of which have adverse effects on platelet function. Although narcotics may precipitate carbon dioxide narcosis, their deleterious effect of respiratory depression can be readily reversed with naloxone. However, anti-inflammatory agents, with their concomitant antiplatelet effects, may predispose to profuse bleeding during anticoagulant or thrombolytic therapy. Such bleeding can be exceedingly difficult to control.

Fever often accompanies PE and not only should be suppressed with acetaminophen but should also lead to a search for accompanying infection, particularly pneumonia. Treatment with antipyretics will make the febrile patient comfortable and will lessen

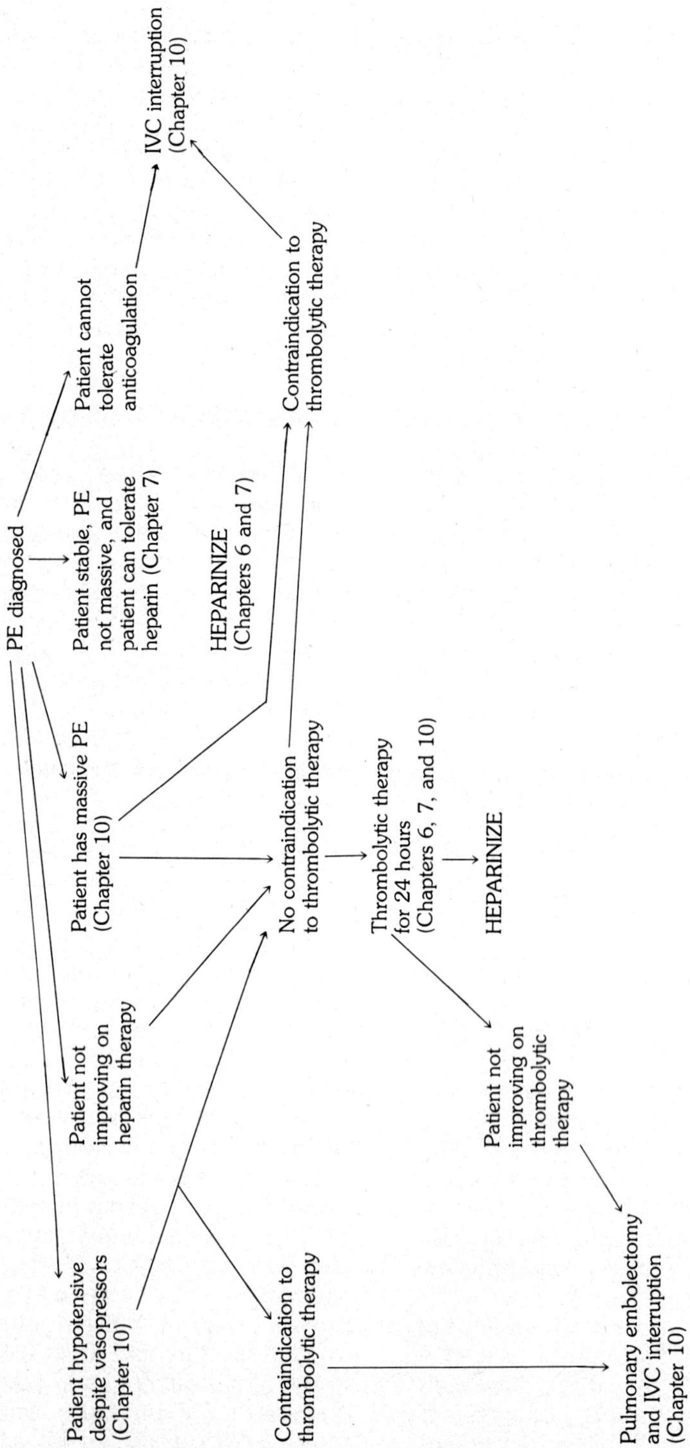


***Figure 7–1.*** Initial therapeutic strategy for PE.

potentially adverse cardiovascular effects of the associated tachycardia.

## OPTIMAL DURATION OF PE AND DVT THERAPY

Chronic anticoagulation is prescribed in PE and DVT for the purpose of averting recurrent venous thromboembolism. Although PE patients often receive chronic warfarin therapy for six months, the optimal duration and optimal intensity of oral anticoagulation are unknown. In patients who have experienced a transient risk factor for PE, such as an operation, the utility of continuing anticoagulation indefinitely is probably low. However, for patients with an irreversible risk factor (e.g., metastatic cancer) or with a risk factor that is not easily modified (e.g., massive obesity), a stronger case can be made for continuing anticoagulants indefinitely.

In phase II of the Urokinase Pulmonary Embolism Trial, 26 per cent of the patients had experienced PE previously.[46] In most, the earlier episode had occurred within a month of the index episode. However, in one-fifth of patients, the previous episode had occurred more than six months earlier. This latter finding raises questions about the advisability of routinely discontinuing oral anticoagulant therapy six months after the occurrence of PE and highlights the need for particular vigilance regarding potential PE recurrence during the month after initial diagnosis.

Recurrent PE can lead to chronic, persistent pulmonary artery clot,[47] with attendant pulmonary hypertension and cor pulmonale.[48] This major complication of PE occurs most often when the diagnosis of PE is initially overlooked and anticoagulation is withheld for months or years.[49] Under rare circumstances, chronic obstruction of the pulmonary arteries can also occur despite prompt administration of anticoagulation.[50] Chronic PE that is refractory to anticoagulants and thrombolytic agents can be managed with thromboendarterectomy (see Chapter 15).

For DVT patients, three months of anticoagulation is the conventional approach. However, as with PE, the optimal duration of anticoagulation is unknown. A study by Hull and colleagues showed that among patients in whom DVT recurred after three months of anticoagulation, 18 of 89 (20 per cent) experienced *another* recurrence (i.e., a third episode) of DVT.[51] Of these 18 patients, five had concomitant PE that was fatal in all but one patient. These findings suggest that patients with a single recurrence of DVT should be treated with anticoagulants for much longer than the traditional three-month period.

### Potential Detection of Occult Malignancy

It appears that occult malignancy is associated with both PE[68] and DVT.[69] In a case-control study of 129 patients with angiographically proven PE, the frequency of cancer being diagnosed before PE was 12 per cent, compared with 10 per cent in a control group without PE (p = NS). The controls consisted of patients who underwent pulmonary angiography for suspected PE but who had normal pulmonary angiograms. During the two years after pulmonary angiography, cancer was diagnosed in 13 patients with PE, in contrast to no diagnoses of cancer among the control group ($p < 0.001$). The presence of other known risk factors for venous thromboembolism—bedrest, pregnancy, oral contraceptive use, leg trauma, recent surgery, congestive heart failure, gynecologic or prostatic disease—had no impact on the incidence of occult malignancy. In 23 cases without apparent risk factors, 9 per cent were diagnosed as having cancer within two years of angiography; of 90 cases with at least one known venous thromboembolism risk factor (excluding cancer) at the time of PE diagnosis, 12 per cent were found to have cancer in the subsequent two years.

Similar findings were obtained in a study of 420 patients with DVT documented by impedance plethysmography and 1120 controls with negative impedance studies. Over a five-year follow-up period, 8 per cent with DVT developed cancer, compared with 3 per cent of controls ($p < 0.001$). These findings suggest that PE and DVT patients who do not have cancer at the time of diagnosis should be followed up with particular attention to symptoms or signs suggestive of cancer.

## NEW THERAPEUTIC OPTIONS IN THE MANAGEMENT OF DVT

### Embolic Risk

It appears that the risk of embolism depends on the location of DVT and that proximal thigh vein thrombi are more ominous than distal calf vein thrombi. In a study in which all DVT patients underwent lung scanning (regardless of symptoms or signs), none of 21 patients had positive lung scans in the presence of DVT limited to the calf.[52] However, of 15 patients with both thigh and calf vein thrombosis, eight had evidence of PE on lung scan. This suggests that in the future, patients with DVT may be treated heterogeneously, according to the location of the clot. For instance, patients with small thrombi limited to calf veins may be followed without anticoagulant treatment unless proximal thigh vein thrombi are identified on serial imaging studies.

### Fixed Low-Dose Subcutaneous Heparin

In treating DVT patients with conventional doses of warfarin, it is evident that bleeding complications occur frequently despite scrupulous surveillance. For this reason, investigators have searched for a suitable alternative strategy for managing these patients. Hull and coworkers have been in the forefront of designing and testing potential alternatives.[53–55] In 1979, they tested conventional warfarin therapy against fixed low-dose subcutaneous heparin (5000 units every 12 hours) to prevent recurrent DVT.[53] Of 33 patients receiving standard warfarin therapy, with prothrombin times adjusted between 1.5 and 2 times the control value, none had recurrences of DVT. In contrast, among 35 patients receiving low-dose subcutaneous heparin, DVT recurred in nine. Unfortunately, bleeding complications developed in seven patients receiving warfarin, even though in six of these seven patients, the prothrombin time was between 1.5 and 2 times the control value within three days prior to bleeding and at the time of bleeding. In the low-dose heparin group, no patient experienced bleeding complications. Thus, although warfarin was more effective than low-dose subcutaneous heparin in preventing recurrent DVT, this benefit was attenuated by the associated risk of bleeding with warfarin therapy.

### Adjusted-Dose Subcutaneous Heparin

In a follow-up study, Hull and coworkers compared warfarin to *adjusted* subcutaneous heparin therapy for prevention of recurrent proximal DVT.[54] They administered adjusted doses of subcutaneous heparin, given every 12 hours, so that the midinterval PTT measured six hours after injection would approximate 1½ times the control value. The average dose that achieved this effect was 10,000 units per injection. After initial adjustment, the subcutaneous heparin dose was fixed, and no further tests were performed to monitor subcutaneous heparin administration. Treatment with either warfarin or adjusted subcutaneous heparin was continued for 12 weeks. One of the 53 patients who received warfarin and two of the 53 patients who received heparin had new episodes of DVT. This difference was not significant. However, nine patients taking warfarin had bleeding complications compared with one patient taking heparin. No heparin-associated thrombocytopenia or osteopenia was observed. These data suggest that adjusted-dose subcutaneous heparin therapy provides an effective alternative to warfarin and is associated with a lower risk of bleeding.

Despite these promising results with adjusted doses of subcutaneous heparin, there are several disadvantages to long-term therapy with this agent. First, heparin is more expensive than warfarin. Second, subcutaneous administration of heparin is associated with the discomfort of several daily injections. Third, heparin, unlike warfarin, is associated with thrombocytopenia.[56–58] Although heparin-associated thrombocytopenia is usually reported with intravenous administration of heparin, especially bovine-lung heparin,[56, 58] this complication can also occur with subcutaneous heparin administration.[57] Other complications of long-term heparin therapy are reviewed in Chapter 6. Nevertheless, the use of adjusted-dose subcutaneous heparin to treat DVT is appealing for therapy during pregnancy.[59]

### Less Intensive Warfarin Therapy

Because adjusted subcutaneous heparin therapy is not a panacea, Hull and coworkers undertook a study of different intensities of warfarin therapy in the treatment of proximal DVT.[55] After seven days of full-dose intravenous heparin, 96 patients were randomized to either standard or low-dose warfarin therapy. In the conventionally treated group, the prothrombin time averaged 19 seconds, compared with 15 seconds in the less intensely treated group. More intensely treated patients took an average of 6 mg of warfarin daily, whereas the low-dose group averaged 5 mg. Recurrent DVT was detected in one patient from each group during the 12-week trial. However, bleeding complications occurred more frequently in the group receiving standard warfarin therapy (11 of 49 patients) compared with the low-dose warfarin group (two of 47 patients). These data suggest that less intensive warfarin therapy is effective for treating proximal DVT and is associated with a reduced risk of hemorrhage compared with standard dose warfarin. Nevertheless, one should note that the difference in warfarin dosage between the two groups was only 1 mg per day.

With the publication of these studies by Hull and coworkers, the therapeutic options for treating DVT have increased. Figure 7–2 summarizes the strategies available for managing DVT.

As stated earlier, the optimal duration for anticoagulation is unknown. In patients who have a risk factor for thrombosis that is not transient (e.g., antithrombin III deficiency or cancer), chronic anticoagulation is warranted. For patients with a transient risk factor (e.g., operation), three months of anticoagulation may be reasonable. However, for any patient who demonstrates *recurrent* DVT, anticoagulation should probably be undertaken for at least a year even if no specific risk factor can be identified.

## ADJUNCTIVE THERAPY FOR DVT

### Leg Pain and Swelling

For those patients who experience leg pain and swelling, bedrest in the Trendelenburg position (head down and legs elevated) is usually advisable during the initial treatment. However, after leg swelling subsides, these patients should be mobilized and should ambulate while wearing elastic stockings or bandages. There is no evidence to support the notion that ambulation will precipitate PE in patients with DVT.

### Management of the Postphlebitic Syndrome (PPS)

After the occurrence of DVT, venous outflow can be blocked by damaged venous valves and result in inadequate tissue perfusion. The most frequent symptoms are leg pain and swelling. Incompetent venous valves can cause signs of PPS, including ankle and leg edema, pigmentation abnormalities (i.e., stasis dermatitis), and leg ulceration. To evaluate the long-term sequelae of DVT, Strandness and coworkers conducted a prospective long-term study of DVT patients with an average follow-up of 39 months.[60] Pain or swelling was noted by 67 per cent of patients. Limb measurements were made routinely at the calf and thigh. In 59 per cent of patients, circumference increased by 1 cm or more; pigmentation abnormalities developed in 23 per cent, and ulceration occurred in 5 per cent.

Edema due to PPS can usually be managed with graded elastic support stockings or (ACE®) elastic bandages. The pruritus associated with stasis dermatitis can usually be treated successfully with oral antihistamines. In most instances, stasis dermatitis will occur without cellulitis, even when the leg appears warm, reddened, and swollen. Therefore, antibiotics should be withheld unless the patient manifests leg pain, fever, and leukocytosis. (Only rarely will a bacterial pathogen be identified, even if cellulitis accompanies stasis dermatitis.)

Small stasis ulcers can usually be managed by assiduous application of "wet-to-dry" dressings. These consist of topical gauzes treated with saline or with 3% hydrogen peroxide. Dressings are placed over the ulcer and are removed several hours later, after drying. Larger stasis ulcers may require debridement and possibly skin grafting. In patients with severe refractory PPS, autologous vein valve transplantation can be considered.[61, 62] This procedure involves inserting a 2-cm segment of brachial vein that contains a normal venous valve into the superficial femoral vein. Half of the patients undergoing vein valve transplantation have reported healing of stasis ulcers, and in almost all cases, leg discomfort has been reduced.

## VENOUS THROMBOSIS OF THE UPPER EXTREMITIES

Upper extremity venous thrombosis is uncommon and probably represents less than 1 per cent of all cases of peripheral venous thrombosis. The literature on this subject is sparse and essentially consists of case reports and case series. In the four descriptive studies[63–66] summarized in Table 7–4, pulmonary embolism occurred rarely. Nevertheless, our understanding of upper extremity

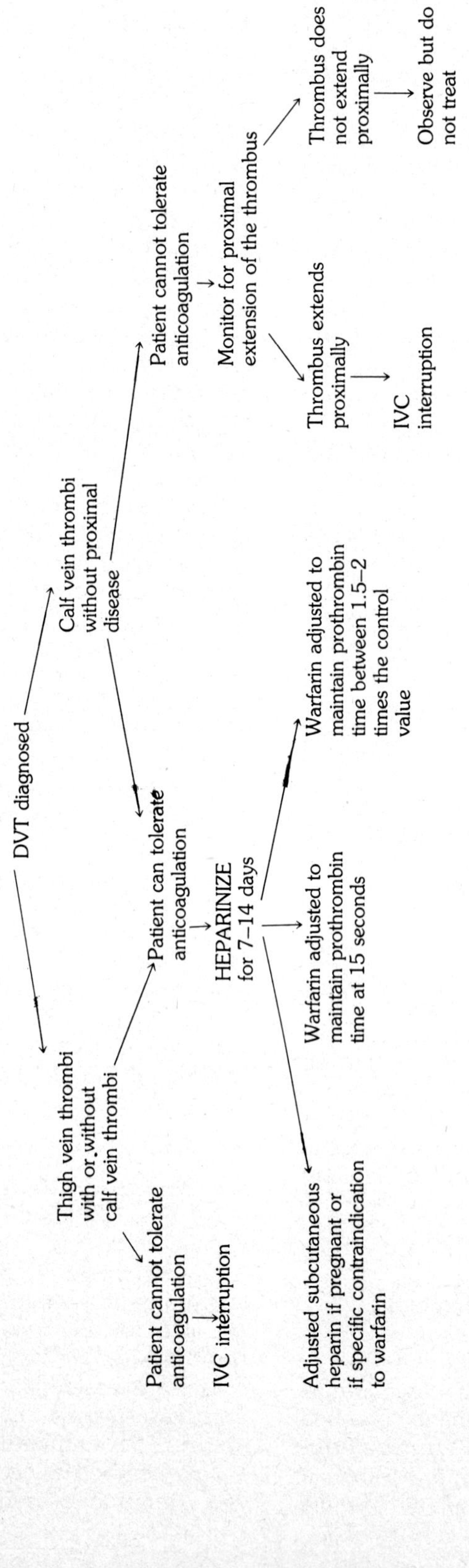


***Figure 7–2.*** Strategies for managing DVT.

*Table 7–4.* Upper Extremity Venous Thrombosis

| Reference | Number of Cases | Number with PE (%) |
|---|---|---|
| Swinton et al.[63] | 23 | 2 (8) |
| Tilney et al.[64] | 48 | 0 (0) |
| Campbell et al.[65] | 25 | 2 (8) |
| Prescott and Tikoff[66] | 12 | 1 (8) |

thrombosis and its relation to pulmonary embolism is limited.

*Thrombophlebitis migrans* involves superficial veins and often occurs in the upper extremity. This condition tends to be migratory and resistant to anticoagulation. It may appear months or years before symptoms and signs of malignancy become apparent.[70, 71]

## SUMMARY

Although most patients with venous thromboembolism are currently not treated with thrombolytic agents, this practice may change over the next few years, as physicians and nurses become more familiar with these drugs in the treatment of myocardial infarction. Furthermore, tPA may prove to lyse venous clots with substantially fewer hemorrhagic complications than occur with streptokinase or urokinase.

The optimal duration of treatment for PE and DVT will come under increasing scrutiny. It is likely that for proximal DVT and for PE, certain patients should be treated for much longer than the conventional three to six months. An intriguing prospect is the use of less intensive warfarin therapy in patients with proximal DVT. This practice should allow the effectiveness of conventional warfarin to be maintained but should reduce bleeding complications. It will be important to test the results of the studies by Hull and coworkers in other patient populations. Further, it would be logical to extend the less intensive warfarin protocol as designed for proximal DVT to investigations involving patients with PE.

## REFERENCES

1. Alpert, J. S., Smith, R., Carlson, C. J., et al.: Mortality in patients treated for pulmonary embolism. J.A.M.A., *236*:1477, 1976.
2. Dalen, J. E., Banas, J. S., Jr., Brooks, H. L., et al.: Resolution rate of acute pulmonary embolism in man. New Engl. J. Med., *280*:1194, 1969.
3. Barritt, D. W., and Jordan, S. D.: Anticoagulant drugs in the treatment of pulmonary embolism: A controlled trial. Lancet, *1*:1309, 1960.
4. Bauer, G.: Thrombosis: Early diagnosis and abortive treatment with heparin. Lancet, *1*:447, 1946.
5. Moore, F. D., Jr., Osteen, R. T., Karp, D. D., et al.: Anticoagulants, venous thromboembolism, and the cancer patient. Arch. Surg., *116*:405, 1981.
6. Marder, V. J., Soulen, R. L., Atichartakarn, V., et al.: Quantitative venographic assessment of deep vein thrombosis in the evaluation of streptokinase and heparin therapy. J. Lab. Clin. Med., *89*:1018, 1977.
7. The Urokinase Pulmonary Embolism Trial: A National Cooperative Study. Circulation, *47*:II–38, 1973.
8. Basu, D., Gallus, A., Hirsh, J., et al.: A prospective study of the value of monitoring heparin treatment with the activated partial thromboplastin time. New Engl. J. Med., *287*:324, 1972.
9. Deykin, D.: Regulation of heparin therapy. New Engl. J. Med., *287*:355, 1972.
10. Wilson, J. E. III, Bynum, L. J., and Parkey, R. W.: Heparin therapy in venous thromboembolism. Am. J. Med., *70*:808, 1981.
11. Andersson, G., Fagrell, B., Holmgren, K., et al.: Subcutaneous administration of heparin: A randomised comparison with intravenous administration of heparin to patients with deep-vein thrombosis. Thromb. Res., *27*:631, 1982.
12. Salzman, E. W., Deykin, D., Shapiro, R. M., et al.: Management of heparin therapy: Controlled prospective trial. New Engl. J. Med., *292*:1046, 1975.
13. Glazier, R. L., and Crowell, E. B.: Randomized prospective trial of continuous vs intermittent heparin therapy. J.A.M.A., *236*:1365, 1976.
14. Mant, M. J., O'Brien, B. D., Thong, K. L., et al.: Haemorrhagic complications of heparin therapy. Lancet, *1*:1133, 1977.
15. Wilson, J. R., and Lampman, J.: Heparin therapy: A randomized prospective study. Am. Heart J., *97*:155, 1979.
16. Sasahara, A. A., Sharma, G. V. R. K., McIntyre, K. M., et al.: A national cooperative trial of thrombolysis in pulmonary embolism: Phase I results of urokinase therapy. J. Louisiana State Med. Soc., *124*:130, 1972.
17. Tibbutt, D. A., Davies, J. A., Anderson, J. A., et al.: Comparison by controlled clinical trial of streptokinase and heparin in treatment of life-threatening pulmonary embolism. Br. Med. J., *1*:343, 1974.
18. Ly, B., Arnesen, J., Eie, H., et al.: A controlled clinical trial of streptokinase and heparin in the treatment of major pulmonary embolism. Acta Med. Scand., *203*:465, 1978.
19. Sharma, G. V. R. K., Burleson, V. A., and Sasahara, A. A.: Effect of thrombolytic therapy on pulmonary-capillary blood volume in patients with pulmonary embolism. New Engl. J. Med., *303*:842, 1980.
20. Fratantoni, J. C., Ness, P., and Simon, T. L.: Thrombolytic therapy: Current status. New Engl. J. Med., *293*:1073, 1975.
21. Marder, V. J.: The use of thrombolytic agents: Choice of patient, drug administration, laboratory monitoring. Ann. Intern. Med., *90*:802, 1979.
22. Bell, W. R., and Meek, A. G.: Guidelines for the use of thrombolytic agents. New Engl. J. Med., *301*:1266, 1979.
23. Sharma, G. V. R. K., Cella, G., Parisi, A. F., et al.: Thrombolytic therapy. New Engl. J. Med., *306*:1268, 1982.

24. Thrombolytic Therapy in Thrombosis: A National Institutes of Health Consensus Development Conference. Ann. Intern. Med., *93*:141, 1980.
25. Marder, V. J.: Are we using fibrinolytic agents often enough? Ann. Intern. Med., *93*:136, 1980.
26. Schrier, S. L.: Thrombolytic therapy. Ann. Intern. Med., *93*:629, 1980.
27. Sasahara, A. A.: The case for fibrinolytic therapy. J. Cardiovasc. Med., *5*:794, 1980.
28. Dalen, J. E.: The case against fibrinolytic therapy. J. Cardiovasc. Med., *5*:799, 1980.
29. Robertson, B. R., Nilsson, I. M., and Nylander, G.: Value of streptokinase and heparin in treatment of acute deep venous thrombosis: A coded investigation. Acta Chir. Scand., *134*:203, 1968.
30. Kakkar, V. V., Flanc, C., Howe, C. T., et al.: Treatment of deep vein thrombosis. A trial of heparin, streptokinase, and arvin. Br. Med. J., *1*:806, 1969.
31. Robertson, B. R., Nilsson, I. M., and Nylander, G.: Thrombolytic effect of streptokinase as evaluated by phlebography of deep venous thrombi of the leg. Acta Chir. Scand., *136*:173, 1970.
32. Tsapogas, M. J., Peabody, R. A., Wu, K. T., et al.: Controlled study of thrombolytic therapy in deep vein thrombosis. Surgery, *74*:973, 1973.
33. Porter, J. M., Seaman, A. J., Common, H. H., et al.: Comparison of heparin and streptokinase in the treatment of venous thrombosis. Am. Surg., *41*:511, 1975.
34. Elliot, M. S., Immelman, E. J., Jeffery, P., et al.: A comparative randomized trial of heparin versus streptokinase in the treatment of acute proximal venous thrombosis: An interim report of a prospective trial. Br. J. Surg., *66*:838, 1979.
35. Goldhaber, S. Z., Buring, J. E., Lipnick, R. J., et al.: Pooled analyses of randomized trials of streptokinase and heparin in phlebographically documented acute deep venous thrombosis. Am. J. Med., *76*:393, 1984.
36. Wiman, B., and Collen, D.: Molecular mechanism of physiological fibrinolysis. Nature, *272*:549, 1978.
37. Collen, D.: On the regulation and control of fibrinolysis. Edward Kowalski Memorial Lecture. Thromb. Haemost., *43*:77, 1980.
38. Rijken, D. C., and Collen, D.: Purification and characterization of the plasminogen activator secreted by human melanoma cells in culture. J. Biol. Chem., *256*:7035, 1981.
39. Collen, D., Rijken, D. C., van Damme, J., et al.: Purification of human tissue-type plasminogen activator in centigram quantities from human melanoma cell culture fluid and its conditioning for use in vivo. Thromb. Haemost., *48*:294, 1982.
40. Pennica, D., Holmes, W. E., Kohr, W. J., et al.: Cloning and expression of human tissue-type plasminogen activator cDNA in *E. coli*. Nature, *301*:214, 1983.
41. Korninger, C., Stassen, J. M., and Collen, D.: Turnover of human extrinsic (tissue-type) plasminogen activator in rabbits. Thromb. Haemost., *46*:658, 1981.
42. Van de Werf, F., Bergmann, S. R., Fox, K. A. A., et al.: Coronary thrombolysis with human tissue-type plasminogen activator produced by recombinant DNA technology. Circulation, *68*:III-185, 1983 (abstract).
43. Gold, H. K., Fallon, J. T., Yasuda, T., et al.: Coronary thrombolysis with recombinant human tissue plasminogen activator. Circulation, *68*:III–38, 1983 (abstract).
44. Bergmann, S. R., Fox, K. A. A., Rand, A. L., et al.: Recovery of metabolism and perfusion assessed with PET after coronary thrombolysis with plasminogen activator. Circulation, *68*:III–38, 1983 (abstract).
45. Bergmann, S. R., Fox, K. A. A., Ter-Pogossian, M. M., et al.: Clot-selective coronary thrombolysis with tissue-type plasminogen activator. Science, *220*:1181, 1983.
46. Bell, W. R., Simon, T. L., and DeMets, D. L.: The clinical features of submassive and massive pulmonary emboli. Am. J. Med., *62*:355, 1977.
47. Shuck, J. W., Walder, J. S., Kam, T. H., et al.: Chronic persistent pulmonary embolism: Report of three cases. Am. J. Med., *69*:790, 1980.
48. Sutton, G. C., Hall, R. J. C., and Kerr, I. H.: Clinical course and late prognosis of treated subacute massive, acute minor, and chronic pulmonary thromboembolism. Br. Heart J., *39*:1135, 1977.
49. Moser, K. M., Spragg, R. G., Utley, J., et al.: Chronic thrombotic obstruction of major pulmonary arteries: Results of thromboendarterectomy in 15 patients. Ann. Intern. Med., *99*:299, 1983.
50. Hughes, R. L., Mann, S., Smith, L. H., et al.: Recurring pulmonary emboli: Clinical conference in pulmonary disease from Northwestern University Medical School, Chicago. Chest, *81*:230, 1982.
51. Hull, R., Carter, C. J., Jay, R. M, et al.: The diagnosis of acute, recurrent, deep-vein thrombosis: A diagnostic challenge. Circulation, *67*:901, 1983.
52. Moser, K. M., and LeMoine, J. R.: Is embolic risk conditioned by location of deep venous thrombosis? Ann. Intern. Med., *94*:439, 1981.
53. Hull, R., Delmore, T., Genton, E., et al.: Warfarin sodium versus low-dose heparin in the long-term treatment of venous thrombosis. New Engl. J. Med., *301*:855, 1979.
54. Hull, R., Delmore, T., Carter, C., et al.: Adjusted subcutaneous heparin versus warfarin sodium in the long-term treatment of venous thrombosis. New Engl. J. Med., *306*:189, 1982.
55. Hull, R., Hirsh, J., Jay, R., et al.: Different intensities of oral anticoagulant therapy in the treatment of proximal-vein thrombosis. New Engl. J. Med., *307*:1676, 1982.
56. Bell, W. R., Tomasulo, P. A., Alving, B. M., et al.: Thrombocytopenia occurring during the administration of heparin: A prospective study in 52 patients. Ann. Intern. Med., *85*:155, 1976.
57. Cines, D. B., Kaywin, P., Bina, M., et al.: Heparin-associated thrombocytopenia. New Engl. J. Med., *303*:788, 1980.
58. Bell, W. R., and Royall, R. M.: Heparin-associated thrombocytopenia: A comparison of three heparin preparations. New Engl. J. Med., *303*:902, 1980.
59. Gurewich, V.: Managing anticoagulant therapy during pregnancy. J. Cardiovasc. Med., *9*:131, 1984.
60. Strandness, D. E., Jr., Langlois, Y., Cramer, M., et al.: Long-term sequelae of acute venous thrombosis. J.A.M.A., *250*:1289, 1983.
61. Taheri, S. A., Lazar, L., Elias, S. M., et al.: Vein valve transplant. Surgery, *91*:28, 1982.
62. Taheri, S. A., Lazar, L., and Elias, S.: Status of vein valve transplant after 12 months. Arch. Surg., *117*:1313, 1982.
63. Swinton, N. W., Jr., Edgett, J. W., Jr., and Hall, R. J.: Primary subclavian-axillary vein thrombosis. Circulation, *38*:737, 1968.
64. Tilney, N. L., Griffiths, H. J. G., and Edwards, E. A.: Natural history of major venous thrombosis of the upper extremity. Arch. Surg., *101*:792, 1970.

65. Campbell, C. B., Chandler, J. G., Tegtmeyer, C. J., et al.: Axillary, subclavian, and brachiocephalic vein obstruction. Surgery, *82*:816, 1977.
66. Prescott, S. M., and Tikoff, G.: Deep venous thrombosis of the upper extremity: A reappraisal. Circulation, *59*:350, 1979.
67. Urokinase Pulmonary Embolism Trial Study Group: Urokinase-streptokinase embolism trial: Phase 2 results. J.A.M.A., *229*:1606, 1974.
68. Gore, J. M., Appelbaum, J. S., Greene, H. L., et al.: Occult cancer in patients with acute pulmonary embolism. Ann. Intern. Med., *96*:556, 1982.
69. Goldberg, R. J., Seneff, M., Gore J. M., et al.: Association between deep venous thrombosis and occult malignancy. (Personal communication)
70. Greenberg, E., Divertie, M. B., and Woolner, L. B.: A review of unusual systemic manifestations associated with carcinoma. Am. J. Med., *36*:106, 1964.
71. Lieberman, J. S., Borrero, J., Urdaneta, E., et al.: Thrombophlebitis and cancer. J.A.M.A., *177*:542, 1961.
72. Van de Werf, F., Bergmann, S. R., Fox, K. A. A., et al.: Coronary thrombolysis in dogs with intravenously administered human tissue-type plasminogen activator produced by recombinant DNA technology. Circulation, *69*:605, 1984.
73. Van de Werf, F., Ludbrook, P. A., Bergmann, S. R., et al.: Coronary thrombolysis with tissue-type plasminogen activator in patients with evolving myocardial infarction. New Engl. J. Med., *310*:609, 1984.
74. Van de Werf, F., Bergmann, S. R., Fox, K. A. A., et al.: Coronary thrombolysis with intravenously administered human tissue–type plasminogen activator produced by recombinant DNA technology. Circulation, *69*:605, 1984.
75. Marder, V. J., Butler, F. O., and Barlow, G. H.: Antifibrinolytic therapy. *In* Colman, R. W., Hirsh, J., J. Marder, V. J., et al. (Eds.): Hemostasis and Thrombosis: Basic Principles and Clinical Practice. J. B. Lippincott Co., Philadelphia, 1982, p. 644.

CHAPTER 8

# PREVENTION OF VENOUS THROMBOEMBOLISM

SAMUEL Z. GOLDHABER, M.D.

Clearly, prevention of deep venous thrombosis (DVT) and pulmonary embolism (PE) is preferable to treatment of these conditions. In general, the focus has been on in-hospital prophylaxis, because immobilized and postoperative patients are particularly susceptible to DVT, and this setting is most suitable for carrying out prophylactic measures. Although DVT is frequent among patients hospitalized for medical problems such as myocardial infarction, congestive heart failure, and stroke, the prevention of postoperative DVT and PE has been much more thoroughly investigated than has prophylaxis among medical patients. Important advances have been made in achieving prophylaxis in the general surgical population. Yet the complications of DVT and PE remain particularly vexing for patients undergoing orthopedic surgery, especially operations on the hip.

This chapter will survey the frequency of DVT and PE with and without pharmacologic prophylactic measures, such as low-dose heparin, antiplatelet agents, and dextran, and nonpharmacologic measures, such as the use of graded compression stockings or the intermittent compression or electrical stimulation of calf muscles. Studies on the prevention of postoperative venous thromboembolism will be reviewed first, followed by a discussion of studies of DVT and PE in medical patients. In most of these studies, the focus is on DVT rather than on PE, probably because DVT occurs much more frequently and can—even without PE—be an important source of morbidity due to chronic venous insufficiency with its attendant leg pain, swelling, and, ultimately, ulceration.

When reviewing any study of DVT, one should surmise carefully the method used to identify patients with this condition. For example, $^{125}$I-labeled fibrinogen leg scanning is a highly sensitive test for detecting calf vein thrombosis but is relatively insensitive for detecting the clinically more important proximal thigh and pelvic vein thrombi, which are much more likely to embolize to the lungs than are calf vein thrombi. Phlebography remains the most accurate means of diagnosing DVT.

The tables in this chapter cite trials that vary greatly in quality. Although some trials were randomized, others were not. Because of the diversity in study designs, the results of these investigations are not meant to be pooled; rather, they have been included to provide an overview of the literature concerning the prevention of DVT and PE.

## POSTOPERATIVE PROPHYLAXIS OF NONORTHOPEDIC PATIENTS

### Low-Dose Heparin

Low-dose heparin enhances the activity of antithrombin III, a substance that inactivates the small amount of factor Xa required to trigger the conversion of prothrombin to thrombin. Thus, in the absence of active thrombosis, a small amount of heparin-enhanced antithrombin III activity may prevent the generation of thrombin. However, when thrombosis is active, thrombin generation cannot be prevented by low-dose heparin. (Details of the mechanisms and utilization of heparin were described in Chapters 3 and 6, respectively.)

## Prevention of Postoperative DVT

In the early 1970s, many studies demonstrated the efficacy of low-dose subcutaneous heparin in preventing postoperative DVT after nonorthopedic surgery (Table 8–1). In these trials, DVT was diagnosed by means of leg scanning with $^{125}$I-labeled fibrinogen. For example, in 1972, Kakkar and coworkers published the results of a double-blind, randomized trial involving 78 patients over the age of 40 years who underwent major nonorthopedic surgery.[1] Treatment consisted of 5000 units of calcium heparin injected subcutaneously two hours before operation and every 12 hours thereafter for seven days. The control patients received a placebo solution

***Table 8–1.*** Thromboprophylactic Effect of Low-Dose Heparin in Nonorthopedic Surgery*

| Reference | Patient Population | Number of Patients | Frequency of Thrombosis (%) *Controls* | *Low-Dose Heparin* | Significance |
|---|---|---|---|---|---|
| Abernethy and Hartsuck[4] | General surgery | 125 | 5 | 6 | NS |
| Ansay et al.[5] | General surgery | 50 | 63 | 26 | $p < 0.05$ |
| Ballard et al.[6] | Gynecology | 110 | 29 | 4 | $p < 0.01$ |
| Bergqvist and Hallböök[7] | General surgery | 97 | 27 | 13 | $p < 0.05$ |
| Cerrato et al.[8] | Neurosurgery | 100 | 34 | 6 | $p < 0.005$ |
| Clarke-Pearson et al.[9] | Gynecologic malignancy | 185 | 12 | 15 | NS |
| Coe et al.[10] | Urology | 52 | 25 | 21 | NS |
| Covey et al.[11] | General surgery | 105 | 10 | 8 | NS |
| Gallus et al.[2] | General surgery | 209 | 15 | 1 | $p < 0.001$ |
| Gallus et al.[12] | General surgery | 782 | 16 | 4 | $p < 0.05$ |
| Gordon-Smith et al.[13] | General surgery | 150 | 42 | 14[a] | $p < 0.003$ |
| | | | | 8[b] | $p < 0.001$ |
| Groote Schuur Hosp.[14] | Abdominal surgery | 199 | 27 | 12 | $p < 0.007$ |
| Gruber et al.[15] | General surgery | 194 | 36 | 13 | $p < 0.005$ |
| Hedlund and Blombäck[16] | Urology | 59 | 46 | 21 | NS |
| Int. Multicentre Trial[17] | General surgery | 1292 | 25 | 8 | $p < 0.005$ |
| Jackaman et al.[18] | Thorax surgery | 183 | 51 | 28 | $p < 0.005$ |
| Joffe[19] | General surgery | 120 | 51 | 9 | $p < 0.0005$ |
| Kakkar et al.[1] | General surgery | 78 | 42 | 8 | $p < 0.001$ |
| Kettunen et al.[20] | General surgery | 200 | 41 | 8 | $p < 0.001$ |
| Kraytman et al.[21] | General surgery | 50 | 63 | 26 | $p < 0.05$ |
| Kutnowski et al.[22] | Urology | 47 | 36 | 9 | $p < 0.05$ |
| Lahnborg et al.[3] | Abdominal surgery | 112 | 20 | 5 | $p < 0.05$ |
| Lawrence et al.[23] | Abdominal surgery | 242 | 17 | 7 | $p < 0.05$ |
| Multi-Unit Contr. Trial[24] | General surgery | 160 | 43 | 15 | $p < 0.05$ |
| | Gynecology | 55 | 14 | 0 | $p < 0.05$ |
| | Thorax surgery | 38 | 44 | 15 | $p < 0.05$ |
| Nicolaides et al.[25] | General surgery | 251 | 24 | 1 | $p < 0.0001$ |
| Plante et al.[26] | General surgery | 108 | 21 | 7 | $p < 0.05$ |
| Rem et al.[27] | General surgery, urology | 178 | 36 | 13 | $p < 0.001$ |
| Rosenberg et al.[28] | General surgery | 154 | 44 | 7 | $p < 0.001$ |
| Sebeseri et al.[29] | Urology | 65 | 58 | 12 | $p < 0.01$ |
| Strand et al.[30] | General surgery | 100 | 20 | 6 | $p < 0.05$ |
| Taberner et al.[31] | Gynecology | 57 | 23 | 6 | $p < 0.05$ |
| Törngren and Forsberg[32] | Abdominal surgery | 124 | 33 | 16 | $p < 0.05$ |
| Williams[33] | Abdominal surgery | 44 | 33 | 0 | $p < 0.02$ |
| Wu et al.[34] | Abdominal surgery | 88 | 14 | 0 | $p < 0.01$ |

*The $^{125}$I-fibrinogen test was used to detect DVT.

[a]In total, three doses of low-dose heparin.

[b]Low-dose heparin for five days.

Modified from Bergqvist, D.: Postoperative Thromboembolism: Frequency, Etiology, Prophylaxis. Springer-Verlag, New York, 1983, p. 98.

of gelatin having the same consistency as the heparin. Randomization provided two groups of patients who were well-matched for age and other risk factors predisposing to DVT. Preoperative leg scanning was accomplished with $^{125}$I-fibrinogen and was repeated during the first 10 postoperative days. DVT was diagnosed if the counts at any site differed by 20% or more from those at an adjacent point on the same leg or at the same position on the opposite limb and if this difference persisted or increased within the next 24 hours. DVT developed in 17 of the 39 placebo-treated controls (42%) compared with only three of 39 heparin-treated patients (8 per cent) ($p<0.001$). No patient experienced PE.

These results in nonorthopedic surgical patients were gratifying. However, in the same study, an additional group of 50 consecutive patients with hip fractures was not randomized and all were treated with the same regimen of low-dose heparin prior to repair. DVT was diagnosed in 22 of these 50 orthopedic patients (44 per cent). In two of these 22 patients, DVT developed one to two days after heparin was discontinued. In the remaining 20 patients, DVT developed during the heparin regimen. Thus, low-dose heparin appeared to prevent DVT in nonorthopedic surgical patients but offered no apparent benefit to patients undergoing hip surgery. Excessive blood loss in the heparin-treated patients was not a major problem.

Gallus and coworkers[2] administered low-dose subcutaneous heparin every eight hours in a randomized study of 209 general surgical patients and achieved even better results in their treated group than did Kakkar and coworkers.[1] Both groups of investigators gave the first dose of subcutaneous heparin two hours preoperatively. Using $^{125}$I-fibrinogen leg scanning, Gallus and coworkers identified 16 patients (15 per cent) with DVT in the placebo group compared with only one patient (1 per cent) with DVT in the heparin group. With this more aggressive regimen (i.e., heparin every eight rather than every 12 hours), the patients treated with heparin had a significantly higher transfusion requirement (1635 vs. 1117 ml) and a slightly greater decrease in postoperative hematocrit (6.5 vs. 5.1%). However, excessive bleeding in the heparin-treated patients did not seem to be a clinically important problem.

These two studies[1, 2] and many others cited in Table 8–1 provide convincing evidence that low-dose subcutaneous heparin in nonorthopedic surgical patients can significantly reduce the frequency of DVT as assessed by fibrinogen scanning. However, the thrombi diagnosed by this method tend to localize in the calf rather than the thigh. Because calf vein thrombi are less likely to embolize to the lungs than thigh and pelvic vein thrombi,[181] the clinical implications of reducing calf vein thrombi are uncertain. The most important issue is whether low-dose subcutaneous heparin can reduce the frequency of PE—especially *fatal* PE—among postoperative patients.

### Prevention of Postoperative PE

Because PE is uncommon, a large-scale multicenter trial is needed to assess potential differences in mortality between treated patients and controls. For example, a single-institution study such as that by Lahnborg and coworkers[3] showed a significant reduction in *nonfatal* PE among 112 postoperative nonorthopedic patients treated with heparin compared with control subjects. The treatment regimen was 5000 units of subcutaneous sodium heparin two to five hours preoperatively followed by twice-daily administration for 4½ days. All patients underwent pre- and postoperative $^{125}$I-fibrinogen scanning and postoperative lung scanning. Of 54 controls, 19 (35 per cent) had isolated PE, with no DVT detected on $^{125}$I-fibrinogen scanning, whereas only eight of 58 heparin-treated patients (14 per cent) had isolated PE. No patient died during the trial.

It should be noted that the frequency of diagnosed PE was extremely high in both groups of patients, for which there are two possible explanations. First, the investigators who reviewed the lung scans may have "overcalled" PE in both groups of patients. (Criteria for positive lung scans were not stated; however, the radiologists did base their decisions on interobserver agreement.) Second, lung scanning was performed with $^{99m}$Tc-ferric hydroxide rather than the more commonly used $^{99m}$Tc-macroaggregated human serum albumin. It is conceivable that the former agent is associated with more perfusion defects than the more frequently employed macroaggregated albumin. Nevertheless, even in a study with an extremely high frequency of PE and with a significant reduction in *nonfatal* PE, no difference in *fatal* PE could be demonstrated because no patient died in either group. These results provide further rationale for a large-scale multicenter randomized trial of low-dose subcutaneous heparin to examine reduction in fatal PE as a primary endpoint.

Sagar and coworkers[35] conducted a multicenter randomized controlled trial of nonorthopedic surgery patients in which the primary endpoint was to determine whether prophylactic low-dose heparin decreased the frequency of postoperative fatal PE. Patients in the treatment group received 5000 units of sodium heparin subcutaneously two hours preoperatively and then every 12 hours for five days. There were eight deaths due to PE in the control group of 236 patients but none in the 264 heparin-treated patients ($p<0.01$). This study had two problems, however: (1) No definition of fatal PE was given; although 60 of the 66 patients who died from any cause in this study were autopsied, the number of patients autopsied among the eight who were classified as having died from fatal PE and the criteria for pathologic classification at autopsy were not stated. (2) The 4 per cent frequency of fatal PE among the 500 patients is much higher than would be expected among most populations of general surgical patients.

In a larger double-blind randomized study of 1296 patients, Kiil and coworkers[36] assessed the use of low-dose heparin for the prevention of postoperative DVT and PE. Treated patients received 5000 units of subcutaneous sodium heparin on the evening before surgery, followed by the same dose of heparin every 12 hours thereafter for seven days or until discharge, whichever was earlier. Among the 95 postoperative patients who died during the study, the autopsy rate was 82 per cent. Only massive PE judged by the pathologist to be the cause of death was classified as fatal PE. Nonfatal PE was diagnosed by either (1) a ventilation perfusion mismatch on lung scanning or (2) clinical symptoms of PE with phlebographically documented DVT. With regard to autopsy-proven fatal PE, no significant difference could be detected between treated and control patients. However, when the numbers of nonfatal and fatal PE are combined, the results in favor of low-dose heparin become more significant. Overall, 13 patients in the control group had fatal or nonfatal PE, compared with five patients in the heparin-treated group. Within the first postoperative week, nine control patients had fatal or nonfatal PE, compared with one patient in the heparin-treated group. Interestingly, there were more complications from bleeding in the control group. Thus, even in a study that recruited more than 1000 patients, a statistically significant difference in terms of preventing fatal PE could not be demonstrated.

### The International Multicentre Trial

The most comprehensive trial of low-dose heparin in postoperative prophylaxis against fatal PE was organized by Kakkar and is known as the International Multicentre Trial.[17] The results of this study, published in 1975, provide a foundation for current recommendations concerning postoperative prophylaxis. The study was carried out in 28 centers in a randomized controlled design. Eligible patients were over age 40 years and were scheduled to undergo elective major surgery. Those undergoing emergency surgery and those receiving anticoagulant therapy were excluded.

Patients in the treatment group received 5000 units of subcutaneous calcium heparin two hours preoperatively and every eight hours thereafter for seven days. If a patient was still confined to bed at the end of this period, the therapeutic regimen was continued until the patient became ambulatory. Control patients did not receive any specific prophylaxis. Thus, the study was neither single- nor double-blind. Randomization provided treatment and control groups that were well-matched for baseline characteristics.

Each center's pathologist was asked to record causes of death. Uniform criteria were established for determining that PE was the cause of death, i.e., if necropsy revealed massive fresh emboli in the pulmonary trunk, in the main pulmonary artery, or in at least two lobar arteries, *and* if no other possible cause of death was found. However, no group of pathologists reviewed all autopsy findings to make sure that these criteria were followed closely. Gruber and his colleagues from the University of Basel participated in the trial but subsequently criticized these criteria as being too narrow.[15] They believed that (1) multiple peripheral PE could also cause death and (2) PE that contributed to but did not primarily cause death should also be accounted for in the analyses.

Of 2076 patients in the control group, 100 died during the postoperative period, 72 per cent of whom were autopsied. Of 2045 patients in the heparin group, 80 died postoperatively, 66 per cent of whom were autopsied. Of the 72 autopsied control subjects, 16 died of PE; in contrast, only two of the 53 autopsied patients in the heparin group died of PE ($p<0.005$). With regard to patients who died with PE that was deemed at autopsy not to be the cause of death, six were from the control group and three from the heparin group. These data provide strong evidence for the efficacy of low-dose subcutaneous heparin in preventing fatal postoperative PE. Presumably, the mechanism involves prevention of DVT that would subsequently embolize to the lungs. To detect DVT, 10 of the 28 centers performed $^{125}$I-fibrinogen leg scanning on 667 control subjects and 625 heparin-treated patients. DVT was diagnosed in 25 per cent of the controls but in only 8 per cent of the heparin-treated patients ($p<0.005$). At autopsy, DVT was diagnosed in 24 controls and in six patients in the heparin group.

More bleeding occurred among heparin-treated patients. This seemed to be a cause of excess morbidity (117 wound hematomas in controls vs. 158 in heparin-treated patients) without causing an increase in the number of deaths due to hemorrhage (five controls vs. four heparin-treated patients).

Despite these powerful results, there are several valid criticisms of the International Multicentre Trial. First, neither the patients nor the physicians were blinded to treatment group. Second, the principle of "once randomized always analyzed" was not adhered to; 8 per cent of the patients who were entered into the trial were not followed. Third, no attempt was made to classify cause of death among nonautopsied patients.

In addition to these criticisms, two additional points should be noted: (1) Although 4 per cent of the patients in this trial underwent total hip replacement, no differences could be found between the two treatment groups (see Table 8–10); and (2) the total postoperative mortality was not significantly reduced among heparin-treated patients. Nevertheless, such a large-scale study is not likely to be repeated, and the results among general surgical patients appear to be valid, at least qualitatively. A more recent study investigating the efficacy of low-dose heparin in preventing both nonfatal and fatal PE has been hampered by the paucity of patients enrolled.[14] Thus, despite the limitations of the International Multicentre Trial, the results do appear to support the concept that low-dose heparin is effective in preventing postoperative fatal PE among patients undergoing elective general surgery.

After the publication of this trial, the use of prophylactic low-dose heparin in general surgical patients was endorsed by the Council on Thrombosis of the American Heart Association (AHA).[37] Based on the rate of fatal PE in the international trial, the Council stated that prophylactic fixed low doses of heparin might prevent fatal PE in 4000 general surgical patients annually.[38] The Council recommended a slightly less rigorous regimen of subcutaneous heparin: 5000 units every 12 hours instead of every eight hours. The specific recommendations are for patients over age 40 years and are shown in Table 8–2.

### Ultra-Low–Dose Intravenous Heparin

The discomfort of subcutaneous injections and the occasional associated increase in the frequency of wound hematomas prompted Negus and coworkers[39] to administer ultra-low–dose heparin in an attempt to prevent postoperative DVT in general surgical patients. These investigators had previously observed that intravenous heparin, in the ultra-low dose of 1 unit/kg/hour, reduced the postoperative increase in platelet adhesiveness to preoperative levels.[40] Therefore, they undertook a double-blind, randomized trial of 95 patients and compared sodium heparin (1 unit/kg/hour intravenously) with normal saline. The solutions were administered with constant infusion pumps. Infusion was started immediately after the induction of anesthesia and continued as long as the patient required intravenous fluid, within the limits of two to five days. DVT was diagnosed by $^{125}$I-fibrinogen leg scanning in 22 per cent of the saline-treated controls, compared with 4 per cent of the patients treated with ultra-low–dose intravenous heparin. Small wound hematomas occurred in two patients on heparin and in one on saline. There were no significant differences in postoperative bleeding or in blood transfusion requirements. This method of prophylaxis appears promising and merits further investigation.

### Dextran

Dextran is a glucose polymer produced when certain strains of bacteria react with sucrose. Originally, it was introduced for use as a plasma expander. It has also been used for thromboembolism prophylaxis because it reportedly impairs platelet function by caus-

***Table 8–5.*** Thromboprophylactic Effect of Compression Stockings

| Reference | Number of Patients | Type of Stocking | Method[a] | Frequency of Thrombosis (%) Controls | Treatment | Significance |
|---|---|---|---|---|---|---|
| Barnes et al.[b,c 64] | 18 | TED | A | 50 | 0 | $p = 0.029$ |
| Bolton[65] | 142 | TED | A | 38 | 12 | $p < 0.05$ |
| Browse et al.[66] | 90 | Tubigrip | B | 29 | 24 | NS |
| Holford[67] | 95 | TED | A | 49 | 23 | $p < 0.025$ |
| Ishak and Morley[d 68] | 76 | TED | A | 54 | 20 | $p < 0.01$ |
| Rosengarten et al.[70] | 50 | Tubigrip | A | 32 | 32 | NS |
| Scurr et al.[71] | 76 | TED | B | 37 | 11 | $p < 0.01$ |

[a]Method A: The study included two patient groups—one treated and one as control.
Method B: The study included one patient group, with one leg used as control. Armitage's sequential analysis was used for the statistical calculations.
[b]Ultrasound diagnosis.
[c]Barnes et al. have studied hip surgery patients.
[d]Phlebography used to establish diagnosis. Patients also received dextran 70 in an uncontrolled manner.
Modified from Bergqvist, D.: Postoperative Thromboembolism: Frequency, Etiology, Prophylaxis. Springer-Verlag, New York, 1983, p. 67.

periences represent a true increase in reaction frequency or only improved reporting. Examination of the manufacturing and testing records revealed no product aberrations. In the near future, the FDA is planning to launch an overall review of the indications for dextran therapy. Clinicians and pharmacists who encounter adverse reactions to dextran are encouraged to report their findings to the National Center for Drugs and Biologics, 8800 Rockville Pike, Bethesda, MD 20205; telephone (301) 443-5410.

One manufacturer has recently developed a very low molecular weight product known as dextran 1.[69] In clinical trials, administering 20 ml of dextran 1 intravenously 2 minutes before infusion of dextran 40 or 70 significantly decreased the incidence of *severe* (but not mild or moderate) adverse reactions. Dextran 1 will soon be distributed with dextran 40 and 70.

## Nonpharmacologic Prophylaxis

Because of potential adverse effects from pharmacologic postoperative prophylaxis of DVT and PE, there has been increasing use of nonpharmacologic postoperative prophylaxis. The three major methods of nonpharmacologic prophylaxis have been: (1) compression stockings (Table 8–5), (2) electrical stimulation of calf muscles (Table 8–6), and (3) intermittent compression of calf muscles (Table 8–7).

Evidence of the efficacy of standard elastic compression stockings (e.g., Tubigrip stockings) to prevent postoperative DVT has been conflicting. Although earlier studies that relied on a clinical diagnosis of DVT showed that these stockings had a favorable effect,[97–99] more recent studies utilizing $^{125}$I-fibrinogen scanning have not found that they provide a benefit.[66, 70] Because of the concern that

***Table 8–6.*** Thromboprophylactic Effect of Electrical Stimulation of Calf Muscles

| Reference | Number of Patients | Method[a] | Frequency of Thrombosis (%) Controls | Treated | Significance |
|---|---|---|---|---|---|
| Becker and Schampi[44] | 74 | A | 31 | 5 | $p < 0.01$ |
| Browse and Negus[72] | 110 | B | 21 | 8 | $p < 0.01$ |
| Dejode et al.[73] | 64 | B | 15 | 13 | NS |
| Lindström[63] | 77 | A | 30 | 14 | NS |
| Nicolaides et al.[74] | 116 | A | 22 | 2 | $p < 0.0003$ |
| Pollock et al.[75] | 229 | A | 41 | 32 | NS |
| Pollock[76] | 194 | A | 35 | 16 | $p < 0.05$ |
| Rosenberg et al.[28] | 139 | A | 44 | 28 | NS |

[a]Method A: The study included two patient groups—one treated and one as control.
Method B: The study included one patient group, with one leg used as control. Armitage's sequential analysis was used for the statistical calculation.
Modified from Bergqvist, D.: Postoperative Thromboembolism: Frequency, Etiology, Prophylaxis. Springer-Verlag, New York, 1983, p. 69.

***Table 8–7.*** Thromboprophylactic Effect of Intermittent Calf Muscle Compression

| Reference | Number of Patients | Pump Type* | Start of Pumping | Duration of Pumping | Frequency of Thrombosis (%) *Controls* | *Treated* | Significance | Comments |
|---|---|---|---|---|---|---|---|---|
| Browse et al.[77] | 100 | II | Preop. | Approx. 1 hour postop. | 34 | 24 | NS | General surgery, test group both dextran 70 and pump |
| Butson[78] | 119 | III | Intraop. | 24–48 h | 7.0 | 9.7 | NS | General surgery |
| Calnan and Allenby[79] | 100 | II | Intraop. | Intraop. | 30 | 12 | S | General surgery |
| Clark et al.[80] | 37 | II | Intraop. | 17–23 h | 20 | 0 | S | General surgery |
| Clarke-Pearson et al.[179] | 107 | III | Intraop. | 5 days | 35 | 13 | S | Gynecologic malignancy |
| Coe et al.[10] | 53 | III | Intraop. | Hospitalization | 25 | 7 | S | Urology |
| Collins et al.[81] | 94 | III | Intraop. | ≤ 17 days | 29 | 15 | S | Neurosurgery |
| Cranley et al.[82] | 195 | III | Postop. | ? | 12 | 9 | NS | Elective hip surgery, uncontrolled heparin administration |
| Gallus and Darby[83] | 78 | III | Intraop. | 7 days | 53 | 32 | NS | Elective hip surgery |
| Harris et al.[84] | 56 | III | Intraop. | 4–5 days | 30 | 50 | NS | Elective hip surgery, control group warfarin |
| Hills et al.[85] | 73 | II | Intraop. | Incl. day 1 | 39 | 3 | S | General surgery |
| Knight and Dawson[86] | 128 | II | Preop. | 24 hours | 32 | 14 | S | General surgery |
| Lee et al.[87] | 42 | III | Intraop. | Until ambulation | 39 | 0 | S | Hip joint surgery |
| Pedegana et al.[88] | 100 | III | Intraop. | 4 days | 17 | 0 | S | Elective hip surgery control group, elastic stocking |
| Roberts and Cotton[89] | 99 | I | Intraop. | Intraop. | 26 | 6 | S | General surgery in cancer patients |
| Roberts and Cotton[90] | 84 | I | Intraop. | Intraop. | 26 | 18 | NS | General surgery, control group both heparin and pump |
| Sabri et al.[91] | 39 | I | Intraop. | Intraop. | 28 | 5 | S | General surgery |
| Skillman et al.[92] | 95 | III | Intraop. | Hospitalization | 25 | 9 | S | Neurosurgery |
| Takkunen[93] | 70 | [a] | Intraop. | Intraop. | 13 | 14 | NS | General surgery |
| Turpie[94] | 128 | III | Postop. | 5 days | 19 | 2 | S | Neurosurgery |
| Turpie et al.[95] | 129 | [b] | Postop. | 14 days | 23 | 6 | S | Neurosurgery |
| Zelikovski et al.[96] | 43 | [c] | Intraop. | 24 hours | 50 | 4.3 | S | Neurosurgery |

[a]Angiomat. Each cycle = 10 sec with a frequency of 3 min; rapid inflation and rapid deflation; pressure 40 mm Hg.
[b]Rapid sequential inflation of a series of isolated segments; maximum pressure = 50 mm Hg maintained for 5 sec; rapid deflation.
[c]Sequential pump with four segments and a pressure of 50 mm Hg.
*I = Inflation at 8 mm Hg/sec to 40 mm Hg, followed by abrupt deflation (Parke, Davis and Co.); II = gradual inflation to 40 mm Hg for 1 min, followed by deflation for 1 min (Flowtron-Aire Ltd.); III = inflation to 40 mm Hg for 12 sec, followed by deflation for 48 sec (PED-90).
Modified from Bergqvist, D.: Postoperative Thromboembolism: Frequency, Etiology, Prophylaxis. Springer-Verlag, New York, 1983, p. 74.

standard elastic compression stockings might have a tourniquet effect that would actually promote stasis and DVT, a *graded elastic compression stocking* was developed. The most popular type is called a TED (*t*hromboembolism *d*eterrent) stocking. Pressure exerted by the TED stocking is graded: 18 mm Hg at the ankle, 14 mm Hg at mid-calf, 8 mm Hg in the popliteal region, 10 mm Hg at the lower thigh, and 8 mm Hg at the upper thigh. The stocking is manufactured in nine sizes and is classified in length as short, regular, and long and in circumference as small, medium, and large.[71] Most studies evaluating TED stockings for the postoperative prevention of DVT have yielded positive results (see Table 8–5). Nevertheless, although TED stockings appear to afford some protection, DVT still developed in 11 to 23 per cent of patients who wore them (excluding the study by Barnes and coworkers,[64] in which ultrasound was used to establish the diagnosis of DVT).

Some investigators have employed *electrical stimulation of calf muscles* in order to prevent DVT, with mixed results (see Table 8–6). Surface skin electrodes are placed over calf muscles, and muscle contraction is induced by repeated electrical stimulation. As might be expected, this method is impractical, and because of the associated discomfort, it cannot be used readily in the fully conscious patient.[100]

*Intermittent calf muscle compression* has become an increasingly popular method of nonpharmacologic prophylaxis of postoperative DVT. Most studies of this technique have shown a favorable effect in preventing postoperative DVT (see Table 8–7). However, the duration of compression, type of compression, and time when thrombi were diagnosed vary substantially among the different studies. Intermittent calf muscle compression is begun either at the time of surgery or in the immediate postoperative period (Fig. 8–1) and is continued until the patient is fully ambulatory. Some of these devices can be worn under partial plaster casts.[101] In nonorthopedic operations in which bleeding must be minimized (e.g., neurosurgery) or in which low-dose heparin has been used with mixed results (e.g., open prostatectomy), intermittent calf muscle compression may be the prophylactic method of choice.

## POSTOPERATIVE PROPHYLAXIS OF ORTHOPEDIC PATIENTS

### Fixed Low-Dose Heparin

Achieving effective prophylaxis against DVT and PE among orthopedic patients continues to be a vexing problem. These patients, especially those undergoing hip surgery, are more likely to develop DVT and PE than are general surgical patients. There is a high frequency of both DVT (Tables 8–8 and 8–9) and fatal PE (Table 8–10) regardless of whether the hip surgery is performed to repair a fracture or is elective. Orthopedic patients also appear to be more refractory to conventional low-dose heparin prophylaxis than general surgical patients. Even when the reduction in DVT is statistically significant among patients treated with low-dose heparin, the overall frequency of DVT among treated patients usually remains high (Table 8–11). For this reason, standard low-dose

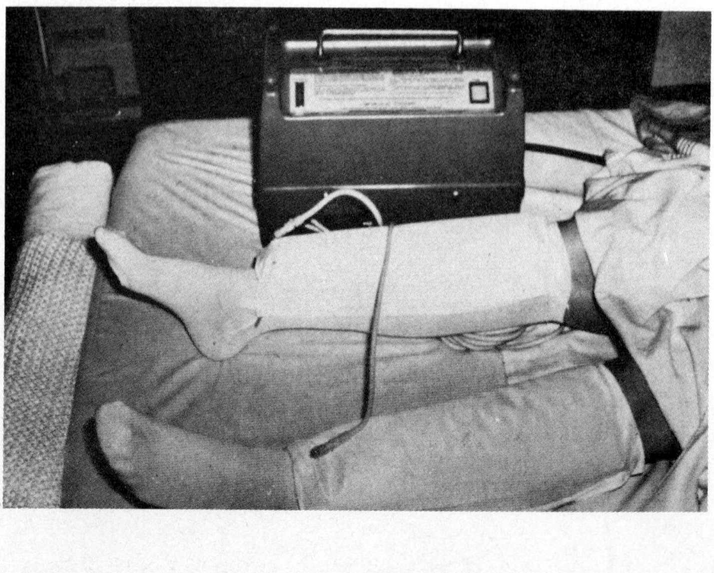

***Figure 8–1.*** Calf compressor designed to prevent thromboembolism. Inflatable stockings extending to just below the knee are fitted to both legs immediately after surgery. Inflation of a pneumatic bladder contained in a pouch inserted in the front and sides of each stocking allows intermittent compression of the calf by increasing circumferential tension on the stocking. In this particular model, an electrical compression pump inflates the bladder in the anterior pouch to achieve a skin pressure of 50 mm Hg over a period of five seconds. This pressure is maintained for an additional 15 seconds for a total inflation time of 20 seconds. The bladder is then deflated for 60 seconds. (Reprinted with permission from Hirsh, J.: Choosing the best of old and new ways to prevent venous thrombosis. J. Cardiovasc. Med., *6*:693, 1981.)

***Table 8–8.*** Frequency of DVT in Patients Who Underwent Surgery for Hip Fracture Without Prophylaxis*

| Reference | Time of Phlebography | Number of Patients | Number of Patients with DVT: *Total* | *Fractured Leg* | *Healthy Leg* |
|---|---|---|---|---|---|
| Ahlberg et al.[43] | 2–10 months | 45 | 16 | 16 | — |
| Borgström et al.[102] | 3–4 weeks | 23 | 13 | 13 | — |
| Culver et al.[103] | Within 4 weeks | 100 | 40 | 40 | — |
| Freeark et al.[104] | On average 12 days postoperatively | 70 | 29 | 29 | — |
| Hamilton et al.[105] | 5–12 days | 38 | 18 | 18 | 10 |
| Johnsson et al.[53] | Within 3 months | 25 | 13 | 13 | — |
| Myhre and Holen[55] | 21 days | 55 | 20 | 20 | — |
| Smyrnis et al.[106] | 6–10 days | 58 | 35 | 26 | 15 |
| Stevens et al.[107] | 9–21 days | 71 | ? | 21 | 13 |

*Diagnosis by phlebography.
Modified from Bergqvist, D.: Postoperative Thromboembolism: Frequency, Etiology, Prophylaxis. Springer-Verlag, New York, 1983, p. 17.

***Table 8–9.*** Frequency of DVT in Patients Who Underwent Elective Surgery of the Hip Without Prophylaxis*

| Reference | Time of Phlebography | Number of Patients | Number of Patients with DVT: *Total* | *Operated Leg* | *Healthy Leg* |
|---|---|---|---|---|---|
| Bergqvist et al.[108] | 21 days | 20 | 12 | 10 | 6 |
| Evarts and Feil[60] | 10 days | 56 | 30 | 30 | — |
| Soreff et al.[109] | 12–14 days | 14 | 5 | 5 | — |
| Stamatakis et al.[110] | ? | 160 | 81 | 81 | — |

*Diagnosis by phlebography.
Modified from Bergqvist, D.: Postoperative Thromboembolism: Frequency, Etiology, Prophylaxis. Springer-Verlag, New York, 1983, p. 18.

***Table 8–10.*** Frequency of Fatal Pulmonary Embolism in Patients Who Underwent Hip Surgery*

| Reference | Number of Patients | Number of Cases of Fatal PE | Reference | Number of Patients | Number of Cases of Fatal PE |
|---|---|---|---|---|---|
| ***Hip Fracture Surgery*** | | | ***Elective Hip Surgery*** | | |
| Ahlberg et al.[43] | 45 | 2 | Bergqvist et al.[45] | 71 | 2 |
| Barrie et al.[111] | 25 | 3 | D'Ambrosia et al.[121] | 99 | 1 |
| Borgström et al.[102] | 29 | 2 | Morris et al.[122] | 32 | 1 |
| Dolk and Westerborn[112] | 282 | 7 | Sagar et al.[123] | 32 | 1 |
| Edwards et al.[113] | 31 | 4 | Schöndorf[124] | 15 | 1 |
| Eskeland et al.[114] | 100 | 7 | | | |
| Galasko et al.[115] | 50 | 2 | | | |
| Hansen et al.[116] | 50 | 2 | | | |
| Morris and Mitchell[117] | 80 | 6 | | | |
| Moskovitz et al.[118] | 23 | 1 | | | |
| Myhre and Holen[55] | 55 | 2 | | | |
| Sevitt and Gallagher[119] | 150 | 15 | | | |
| Zekert et al.[120] | 120 | 8 | | | |

*Patients did not receive any form of prophylaxis against thromboembolism. The diagnosis is based on autopsy findings.
Modified from Bergqvist, D.: Postoperative Thromboembolism: Frequency, Etiology, Prophylaxis. Springer-Verlag, New York, 1983, p. 27.

***Table 8–11.*** Thromboprophylactic Effect of Low-Dose Heparin in Orthopedic Surgery*

| Reference | Number of Patients | Frequency of Thrombosis (%) *Control* | *Low-Dose Heparin* | Significance |
|---|---|---|---|---|
| ***Hip Fracture Surgery*** | | | | |
| Bergqvist et al.[45] | 50 | 91 | 63 | $p < 0.05$ |
| Checketts and Bradley[125] | 51 | 50 | 68 | NS |
| Galasko et al.[115] | 100 | 46 | 16 | $p < 0.001$ |
| Gallus et al.[2] | 46 | 48 | 13 | $p < 0.012$ |
| Lawrence et al.[23] | 50 | 48 | 0 | $p < 0.0005$ |
| Morris and Mitchell[126] | 48 | 67 | 50 | NS |
| Moskovitz et al.[118] | 51 | 39 | 41 | NS |
| Schöndorf[124] | 45 | 60 | 33 | NS |
| Xabregas et al.[127] | 100 | 48 | 0 | $p < 0.0005$ |
| ***Elective Hip Surgery*** | | | | |
| Bergqvist et al.[45] | 143 | 63 | 48 | NS |
| Dechavanne et al.[128] | 40 | 40 | 5 | $p < 0.025$ |
| Dechavanne et al.[129] | 54 | 48 | 7 | $p < 0.01$ |
| de Mourgues et al.[130] | 158 | 59 | 12 | $p < 0.001$ |
| Hampson et al.[131] | 100 | 54 | 46 | NS |
| Hume et al.[132] | 23 | 73 | 50 | NS |
| Lowe[133]† | 94 | 33 | 14 | $p < 0.05$ |
| Mannucci et al.[134] | 143 | 49 | 20 | $p < 0.005$ |
| Morris et al.[122]‡ | 59 | 50 | 11 | $p < 0.005$ |
| Moskovitz et al.[118] | 67 | 59 | 23 | $p < 0.003$ |
| Sagar et al.[123] | 57 | 69 | 32 | $p < 0.01$ |
| Venous Thromb. Clin. Study Group[135] | 64 | 37 | 7 | $p < 0.0046$ |
| ***Other Orthopedic Surgery*** | | | | |
| Abraham-Inpijn and Vreeken[136] | 25 | 46 | 8 | $p < 0.05$ |
| Gallus et al.[12] | 38 | 25 | 0 | $p < 0.05$ |
| Protoulis et al.[137] | 80 | 53 | 25 | $p < 0.01$ |

*All patients were screened for DVT with $^{125}$I-fibrinogen leg scanning, except for the study by Galesko et al., in which a combination of clinical diagnosis and phlebography was used.
†Dose individualized according to plasma heparin level.
‡Certain patients in both groups also received dextran.
Modified from Bergqvist, D.: Postoperative Thromboembolism: Frequency, Etiology, Prophylaxis. Springer-Verlag, New York, 1983, p. 100.

heparin prophylaxis is referred to in the recommendations issued by the Council on Thrombosis of the AHA as being "of limited value" for repair of femoral fracture and for hip and knee joint reconstruction.[37]

The trial by Sagar and coworkers[123] illustrates some of the benefits as well as limitations of low-dose heparin prophylaxis among orthopedic patients. The study population consisted of patients scheduled to undergo elective total hip replacement. Randomization to heparin prophylaxis or to the control group was carried out using sealed envelopes. Prior to surgery, all patients underwent $^{125}$I-fibrinogen leg scanning. Because this test is unable to differentiate between extracellular fibrin extravasation from the operative site and intravascular fibrin deposition due to thrombus formation, ascending phlebography was performed whenever a scan was found to be positive. All patients received routine physiotherapy. The low-dose heparin group received 5000 units of calcium heparin subcutaneously 2 hours preoperatively and then postoperatively every 8 hours for the next 10 days. The control group did not receive placebo injections; thus, neither patients nor staff members were blinded to treatment assignment. DVT developed in 22 of 32 controls (69 per cent) compared with eight of 25 of the treated patients (32 per cent) ($p<0.01$). There was no significant difference in blood loss or wound hematoma formation between the two groups. Thus, although the patients treated with low-dose heparin appeared to benefit from this form of prophylaxis, they still showed a high frequency of DVT (32 per cent).

After hip surgery, the use of fibrinogen leg scanning has been found to underestimate the true frequency of DVT as assessed by phlebography. Harris and coworkers[138] compared fibrinogen scanning and phlebography in 142 limbs of 83 patients without known prior DVT who underwent total hip replacement. With phlebography used as the standard, a positive fibrinogen scan in a site away from the hip wound was a highly sensitive test and represented a fresh thrombus in 25 of 29 patients (86 per cent). However, fibrinogen leg scanning failed to detect half of the venographically demonstrated thrombi. Of 51 fresh thrombi demonstrated on phlebography, only 25 were initially detected on the fibrinogen scan. In two studies[61, 139] of total hip replacement that required patients to undergo phlebography, no beneficial effect of fixed low-dose subcutaneous heparin was demonstrated. In an early study by Harris and coworkers,[61] 55 per cent of patients receiving low-dose heparin had phlebographically confirmed DVT, and in a later study by Kakkar and coworkers,[139] venographically proven DVT developed in 72 per cent of patients on low-dose heparin. However, regardless of whether the less sensitive fibrinogen leg scanning technique or the more accurate venographic technique is used, fixed low-dose heparin appears to confer little protection against DVT in orthopedic patients, even when the results achieve statistical significance (see Table 8–11).

### Adjusted Low-Dose Heparin

Despite the disappointing results with fixed low-dose heparin prophylaxis among orthopedic patients, the use of subcutaneous heparin prophylaxis is appealing because of its relative simplicity of application, low cost, and usual lack of serious adverse effects such as major hemorrhage. As early as 1960, Sharnoff and coworkers[140] utilized the concept of *adjusted* (rather than fixed) low doses of subcutaneous heparin, based on an individual's clotting time, to prevent DVT in patients with hip fracture. However, adjusted low doses of subcutaneous heparin did not gain widespread acceptance, probably because the extra laboratory work was perceived as cumbersome and because no controlled prospective trial had shown this approach to be effective. In 1982, Poller and coworkers[141] suggested that adjusted doses of subcutaneous heparin might provide more effective DVT prophylaxis than a fixed dosage schedule. They studied 55 patients undergoing hip fracture repair or elective total hip replacement and randomized these patients to a fixed dosage schedule of 5000 units subcutaneously every eight hours or to an adjusted dose regimen. Their goal in the latter group was to prolong the PTT to 50 seconds (the normal range observed in their laboratory being 38 to 45 seconds). There were 30 patients in the fixed-dose group, and fibrinogen leg scanning detected DVT in six. Of 25 patients in the adjusted-dose group, three developed DVT. Although this difference did not achieve statistical significance, it suggested that the adjusted dose approach merited further study.

In 1983, researchers from Lausanne, Switzerland, published a study with favorable results in which adjusted doses of subcutaneous heparin effectively prevented DVT after elective total hip replacement.[142] In this protocol, all patients were instructed to avoid aspirin and other nonsteroidal anti-inflammatory drugs for the two weeks prior to admission. Of 96 patients randomized, 17 were then excluded from the study or from the evaluation because of cardiac or respiratory failure, sepsis, protocol violations, or the patient's refusal to continue the study. Unfortunately, these patients were not included in end-point or follow-up evaluation. This approach runs counter to accepted clinical trial methodology in which a patient who is "once randomized" is then "always analyzed." Of the 79 patients remaining in the study, 41 were assigned to fixed low-dose subcutaneous heparin (3500 units every eight hours), and 38 patients received adjusted-dose subcutaneous heparin. Heparin prophylaxis began two days preoperatively. In the adjusted-dose group, PTT was measured two and six hours after the morning injection on the two preoperative days, when the patient left the operating room, and every two days postoperatively. Heparin dosage was increased when the six-hour postinjection PTT was less than 31.5 seconds and was decreased when this value was more than 36 seconds. The primary end-point of the study was prevention of DVT. All patients underwent venography of the operated leg between the 7th and 9th postoperative days, or sooner if clinical signs or symptoms suggested DVT. Those with DVT were treated with full heparinization followed by oral anticoagulation. Those with negative venograms received prophylactic oral acenocoumarol for two months. Administration of low-dose heparin to those without DVT was continued simultaneously with oral anticoagulation until the prothrombin time was in the 25 to 35% range (usually the 11th to 14th postoperative day).

DVT developed in 16 of the 41 patients who received fixed doses of heparin (39 per cent) but in only five of the 38 who received adjusted doses (13 per cent) ($p<0.01$). There were no significant differences between the two groups in total heparin dosage, blood loss, or incidence of wound hematomas. Of interest was that those given adjusted doses required increasingly larger amounts of heparin throughout the first postoperative week to maintain the PTT within the desired range. This suggests that hip surgery induces an increasingly hypercoagulable state in which greater and greater heparin doses are needed in the later postoperative period to reduce the risk of DVT. One major flaw of this study appears to be the exclusion of 17 patients from analysis after randomization. However, if these results can be confirmed by other investigators, adjusted subcutaneous heparin would seem worthwhile for prophylaxis against DVT during total hip replacement.[143]

### Dextran

Dextran (see Tables 8–3 and 8–4) has afforded limited success in studies of DVT prophylaxis among orthopedic patients. Many patients undergoing hip replacement are elderly and have cardiac dysfunction, and dextran can precipitate pulmonary edema in this patient population. Furthermore, dextran is associated with a high rate of allergic reactions. Overall, its use for DVT prophylaxis among orthopedic patients should be reserved for special situations in which other agents are considered too risky (e.g., warfarin) or relatively ineffective (e.g., aspirin in women).

### Aspirin

The results of aspirin prophylaxis against DVT among hip surgery patients have been mixed. In some instances, aspirin has failed to show any beneficial effect.[144] In other instances, the beneficial effect was limited to men.[145] Of concern is that even when aspirin does show a protective effect, the frequency of phlebographically diagnosed DVT among aspirin-treated patients remains high (17 per cent among men treated with aspirin in the 1977 study by Harris and coworkers[145]). More disturbing is the lack of consistency of a protective effect with aspirin, even when the same investigators study the problem. In 1982, Harris and coworkers[146] administered the same dose of aspirin (600 mg twice daily) to men undergoing total hip replacement as was used in their previous study.[145] Phlebographically diagnosed DVT occurred in 32 per cent of the men on this regimen. Thus, aspirin may provide some protection when compared with no drug therapy among controls. However, the high frequency of DVT noted among aspirin-treated men undergoing total hip replacement remains disconcerting.

### Warfarin

Warfarin has been used to prevent DVT in patients undergoing hip surgery.[55, 61, 105, 117, 132, 147–150, 183] Although this drug was effective in some studies,[55, 105, 117, 148] the frequency of DVT even in "successful" studies ranged from 9 to 31 per cent. Warfarin obviously has the potential disadvantage of precipitating major hemorrhage. In addition, frequent laboratory assay of the prothrombin time is necessary. Despite these drawbacks, in the patient at high risk for DVT or PE (e.g., a patient with prior DVT or PE), warfarin may be the most appropriate agent in the setting of hip surgery.

### Nonpharmacologic Methods

Among patients undergoing hip surgery, the use of graded compression stockings has had mixed results.[64, 68] Intermittent calf muscle compression has been found to have both a positive effect[87, 88] and no effect[82–84] in reducing the frequency of DVT. At this time, nonpharmacologic methods of DVT prophylaxis cannot be relied upon for hip surgery patients.

### Caval Interruption

Interruption of the inferior vena cava with a device such as the transvenous Kimray-Greenfield filter (see Chapter 10) should be considered in the high-risk orthopedic patient who is unable to tolerate anticoagulation. For instance, a patient with a prior PE and an active duodenal ulcer who needs repair of a hip fracture might be a suitable candidate for caval interruption.

## MEDICAL PATIENTS

Most studies of prophylaxis against DVT and PE have been conducted among postoperative patients. However, medical patients are also susceptible to these conditions. General medical patients are frequently immobilized for prolonged periods; those who have cancer are likely to be in a hypercoagulable state.

### Myocardial Infarction

The statistical technique of "pooling" (see Chapter 1 and Figure 1–1) has been used to demonstrate a reduction in mortality among myocardial infarction (MI) patients treated with systemic ("full") anticoagulation.[151] The results of some studies in which no reduction in mortality was observed may have appeared "negative" because of an inadequate sample size and the beta (or Type II) error.[152] Even among studies showing no difference in overall mortality, there was usually a reduction in the frequency of peripheral arterial and pulmonary embolization.[153–155] When interpreting these results, one should note that these trials were carried out at a time when routine hospitalization for MI lasted three weeks or longer. One could argue that such results are no longer valid in the current era of predischarge exercise testing and 10- to 12-day hospitalizations for patients with uncomplicated MIs.

In the late 1960s and early 1970s, systemic ("full") anticoagulation was studied primarily to determine whether such therapy would reduce the frequency of DVT. Heparinization appeared efficacious against DVT in both controlled[156, 157] and uncontrolled[158] studies. Similar beneficial results were found in most[2, 159–161] but not all[162] studies of fixed low-dose subcutaneous heparin.

With the renewed interest in thrombolytic therapy for MI patients,[163, 182] the issue of heparin anticoagulation to prevent DVT and PE has become a secondary concern. An increasing number of MI patients are being treated with intracoronary or intravenous thrombolytic agents. Both routes of administration produce a systemic lytic state. After cessation of thrombolytic therapy, the threat of restenosis within the coronary circulation has prompted the administration of systemic heparin. Thus, in an effort to lyse coronary thrombi and prevent their recurrence, systemic anticoagulation is being utilized with increasing frequency after thrombolytic therapy. On the basis of previous studies, one can expect the frequency of DVT and PE to diminish as the use of systemic anticoagulation becomes more widespread.

It is difficult to study DVT prophylaxis in immobilized patients with *unstable angina* because, in general, these patients are being stabilized expeditiously and will be referred promptly for cardiac catheterization and bypass surgery. Salzman and coworkers[164] abandoned a protocol to study such patients because "patient accession was insufficient." Nevertheless, they found some interesting trends that approached but did not attain statistical significance. Those patients treated with intermittent calf muscle compression or fixed low-dose heparin (5000 units subcutaneously every 12 hours) had fewer episodes of venous thromboembolism than did controls treated with graded compression stockings.

### Stroke

DVT during hospitalization for stroke is common[165] and can lead to PE.[166] The frequency of DVT can be reduced with low-dose subcutaneous heparin.[167] However, before instituting even low-dose heparin therapy, the physician should exclude the possibility of hemorrhage by means of computed tomography and, if warranted, lumbar puncture. For those patients found to have hemorrhagic stroke, intermittent calf muscle compression would appear useful based on results among neurosurgical patients.

Patients with spinal cord injury have been studied for DVT prevention with elastic stocking compression,[168] systemic anticoagulation,[169] and fixed low-dose heparin.[170, 171] These trials[168–171] have involved small numbers of patients and have not been randomized or controlled.

### General Medical Patients

A study of general medical in-patients, which excluded those with MI or stroke, demonstrated a 31 per cent reduction in mortality among the group treated with prophylactic fixed low-dose sodium heparin (5000 units subcutaneously every 12 hours).[172] This trial had two major limitations: (1) it was neither single- nor double-blind and (2) decisions regarding patient eligibility were open to bias, because treatment assignment was known by those who applied the exclusion criteria. Despite these drawbacks, the results were analyzed appropriately, according to the principle of "intention to treat."

## OTHER PROPHYLACTIC MODALITIES

### Dihydroergotamine

Dihydroergotamine is a parenterally administered potent venoconstrictor that affects arterial vessels only slightly. In combination with fixed low-dose heparin, dihydroergotamine has reduced the frequency of phlebographically proven DVT among hip surgery patients from 72 per cent (in the group treated with only fixed low-dose heparin) to 24 per cent (among those treated with both medications).[139] These favorable results need confirmation with additional studies.

### Ancrod

Ancrod is a defibrinating enzyme obtained from the Malayan pit viper. Because it reduces plasma fibrinogen, blood viscosity decreases. Randomized double-blind controlled trials using subcutaneous ancrod and saline placebo have demonstrated ancrod's efficacy in preventing DVT after hip surgery, with radiologic assessment by fibrinogen leg scanning[173] or phlebography.[174]

### Lidocaine

Lidocaine has been shown experimentally to inhibit adhesion of white blood cells to endothelium. Consequently, it was postulated that lidocaine might prevent endothelial damage after operative trauma to venous endothelium. To test this hypothesis, lidocaine or a control infusion of 5% dextrose was administered to 28 elective hip surgery patients in a randomized trial.[175] The loading dose of lidocaine was 1 mg/kg followed by a 2 mg/minute infusion for six days. This is the usual dose administered for ventricular arrhythmia prophylaxis during suspected acute MI. In the DVT prophylaxis study, all patients were assessed phlebographically. The study was terminated prematurely because of the striking difference in results between the two groups. On the 6th postoperative day, the frequency of DVT among controls was 78 per cent, compared with a 14 per cent frequency among lidocaine-treated patients. By the 14th postoperative day, eight days after cessation of lidocaine, the frequency of DVT among patients previously treated with lidocaine rose to 53 per cent. Thus, lidocaine appeared efficacious in preventing DVT among elective hip surgery patients. However, these results require further validation.

### Two-Step Warfarin Therapy

A two-step warfarin regimen has been described for use in patients undergoing elective total hip or knee replacement.[176] Ten to 14 days preoperatively, a low dose of warfarin was given to prolong the prothrombin time by 1.5 to 3.0 seconds compared with the control value. Immediately after surgery, the warfarin dose was increased to prolong the prothrombin time to 1.5 times the control. In a randomized controlled trial, the frequency of venographically documented DVT was 21 per cent among two-step warfarin patients, compared with 51 per cent among those treated with dextran 40 ($<0.005$). There was no difference in the frequency of bleeding between the two groups. Although the decrease in DVT was significant among warfarin-treated patients, a failure rate of 21 per cent is still substantial.

## RECOMMENDED APPROACH

Despite the multitude of studies that have been carried out, many aspects of DVT and PE prophylaxis remain unresolved. The most convincing results of effective prophylaxis have been seen among general surgical patients undergoing thoracic or abdominal operations. Certainly, postoperative prophylaxis for these patients would be cost effective.[177] Efforts at prophylaxis have been least successful among patients undergoing elective or emergency hip surgery. The least studied group of patients has been the general medical population.

Except for its application among orthopedic surgery patients, it appears that enthusiasm for DVT/PE prophylaxis has waned during the past decade. Many physicians, both medical and surgical, rely solely on early ambulation and graded compression stockings to prevent these complications. However, the dearth of diagnoses of DVT/PE may lead to a false sense of security, because in most patients, DVT and often PE will go undetected clinically unless these conditions are actively sought. Thus, an increasingly lax attitude toward prophylaxis is probably injudicious.

In order to recommend an approach to

prophylaxis, one can examine the studies conducted to date and make biologically plausible assumptions in situations in which uncertainty persists.[178] The summary table on this page presents an approach to DVT/PE prophylaxis that progresses from secure guidelines for general abdominothoracic surgery to reasonable conjecture for general medical patients. The reader is advised not to construe these recommendations as fiat. Each individual patient's risk for venous thrombosis must be weighed against the risks (most often bleeding) associated with a particular prophylactic maneuver.

The most carefully documented guidelines are those proposed by the AHA for thoracic and abdominal surgery patients. It is usually reasonable to combine the AHA recommendations for fixed low-dose subcutaneous heparin with the routine use of graded compression stockings. For patients at higher risk of thrombosis, the daily heparin dosage can be increased and intermittent calf muscle compression can be substituted for graded compression stockings. Although low-dose subcutaneous heparin can help prevent venous thromboembolism among general surgery patients, its acceptance has been limited somewhat by the unfounded fear that this approach induces a high rate of bleeding complications.[180]

For patients undergoing eye surgery, neurosurgery, or open prostatectomy, bleeding must be minimized and therefore the use of heparin is generally contraindicated. Intermittent calf muscle compression has been shown to be effective in preventing DVT among these surgical patients. Although the original devices were cumbersome and unsuited for routine use, newer devices are much less unwieldy and have become more acceptable to both patients and nursing staff.[180] For especially high-risk patients, dextran can be administered as well.

No prophylactic regimen has proven satisfactory for patients undergoing hip surgery. The administration of adjusted doses of subcutaneous heparin appears promising but

An Approach to Prophylaxis

| Type of Operation or Condition | Usual-Risk Patient | High-Risk Patient (e.g., Prior DVT or PE) |
|---|---|---|
| General abdominothoracic surgery | Fixed low-dose heparin, 5000 units SC q12h starting 2 hours preoperatively (per AHA guidelines) PLUS Graded compression stockings | Increase frequency of heparin dosage to 5000 units SC q8h. Substitute intermittent calf muscle compression for graded compression stockings |
| Eye or neurosurgery; open prostatectomy (N.B.: Bleeding must be minimized in these operations) | Intermittent calf muscle compression | (?) Add dextran |
| Hip surgery | (?) Adjusted doses of SC heparin (needs confirmation) OR (?) Aspirin in men (high failure rate of 17 to 32%) OR (?) Dextran (special situations only—see text) | Substitute warfarin OR Caval interruption |
| General (non-MI) medical patients, including nonhemorrhagic stroke (See text for discussion of MI patients) | Fixed low-dose heparin 5000 units SC q12h, PLUS Graded compression stockings | Increase frequency of heparin dosage to 5000 units SC q8h OR "Full" anticoagulation, with continuous infusion heparin overlapping with therapeutic doses of warfarin |
| Hemorrhagic stroke | Intermittent calf muscle compression | (?) Add dextran |

needs further study. Results with aspirin have been poor in women and, at best, mixed in men. Dextran reduces the frequency of DVT but may not be safer than warfarin. Thus, DVT prophylaxis in this group of patients must be investigated further. Despite insufficient evidence of its benefit, adjusted doses of subcutaneous heparin may be the most prudent option among usual-risk patients undergoing hip surgery. Warfarin should be considered for those orthopedic patients at particularly high risk for DVT or PE, such as those who have sustained prior episodes of venous thromboembolism. If warfarin cannot be tolerated, prophylactic caval interruption can be considered in high-risk patients.

Although few studies have been carried out among the general medical population, most of these patients would probably benefit from DVT prophylaxis with fixed low-dose heparin. Concomitant use of graded compression stockings poses no increased risk and would seem prudent. For medical patients at high risk, the total daily dose of subcutaneous heparin can be increased, if appropriate. However, some medical patients, such as those with hemorrhagic stroke, cannot tolerate any anticoagulation. Such patients are at risk for DVT and should generally receive prophylaxis similar to that for neurosurgical patients. This would usually entail intermittent calf muscle compression.

Despite our most zealous efforts at prophylaxis, DVT and PE will ensue in some instances. To minimize the adverse impact of these complications, constant vigilance is required to expedite accurate diagnosis and effective treatment.

## REFERENCES


1. Kakkar, V. V., Corrigan, T., Spindler, J., et al.: Efficacy of low doses of heparin in prevention of deep-vein thrombosis after major surgery: A double blind, randomized trial. Lancet, 2:101, 1972.
2. Gallus, A. S., Hirsh, J., Tuttle, R. J., et al.: Small subcutaneous doses of heparin in prevention of venous thrombosis. New Engl. J. Med., *288*:545, 1973.
3. Lahnborg, G., Bergstrom, K., Friman, L., et al.: Effect of low-dose heparin on incidence of postoperative pulmonary embolism detected by photoscanning. Lancet, *1*:329, 1974.
4. Abernethy, E. A., and Hartsuck, J. M.: Postoperative pulmonary embolism. A prospective study utilizing low dose heparin. Am. J. Surg., *128*:739, 1974.
5. Ansay, J., Fastrez, R., Kutnowski, M., et al.: Prévention des thromboses veineuses profondes postopératoires par l'héparine sous-cutanée à faibles doses. Ann. Chir., *31*:263, 1977.
6. Ballard, R. M., Bradley-Watson, P. J., Johnstone, F. D., et al.: Low doses of subcutaneous heparin in the prevention of deep vein thrombosis after gynaecological surgery. J. Obstet. Gynaecol. Brit. Commonw., *80*:469, 1973.
7. Bergqvist, D., and Hallböök, T.: Prophylaxis of postoperative venous thrombosis in a controlled trial comparing dextran 70 and low-dose heparin. World J. Surg., *4*:239, 1980.
8. Cerrato, D., Ariano, C., and Fiacchino, F.: Deep vein thrombosis and low-dose heparin prophylaxis in neurosurgical patients. J. Neurosurg., *49*:378, 1978.
9. Clarke-Pearson, D. L., Coleman, R. E., Synan, I. S., et al.: Venous thromboembolism prophylaxis in gynecologic oncology: A prospective, controlled trial of low-dose heparin. Am. J. Obstet. Gynecol., *145*:606, 1983.
10. Coe, N. P., Collins, R. E. C., Klein, L. A., et al. Prevention of deep vein thrombosis in urological patients: A controlled, randomized trial of low-dose heparin and external pneumatic compression boots. Surgery, *83*:230, 1978.
11. Covey, T. H., Sherman, L., and Baue, A. E.: Low-dose heparin in postoperative patients. A prospective coded study. Arch. Surg., *110*:1021, 1975.
12. Gallus, A. S., Hirsh, J., O'Brien, S. E., et al.: Prevention of venous thrombosis with small, subcutaneous doses of heparin. J.A.M.A., *235*:1980, 1976.
13. Gordon-Smith, I. C., Grundy, D. J., Le Quesne, L. P., et al.: Controlled trial of two regimens of subcutaneous heparin in prevention of postoperative deep-vein thrombosis. Lancet, *1*:1133, 1972.
14. Groote Schuur Hospital Thromboembolus Study Group: Failure of low-dose heparin to prevent significant thromboembolic complications in high-risk surgical patients. Interim report of a prospective trial. Br. Med. J., *1*:1447, 1979.
15. Gruber, U. F., Duckert, F., Fridrich, R., et al.: Prevention of postoperative thromboembolism by dextran 40, low doses of heparin, or xantinol nicotinate. Lancet, *1*:207, 1977.
16. Hedlund, P. O., and Blombäck, M.: The effect of prophylaxis with low dose heparin on blood coagulation parameters. A double blind study in connection with transvesical prostatectomy. Thromb. Haemost., *41*:337, 1979.
17. An International Multicentre Trial: Prevention of fatal postoperative pulmonary embolism by low doses of heparin. Lancet, 2:45, 1975.
18. Jackaman, F. R., Perry, B. J., and Siddons, H.: Deep vein thrombosis after thoracotomy. Thorax, *33*:761, 1978.
19. Joffe, S.: Drug prevention of post-operative deep vein thrombosis. A comparative study of calcium heparinate and sodium pentosan polysulphate. Arch. Surg., *111*:37, 1976.
20. Kettunen, K., Poikolainen, E., Karjalainen, P., et al.: Prophylaxis of deep-vein thrombosis with small doses of subcutaneous heparin. (In Finnish). Duodecim, *90*:834, 1974.
21. Kraytman, M., Kutnowski, M., Ansay, J., et al.: Prophylaxie par l'héparine sous-cutanée à faibles doses des thromboses veineuses postopératoires. Acta Chir. Belg., *5*:519, 1976.
22. Kutnowski, M., Vandendris, M., Steinberger, R., et

al.: Prevention of postoperative deep-vein thrombosis by low-dose heparin in urological surgery. A double-blind, randomised study. Urol. Res., *5*:123, 1977.
23. Lawrence, J. D., Xabregas, A., Gray, L., et al.: Seasonal variation in the incidence of deep vein thrombosis. Br. J. Surg. *64*:777, 1977.
24. A multi-unit controlled trial: Heparin versus dextran in the prevention of deep-vein thrombosis. Lancet, *2*:118, 1974.
25. Nicolaides, A. N., Dupont, A. N., Desai, S., et al.: Small doses of subcutaneous sodium heparin in preventing deep venous thrombosis after major surgery. Lancet, *2*:890, 1972.
26. Plante, J., Boneu, B., Vaysse, C., et al.: Dipyridamole-aspirin versus low doses of heparin in the prophylaxis of deep venous thrombosis in abdominal surgery. Thromb. Res., *13*:399, 1979.
27. Rem, J., Duckert, F., Fridrich, R., et al.: Subkutane klein heparindosen zur thromboseprophylaxe in der allgemeinen chirurgie und urologie. Schweiz. Med. Wschr., *105*:827, 1975.
28. Rosenberg, I. L., Evans, M., and Pollock, A. V.: Prophylaxis of postoperative leg vein thrombosis by low dose subcutaneous heparin or preoperative calf muscle stimulation: A controlled clinical trial. Br. Med. J., *1*:649, 1975.
29. Sebeseri, O., Kummer, H., and Zingg, E.: Controlled prevention of post-operative thrombosis in urological diseases with depot heparin. Eur. Urol. *1*:229, 1975.
30. Strand, L., Bank-Mikkelsen, O. K., and Lindewald, H.: Small heparin doses as prophylaxis against deep-vein thrombosis in the major surgery. Acta Chir. Scand., *141*:624, 1975.
31. Taberner, D. A., Poller, L., Burslem, R. W., et al.: Oral anticoagulants controlled by the British comparative thromboplastin versus low-dose heparin in prophylaxis of deep vein thrombosis. Br. Med. J., *1*:272, 1978.
32. Törngren, S., and Forsberg, K.: Concentrated or diluted heparin prophylaxis of postoperative deep venous thrombosis. Acta Chir. Scand., *144*:283, 1978.
33. Williams, H. T.: Prevention of postoperative deep-vein thrombosis with perioperative subcutaneous heparin. Lancet, *2*:950, 1971.
34. Wu, T. K., Tsapogas, M. J., and Jordan, F. R.: Prophylaxis of deep venous thrombosis by hydroxychloroquine sulfate and heparin. Surg. Gynecol. Obstet. *145*:714, 1977.
35. Sagar, S., Massey, J., and Sanderson, J. M.: Low dose heparin prophylaxis against fatal pulmonary embolism. Br. Med. J., *4*:257, 1975.
36. Kiil, J., Kiil, J., Axelsen, F., et al.: Prophylaxis against postoperative pulmonary embolism and deep-vein thrombosis by low-dose heparin. Lancet, *1*:1115, 1978.
37. Council on Thrombosis of the American Heart Association: Prevention of venous thromboembolism in surgical patients by low-dose heparin. Circulation, *55*:423A, 1977.
38. Sherry, S.: Low-dose heparin prophylaxis for postoperative venous thromboembolism. New Engl. J. Med., *293*:300, 1975.
39. Negus, D., Friedgood, A., Cox, S. J., et al.: Ultralow dose intravenous heparin in the prevention of postoperative deep-vein thrombosis. Lancet, *1*:891, 1980.
40. Negus, D., Pinto, D. J., and Slack, W. W.: Effect of small doses of heparin on platelet adhesiveness and lipoprotein-lipase activity before and after surgery. Lancet, *1*:1202, 1971.
41. Hirsh, J., Genton, E., and Hull, R.: Venous Thromboembolism. Grune and Stratton, New York, 1981, p. 225.
42. Bergqvist, D.: Postoperative Thromboembolism: Frequency, Etiology, Prophylaxis. Springer-Verlag, New York, 1983, p. 129.
43. Ahlberg, Å., Nylander, G., Robertson, B., et al.: Dextran in prophylaxis of thrombosis in fractures of the hip. Acta Chir. Scand. [Suppl.], *387*:83, 1968.
44. Becker, J., and Schampi, B.: The incidence of postoperative venous thrombosis of the legs. A comparative study on the prophylactic effect of dextran 70 and electrical calf muscle stimulation. Acta Chir. Scand., *139*:357, 1973.
45. Bergqvist, D., Efsing, H. O., Hallböök, T., et al.: Thromboembolism after elective and posttraumatic hip surgery. A controlled prophylactic trial with dextran and low-dose heparin. Acta Chir. Scand., *145*:213, 1979.
46. Bonnar, J., and Walsh, J.: Prevention of thrombosis after pelvic surgery by British dextran 70. Lancet, *1*:614, 1972.
47. Carter, A. E., and Eban, R.: The prevention of postoperative deep venous thrombosis with dextran 70. Br. J. Surg., *60*:681, 1973.
48. Daniel, W. J., Moore, A. R., and Flanc, C.: Prophylaxis of deep vein thrombosis (DVT) with dextran 70 in patients with a fractured neck of the femur. Aust. N.Z. J. Surg., *41*:289, 1972 (abstract).
49. Harper, D. R., Dhall, D. P., and Woodruff, P. W. H.: Prophylaxis in iliofemoral venous thrombosis. The major amputee as a clinical research model. Br. J. Surg., *60*:831, 1973.
50. Hedlund, P. O.: Postoperative venous thrombosis in benign prostatic disease. A study of 316 patients using the I-125-fibrinogen uptake test. Scand. J. Urol. Nephrol. [Suppl.], *27*:1, 1975.
51. Hurson, B., Ennis, J. T., Corrigan, T. P., et al.: Dextran prophylaxis in total hip replacement: A scintigraphic evaluation of the incidence of deep vein thrombosis and pulmonary embolus. Ir. J. Med. Sci., *148*:140, 1979.
52. Huttunen, H., Mattila, M. A. K., Alhava, E. M., et al.: Preoperative infusion of dextran 70 and dextran 40 in the prevention of postoperative deep venous thrombosis as confirmed by the I-125-fibrinogen uptake method. Ann. Chir. Gynaecol., *66*:79, 1977.
53. Johnsson, S. R., Bygdeman, S., and Eliasson, R.: Effect of dextran on postoperative thrombosis. Acta Chir. Scand. [Suppl.], *387*:80, 1968.
54. Kline, A., Hughes, L. E., Campbell, H., et al.: Dextran 70 in prophylaxis of thromboembolic disease after surgery: A clinically oriented randomized double-blind trial. Br. Med. J., *2*:109, 1975.
55. Myhre, H. O., and Holen, A.: Thrombosis prophylaxis. Dextran or sodium warfarin? A clinical study. (In Norwegian). Nord. Med., *82*:1534, 1969.
56. Renney, J. T. G., Kakkar, V. V., and Nicolaides, A. N.: The prevention of postoperative deep vein thrombosis, comparing dextran-70 and intensive physiotherapy. Br. J. Surg., *57*:388, 1979 (abstract).
57. Sechas, M., Papachristodoulou, A., Mandalaki, T., et al.: Prophylaxis of postoperative venous thrombosis of the lower extremities. *In* Louros, N. C., and Le Vay, D. (Eds.): Proceedings of the Biennial World Congress of the International College of Surgeons. Excerpta Medica, Amsterdam-Oxford, 1977, p. 946.

58. Stephenson, C. B. S., Wallace, J. C., and Vaughan, J. V.: Dextran 70 in the prevention of postoperative deep-vein thrombosis with observations on pulmonary embolism: Report on a pilot study. N.Z. Med J., *77*:302, 1973.
59. Bergman, B., Bergqvist, D., and Dahlgren, S.: The incidence of venous thrombosis in the lower limbs following elective gallbladder surgery. A study with the I-125-fibrinogen test. Upsala J. Med. Sci., *80*:41, 1975.
60. Evarts, C. M., and Feil, E. J.: Prevention of thromboembolic disease after elective surgery in the hip. J. Bone Joint Surg. [Am.], *53*:1271, 1971.
61. Harris, W. H., Salzman, E., Athanasoulis, C., et al.: Comparison of warfarin, low-molecular-weight dextran, aspirin, and subcutaneous heparin in prevention of venous thromboembolism following total hip replacement. J. Bone Joint Surg. [Am.], *56*:1552, 1974.
62. Hutter, O., Duckert, F., Fridrich, R., et al.: Dextran 40 zur prophylaxe tiefer venenthrombosen in der chirurgie. Dtsch. Med. Wschr., *101*:1834, 1976.
63. Lindström, B.: On the prophylaxis of postoperative thromboembolism in general surgery. The importance of venous pooling in the calves. Thesis, University of Göteborg, 1982. Cited in Bergqvist, D.: Postoperative Thromboembolism: Frequency, Etiology, Prophylaxis. Springer-Verlag, New York, 1983.
64. Barnes, R. W., Brand, R. A., Clarke, W., et al.: Efficacy of graded-compression antiembolism stockings in patients undergoing total hip arthroplasty. Clin. Orthop. Rel. Res., *132*:61, 1978.
65. Bolton, J.: The prevention of post-operative deep venous thrombosis by graduated compression stockings. Scot. Med. J., *23*:333, 1978.
66. Browse, N. L., Jackson, B. T., Mayo, M. E., et al.: The value of mechanical methods of preventing postoperative calf vein thrombosis. Br. J. Surg., *61*:219, 1974.
67. Holford, C. P.: Graded compression for preventing deep venous thrombosis. Br. Med. J., *2*:969, 1976.
68. Ishak, M. A., and Morley, K. D.: Deep venous thrombosis after total hip arthroplasty: A prospective controlled study to determine the prophylactic effect of graded pressure stockings. Br. J. Surg., *68*:429, 1981.
69. Users reminded about adverse reactions to dextran. FDA Drug Bulletin, *13*:23, 1983.
70. Rosengarten, D. S., and Laird, J.: The effect of leg elevation on the incidence of deep vein thrombosis after operation. Br. J. Surg., *58*:182, 1971.
71. Scurr, J. H., Ibrahim, S. Z., Faber, R. G., et al.: The efficacy of graduated compression stockings in the prevention of deep vein thrombosis. Br. J. Surg., *64*:371, 1977.
72. Browse, N. L., and Negus, D.: Prevention of postoperative leg vein thrombosis by electrical muscle stimulation. An evaluation with I-125-fibrinogen. Br. Med. J., *3*:615, 1970.
73. Dejode, L. R., Khurshid, M., and Walther, W. W.: The influence of electrical stimulation of the leg during surgical operations on the subsequent development of deep-vein thrombosis. Br. J. Surg., *60*:31, 1973.
74. Nicolaides, A. N., Kakkar, V. V., Field, E. S., et al.: Soleal veins, stasis and prevention of deep vein thrombosis. *In* Kakkar, V. V., and Jouhar, A. J. (Eds.): Thromboembolism: Diagnosis and treatment. Churchill Livingstone, London, 1972, p. 56.
75. Pollock, A. V., Rosenberg, I. L., and Evans, M.: Prevention of postoperative leg vein thrombosis: A comparison of low-dose heparin and electrical calf stimulation. *In* Kakkar, V. V., and Thomas, D. P. (Eds.): Heparin. Chemistry and Clinical Usage. Academic Press, London, 1976, p. 349.
76. Pollock, A. V.: Calf-muscle stimulation as a prophylactic method against deep vein thrombosis. Triangle, *16*:41, 1977.
77. Browse, N. L., Clemenson, G., Bateman, N. T., et al.: Effect of intravenous dextran 70 and pneumatic leg compression on incidence of postoperative pulmonary embolism. Br. Med. J., *2*:1281, 1976.
78. Butson, A. R. C.: Intermittent pneumatic calf compression for prevention of deep venous thrombosis in general abdominal surgery. Am. J. Surg., *142*:525, 1981.
79. Calnan, J. S., and Allenby, F.: The prevention of deep vein thrombosis after surgery. Br. J. Anaesth., *47*:151, 1975.
80. Clark, W. B., MacGregor, A. B., Prescott, R. J., et al.: Pneumatic compression of the calf and postoperative deep vein thrombosis. Lancet, *2*:5, 1974.
81. Collins, R., Coe, N., Goldstein, E., et al.: External pneumatic compression of the legs to prevent venous thromboembolism in neurosurgical patients. Thromb. Haemost., *38*:196, 1977 (abstract).
82. Cranley, J. J., Canos, A. J., and Mahalingam, K.: Noninvasive diagnosis and prophylaxis of deep venous thrombosis of the lower extremities. *In* Madden, J., and Hume, M. (Eds.): Venous Thromboembolism. Prevention and Treatment. Appleton-Century-Crofts, New York, 1976, p. 131.
83. Gallus, A., and Darby, T.: Intermittent calf compression; a randomized trial in elective hip replacement. Thromb. Haemost., *46*:93, 1981 (abstract).
84. Harris, W. H., Raines, J. K., Athanasoulis, C., et al.: External pneumatic compression versus warfarin in reducing thrombosis in high-risk patients. *In* Madden, J., and Hume, M. (Eds.): Venous Thromboembolism. Prevention and Treatment. Appleton-Century-Crofts, New York, 1976, p. 51.
85. Hills, N. H., Pflug, J. J., Jeyasingh, K., et al.: Prevention of deep vein thrombosis by intermittent pneumatic compression of calf. Br. Med. J., *1*:131, 1972.
86. Knight, M. T. N., and Dawson, R.: Effect of intermittent compression of the arms on deep venous thrombosis in the legs. Lancet, *2*:1265, 1976.
87. Lee, B. Y., Trainer, F. S., Kavner, D., et al.: Noninvasive prevention of thrombosis of deep veins of the thigh using intermittent pneumatic compression. Surg. Gynecol. Obstet., *142*:705, 1976.
88. Pedegana, L. R., Burgess, E. M., Moore, A. J., et al.: Prevention of thromboembolic disease by external pneumatic compression in patients undergoing total hip arthroplasty. Clin. Orthop. Rel. Res., *128*:190, 1977.
89. Roberts, V. C., and Cotton, L. T.: Prevention of postoperative deep vein thrombosis in patients with malignant disease. Br. Med. J., *1*:358, 1974.
90. Roberts, V. C., and Cotton, L. T.: Failure of low-dose heparin to improve efficacy of peroperative intermittent calf compression in preventing postoperative deep vein thrombosis. Br. Med. J., *3*:458, 1975.
91. Sabri, S., Roberts, V. C., and Cotton, L. T.: Prevention of early postoperative deep vein thrombo-

sis by intermittent compression of the leg during surgery. Br. Med. J., *4*:394, 1971.

92. Skillman, J. J., Collins, R. E. C., Coe, N. P., et al.: Prevention of deep vein thrombosis in neurosurgical patients: A controlled, randomized trial of external pneumatic compression boots. Surgery, *83*:354, 1978.
93. Takkunen, O.: The effect of different modes of artificial ventilation and of some prophylactic means on the incidence of postoperative deep vein thrombosis. Ann. Chir. Gynaecol. [Suppl.] *191*:1, 1975.
94. Turpie, A. G. G.: Nonpharmacologic prophylaxis against venous thrombosis: Prevention of venous thrombosis in neurosurgical patients with intermittent calf compression. *In* Madden, J., and Hume, M. (Eds.): Venous Thromboembolism. Prevention and Treatment. Appleton-Century-Crofts, New York, 1976, p. 165.
95. Turpie, A. G. G., Delmore, T., Hirsh, J., et al.: Prevention of venous thrombosis by intermittent sequential calf compression in patients with intracranial disease. Thromb. Res., *15*:611, 1979.
96. Zelikovski, A., Zucker, G., Eliashiv, A., et al.: A new sequential pneumatic device for the prevention of deep vein thrombosis. J. Neurosurg., *54*:652, 1981.
97. Wilkins, R. W., Mixter, G., Jr., Stanton, J. R., et al.: Elastic stockings in the prevention of pulmonary embolism: A preliminary report. New Engl. J. Med., *246*:360, 1952.
98. Wilkins, R. W., and Stanton, J. R.: Elastic stockings in the prevention of pulmonary embolism. New Engl. J. Med., *248*:1087, 1953.
99. Makin, G. S.: A clinical trial of "Tubigrip" to prevent deep venous thrombosis. Br. J. Surg., *56*:373, 1969.
100. Hirsh, J., Genton, E., and Hull, R.: Venous Thromboembolism. Grune and Stratton, New York, 1981, p. 218.
101. Hirsh, J.: Choosing the best of old and new ways to prevent venous thrombosis. J. Cardiovasc. Med., *6*:691, 1981.
102. Borgström, S., Greitz, T., van der Linden, W., et al.: Anticoagulant prophylaxis of venous thrombosis in patients with fractured neck of the femur. A controlled clinical trial using venous phlebography. Acta Chir. Scand., *129*:500, 1965.
103. Culver, D., Crawford, J. S., Gardiner, J. H., et al.: Venous thrombosis after fractures of the upper end of the femur. A study of incidence and site. J. Bone Joint Surg., *52B*:61, 1970.
104. Freeark, R., Boswick, J., and Fardin, R.: Posttraumatic venous thrombosis. Arch. Surg., *95*:567, 1967.
105. Hamilton, H. W., Crawford, J. S., Gardiner, J. H., et al.: Venous thrombosis in patients with fracture of the upper end of the femur. A phlebographic study of the effect of prophylactic anticoagulation. J. Bone Joint Surg., *52B*:268, 1970.
106. Smyrnis, S. A., Kolios, A. S., and Agnantis, J. K.: Deep-vein thrombosis in patients with fracture of the upper part of the femur. A phlebographic study. Br. J. Surg., *60*:447, 1973.
107. Stevens, J., Fardin, R., and Freeark, R. J.: Lower extremity thrombophlebitis in patients with femoral neck fractures. A venographic investigation and a review of the early and late significance of the findings. J. Trauma, *8*:527, 1968.
108. Bergqvist, D., Elvelin, R., Eriksson, U., et al.: Thrombosis following hip arthroplasty. A study using phlebography and I-125-fibrinogen test. Acta Orthop. Scand., *47*:549, 1976.
109. Soreff, J., Johnsson, H., Diener, L., et al.: Acetylsalicylic acid in a trial to diminish thromboembolic complications after elective hip surgery. Acta Orthop. Scand., *46*:246, 1975.
110. Stamatakis, J. D., Kakkar, V. V., Sagar, S., et al.: Femoral vein thrombosis and total hip replacement. Br. Med. J., *2*:223, 1977.
111. Barrie, W. W., Wood, E. H., Crumlish, P., et al.: Low-dosage ancrod for prevention of thrombotic complications after surgery for fractured neck of femur. Br. Med. J., *4*:130, 1974.
112. Dolk, T., and Westerborn, O.: Complications and mortality in patients with hip fracture. (In Swedish). Läkartidningen, *74*:3654, 1977.
113. Edwards, D. H., Steel, W. M., and Bentley, G.: Prophylaxis with dextran 70 against thrombosis in patients with fractures of the upper end of the femur. Injury, *6*:250, 1975.
114. Esekland, G., Solheim, K., and Skjörten, F.: Anticoagulant prophylaxis, thromboembolism and mortality in elderly patients with hip fractures. A controlled clinical trial. Acta Chir. Scand., *131*:16, 1966.
115. Galasko, C. S. B., Edwards, D. H., Fearn, C. B. D. A., et al.: The value of low dosage heparin for the prophylaxis of thromboembolism in patients with transcervical and intertrochanteric femoral fractures. Acta Orthop. Scand., *47*:276, 1976.
116. Hansen, E. H., Jessing, P., Lindewald, H., et al.: Hydroxychloroquine sulphate in prevention of deep venous thrombosis following fracture of the hip, pelvis, or thoracolumbar spine. J. Bone Joint Surg., *58A*:1089, 1976.
117. Morris, G. K., and Mitchell, J. R. A.: Warfarin sodium in prevention of deep venous thrombosis and pulmonary embolism in patients with fractured neck of femur. Lancet, *2*:869, 1976.
118. Moskovitz, P. A., Ellenberg, S. S., Feffer, H. L., et al.: Low-dose heparin for prevention of venous thromboembolism in total hip arthroplasty and surgical repair of hip fractures. J. Bone Joint Surg. (Am.), *60A*:1065, 1978.
119. Sevitt, S., and Gallagher, N. G.: Prevention of venous thrombosis and pulmonary embolism in injured patients. A trial of anticoagulant prophylaxis with phenidone in middle-aged and elderly patients with fractured necks of femur. Lancet, *2*:981, 1959.
120. Zekert, F., Kohn, P., Vormittag, E., et al.: Thromboembolieprophylaxe mit acetylsalicylsäure bei operationen wegen hüftgelelenksnaher frakturen. Mschr. Unfallheilkd., *77*:97, 1974.
121. D'Ambrosia, R. D., Lipscomb, P. R., McClain, E. J., et al.: Prophylactic anticoagulation in total hip replacement. Surg. Gynecol. Obstet., *140*:523, 1975.
122. Morris, G. K., Henry, A. P. J., and Preston, B. J.: Prevention of deep-vein thrombosis by low-dose heparin in patients undergoing total hip replacement. Lancet, *2*:797, 1974.
123. Sagar, S., Stamatakis, J. D., Higgins, A. F., et al.: Efficacy of low-dose heparin in prevention of extensive deep-vein thrombosis in patients undergoing total-hip replacement. Lancet, *1*:1151, 1976.
124. Schöndorf, T. H.: Thromboembolieprophylaxe mit heparin bei elektiven hüftgelenksoperationen. Deutsch. Med. Wschr., *103*:1877, 1978.
125. Checketts, R. G., and Bradley, J. G.: Low-dose

heparin in femoral neck fractures. Injury, 6:42, 1974.
126. Morris, G. K., and Mitchell, J. R. A.: Preventing venous thromboembolism in elderly patients with hip fractures: Studies of low-dose heparin, dipyridamole, aspirin, and flurbiprofen. Br. Med. J., *1*:535, 1977.
127. Xabregas, A., Gray, L., and Ham, J. M.: Heparin prophylaxis of deep vein thrombosis in patients with a fractured neck of the femur. Med. J. Aust., *1*:620, 1978.
128. Dechavanne, M., Ville, D., Viala, J. J., et al.: Controlled trial of platelet anti-aggregating agents and subcutaneous heparin in prevention of postoperative deep vein thrombosis in high risk patients. Haemostasis, *4*:94, 1975.
129. Dechavanne, M., Saudin, F., Viala, J. J., et al.: Prévention des thromboses veineuses. Succès de l'héparine à fortes doses lors des coxarthroses. Nouv. Presse Med., *3*:1317, 1974.
130. de Mourgues, G., Pagnier, F., Clermont, N., et al.: Étude de l'efficacité de l'héparin sous-cutanée utilisée selon deux protocoles dans la prévention de la thrombose veineuse postopératoire après prothèse totale de hanche. Rev. Chir. Orthop., *65*:74, 1979.
131. Hampson, W. G. J., Harris, F. C., Lucas, H. K., et al.: Failure of low-dose heparin to prevent deep-vein thrombosis after hip-replacement arthroplasty. Lancet, *2*:795, 1974.
132. Hume, M., Kuriakose, T. X., Zuch, L., et al.: I-125-fibrinogen and the prevention of venous thrombosis. Arch. Surg., *107*:803, 1973.
133. Lowe, L. W.: Venous thrombosis and embolism. J. Bone Joint Surg. [Br.], *63B*:155, 1981.
134. Mannucci, P. M., Citterio, L. E., and Panajotopoulos, N.: Low-dose heparin and deep-vein thrombosis after total hip replacement. Thromb. Haemost., *36*:157, 1976.
135. Venous Thrombosis Clinical Study Group: Small doses of subcutaneous sodium heparin in the prevention of deep vein thrombosis after elective hip operations. Br. J. Surg., *62*:348, 1975.
136. Abraham-Inpijn, L., and Vreeken, J.: Effect of low-dose heparin on incidence of postoperative thrombosis in orthopaedic patients. Arch. Chir. Neerl., *27*:63, 1975.
137. Protoulis, C., Bouvier, C., Vaucher, J., et al.: Incidence et prévention de la thrombose veineuse profonde dans la chirurgie de la hanche. Schweitz. Rundschau. Med., *65*:1298, 1976.
138. Harris, W. H., Salzman, E., Athanasoulis, C., et al.: Comparison of I-125-fibrinogen count scanning with phlebography for detection of venous thrombi after elective hip surgery. New Engl. J. Med., *292*:665, 1975.
139. Kakkar, V. V., Stamatakis, J., Bentley, P. G., et al.: Prophylaxis for postoperative deep-vein thrombosis. Synergistic effect of heparin and dihydroergotamine. J.A.M.A., *241*:39, 1979.
140. Sharnoff, J. G., Rosen, R. L., Sadler, A. H., et al.: Prevention of fatal pulmonary thromboembolism by heparin prophylaxis after surgery for hip fractures. J. Bone Joint Surg., *58A*:913, 1976.
141. Poller, L., Taberner, D. A., Sandilands, D. G., et al.: An evaluation of APTT monitoring of low-dose heparin dosage in hip surgery. Thromb. Haemost., *47*:50, 1982.
142. Leyvraz, P. F., Richard, J., Bachmann, F., et al.: Adjusted versus fixed-dose subcutaneous heparin in the prevention of deep-vein thrombosis after total hip replacement. New Engl. J. Med., *309*:954, 1983.
143. Salzman, E. W.: Progress in preventing venous thromboembolism. New Engl. J. Med., *309*:980, 1983.
144. Stamatakis, J. D., Kakkar, V. V., Lawrence, D., et al.: Failure of aspirin to prevent postoperative deep vein thrombosis in patients undergoing total hip replacement. Br. Med. J., *1*:1031, 1978.
145. Harris, W. H., Salzman, E. W., Athanasoulis, C. A., et al.: Aspirin prophylaxis of venous thromboembolism after total hip replacement. New Engl. J. Med., *297*:1246, 1977.
146. Harris, W., Athanasoulis, C. A., Waltman, A. C., et al.: High and low-dose aspirin prophylaxis against venous thromboembolic disease in total hip replacement. J. Bone Joint Surg., *64A*:63, 1982.
147. Bergqvist, D., and Dahlgren, S.: Leg vein thrombosis diagnosed by I-125-fibrinogen test in patients with fracture of the hip: A study of the effect of early prophylaxis with dicoumarol or dextran 70. Vasa, 2:121, 1973.
148. Borgström, S.: Investigation of the effect of dicumarol and early ambulation in the prevention of postoperative thrombo-embolism in a surgical material strongly disposed to thrombosis. Acta Chir. Scand. [Suppl.], *150*:5, 1950.
149. Bronge, A., Dahlgren, S., and Lindquist, B.: Prophylaxis against thrombosis in femoral neck fractures—a comparison between dextran 70 and dicumarol. Acta Chir. Scand., *137*:29, 1971.
150. Pinto, D. J.: Controlled trial of an anticoagulant (warfarin-sodium) in the prevention of venous thrombosis following hip surgery. Br. J. Surg., *57*:349, 1970.
151. Chalmers, T. C., Matta, R. J., Smith, H., Jr., et al.: Evidence favoring the use of anticoagulants in the hospital phase of acute myocardial infarction. New Engl. J. Med., *297*:1091, 1977.
152. Freiman, J. A., Chalmers, T. C., Smith, H., Jr., et al.: The importance of beta, the type II error and sample size in the design and interpretation of the randomized control trial: Survey of 71 "negative" trials. New Engl. J. Med., *299*:690, 1978.
153. Frishman, W. H., and Ribner, H. S.: Anticoagulation in myocardial infarction: Modern approach to an old problem. Am. J. Cardiol., *43*:1207, 1979.
154. Hilden, T., Iversen, K., Raaschou, F., et al.: Anticoagulants in acute myocardial infarction. Lancet, *2*:327, 1961.
155. Veterans Administration Cooperative Clinical Trial: Anticoagulants in acute myocardial infarction. J.A.M.A., *225*:724, 1973.
156. Handley, A. J., Emerson, P. A., and Fleming, P. R.: Heparin in the prevention of deep vein thrombosis after myocardial infarction. Br. Med. J., *2*:436, 1972.
157. Wray, R., Maurer, B., and Shillingford, J.: Prophylactic anticoagulant therapy in the prevention of calf-vein thrombosis after myocardial infarction. New Engl. J. Med., *288*:815, 1973.
158. Nicolaides, A. N., Kakkar, V. V., Renney, J. T. G., et al.: Myocardial infarction and deep-vein thrombosis. Br. Med. J., *1*:432, 1971.
159. Steffensen, K. A.: Coronary occlusion treated with small doses of heparin. Acta Med. Scand., *186*:519, 1969.
160. Warlow, C., Beattie, A. G., Terry, G., et al.: A

double-blind trial of low doses of subcutaneous heparin in the prevention of deep-vein thrombosis after myocardial infarction. Lancet, *2*:934, 1973.
161. Emerson, P. A., and Marks, P.: Preventing thromboembolism after myocardial infarction: Effect of low-dose heparin or smoking. Br. Med. J., *1*:18, 1977.
162. Handley, A. J.: Low-dose heparin after myocardial infarction. Lancet, *2*:623, 1972.
163. Stampfer, M. J., Goldhaber, S. Z., Yusuf, S., et al.: Effect of intravenous streptokinase on acute myocardial infarction: Pooled results from randomized trials. New Engl. J. Med., *307*:1180, 1982.
164. Salzman, E. W., Sobel, M., Lewis, J., et al.: Prevention of venous thromboembolism in unstable angina pectoris. New Engl. J. Med., *306*:991, 1982.
165. Warlow, C., Ogston, D., and Douglas, A. S.: Deep venous thrombosis of the legs after strokes: Incidence and predisposing factors. Br. Med. J., *1*:1178, 1976.
166. Warlow, C., Ogston, D., and Douglas, A. S.: Deep venous thrombosis of the legs after strokes: Natural history. Br. Med. J., *1*:1180, 1976.
167. McCarthy, S. T., Turner, J. J., Robertson, D., et al.: Low-dose heparin as a prophylaxis against deep-vein thrombosis after acute stroke. Lancet, *2*:800, 1977.
168. van Hove, E.: Prevention of thrombophlebitis in spinal injury patients. Paraplegia, *16*:332, 1978–1979.
169. Perkash, A.: Experience with the management of deep vein thrombosis in patients with spinal cord injury. Part II: A critical evaluation of the anticoagulant therapy. Paraplegia, *18*:2, 1980.
170. Casas, E. R., Sánchez, M. P., Arias, C. R., et al.: Prophylaxis of venous thrombosis and pulmonary embolism in patients with acute traumatic spinal cord lesions. Paraplegia, *15*:209, 1977–1978.
171. Watson, N.: Anti-coagulant therapy in the prevention of venous thrombosis and pulmonary embolism in the spinal cord injury. Paraplegia, *16*:265, 1978–1979.
172. Halkin, H., Goldberg, J., Modan, M., et al.: Reduction of mortality in general medical in-patients by low-dose heparin prophylaxis. Ann. Intern. Med., *96*:561, 1982.
173. Lowe, G. D. O., Campbell, A. F., Meek, D. R., et al.: Subcutaneous ancrod in prevention of deep-vein thrombosis after operation for fractured neck of femur. Lancet, *2*:698, 1978.
174. Belch, J. J. F., Meek, D. R., Lowe, G. D. O., et al.: Subcutaneous ancrod in prevention of deep vein thrombosis after hip replacement surgery. Thromb. Res., *25*:23, 1982.
175. Cooke, E. D., Bowcock, S. A., Lloyd, M. J., et al.: Intravenous lignocaine in prevention of deep venous thrombosis after elective hip surgery. Lancet, *2*:797, 1977.
176. Francis, C. W., Marder, V. J., Evarts, M., et al.: Two-step warfarin therapy: Prevention of postoperative venous thrombosis without excessive bleeding. J.A.M.A., *249*:374, 1983.
177. Salzman, E. W., and Davies, G. C.: Prophylaxis of venous thromboembolism. Analysis of cost effectiveness. Ann. Surg., *191*:207, 1980.
178. Goldhaber, S. Z., and Smith, T. W.: Prophylaxis of deep venous thrombosis and pulmonary embolism. Lifeline, *2*:1, 1984.
179. Clarke-Pearson, D. L., Synan, I. S., Hinshaw, W. M., et al.: Prevention of postoperative venous thromboembolism by external pneumatic calf compression in patients with gynecologic malignancy. Obstet. Gynecol., *63*:92, 1984.
180. Hull, R. D., and Hirsh, J.: Preventing venous thromboembolism. J. Cardiovasc. Med., *9*:63, 1984.
181. Moser, K. M., and LeMoine, J. R.: Is embolic risk conditioned by location of deep venous thrombosis? Ann. Intern. Med., *94*:439, 1981.
182. Swan, H. J. C.: Thrombolysis in acute evolving myocardial infarction: A new potential for myocardial salvage. New Engl. J. Med., *308*:1354, 1983.
183. Bergqvist, E., Bergqvist, D., Bronge, A., et al.: An evaluation of early thrombosis prophylaxis following fracture of the femoral neck: A comparison between dextran and dicoumarol. Acta Chir. Scand., *138*:689, 1972.

# PART III

# SPECIAL CLINICAL TOPICS

CHAPTER 9

# THE HYPERCOAGULABLE STATE

RICHARD B. STEAD, M.D.

The definition and recognition of the hypercoagulable state have been nebulous, in part because of our incomplete understanding of the hemostatic system and in part because there is no single laboratory abnormality that can define the condition. In fact, the hypercoagulable syndrome has many different etiologies but can be arbitrarily divided into two categories: (1) primary hypercoagulable disorders, which are usually inherited, well-defined quantitative or qualitative abnormalities of a particular component of the hemostatic system and (2) the secondary hypercoagulable states such as pregnancy and malignancy, which are common and, at present, appear to be multifactorial, i.e., not usually recognized to be caused by a single, specific abnormality. This chapter will review the clinical and laboratory approach to the suspected hypercoagulable patient and discuss the recognized primary and secondary hypercoagulable disorders (Table 9–1).

***Table 9–1.*** Hypercoagulable Disorders

**Primary**

1. Antithrombin III deficiencies (congenital or acquired)
2. Protein C deficiency
3. Abnormal fibrinogen
4. Decreased or abnormal plasminogen
5. Vascular plasminogen activator deficiency
6. Plasminogen activator inhibitor
7. ? Factor XII deficiency
8. Homocystinuria

**Secondary**

1. Immobilization
2. Postoperative state
3. Malignancy
4. Pregnancy
5. Oral contraceptives and estrogens
6. Nephrotic syndrome
7. Other drugs: heparin, EACA, prothrombin complex concentrates (Proplex®, Konyne®)
8. "Lupus-like anticoagulant"
9. Platelet disorders: e.g., myeloproliferative disorders, paroxysmal nocturnal hemoglobinuria, diabetes mellitus, hypercholesterolemia (?)
10. "Hyperviscosity": e.g., Waldenström's macroglobulinemia, polycythemia
11. Prosthetic surfaces

## THE HYPERCOAGULABLE STATE DEFINED

In the broadest sense, the hypercoagulable state can be thought of as the regulation of hemostasis or thrombosis gone awry, predisposing the patient to unusual, frequent, or recurring thrombotic events. Operationally, it can be defined as any laboratory or clinical abnormality that is pathogenically associated with an increased tendency to develop thrombosis.[1] One must try to distinguish between laboratory abnormalities that are causally related to the thrombosis and those that are markers of ongoing coagulation activity or even of an underlying disease.[1–3] Table 9–2 lists examples of various defects at each level of the hemostatic mechanism that have been associated with an enhanced thrombotic tendency.

It may seem perplexing that the hypercoagulable state may exist subclinically for years. In general, a hypercoagulable disorder is *permissive* of enhanced thrombosis but does not necessarily *initiate* the thrombosis. A clinical event or condition that will initiate the thrombosis and trigger the clinically apparent episode may sometimes be required. Because triggers of sufficient magnitude are not al-

***Table 9–2.*** Defects in the Hemostatic System Associated with the Hypercoagulable State

| Defective Hemostatic Component | Example |
|---|---|
| Abnormalities in blood flow | Sickle cell anemia<br>Waldenström's macroglobulinemia<br>Venous stasis |
| Abnormal vessel wall | Prosthetic heart valves; shunts<br>Homocystinuria (?) |
| Platelet abnormalities | |
| Elevated platelet count (>$10^6$/$mm^3$) | Usually not, but may be in patients with myeloproliferative disorders, especially after splenectomy |
| Qualitative platelet defects | Myeloproliferative disorders<br>Diabetes mellitus<br>Hypercholesterolemia |
| Abnormal clotting factors | Factor XII deficiency |
| Abnormal or deficient inhibitors | Antithrombin III deficiency (qualitative or quantitative)<br>Protein C deficiency |
| Circulating, activated clotting factors | Malignancy<br>Disseminated intravascular coagulation (DIC)<br>Liver disease |
| Abnormal fibrinolysis | Dysfibrinogenemia (usually more susceptible to bleeding but some examples of resistance to fibrinolysis)<br>Diminished release of vascular plasminogen activator<br>Qualitative or quantitative decrease in plasminogen |

ways present, the occurrence of thrombotic events tends to be episodic. Thus, the clinical recognition of the hypercoagulable state may depend not only on the underlying hemostatic defect but also on the presence and magnitude of an initiating factor.[4] For example, healthy young women taking oral contraceptives have a very low risk for thrombosis under ordinary circumstances. However, when an initiator of hemostasis such as abdominal surgery is superimposed on a mild secondary hypercoagulable state induced by oral contraceptives, the risk of pulmonary embolism may increase sixfold compared with matched controls.[5]

## APPROACH TO THE PATIENT: WHEN TO SUSPECT A PRIMARY HYPERCOAGULABLE DISORDER

There are several difficult questions in approaching patients with recurrent thromboembolic disease. When should one suspect a primary hypercoagulable state—on the first, second, third, or subsequent episode? How well must the recurrence be documented? Was the preceding episode adequately treated? The presence of one or more of the clinical features noted in Table 9–3 should raise the index of suspicion of a primary hypercoagulable disorder.

The history is the most important factor in determining how far to proceed in the evaluation of the patient: *the personal and family histories are much more important than any single laboratory test currently available.* The intensity of the laboratory evaluation should be dictated by the extent and number of features listed in Table 9–3. A striking family history of thromboembolic events diagnosed by objective criteria is a most important factor that should suggest a primary hypercoagulable disorder. Early age of onset may also be a very reliable indicator. Although multiple recurrences should raise the index of suspicion, it should be noted that deep venous thrombosis (DVT) often tends to be a recurrent disease even in the absence of any established hypercoagulable disorder. Two surgical studies[6, 7] have shown that the history of previous venous thrombosis increases the risk of postoperative DVT by almost threefold. Recurrences should be diagnosed objectively, preferably by radiographic methods, because clinical diagnosis is notoriously unreliable. Furthermore, as noted later in this chapter, thromboembolic disease is relatively common in hospitalized patients, especially those who are post partum, have undergone surgery, or have a malignancy or congestive heart failure. The presence of the first or even second or possibly third episode in one of these settings should not *necessarily* mandate an exhaustive evaluation for the presence of a primary hypercoagulable disorder. However, if other features listed in Table 9–3 are present, such an assessment may be indicated.

In evaluating an apparent failure of conventional therapy, one must be careful to note such factors as the adequacy of patient compliance and the monitoring of therapy as well as the presence of an underlying systemic disease. A patient with recurrent DVT

***Table 9–3.*** When to Suspect Primary Hypercoagulable Disorders: Clinical Features

| |
|---|
| Strong family history of "idiopathic" thromboembolism |
| Onset at an early age (less than age 35) |
| Two or more *well-documented* recurrences |
| Refractory to conventional therapy or early recurrence following discontinuation of prolonged therapy |
| Absence of other predisposing systemic disease, e.g., malignancy |
| Unusual location or presentation, e.g., mesenteric or axillary vein thrombosis; DVT *early* in pregnancy |

should be evaluated for the presence of an underlying disease that may be associated with thrombosis, including vasculitis, diabetes, hyperlipidemia, occult malignancy, or myeloproliferative disorder. Every effort should be made to identify and *treat* underlying systemic disorders that may predispose to thrombosis before an exhaustive evaluation for a primary hypercoagulable disorder is undertaken. By definition, it is difficult, if not impossible, to diagnose a primary hypercoagulable disorder in the presence of a systemic disease that predisposes to thrombosis. The location or presentation of the thrombosis is less likely to be helpful. More often than not, primary hypercoagulable disorders will demonstrate a typical presentation of DVT in the lower extremities or of pulmonary emboli. Although an unusual thrombotic event such as mesenteric vein thrombosis may be a feature of antithrombin III deficiency, this is not the most common presentation.

## LABORATORY EVALUATION

If the history is strongly suggestive of a hypercoagulable disorder, one must consider which laboratory tests to perform. Laboratory tests for the evaluation of patients suspected of having a hypercoagulable disorder fall into two general categories: (1) nonspecific tests (Table 9–4), which either (a) reflect transient responses to trauma or inflammation but neither specifically predict nor detect thrombosis or (b) reflect the activation of platelets or coagulation enzymes and may detect clinical or subclinical thrombosis but do not identify specific disorders; and (2) specific tests (Table 9–5), which identify underlying specific primary hypercoagulable disorders and predict those patients who are at high risk for recurrent thromboembolic events but do not detect ongoing thrombosis.

The first group of tests (Table 9–4A), which neither specifically detects nor predicts thrombosis, may be abnormal in parallel with other acute phase reactants, coincident with the thrombotic process itself or due to an underlying disease. Examples include elevation of the platelet count and elevations in levels of certain unactivated clotting factors: factor VII, VIII, V, and fibrinogen (factor I). Such inactive clotting factors (zymogens) must be enzymatically activated to participate in coagulation reactions and normally circulate in vast excess of physiologic requirements. Elevated levels of these inactive precursors do not necessarily confer an elevated risk for thrombosis nor do they specifically detect thrombotic disease.[1–2]

Tests that may detect clinical or subclinical thrombosis (Table 9–4B) include a group of readily available tests such as fibrin split products, platelet hyperaggregability, and platelet products such as thromboxane $B_2$ ($TxB_2$) (the metabolically stable breakdown product of thromboxane $A_2$), platelet factor 4 (PF4), and beta thromboglobulin (βTG). Un-

***Table 9–4.*** Nonspecific Tests Available for the Laboratory Evaluation of the Suspected Hypercoagulable Patient

A. Tests that detect transient responses to trauma and inflammation

- Elevated levels of "unactivated" clotting factors: fibrinogen, factors V, VII, VIII
- Elevated platelet count
- Reduced levels of antithrombin III
- Reduced fibrinolytic activity
  - Prolonged euglobulin lysis time
  - Elevated antiplasmin time

B. Tests that detect clinical or subclinical thrombosis

- Platelet activation or release
  - Shortened platelet survival
  - Elevated thromboxane $B_2$ ($TxB_2$)
  - Elevated platelet factor 4 (PF4)
  - Elevated beta thromboglobulin (βTG)
  - Elevated circulating platelet aggregates
  - Spontaneous or hyperreactive platelet aggregation
- Activation of coagulation enzymes
  - Fibrin formation
  - Elevated fibrin split products (FSPs)
  - Elevated fibrin monomer complexes
  - Increased fibrinogen turnover
  - Elevated fibrinopeptide A (FPA)
  - Elevated fibrin (fibrinogen fragment E)
- Thrombin generation
  - Elevated $F_{1+2}$ fragment
  - Elevated thrombin:antithrombin complexes
- Plasmin:antiplasmin complexes

***Table 9–5.*** Specific Tests Available for Laboratory Evaluation of the Suspected Hypercoagulable Patient

| Condition | Assay | Comments |
|---|---|---|
| Abnormal or deficient inhibitors of coagulation | | |
| 1. AT III deficiency[14, 16] | Immunologic<br>Functional | Assay widely (commercially) available; warfarin may elevate levels and heparin may decrease levels. Depressed levels may be associated with secondary hypercoagulable state |
| 2. Protein C deficiency[17] | Immunologic<br>Functional | Assay not readily available; must be measured off anticoagulants or normalized for anticoagulant effect |
| Defective fibrinolysis | | |
| 1. Defective release of plasminogen activator[22, 23] | Functional | Assay not widely available |
| 2. Factor XII deficiency[26] | Functional | PTT prolonged; assay widely available |
| 3. Plasminogen activator inhibitor[25] | Functional | Impaired fibrinolysis |
| 4. Abnormal fibrinogen (dysfibrinogenemia)[24] | Functional | Usually associated with bleeding but may be associated with thrombosis |
| 5. Abnormal plasminogen[19–21] | Immunologic<br>Functional | Assay not widely available |
| Other | | |
| 1. Homocystinuria[28] | Biochemical | Arterial and venous events commonly associated with endothelial damage |
| 2. Myeloproliferative disease[29, 30] | | Usually associated with bleeding, but may be associated with thrombosis. No assay available, clinical features of myeloproliferative disease apparent (e.g., splenomegaly, abnormal CBC, platelet count, karyotype, LAP score) |
| 3. "Lupus-like anticoagulant"[27] | Functional | PTT prolonged; assay widely available. May be associated with a secondary hypercoagulable state |

fortunately, all of the currently available tests suffer from a lack of sensitivity or specificity and are probably not clinically useful, though they may have certain applications in clinical research.[2, 3]

A new generation of tests is being developed (Fig. 9–1) that measure biochemical markers of the coagulation reactions central to the formation of fibrin.[2] When Xa enzymatically activates prothrombin (factor II), it releases a peptide activation fragment $F_{1+2}$ as well as thrombin (factor IIa). Free thrombin acts on fibrinogen (factor I) to form fibrin, the protein substance of clot, with the release of small peptide fragments, fibrinopeptides A and B (FPA, FPB). Thrombin is physiologically neutralized by antithrombin III, forming a thrombin:antithrombin complex (T:AT). New radioimmunoassays can detect thrombin generation ($F_{1+2}$, T:AT)[8, 9] and fibrin formation (FPA)[10] at nanomolar levels. Such assays show promise for detecting clinical or subclinical thrombosis.[11–13] Unfortunately, the high sensitivity of these assays may be offset by problems with specificity. For example, elevations may be seen with sepsis, malignancy, and vasculitis. They may also be subject to artifacts of venipuncture and processing. It is hoped that refinements in such assays may prove clinically useful in detecting thrombosis or as screening tests to determine which patients may be "prethrombotic" or hypercoagulable. At the moment, however, these assays are available only on a research basis.

Specific biochemical, functional, or immunologic assays have been developed to detect each of the recognized primary hypercoagulable disorders as well as the "lupus-like anticoagulant" (see Table 9–1). Except for antithrombin III, which is a widely available assay, each of the other assays is performed on a research basis in one or more specialized research laboratories. Table 9–1 lists the presently recognized primary hypercoagulable disorders that seem likely to be *causally* related to recurrent or familial thromboembolic disease. The nature and limitations of currently available assays are outlined in Table 9–5. Most of the tests for these disorders are not readily available and may require attention to such other factors as processing of samples and drugs that the patient may be receiving, including anticoagulants. It should be noted that additional hypercoagulable disorders are being described with increasing frequency.

The evaluation of such patients can be frustrating, even to the hematologist, for a variety of reasons. There are currently no

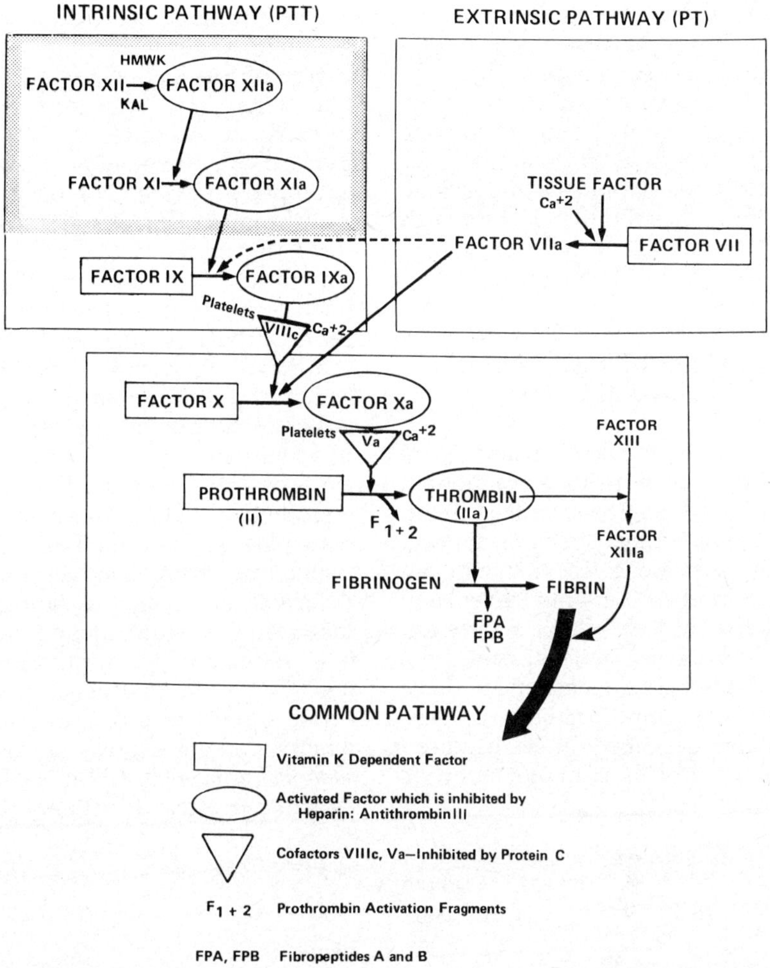


***Figure 9–1.*** Relationship of prothrombin activation fragments ($F_{1+2}$) and fibrinopeptides A and B (FPA and FPB) to thrombin and fibrinogen. (See text for details.)

clinically available, reliable screening tests to determine which patients should be investigated. The history, in particular the features listed in Table 9–3, is still the best screening test. Once a patient is strongly suspected of a primary hypercoagulable disorder—*and more common secondary causes have been thoroughly considered and excluded*—the task of ruling out each of the known primary disorders begins. Given the wide availability of the assay and the known frequency of the disease, a functional assay for antithrombin III should be performed. One may then systematically exclude each of the other disorders, but the order of evaluation is somewhat arbitrary. This is because these disorders (see Table 9–5) cannot be distinguished on clinical grounds except for the relatively unusual physiognomy and the occurrence of both arterial and venous events in homocystinuria.[31] Furthermore, neither normal populations nor large numbers of patients with thromboembolic disease have been systematically surveyed for most of these disorders; thus, little can be said about their relative frequency.

Those patients and their families who, based on their history, appear to have a very high likelihood of a primary hypercoagulable disorder may require a difficult and time-consuming evaluation. An evaluation of appropriate patients can have critical therapeutic implications for the patient and family in defining the duration of anticoagulant therapy as well as in the consideration of new modes of therapy, such as antithrombin III replacement. Only a thorough evaluation of such patients will define the true frequency of these defects and uncover new abnormalities that will help to increase our understanding of the hemostatic system. It is expected that many of these assays will become more widely available over the next several years, making the evaluation of the hypercoagulable patient a less formidable task.

Patients with a documented primary hypercoagulable disorder may require lifelong anticoagulation, usually with oral anticoagulants. Such decisions should be individualized, taking into consideration factors such as the clinical history of thrombosis and an assessment of the risk of hemorrhage.

## PRIMARY HYPERCOAGULABLE DISORDERS

The primary hypercoagulable disorders are rare inherited defects of a single component of the hemostatic system that manifest themselves by recurrent thrombosis, often starting at an early age. At present, less than a dozen such defects and their variants have been described, each of which affects a different component of the hemostatic system (Fig. 9–2) (see also Table 9–1). At least one of these primary disorders, antithrombin III deficiency, has been described in an acquired form, owing to protein losses in the nephrotic syndrome.[14, 32]

**Antithrombin III Deficiency.** Qualitative or quantitative defects of this important inhibitor of coagulation are by far the most well known and best characterized of the primary hypercoagulable disorders and the only ones that most coagulation laboratories are equipped to screen for on a routine basis. Antithrombin III (AT III) is the major inhibitor of thrombin in plasma. AT III not only complexes with and inactivates thrombin (factor IIa), but also inactivates the other serine proteases such as factors XIIIa, XIa, IXa, Xa, and plasmin. Heparin catalyzes this action of antithrombin III in vitro. Not only is heparin a potent catalyst of antithrombin III activity in vitro, but there is recent in vivo evidence of a heparin-like substance on the endothelial surface, termed heparan, that may play an important physiologic role in regulating thrombosis (Fig. 9–3).[154] AT III deficiency is really a family of diseases that result in either quantitative or qualitative reduction in antithrombin III activity.[14, 15, 148, 149] It appears that some families express low levels of a *normal gene product,* whereas others express normal levels of an *abnormal gene product.*[148] It is therefore important to perform a functional (biologic) assay

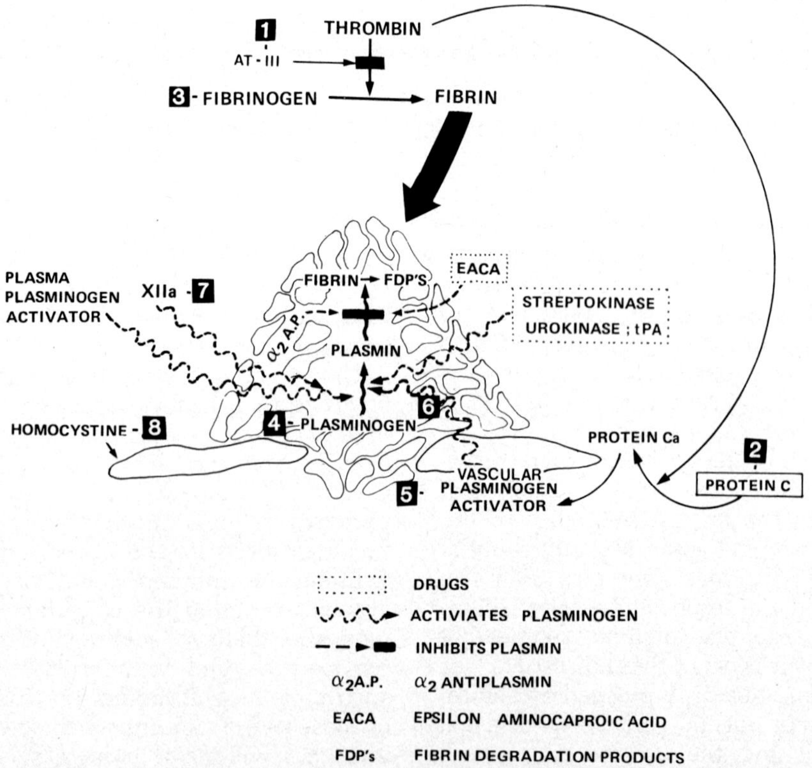


*Figure 9–2.* Elements of the hemostatic system that have been associated with primary hypercoagulable disorders. (See text for details.)

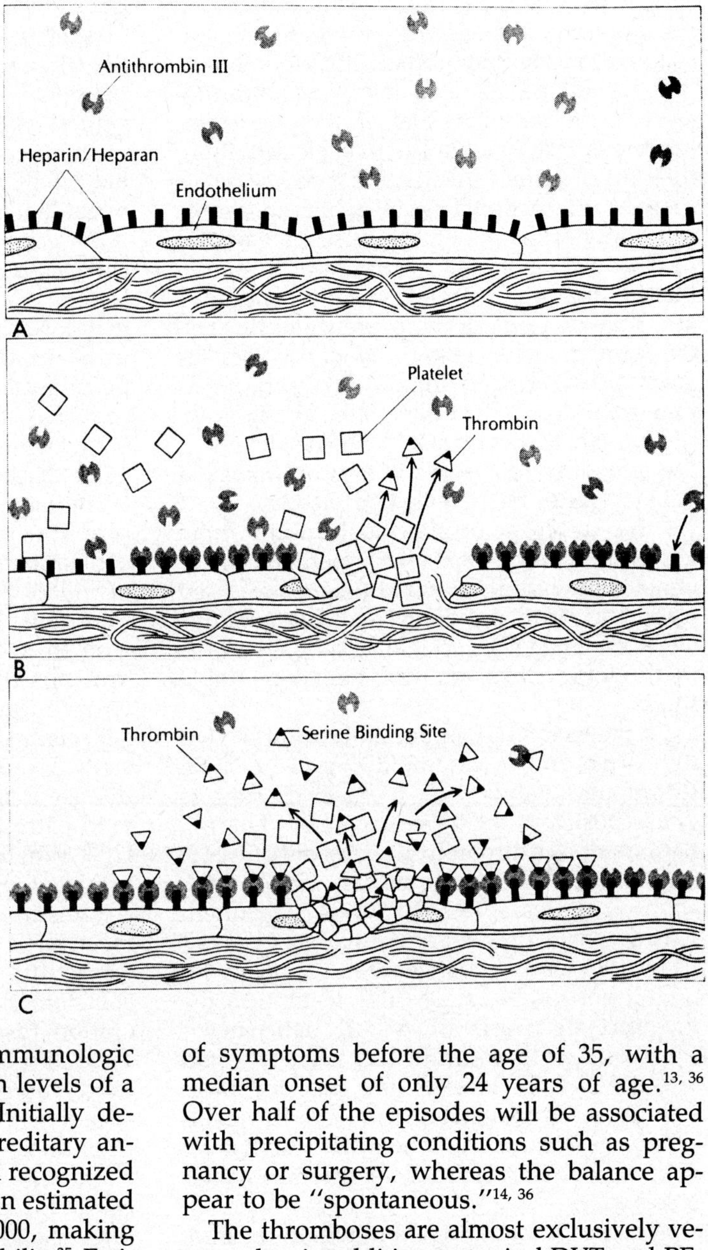


*Figure 9–3.* Physiologic role of antithrombin III (AT III). Although AT III inhibits thrombin in the circulation, its most important physiologic role may be on the endothelial cell surface, where it attaches to and becomes activated by heparin-like molecules (heparan) (*A* and *B*). AT III prevents excessive propagation of thrombus formation by neutralizing thrombin near the site of vascular wall injury (*C*). Congenital or acquired deficiency of AT III leads to reduced inhibition of thrombin and a hypercoagulable state. (Reprinted with permission from Bussel, J. B.: Circulating Anticoagulants: Physiologic and Pathophysiologic. Hospital Practice, *18*:2, 1983. Drawing by Alan D. Iselin.)

for antithrombin III, because immunologic assays may detect normal or high levels of a dysfunctional antithrombin.[14, 16] Initially described by Egeberg in 1965,[33] hereditary antithrombin III deficiency has been recognized in hundreds of patients and has an estimated prevalence of 1 in 5000 to 1 in 2000, making it at least as common as hemophilia.[35] Estimates of the prevalence of AT III deficiency in patients hospitalized for DVT or PE range as high as 2 to 3 per cent.[14, 34, 35] It is inherited in an autosomal manner, males and females being about equally affected. The homozygous state has not been described.

There is considerable heterogeneity, not only in the precise molecular basis of this disease but also in the clinical severity, even within a given family, which often cannot be explained by antithrombin III levels. At least 85 per cent of affected individuals can expect to have at least one thrombotic event before the age of 60.[14, 36] The majority have the onset of symptoms before the age of 35, with a median onset of only 24 years of age.[13, 36] Over half of the episodes will be associated with precipitating conditions such as pregnancy or surgery, whereas the balance appear to be "spontaneous."[14, 36]

The thromboses are almost exclusively venous, but in addition to typical DVT and PE, unusual thrombotic events such as mesenteric or axillary vein thrombosis or DVT *early* in pregnancy may occur. (Pregnancy itself is associated with an increased incidence of thromboembolic events, but these are primarily in the puerperium.)

Affected persons have reduced levels of plasma antithrombin III, approximately 40 to 60 per cent of normal, but levels of less than 75 per cent of normal may be associated with an increased risk of thrombosis.[14] The accurate diagnosis of AT III deficiency depends on the limitations of the assays[14, 16] used and when the measurements are made. AT III *antigen* may be measured most accurately by the immunoelectrophoresis method of Laurell, although other radial diffusion immunologic assays are available. The immunologic assays are, in general, easier to perform, but they do not assess the biologic activity of the antithrombin III that is present. This requires a functional assay, which measures the ability of the patient's plasma (not serum) to neutralize a standard amount of thrombin (factor IIa) or Xa under specific conditions and may be done in the presence of heparin (heparin cofactor assay). Heparin cofactor assays and crossed immunoelectrophoresis may help detect dysfunctional or variant antithrombin III molecules.[148, 149] The details of the laboratory diagnosis of antithrombin deficiency have been reviewed elsewhere.[14, 16] As the structure of abnormal antithrombin genes is characterized, new methods of diagnosis (including prenatal diagnosis) based upon the structural analysis of the patient's DNA may become feasible, analogous to the methodology in diagnosing hemoglobinopathies.

In practice, it is important to know that the drugs most commonly used to treat thrombotic events may themselves lead to "false-positive" or "false-negative" determinations of antithrombin III deficiency. Acute thrombosis itself may be associated with slightly depressed AT III levels. Treatment with heparin may temporarily *lower* the AT III level by 10 to 15 per cent[14] in patients with ongoing thrombosis, possibly leading to the incorrect diagnosis of AT III deficiency.[37] Treatment with warfarin has been reported to raise AT III levels;[37] the mechanism is unknown. If possible, the AT III levels should be determined when the patient is off anticoagulants, well after the thrombosis has resolved.

Because the anticoagulant activity of heparin is dependent on the interaction with antithrombin III, higher doses of heparin may be required for effective anticoagulation. In practice, most patients with AT III deficiency can be treated successfully with heparin followed by warfarin. Oral anticoagulant therapy, which is not dependent on antithrombin III, is effective and may be required for prolonged periods. Lifetime anticoagulation has been recommended for symptomatic family members, but the treatment of asymptomatic affected family members is controversial. AT III concentrates, produced initially by conventional blood fractionation techniques and eventually by recombinant DNA technology, are becoming available. The therapeutic and prophylactic role of such AT III concentrates in the treatment of such patients will have to be carefully defined by clinical trials.

The preceding discussion refers to congenital AT III deficiency, but it should be recognized that acquired AT III deficiency has been reported in a number of conditions. The clinical significance is often not well established.[14] Patients with a nephrotic syndrome may lose significant amounts of AT III in the urine in direct proportion to the level of proteinuria. Levels of AT III below 75 per cent may contribute to the high-risk thrombotic events observed in such patients.[14]

As discussed later in this chapter, AT III levels may be reduced by as much as 15 per cent in women taking oral contraceptive pills containing estrogen. The relative importance of mildly reduced antithrombin III levels is uncertain. It seems prudent, however, that women with known AT III deficiency or previous thromboembolic disease use alternative means of contraception.

**Protein C Deficiency.** A more recently described cause of recurrent thromboembolic disease is a deficiency of another important modulator of the hemostatic system, Protein C.[158] Whereas antithrombin III inhibits the activated factors XIIa, XIa, IXa, and Xa in the coagulation cascade (see Fig. 9–1), Protein C inactivates two other activated clotting factors, VIIIc and Va,[17] which are important cofactors in Xa and thrombin (factor IIa) generation, respectively (see Chapter 3, Fig. 3–8). Thus, Protein C and antithrombin III may exert complementary inhibitory effects. In addition, Protein C appears to activate the fibrinolytic system in vivo[150] (see Fig. 9–2).

Protein C deficiency, with antigenic levels of 40 to 50 per cent of normal, has been reported in several families with a striking history of thromboembolic disease.[18, 151] Patients and their family members tend to present at an early age with recurrent superficial or deep vein thrombophlebitis, often complicated by pulmonary emboli, a presentation similar to antithrombin III deficiency. The incidence of this disorder has not been precisely determined, but family studies strongly suggest an autosomal dominant mode of inheritance.[18] A recent survey in the Western Netherlands has suggested that as many as one per cent of patients with DVT may have Protein C deficiency; the frequency of Protein C deficiency in this population has been estimated at 1 in 16,000.[159] Currently, diagnosis and screening are limited by several factors. At the moment, the immunologic assay is not widely available, and functional assays of Protein C have only recently been described.[160–162] Furthermore, because Protein C synthesis in the liver is vitamin K–dependent, levels are significantly depressed by liver disease and by warfarin. If Protein C levels must be measured while the patient is receiving oral anticoagulants, anticoagulation must be stabilized and the Protein C level interpreted with respect to levels of other known vitamin K–dependent clotting factors.[18, 151]

Further suppression of functional Protein C (a vitamin K–dependent protein) by warfarin might be expected to be detrimental to Protein C–deficient patients. However, in the few Protein C–deficient patients studied to date, warfarin appears to be effective in preventing recurrent thromboembolic episodes.[18, 151, 158] Withdrawal of warfarin can place such patients at risk for recurrent thrombosis. A recent report has implicated Protein C deficiency in the development of warfarin-induced skin necrosis.[163] Whether these preliminary findings will be confirmed among larger series of Protein C–deficient patients is not yet known.

**Defective Fibrinolysis Due to Abnormal Plasminogen or Plasminogen Activators.** Plasmin is the enzyme that degrades the fibrin clot (fibrinolysis) (see Fig. 9–2). Plasminogen is the larger, inactive precursor that circulates in the blood and is trapped within the clot with fibrin. The plasminogen must be activated by a tissue or plasma plasminogen activator, although their exact roles are not well defined at this time. The regulation of plasminogen activation to form plasmin is a complex process facilitated by (1) release of *vascular* (tissue) plasminogen activator from the vessel wall, (2) factor XIIa activation of *plasma* plasminogen activator, and (3) Protein C, which may act by release of vascular plasminogen activator (see Fig. 9–2). This process is physiologically inhibited by plasminogen activator inhibitors including $\alpha_2$ plasmin inhibitor, also termed alpha-2 antiplasmin (see Fig. 9–2). Once formed, the enzyme plasmin cleaves fibrin at specific sites. Potentially, a hypercoagulable state due to diminished fibrinolysis could be due to any of the following abnormalities: (1) deficient or dysfunctional plasminogen activator; (2) an increased inhibitor of fibrinolysis; (3) fibrin that is resistant to plasmin degradation (dysfibrinogenemia); and (4) diminished plasmin/plasminogen (see Fig. 9–2). In fact, defects in each of these biochemical elements have been reported in association with familial thromboembolic disease.

At least two groups have reported families with defective release of *vascular* (tissue) plasminogen activator from the vessel wall.[23, 153] Defects in the activation of a *plasma* plasminogen activator have been suggested in Factor XII–deficient patients.[26] Factor XII (Hageman factor) is most often thought of as the initial factor in the "intrinsic" arm of the coagulation cascade (see Chapter 3, Fig. 3–5). It also appears to have a role in fibrinolysis vis-à-vis its activation of *plasma* plasminogen activator. Factor XII–deficient patients do not have a clinical bleeding disorder[36] but may have a hypercoagulable disorder.[26, 155] Indeed, the index case, Mr. Hageman, died of a massive pulmonary embolism[39] (Fig. 9–4). Deficiency of prekallikrein (Fletcher factor), another contact activation factor, may also be associated with a hypercoagulable state; not enough cases have been observed to confirm this.[155]

Qualitative and quantitative abnormalities of plasminogen have been reported in association with recurrent thromboembolic disease (see Table 9–5). Functional and immunologic assays have been described but are not widely available.[19–21, 152] Most such patients have functional levels that are decreased to a greater extent than the immunologic levels, implying a qualitative defect in the plasminogen molecule.[20, 152] A recently described patient and two asymptomatic family members had markedly decreased im-

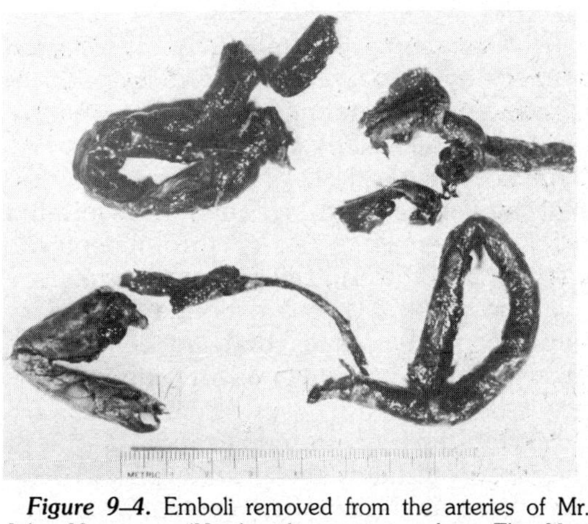

***Figure 9–4.*** Emboli removed from the arteries of Mr. John Hageman. (Used with permission from The New England Journal of Medicine. Photograph courtesy of Drs. Robert J. Busse, Jr., Robert P. Sheon, and Oscar D. Ratnoff.)

munologic *and* functional levels of plasminogen, implying a quantitative defect.[21]

Abnormal fibrinogen (dysfibrinogenemia) has been described most commonly in patients with acquired bleeding disorders (see Table 9–5). However, a few such patients with dysfibrinogenemia appear to be hypercoagulable;[24, 155] in some cases this may be due to resistance of the abnormal fibrin to degradation by plasmin.

**Other Disorders.** Disorders of platelets and the vessel wall may be associated with an increased risk of thromboembolism. Homocystinuria is a rare autosomal recessive disorder that carries a high morbidity and mortality from both arterial and venous thrombosis at an early age.[28, 31] The metabolic disorder causes endothelial cell injury, which is presumably responsible for abnormal platelet–vessel wall interactions as measured by a shortened platelet survival time.

In summary, there are presently only a few well-characterized defects that can be classified as primary hypercoagulable disorders. Except for AT III and Protein C deficiency, there is little information regarding the actual frequency of these disorders. The other disorders may be more common than the few case reports indicate, but screening for them has been limited because the assays are not widely available. Systematic screening of large numbers of normal and affected individuals will be required to place these disorders in their proper perspective.

## SECONDARY HYPERCOAGULABLE STATES

In contrast to the relatively uncommon primary hypercoagulable disorders, with increasingly well defined molecular mechanisms, are the relatively common secondary hypercoagulable states. These secondary hypercoagulable syndromes may be associated with an increased risk of thromboembolic events, but the molecular mechanisms are not known. Table 9–1 lists the secondary hypercoagulable states that are believed to be associated with venous thromboembolic disease.

**Immobilization.** Immobilization is one of the most commonly recognized causes of the hypercoagulable state in such diverse groups as hospitalized patients, paraplegics, stroke victims, and those undergoing prolonged sedentary travel.[40–47] Platelet aggregation may be the initiating event; with prolonged stasis, platelet aggregates may form in the pockets behind the cusps of venous valves, especially if they are incompetent.[48] This may trigger local activation of the coagulation cascade with propagation of the clot favored by the positive feedback loop of platelet aggregation and coagulation activation.

**Postoperative State.** The postoperative state is a complex example of the secondary hypercoagulable state. Orthopedic procedures generally carry an increased risk of venous thromboembolism compared with other operative procedures.[49–56] Certain procedures such as total hip replacement have been shown by intraoperative venography to cause almost complete occlusion of the femoral veins.[4] The frequency of DVT in patients with tibial fractures[49, 50] or those undergoing hip surgery[51–53] is estimated to be as high as 50 per cent by a combination of invasive and noninvasive tests. The frequency of fatal PE complicating hip surgery is high[54–56] (see Table 8–10, page 145).

Other surgical groups are at a somewhat lower but still significant risk. In five series of patients undergoing thoracic or abdominal surgery, the incidence of venous thrombosis, as documented by the sensitive method of $^{125}$I fibrinogen leg scanning, ranged from 14 to 33 per cent.[57–61] A review of five series of over 200 patients undergoing open prostatectomy shows a 35 per cent frequency of venous thrombosis by leg scanning. This compares with a significantly lower frequency in patients undergoing transurethral prostatectomy.[62] Thus, several factors are important in the pathogenesis of postoperative venous thrombosis, including immobilization, local impairment of venous return, and the extent of tissue trauma and coagulation enzyme activation. There are also several other contributing risk factors for postoperative thrombosis, including malignancy, pregnancy, oral contraceptive use, previous venous thrombosis,[6] advanced age, and varicose veins. Patients with primary hypercoagulable disorders are also at increased risk for postoperative thromboembolism.

**Malignancy.** Trousseau recognized the relationship between thrombosis and malignancy in the description of migratory thrombophlebitis in cancer patients.[64] Several postmortem studies have found the frequency of venous thrombosis and pulmonary emboli to be much higher in patients with certain types of cancers,[58, 65] especially adenocarcinoma of the pancreas, lung, stomach, prostate, colon, breast, and uterus. Other prospective studies of surgical patients have confirmed an approximately threefold higher frequency of thromboembolism in those with malignant disease.[6, 66–68]

The presentation of the hypercoagulable state associated with malignancy is highly variable. Five overlapping syndromes have been defined:[69] (1) nonbacterial thrombotic endocarditis; (2) arterial emboli; (3) DIC with or without associated hemorrhage; (4) superficial migratory thrombophlebitis often involving unusual locations such as the upper extremities; and (5) typical deep venous thrombosis and/or pulmonary emboli. This discussion will be confined to the latter two manifestations.

Migratory superficial thrombophlebitis is an otherwise rare disorder that should call attention to the possibility of an occult malignancy; it may antedate the diagnosis of the malignancy by months or years.[70, 71] More recently, Gore and coworkers[72] have drawn attention to the increased frequency of occult malignancy in patients who present with acute pulmonary embolism. These investigators have found an increased frequency of occult malignancy in association with patients who present with DVT (personal communication). Overall, patients with malignancy may demonstrate two striking laboratory features: (1) evidence of an inflammatory response, which includes nonspecific elevations in platelet count, fibrinogen (factor I) and factors V, VIII, IX, and X and (2) evidence of generalized coagulation system activation ranging from subclinical, chronic DIC to fulminant DIC with microangiopathic hemolytic anemia.[72] Indeed, a low platelet count or low fibrinogen level in a patient with malignancy may be the only evidence of chronic DIC.

Chronic DIC, with its predisposition to either thrombosis or hemorrhage, may be due to release from the tumor of a "thromboplastin-like material," such as mucin, which can activate factor X.[68, 73, 74] Promyelocytic leukemia is frequently accompanied by bleeding due to DIC but may also be complicated by thrombotic events. Promyelocyte granules release several proteases,[76] including elastase, which can directly activate factor X,[156] and thromboplastin, which can activate Factor VII.[76]

Laboratory evaluation of the cancer patient with a thrombotic complication should be directed at detecting the presence of DIC, using the following criteria: (1) thrombocytopenia and microangiopathic changes observed on the peripheral blood smear, (2) prolonged PT and/or PTT, (3) hypofibrinogenemia, (4) elevated fibrin split products, and, in the future, (5) elevation of more sensitive parameters of thrombin activation.

The treatment of cancer patients with thromboembolic disease is notoriously difficult because of recurrent thrombosis despite anticoagulation and the high potential for toxicity in patients who may bleed into necrotic tumor and/or have an underlying bleeding diathesis due to DIC. Heparin may be superior to warfarin in the treatment of such patients. In a review by Sack,[69] heparin was successful in treating 80 per cent of cancer patients with thrombosis, although there were recurrences in 50 per cent of the patients when heparin was stopped, despite the use of oral anticoagulants. In fact, warfarin was only effective in preventing recurrences in 20 per cent of such patients. Successful therapy of the underlying malignancy is also associated with a lower incidence of recurrence. However, high-dose combination chemotherapy, with its attendant myelosuppression, may add to the risk of anticoagulation. Malignancy and its treatment are not an absolute contraindication to anticoagulation. Some[77] advocate the use of inferior vena cava interruption in such patients. This may be useful in preventing fatal pulmonary emboli in patients with a documented high risk of bleeding or in those who have clearly failed anticoagulant therapy, but it does not prevent the morbidity of ongoing phlebitis and may exacerbate the postphlebitic syndrome. For these reasons, initial anticoagulation with intravenous heparin followed by dose-adjusted subcutaneous heparin would be particularly attractive, although it has not been evaluated and compared with other alternatives in this setting.

**Pregnancy.** Pregnancy is accompanied by significant changes in the physiologic balance between coagulation and fibrinolysis.[78] It is clear from the increased frequency of both hemorrhagic and thrombotic complications associated with pregnancy that the delicate balance can be readily perturbed in either direction. Important factors may include changes in hormonal balance, venous blood flow, and viscosity.[79] In addition to the risk associated with physiologic changes of pregnancy, the increased risks of thrombotic disease in the postpartum period reflect additional traumatic or surgical factors.

Pregnancy can be viewed as a state of

ongoing placental fibrin deposition manifested as compensated, chronic low-grade DIC. The spiral arteries that supply the maternal blood to the placenta undergo extensive remodeling during pregnancy with replacement of the internal elastic lamina and smooth muscle by fibrin.[78] This extravascular and intravascular fibrin deposition is mediated by thrombin and requires the continuous activation and consumption of clotting factors. Levels of factors XII, X, VIII, and V increase during the third trimester; fibrinogen levels in the third trimester reach twice those in the nonpregnant state.[78] Antithrombin III levels are slightly depressed but not enough to confer an enhanced risk of thrombosis.[14] More importantly, there is biochemical evidence of enhanced thrombin activation during normal pregnancy, which is manifested by elevated $F_{1+2}$, T:AT, and FPA levels[12] (see Fig. 9–1). Coincident with the activation of the coagulation system is a progressive depression in fibrinolytic activity, which is rapidly reversed after delivery of the placenta.[78] There is evidence that the placenta produces an inhibitor of fibrinolysis.[80, 81] Thus, the hemostatic system with ongoing coagulation activation and fibrinolytic depression is poised to cope with the sudden hemostatic challenge of placental separation, in which placental vessels carrying 500 to 800 ml of blood per minute must be clotted off within seconds.[78] The placental bed is rapidly covered by a fibrin mesh requiring 5 to 10 per cent of total body fibrinogen.[82] This combination of coagulation activation, fibrinolytic depression, and the trauma of birth with the release of tissue factor (especially in cesarean section) contributes to the greater risk of pathologic thrombosis in the postpartum period.

There is considerable controversy regarding the risk of thrombosis in the antepartum period.[83–85] The true frequency of thrombotic disease during pregnancy may be significantly underestimated[79] owing to the lack of recognition of subclinical events and the reservations of exposing the fetus to the risks of radiographic procedures. It is possible that antepartum subclinical disease may become manifest during the postpartum period as thrombophlebitis or later as venous insufficiency, postphlebitic syndrome, or pulmonary hypertension.[86] Nevertheless, there is agreement that the first month after delivery carries an increased risk of thromboembolism ranging from 20- to 50-fold.[84, 87]

The treatment of thrombotic disease during pregnancy poses special problems. Heparin, despite its association with increased fetal death, is the preferred anticoagulant during pregnancy, because it does not cross the placenta and does not carry the risks of teratogenicity and fetal intracranial hemorrhage associated with the oral anticoagulants (see Chapter 6). Heparin may be initiated by the intravenous route and continued by intermittent subcutaneous injection throughout pregnancy and the postpartum period, when the risk of recurrence is highest. Heparin is not secreted into human milk. Heparin should be discontinued during labor and resumed two to six hours after delivery.[88]

**Oral Contraceptives and Estrogens.** Most epidemiologic studies indicate that oral contraceptives increase the risk of cardiovascular,[89–92] cerebral vascular,[91–93] and venous thromboembolic events.[96–99] Analysis is complicated by the extreme heterogeneity of oral contraceptive preparations containing estrogens of differing potency and dose combined with a corresponding number of progesterones of varying potency and androgenic and estrogenic activity. Initial case-control studies from Britain[100–102] and the United States[92, 96, 103, 104] have all found that contraceptive users have an increased risk of venous thrombosis compared with controls; the relative risk range is from 2:1 to 11:1. One large prospective trial of 23,000 users and a similar number of controls found an estimated risk of 5:1;[105] however, the study lacked objective diagnostic criteria.

The one study that cast doubt on the risk was a controlled randomized trial of 10,000 women followed for up to eight years.[106] Although no increased risk was found in the oral contraceptive group, there were several major flaws in the study design. This study was unblinded and without objective end points, and almost two-thirds of the potential cases of thrombophlebitis were excluded from the analysis, leaving only 17 clinical events (nine in the oral contraceptive users and eight in the nonusers).

Overall, the weight of evidence strongly favors an increased risk of venous thrombosis in women taking the oral contraceptive pill.[107] Although the absolute risk is still low, there is an increased relative risk, which may be heightened by other risk factors, including duration of use, age, cigarette smoking, parity, and surgery. The risk of thrombotic events appears to be most closely correlated with estrogen dose (potency). Preparations containing more than 50 micrograms of estrogen were associated with an excess risk of thrombotic events.[108] Further evidence of the association of estrogen use and the risk of thrombosis can be found in trials of estrogen suppression of lactation[109] and treatment of prostatic cancer[110, 111] and coronary artery disease.[112] A group of men who participated in the Coronary Drug Project were given estrogen to modify the risk of subsequent myocardial infarction; the increased frequency of PE necessitated the discontinuation of this segment of the trial.

The absence of increased risk of PE in users of postmenopausal estrogen replacement most likely reflects the much lower potency of the conjugated estrogens used to treat these patients. The relative dose used in replacement therapy is between one-fifth and one-tenth of that used in typical "low-estrogen" oral contraceptive pills.[113]

Although most authorities agree on the relative risk, the underlying mechanisms remain enigmatic. Elevated levels of factors VII, IX, X, prothrombin, and fibrinogen are nonspecific and do not contribute to the risk of thrombosis.[114–116] Rather, these and other laboratory abnormalities, including a shortened PTT[117] and PT[118] and thrombocytosis, are probably only markers of a hyperactive coagulation system rather than the causes of it. There is some evidence that platelet hyperaggregability is increased by estrogen.[119] Elevated levels of beta thromboglobulin and platelet factor 4 (PF4), markers of platelet aggregation, are found in plasma of patients treated with estrogen. There is conflicting evidence of reduced[157] or enhanced[118] fibrinolytic activity in oral contraceptive users.

Over the past several years there has been much interest in the effects of oral contraceptives on antithrombin III levels. Several studies in animal models[121, 122] and in women[125–129] taking estrogen-containing oral contraceptives have shown that estrogens decrease antithrombin III activity. Sagar and coworkers[5] found that oral contraceptive use was associated with an increased risk of DVT in women undergoing surgery. They found that the risk correlated with a decrease in antithrombin III level and that AT III levels dropped more in oral contraceptive users than in nonusers. Three out of five women on oral contraceptives with preoperative antithrombin III activities of less than 50 per cent developed DVT. Nevertheless, care must be taken in inferring a causal relationship between low AT III levels induced by oral contraceptives and development of DVT. Other effects of estrogens, such as decreased vascular plasminogen activator levels,[157] increased blood viscosity,[130] and increased distensibility of peripheral veins leading to venous stasis, may also contribute to a hypercoagulable state.

**Other Disorders.** Diabetes[131] and hyperlipidemia[132, 133] have been associated with hyperaggregable platelets; prosthetic devices[134] and vasculitis[135] have been associated with abnormal platelet survival. Certain hematologic disorders may decrease blood fluidity, e.g., Waldenström's macroglobulinemia,[136] polycythemia vera,[29, 137–142] and sickle cell anemia.[143] The myeloproliferative disorders (polycythemia vera, chronic myelogenous leukemia, essential thrombocytosis, myeloid metaplasia, and myelofibrosis) usually are associated with a hemorrhagic tendency, but a proportion of these patients have an increased risk of thrombosis independent of hematocrit, white cell, or platelet count.[29, 30]

Finally, in addition to estrogens, other drugs with direct hemostatic activity have been associated with an increased risk of thrombosis in certain circumstances. Epsilon-aminocaproic acid (EACA; [Amicar®]) is a potent inhibitor of fibrinolysis (see Fig. 9–2). It has been used to control bleeding in subarachnoid hemorrhage, after urologic surgery, after oral surgery in hemophiliacs, and as an antidote to reverse the effects of fibrinolytic agents. EACA inhibits clot dissolution (fibrinolysis) by inhibiting plasmin (see Fig. 9–2). The patients who develop a serious thrombotic process while receiving EACA probably all have an underlying thrombotic tendency, which may be unmasked by EACA's inhibition of fibrinolysis. Disseminated intravascular coagulation (DIC) seems to be the common risk factor[144] in case reports of thrombosis associated with EACA following septic abortion, prostatectomy[146] for prostate carcinoma, and surgical repair of congenital cardiac anomalies.[147]

Prothrombin complex concentrates (Proplex®, Konyne®) containing activated clotting factors have been associated with abnormal thrombotic events. Paradoxically, *heparin* may cause an immune thrombocytopenia, often associated with arterial and venous thromboses (see Chapter 6).

This chapter has focused on the recognition and laboratory evaluation of the hypercoagulable patient, the understanding of the clinical features and pathophysiology of the few currently recognized[10] hypercoagulable disorders, and the variety of clinical conditions that may be associated with a secondary hypercoagulable state. Hopefully, as newer laboratory tests become generally available, the screening, specific diagnosis, and individualized treatment of patients suspected of having hypercoagulable states will be facilitated.

ACKNOWLEDGMENTS: The author acknowledges Drs. A. I. Schafer and R. D. Rosenberg for their stimulating discussions on these topics. Drs. K. A. Bauer, A. I. Schafer, and N. W. Stead kindly reviewed my manuscripts. Special thanks go to my wife, Elizabeth Ryll, for typing Chapters 3, 6, and 9.

## REFERENCES


1. Hirsh, J.: Hypercoagulability. Semin. Hematol., *14*:409, 1977.
2. Hirsh, J.: Blood tests for the diagnosis of venous and arterial thrombosis. Blood, *57*:1, 1981.
3. Lowe, G. D. O.: Laboratory evaluation of hypercoagulability. Clin. Haematol., *10*:407, 1981.
4. Wessler, S.: Hypercoagulability: What cause, what therapy? J. Cardiovasc. Med., *7*:199, 1982.
5. Sagar, S., Thomas, D. P., Stamatakis, J. D., et al.: Oral contraceptives, antithrombin-III activity, and post-operative deep-vein thrombosis. Lancet, *1*:509, 1976.
6. Kakkar, V. V., Howe, C. T., Nicolaides, A. N., et al.: Deep vein thrombosis of the leg: Is there a "high risk" group? Am. J. Surg., *120*:527, 1970.
7. Nicolaides, A. N., and Irving, D.: Clinical factors and the risk of deep vein thrombosis. *In* Nicolaides, A. N. (Ed.): Thromboembolism; Etiology, Advances in Prevention and Management, University Park Press, Baltimore, 1975, p. 193.
8. Lau, H. K., Rosenberg, J. S., Beeler, D. L., et al.: The isolation and characterization of a specific antibody population directed against prothrombin activation fragments $F_2$ and $F_{1+2}$. J. Biol. Chem., *254*:8751, 1979.
9. Lau, H. K., and Rosenberg, R. D.: The isolation and characterization of a specific antibody population directed against the thrombin:antithrombin complex. J. Biol. Chem., *255*:5885, 1980.
10. Nossel, H. L., Yudelman, I., Canfield, R. E., et al.: Measurement of fibrinopeptide A in human blood. J. Clin. Invest., *54*:43, 1974.
11. Yudelman, I., and Greenberg, J.: Factor affecting fibrinopeptide A levels during anticoagulant therapy. Blood, *59*:787, 1982.
12. Bauer, K. A., and Rosenberg, R. D.: Assays for thrombin generation in humans with prethrombotic states. Thromb. Haemost., *50*:159, 1983.
13. Teitel, J. M., Bauer, K. A., Lau, H. K., et al.: Studies of the prothrombin activation pathway utilizing radioimmunoassays for the $F_2/F_{1+2}$ fragment and thrombin:antithrombin complex. Blood, *59*:1086, 1982.
14. Thaler, E., and Lechner, K.: Antithrombin-III deficiency and thromboembolism. Clin. Haematol., *10*:369, 1981.
15. Prochownik, E. V., Antonarakis, S., Bauer, K. A., et al.: Molecular heterogeneity of inherited antithrombin-III deficiency. New Engl. J. Med., *308*:1549, 1983.
16. Farweed, J., Messmore, H. L., Walenga, J. M., et al.: Laboratory evaluation of antithrombin-III: A critical overview of currently available methods for antithrombin-III measurements. Semin. Thromb. Hemost., *8*:288, 1982.
17. Morlar, R. A., Kleiss, A. J., and Griffin, J. H.: Human protein C: Inactivation of factors V and VIII by the activated molecule. An. N.Y. Acad. Sci., *370*:303, 1981.
18. Broekman, A. W., Veltkamp, J. J., and Bertina, R. M.: Congenital Protein C Deficiency and Venous Thromboembolism: A Study of Three Dutch Families. New Engl. J. Med., *309*:341, 1983.
19. Aoki, N., Moroi, M., Sakata, Y., et al.: Abnormal plasminogen: A hereditary molecular abnormality found in a patient with recurrent thrombosis. J. Clin. Invest., *61*(5):1186, 1978.
20. Kazama, M., Tahara, C., Suzuki, Z., et al.: Abnormal plasminogen, a case of recurrent thrombosis. Thromb. Res., *21*:517, 1981.
21. Lottenberg, R., Dolly, F. R., and Kitchens, L.: Pulmonary hypertension and recurrent thromboembolic phenomena associated with hypoplasminogenemia. Clin. Res., *31*:318a, 1983.
22. Campbell, E. E., Shifman, M. A., Pasqua, J. J., et al.: A chromogenic assay for releasable plasminogen activator. Clin. Chem., *28*:1125, 1982.
23. Johanson,L., Hedner, U., and Nilsson, I. M.: A family with thromboembolic disease associated with deficient fibrinolytic activity in vessel wall. Acta Med. Scand., *203*:477, 1978.
24. Al-Mondhiry, H. A. B., Bilezikian, S. B., and Nossel, H. L.: Fibrinogen "New York"—an abnormal fibrinogen associated with thromboembolism: Functional evaluation. Blood, *45*:607, 1975.
25. Isacson, S., and Nilsson, I. M.: Defective fibrinolysis in blood and vein walls in recurrent "idiopathic" venous thrombosis. Acta Chir. Scand., *138*:313. 1972.
26. Dyerberg, J., and Stoffersen, E.: Recurrent thrombosis in a patient with Factor XII deficiency. Acta Hematol., *63*:278, 1980.
27. Mueh, J. R., Herbst, K. D., and Rapaport, I.: Thrombosis in patients with the lupus anticoagulant. Ann. Intern. Med., *92*:156, 1980.
28. Harker, L. A., Slichter, S. J., Scott, C. R., et al.: Homocystinemia: Vascular injury and arterial thrombosis. New Engl. J. Med., *291*:537, 1974.
29. Chievitz, E., and Thiede, T.: Complications and causes of death in polycythemia vera. Acta Med. Scand., *172*:513, 1962.
30. Schafer, A. I.: Deficiency of platelet lipoxygenase activity in myeloproliferative disorders. New Engl. J. Med., *306*:381, 1982.
31. Thompson, A. R., and Harker, L. A.: Manual of Thrombosis and Hemostasis. F. A. Davis, Philadelphia, 1983, p. 142.
32. Kauffman, R. H., Veltkamp, J. J., van Tilberg, N. H., et al.: Acquired antithrombin deficiency and thrombosis in the nephrotic syndrome. Am. J. Med., *65*:607, 1978.
33. Egeberg, O.: Inherited antithrombin deficiency causing thrombophilia. Thromb. Diath. Haemorrh., *13*:516, 1965.
34. Shapiro, S. S., and Anderson, D. B.: Thrombin Inhibition in Normal Plasma. *In* Lundblad, R. L.,

Fenton, J. W., and Mann, K. G. (Eds.): Chemistry and Biology of Thrombin. Ann Arbor Science Publishing, Michigan, 1977, p. 361.
35. Rosenberg, R. D.: Actions and interactions of antithrombin and heparin. New Engl. J. Med., *292*:146, 1975.
36. Filip, D. J., Eckstein, J. D., and Veltkamp, J. J.: Hereditary antithrombin-III deficiency and thromboembolic disease. Am. J. Hematol., *2*:343, 1976.
37. Marciniak, F., Farley, C. H., and DeSimone, P. A.: Familial thrombosis due to antithrombin-III deficiency. Blood, *43*:219, 1974.
38. Colman, R. W.: Contact phase, the Hemophilias and von Willebrand's Disease. *In* Colman, R. W., Hirsh, J., Marder, V. J., et al. (Eds.): Hemostasis and Thrombosis. J. B. Lippincott, Philadelphia, 1982, p. 3.
39. Ratnoff, O. D., Busce, F. J., and Sheon, R. P.: The demise of John Hageman. New Engl. J. Med., *279*:760, 1968.
40. Collins, R. E. C., Field, S., and Castleden, W. N.: Thrombosis of leg arteries after prolonged travel. Br. Med. J., *2*:1478, 1979.
41. Slazman, E. W.: Venous Thromboembolism in Surgical Patients. *In* Sherry, S., Brinkhous, K. M., Genton, E., et al. (Eds.): Thrombosis. National Academy of Sciences, Washington, D.C., 1969, p. 50.
42. Gallus, A. S.: Venous Thromboembolism: Incidence and Clinical Risk Factors. *In* Madden, J. L., and Hume, M., (Eds.): Venous Thromboembolism: Prevention and Treatment. Appleton-Century-Crofts, New York, 1976, p. 1.
43. Gibbs, N. M.: Venous thrombosis of the lower limbs with particular reference to bed-rest. Br. J. Surg., *45*:209, 1957.
44. Sevitt, S., and Gallagher, N.: Venous thrombosis and pulmonary embolism: A clinico-pathological study in injured and burned patients. Br. J. Surg., *48*:475, 1961.
45. Warlow, C., Ogston, D., and Douglas, A. S.: Venous thrombosis following strokes. Lancet, *1*:1305, 1972.
46. Cope, C., Reyes, T., and Skversky, N. J.: Phlebographic analysis of the incidence of thrombosis in hemiplegia. Radiology, *109*:581, 1973.
47. Heatley, R. V., Hughes, L. E., Morgan, A., et al.: Preoperative or postoperative deep-vein thrombosis? Lancet, *1*:437, 1976.
48. Sigel, B., Ipsen, J., and Felix, W. R.: Epidemiology of lower extremity deep venous thrombosis in surgical patients. Ann. Surg., *179*:278, 1974.
49. Hjelmstedt, A., and Bergvall, U.: Incidence of thrombosis in patients with tibial fractures. Acta Chir. Scand., *134*:209, 1968.
50. Cohen, S. H., Erlich, G. E., Kauffman, M. S., et al.: Thrombophlebitis after knee surgery. J. Bone Joint Surg., *55A*(1):106, 1973.
51. Field, E. S., Nicolaides, A. N., Kakkar, W., et al.: Deep vein thrombosis in patients with fractures of the femoral neck. Br. J. Surg., *59*:377, 1972.
52. Hampson, W. G. J., Harris, F. C., Lucas, H. K., et al.: Failure of low-dose heparin to prevent deep vein thrombosis after hip replacement arthroplasty. Lancet, *12*:795, 1974.
53. Hume, M., Turner, R. H., Kuriakose, T. X., et al.: Venous thrombosis after total hip replacement. J. Bone Joint Surg., *58*:933, 1976.
54. Zekert, F.: Thrombosen, Embolien und Aggregationshemmer in der Chirurgie. Schattauer, Stuttgart, 1975.
55. Eskeland, G., Solheim, K., and Skjorten, F.: Anticoagulant prophylaxis, thromboembolism and mortality in elderly patients with hip fractures. Acta Chir. Scand., *131*:16, 1966.
56. Sevitt, S., and Gallagher, N. G.: Prevention of venous thrombosis and pulmonary embolism in injured patients. Lancet, *2*:981, 1959.
57. Smyrnis, S. A., and Kolios, A. S.: Deep vein thrombosis in surgical patients: A phlebographic study. Surgery, *73*:692, 1973.
58. Spriad, S., Antcliffe, A. C., and Martin, P.: Deep vein thrombosis in two district hospitals in Essex. Br. J. Surg., *58*:563, 1971.
59. Gallus, A. S., Hirsh, J., Tuttle, R. J., et al.: Small subcutaneous doses of heparin in prevention of venous thrombosis. New Engl. J. Med., *288*:545, 1973.
60. Nicolaides, A. N., DuPont, P. A., Desai, S., et al.: Small doses of subcutaneous sodium heparin in preventing deep vein thrombosis after major surgery. Lancet, 2:890, 1972.
61. Kakkar, V. V.: The diagnosis of deep vein thrombosis using the $^{125}$I fibrinogen test. Arch. Surg., *104*:152, 1972.
62. Carter, C., and Gent, M.: The Epidemiology of Venous Thrombosis. *In* Colman, R. W., Hirsh, J., Marder, V. J., et al.(Eds.): Hemostasis and Thrombosis. J. B. Lippincott, Philadelphia, 1982, p. 810.
63. Freiman, D. G., Suyemoto, J., and Wessler, S.: Frequency of thromboembolism in man. New Engl. J. Med., *272*:1278, 1965.
64. Trousseau, A.: Phlegmasia alba dolens. Clinique Medical d l'Hotel Dieu de Paris, Vol. 3. Second edition. Balliere, Paris, 1865.
65. Coon, W. W., and Coller, F. A.: Some epidemiologic considerations of thromboembolism. Surg. Gynecol. Obstet., *109*:487, 1959.
66. Walsh, J. J., Bonnar, J., and Wright, F. W.: A study of pulmonary embolism and deep leg vein thrombosis after major gynecological surgery using labelled fibrinogen-phlebography and lung scanning. J. Obstet. Gynaecol. Br. Commonw., *81*:311, 1974.
67. Rosenberg, L., Evans, M., and Pollack, A. V.: Prophylaxis of postoperative leg vein thrombosis by low dose subcutaneous heparin or postoperative calf muscle stimulation: A controlled clinical trial. Br. J. Med., *1*:649, 1975.
68. Pineo, G. F., Brain, M. C., Gallus, A. S., et al.: Tumors, mucous production and hypercoagulability. Ann. N.Y. Acad. Sci., *230*:262, 1974.
69. Sack, G. H., Levin, J., and Bell, W. R.: Trousseau's syndrome and other manifestations of chronic disseminated coagulopathy in patients with neoplasms: Clinical, pathophysiologic and therapeutic features. Medicine, *56*:1, 1977.
70. Greenberg, E., Diverte, M. B., and Woolner, L. B.: A review of unusual systemic manifestations associated with carcinoma. Am. J. Med., *36*:106, 1964.
71. Lieberman, J. S., Borrero, J., Urdaneta, E., et al.: Thrombophlebitis and cancer. JAMA, *177*:542, 1961.
72. Gore, J. M., Appelbaum, J. S., Greene, H. L., et al.: Occult cancer in patients with acute pulmonary embolism. Ann. intern. Med., *96*:556, 1982.
73. Pineo, G. F., Regorczi, F., and Hatton, M. W. C.: The activation of coagulation by extracts of mucin: A possible pathway of intravascular coagulation

accompanying adenocarcinomas. J. Lab. Clin. Med., *82*:255, 1973.
74. Gordon, S. G., Franks, J. J., and Lewis, B.: Cancer procoagulant-A: A factor X activating procoagulant from malignant tissue. Thromb. Res., *6*:127, 1975.
75. Bick, R. L.: Alterations of hemostasis associated with malignancy. Semin. Thromb. Hemost., *5*:1, 1978.
76. Gralnick, H. R., and Abrell, E.: Studies of procoagulant and fibrinolytic activity of promyelocytes in acute promyelocytic leukemia. Br. J. Haematol., *24*:89, 1973.
77. Moore, F. D., Jr., Osteen, R. T., Karp, D. D., et al.: Anticoagulants, venous thromboembolism and cancer patients. Arch. Surg., *116*:405, 1981.
78. Hathaway, W. E., and Bonnar, J.: Perinatal Coagulation. Grune and Stratton, N.Y., 1978, p. 27.
79. Tooke, J. E., and McNicol, G. P.: Thrombotic disorders associated with pregnancy and the pill. Clin. Haematol., *10*:613, 1981.
80. Kwano, T., Morimoto, K., and Uemura, Y.: Urokinase inhibitors in human placenta. Nature, *217*:253, 1968.
81. Walker, J. E., Gow, L., Campbell, D. M., et al.: The inhibition by plasma of urokinase and tissue activator-induced fibrinolysis in pregnancy and the puerperium. Thromb. Haemost., *49*:21, 1983.
82. Ludwig, H.: Uterine haemostase postpartum. Thromb. Diath. Haemorrh., Suppl. *44*:105, 1971.
83. Aapo, L. A., Johnson, M. R., and Juergens, J. L.: Acute deep vein thrombosis associated with pregnancy. Obstet .Gynecol., *28*:553, 1966.
84. Carter, C., and Gent, M.: The Epidemiology of Venous Thrombosis. *In* Colman, R. W., Hirsh, J., Marder, V. J., et al. (Eds.): Hemostasis and Thrombosis. J. B. Lippincott, Philadelphia, 1982, p. 811.
85. Howie, P. W.: Thromboembolism. Clin. Obstet. Gynecol., *4*:397, 1977.
86. Fleischner, F. G.: Recurrent pulmonary embolism and cor pulmonale. New Engl. J. Med., *276*:1213, 1967.
87. Siegel, D. G.: Pregnancy, the puerperium and the steroid contraceptive. Millbank Mem. Fund Q., *50*(Suppl. 2):15, 1972.
88. Graeff, H., and Kuhn, W.: Coagulation Disorders in Obstetrics. W. B. Saunders, Philadelphia, 1980, p. 105.
89. Beral, V.: Cardiovascular disease mortality trends and oral contraceptive use in young women. Lancet, 2:1047, 1976.
90. Kaplan, N. M.: Cardiovascular complications of oral contraceptives. Ann. Rev. Med., *29*:31, 1978.
91. Durand, J. L., and Bressler, R.: Clinical pharmacology of the steroidal oral contraceptives. Adv. Intern. Med., *24*:97, 1979.
92. Stolley, P. D., Tonascia, J. A., Tockman, M. S., et al.: Thrombosis with low-estrogen oral contraceptives. Am. J. Epidemiol., *102*:197, 1975.
93. Collaborative Group for the Study of Stroke in Young Women: Oral contraception and increased risk of cerebral ischemia or thrombosis. New Engl. J. Med., *288*:871, 1973.
94. Collaborative Group for the Study of Stroke in Young Women: Contraceptives and stroke in young women. JAMA, *231*:718, 1975.
95. Ask-Upmark, E., and Bickerstaff, E. R.: Vertebral artery occlusion and oral contraceptives. Br. Med. J., *1*:487, 1976.
96. Boston Collaborative Drug Surveillance Program. Oral contraceptives and venous thromboembolic disease, surgically confirmed gallbladder disease, and breast tumors. Lancet, *1*:1399, 1973.
97. Sartwell, P. E.: Oral contraceptives and thromboembolism: A further report. Am. J. Epidemiol., *94*:192, 1971.
98. Sager, S., Thomas, D. P., Stamatakis, J. D., et al.: Oral contraceptives, antithrombin-III activity, and postoperative deep-vein thrombosis. Lancet, *1*:509, 1976.
99. Vessey, M. P., and Mann, J. I.: Female sex hormones and thrombosis. Br. Med. Bull., *34*:157, 1978.
100. Vessey, M. P., and Doll, R.: Investigation of relation between use of oral contraceptives and thromboembolic disease. Br. Med. J., *2*:199, 1968.
101. Vessey, M. P., and Doll, R.: Investigation of relation between use of oral contraceptives and thromboembolic disease: A further report. Br. Med. J., *2*:651, 1969.
102. Vessey, M. P., Doll, R., Fairbairn, A. S., et al.: Postoperative thromboembolism and use of oral contraceptives. Br. Med. J., *3*:123, 1970.
103. Sartwell, P. E., Masi, A. T., Arthes, F. G., et al.: Thromboembolism and oral contraceptives: An epidemiologic case-control study. Am. J. Epidemiol., *90*:365, 1969.
104. Greene, G. R., and Sartwell, P. E.: Oral contraceptive use in patients with thromboembolism following surgery, trauma or infection. Am. J. Public Health, *62*:680, 1972.
105. Oral Contraceptives and Health: An Interim Report from the Oral Contraception Study of the Royal College of General Practitioners, p. 1. London, Sir Isaac Pitman & Sons, 1974.
106. Fuertes de la Haba, A., Curet, J. O., Pelegrina, I., and Bangdiwala, I.: Thrombophlebitis among oral and non-oral contraceptive users. Obstet. Gynecol., *38*:259, 1971.
107. Carter, C., and Gent, M.: The epidemiology of venous thrombosis. *In* Colman, R. W., Hirsh, J., Marder, V. J., et al. (Eds.): Hemostasis and Thrombosis. J. B. Lippincott, Philadelphia, 1982, p. 816.
108. Colman, R. W., Hirsh, J., Marder, V. J., et al.: Hemostasis and Royal College of General Practitioners. Oral Contraceptives and Health. Pitman Medical, London, 1974.
109. Daniel, D. G., Campbell, H., and Turnbull, A. C.: Puerperal thromboembolism and suppression of lactation. Lancet, *2*:287, 1967.
110. Blackard, C. E., Doe, R. P., Mellinger, G. T., et al.: Incidence of cardiovascular disease and death in patients receiving diethylstilbestrol for carcinoma of the prostate. Cancer, *26*:249, 1970.
111. The Veterans Administration Co-operative Urological Research Group. Treatment and survival of patients with cancer of the prostate. Surg. Gynecol. Obstet., *124*:1011, 1967.
112. Coronary Drug Project Research Group. The coronary drug project. JAMA, *214*:1303, 1970.
113. Judd, H. L. (Moderator): Estrogen replacement therapy: Indications and complications. Ann. Intern. Med., *98*:195, 1983.
114. Meade, T. W., Brozovic, M., Chakrabarti, R., et al.: An epidemiological study of the haemostatic and other effects of oral contraceptives. Br. J. Haematol., *34*:353, 1976.
115. Ambrus, J. L., Niswander, K. R., Courey, N. G., et al.: Progestational agents and blood coagulation. II. Am. J. Obstet. Gynecol., *103*:994, 1969.
116. Poller, L., and Thomson, J. M.: Clotting factors

during oral contraception: Further report. Br. Med. J., *2*:23, 1966.
117. Poller, L., Tabiowo, A., and Thompson, J. M.: Effects of low-dose oral contraceptives on blood coagulation. Br. Med. J., *3*:218, 1968.
118. Boston Collaborative Drug Surveillance Program. Surgically confirmed gallbladder disease, venous thromboembolism, and breast tumors in relation to postmenopausal estrogen therapy. New Engl. J. Med., *290*:15, 1974.
119. Schorer, A. E., Gerrard, J. M., White, J. G., et al.: Oral contraceptive use alters the balance of platelet prostaglandin and thromboxane synthesis. Prostaglandins Med., *1*:5, 1978.
120. Ball, A. P., and McKee, P. A.: Fibrin formation and dissolution in women receiving oral contraceptive drugs. J. Lab. Clin. Med., *89*:751, 1977.
121. Kobayashi ,N., and Takeda, Y.: Effects of a large dose of oestradiol on antithrombin-III metabolism in male and female dogs. Eur. J. Clin. Invest., *7*:373, 1974.
122. Kobayashi, N., and Takeda, Y.: Studies on the effects of estradiol, progesterone, cortisol, thrombophlebitis, and typhoid vaccine on synthesis and catabolism of antithrombin-III in the dog. Thromb. Haemost., *37*:111, 1977.
123. Gitel, S. N., Grieco, A. J., Wessler, S., et al.: The thrombogenicity of G-azauridine. Haemostasis, *8*:54, 1979.
124. Gitel, S. N., Salvati, E. A., Wessler, S., et al.: The effect of total hip replacement and general surgery on antithrombin-III in relation to venous thrombosis. J. Bone Joint Surg. (Am.), *61*:653, 1979.
125. Howie, P. W., Mallinson, A. C., Prentice, C. R. M., et al.: Effect of combined oestrogen-progesterone contraceptives, oestrogen and progesterone on antiplasmin and antithrombin activity. Lancet, *2*:1329, 1974.
126. Conrad, J., Salomon, Y., and Samama, M.: Variations de l'antithrombine-III chez les femmes sous contraception orale. Pathol. Biol. (Paris), *22*:77, 1974.
127. Fagerhol, M. K., Abilgaard, U., Bergsjo, P., et al.: Oral contraceptives and low antithrombin-III concentration. Lancet, *2*:1175, 1970.
128. Peterson, R. A., Krull, P. E., Finley, P., et al.: Changes in antithrombin-III and plasminogen by oral contraceptives. Am. J. Clin. Path., *53*:468, 1970.
129. von Kaulla, E., and von Kaulla, K. N.: Oral contraceptives and low antithrombin-III activity. Lancet, *1*:36, 1970.
130. Aronson, H. B., Magora, F., and Sihenker, J. G.: Effect of oral contraceptives on blood viscosity. Am. J. Obstet. Gynecol., *10*:997, 1971.
131. Colwell, J. A., Halushka, P. V., Sarji, K. E., et al.: Platelet function and diabetes mellitus. Med. Clin. North Am., *62*:753, 1978.
132. Carvalho, A. C. A., Colman, R. W., and Lees, R. S.: Platelet function in hyperlipoproteinemia. New Engl. J. Med., *290*:434, 1974.
133. Shattil, J. S., Bennett, J., Colman, R. W., et al.: Abnormalities of cholesterol-phospholipid composition in platelets and low density lipoproteins of human hyperbetalipoproteinemia. J. Lab. Clin. Med., *89*:341, 1977.
134. Harker, L. A., Hirsh, J., Gent, M., et al.: Critical evaluation of platelet inhibiting drugs in thrombotic disease. Prog. Hematol., *9*:229, 1975.
135. Fauci, S. S., Haynes, B. F., and Katz, P.: The spectrum of vasculitis. Ann. Intern. Med., *89*:660, 1978.
136. Bloch, K. J., and Maki, D. G.: Hyperviscosity syndromes associated with immunoglobulin abnormalities. Semin. Hematol., *10*:113, 1973.
137. Perkins, J., Israels, M., and Wilkinson, J. F.: Polycythemia vera: Clinical studies on a series of 127 patients managed without radiation therapy. Q. J. Med., *33*:499, 1964.
138. Thomas, D. J., Marshall, J., Russell, R. W., et al.: Effect of haematocrit on cerebral blood-flow in man. Lancet, *2*:941, 1977.
139. Zucker, S., and Mielke, C. H.: Classification of thrombocytosis based on platelet function tests: Correlation with hemorrhagic and thrombotic complications. J. Lab. Clin. Med., *80*:385, 1972.
140. Vreeken, J., and van Aken, W. G.: Spontaneous aggregation of blood platelets as a cause of idiopathic thrombosis and recurrent painful toes and fingers. Lancet, *2*:1395, 1971.
141. Preston, F. E., Emmanuel, I. G., Winfield, D. A., et al.: Essential thrombocytopenia and peripheral gangrene. Br. Med. J., *3*:548, 1974.
142. Wu, K. K.: Platelet hyperaggregability and thrombosis in patients with thrombocythemia. Ann. Intern. Med., *88*:7, 1978.
143. Klug, P. P., Lessin, L. S., and Radice, P.: Rheologic aspects of sickle cell disease. Arch. Intern. Med., *133*:577, 1974.
144. Marder, V. J., Butler, F. O., and Barlow, G. H.: Antifibrinolytic Therapy. *In* Colman, R. W., Hirsh, J., Marder, V. J., et al. (Eds.): Hemostasis and Thrombosis. J. B. Lippincott, Philadelphia, 1982, p. 644.
145. Clarkson, A. R., Sage, R. E., and Lawrence, J. R.: Consumption coagulopathy and acute renal failure due to gram negative septicemia after abortion: Complete recovery with heparin therapy. Ann. Intern. Med., *70*:1191, 1969.
146. Chartyan, C., and Purtilo, D.: Glomerular capillary thrombosis and acute renal failure after epsilon-aminocaproic acid therapy. New Engl. J. Med., *280*:1102, 1969.
147. Gralnick, H. R., and Greipp, P.: Thrombosis with epsilon aminocaproic acid therapy. Am. J. Clin. Pathol., *56*:151, 1971.
148. Bauer, K. A., Ashenhurst, J. B., Chediak, J., et al.: Antithrombin "Chicago": A functionally abnormal molecule with increased heparin affinity causing familial thrombophilia. Blood, *62*:1242, 1983.
149. Sas, G., Peto, I., Banhegyi, D., et al.: Heterogeneity of the "classical" antithrombin III deficiency. Thromb. Haemost., *43*:133, 1980.
150. Comp, P. C., and Esmon, C. T.: Generation of fibrinolytic activity by infusion of activated protein C in dogs. J. Clin. Invest., *68*:1221, 1981.
151. Griffin, J. H., Evatt, B., Zimmerman, T. S., et al.: Deficiency of protein C in congenital thrombotic disease. J. Clin. Invest., *68*:1370, 1981.
152. Sakata, Y., and Aoki, N.: Molecular abnormality of plasminogen. J. Biol. Chem., *255*:5442, 1980.
153. Stead, N. W., Bauer, K. A., Kinney, T. R., et al.: Venous thrombosis in a family with defective release of vascular plasminogen activator and elevated plasma factor VIII/von Willebrand's factor. Am. J. Med., *74*:33, 1983.
154. Bussel, J. B.: Circulating anticoagulants: Physiologic and pathologic. Hosp. Prac., *18*:169, 1983.
155. Goodnough, L. T., Saito, H., and Ratnoff, O. D.:

Thrombosis or myocardial infarction in congenital clotting factor abnormalities and chronic thrombocytopenia: A report of 21 patients and a review of 50 previously reported cases. Medicine, *62*:248, 1983.
156. Bauer, K., and Rosenberg, R. D.: Personal communication, 1983.
157. Miller, K. E., and Pizzo, S. V.: Venous and arterial thromboembolic disease in women using oral contraceptives. Am. J. Obstet. Gynecol., *144*:824, 1982.
158. Esmon, C. T.: Protein C: Biochemistry, physiology, and clinical implications. Blood, *62*:1155, 1983.
159. Broekmans, A. W., van der Linden, I. K., Veltkamp, J. J., et al.: Prevalence of isolated protein C deficiency in patients with venous thrombotic disease and in the population. (Abstract.) Thromb. Haemost., *50*:350, 1983.
160. Bertina, R. M., Broekmans, A. W., van Es-Krommenhoek, T., et al.: The use of a functional assay for plasma Protein C in the diagnosis of Protein C deficiency. (Abstract.) Thromb. Haemost., *50*:350, 1983.
161. Comp, P. C., Nixon, R. R., and Esmon, C. T.: Determination of functional levels of Protein C, an antithrombotic protein, using thrombin-thrombomodulin complex. Blood, *63*:15, 1984.
162. Sala, N., Owen, W. G., and Collen, D.: A functional assay of Protein C in human plasma. Blood, *63*:671, 1984.
163. Broekmans, A. W., Bertina, R. M., Hofmann, V., et al.: Protein C and the development of skin necrosis during anticoagulant therapy. Thromb. Haemost., *49*:251, 1983.

CHAPTER 10

# MASSIVE PULMONARY EMBOLISM

PETER M. HOAGLAND, M.D.

This separate chapter devoted to massive pulmonary embolism is justified because the distinction between massive and nonmassive embolism is clinically useful and necessary. The massive embolism, when recognized, requires alterations in management. The first section of this chapter will focus on a clinically useful definition of the massive pulmonary embolism. Following this definition, clues for the recognition of the massive embolism will be presented. Later segments will discuss treatment options, both medical and surgical. Potential medical therapies include high doses of heparin, thrombolytic agents, smooth muscle relaxants, and compounds designed to block the neurohumoral responses to pulmonary embolus. More invasive surgical treatments include embolectomy, artificial cardiopulmonary support, and interruption of the inferior vena cava. As will become quickly apparent, a great deal of clinical judgment is necessary in selecting appropriate patients for these newer therapies, because they are uniformly more hazardous than traditional care but fortunately often more efficacious.

## DEFINITION

A pragmatic definition of the massive pulmonary embolus requires that the afflicted patient be at sufficiently increased risk of an unfavorable outcome with traditional care to justify the added risk and potential benefit of more aggressive therapy. The immediately fatal embolism is certainly massive in terms of its consequences. However, it allows no management options other than prophylaxis. These patients will not be the focus of this chapter.

Unfortunately, very few studies of mortality in pulmonary embolism have been stratified according to the anatomic size of the embolus. However, the relatively high mortality reported for patients with a large embolus (Table 10–1) suggests that, in general, the anatomically large embolus poses a greater threat than a small one. Therefore, the anatomically massive embolus warrants special consideration. Indeed, in the past, the definition of a massive embolism has been purely anatomic. For example, in the National Heart, Lung, and Blood Institute cooperative trials of thrombolytic therapy,[1, 2] *massive* was defined as a significant filling defect in two or more pulmonary lobar arteries. This implies involvement of a minimum of 40 per cent of the pulmonary arterial tree. Others have drawn the line at roughly the same point, defining the anatomically massive embolus as one that involves 40 to 50 per cent or more of the pulmonary vasculature.[3, 4] Angiographic series (Table 10–2) suggest that between 30 per cent and 60 per cent of pulmonary emboli are anatomically massive.

A hemodynamic, rather than an anatomic, stratification of prognosis proves to be even more powerful. Therefore, a hemodynamic rather than an anatomic definition of a massive embolism is chosen here. The hemodynamic consequences of an embolus are a function of three parameters: (1) the size of

***Table 10–1.*** Mortality Studies Stratified by Anatomic Size of Embolus

| Reference | "Small" Embolism Size (Mortality) | "Large" Embolism Size (Mortality) |
|---|---|---|
| McDonald[8] 23 patients with major PE treated with heparin, streptokinase, or surgery | | (6/23 = 24%) |
| Hall[4] 88 patients all >50% obstruction at angiography | | (16/88 = 18%) |
| Alpert[7] 144 angiogramed patients from Peter Bent Brigham Hospital | (4/99 = 4%) | (8/45 = 18%) |
| Phase 1 Cooperative Trials[1]* | (7/71 = 10%) | (6/89 = 6%) |

*Note: The roughly equal mortality between large and small emboli in the Phase 1 trial is a surprise. One possible explanation is that the high frequency of underlying cardiopulmonary disease in those patients with small emboli contributed to an unusually high mortality.

***Table 10–2.*** Percentage of Patients with Anatomically Large Emboli

| Reference | Large* | Less than Large | Total |
|---|---|---|---|
| Phase 1 Cooperative Trials[1] | 89 (56%) | 71 (44%) | 160 |
| Phase 2 Cooperative Trials[2] | 107 (64%) | 60 (36%) | 167 |
| Alpert et al.[7] | 30% | | 144 |

*Usually defined as involvement of two lobar arteries or 40%–50% of pulmonary arterial circulation.

***Table 10–3.*** Mortality Studies Stratified by Hemodynamic Presentation

| Reference | No Clinical Shock (Mortality) | Clinical Shock (Mortality) |
|---|---|---|
| Miller et al.[9] | (2/27 = 7%)<br>embolectomy—10<br>streptokinase—9<br>heparin—8 | (9/41 = 22%)<br>embolectomy—23<br>streptokinase—8<br>heparin—10 |
| Alpert et al.[7] | (6/125 = 5%) | (6/19 = 32%) |
| Phase 1 Cooperative Trials[1] | (8/148 = 5%) | (5/15 = 33%) |

***Table 10–4.*** Mortality from Massive PE Without Shock

| Reference | N | Therapy | Mortality |
|---|---|---|---|
| Phase 1 trial* | 39 | Heparin | 7.7% |
| Phase 2 trial* | 40 | Urokinase | 5.0% |
| Peter Bent Brigham Hospital[7]† | 31 | Heparin or vena caval interruption | 6.0% |
| Miller et al.[9]† | 27 | Heparin, streptokinase, or embolectomy | 7.4% |

*Massive = obstruction of ≥ 40% pulmonary circulation.
†Massive = obstruction of ≥ 50% pulmonary circulation.
Reproduced with permission from Dalen, J. E.: Controversy. The case against fibrinolytic therapy. J. Cardiovasc. Med., 5:799, 1980.

the embolus, (2) underlying cardiopulmonary disease, and (3) the neurohumoral response to the embolus. In autopsy series, among all fatal emboli, whether death occurs suddenly or more slowly, only half meet an anatomic definition of massive.[5] Often the fatal embolus is relatively small but poorly tolerated because of underlying medical disease such as congestive heart failure, chronic lung disease, or prior pulmonary emboli. As Table 10–3 demonstrates, the prognosis of patients with embolism and circulatory insufficiency, shock, or cardiac arrest is particularly grim. This is true regardless of the size of the embolus. Mortality in patients without shock is low, regardless of the size of the embolism. As Table 10–4 demonstrates, the mortality even among patients with an anatomically massive embolism is low (six to eight per cent) if the patients do not demonstrate circulatory insufficiency. Much of the mortality in the nonshock cohort stems from underlying disease rather than the impact of embolism.[6] It is not clear that any clinical-therapeutic decision should be based on anatomy alone.

In summary, a clinically useful definition of a massive pulmonary embolism is neither simply a fatal nor a large embolus but rather an event, not immediately fatal, that places the recipient at an unusually high risk of eventual death. The best predictors of mortality are hemodynamic, not anatomic. Therefore, the massive embolism is one that causes hemodynamic deterioration, especially shock, because the prognosis of such patients under traditional care is particularly poor.[11] This group, as Table 10–5 demonstrates, is about 10 per cent of patients with emboli who survive long enough for angiographic diagnosis.

## CLINICAL AND LABORATORY RECOGNITION OF THE MASSIVE EMBOLUS

### Clinical Clues

To treat a massive embolus, it must first be recognized. Because the massive embolus is the one that causes circulatory decompensation, cardiac arrest must raise the possibility of this condition. No information is available as to what percentage of cardiac arrest is due to pulmonary embolism. It has been estimated from autopsy series that five per cent of sudden deaths are due to pulmonary embolism.[12] Embolism patients who presented with cardiac arrest had a case fatality rate of over 40 per cent in one small series,[9] clearly a grim enough prognosis to justify the diagnosis of a massive embolism.

#### Cardiac Arrest

At the time of cardiac arrest, suspicion of pulmonary embolism should exist if there is an appropriate clinical setting. The epidemiology and pathophysiology of anatomically small and large emboli are similar. The lower portion of Table 10–6 demonstrates the similarities in predisposing factors in anatomically massive and submassive emboli among the patients in the two National Institutes of Health cooperative studies. Table 10–7 summarizes the frequency of coexisting conditions in the 167 patients with emboli of all sizes from the first cooperative study. In addition, one should be aware of some of the unusual situations in which massive embolization has been described (Table 10–8).

In a cardiopulmonary arrest, a second clue in addition to an appropriate clinical setting

***Table 10–5.*** Percentage of Patients with Pulmonary Embolism Who Present with Clinical Signs of Reduced Cardiac Output

| Reference | Per Cent (%) Shock | Comments |
|---|---|---|
| Phase 1 Cooperative Trials[1] | (14/160 = 8%) | 11 anatomically massive |
| Phase 2 Cooperative Trials[2] | (12/167 = 7%) but out of a total of 107 hemodynamically large | All 12 anatomically large |
| McDonald et al.[8] | (13%) | Of "major" PE |
| Stein et al.[10] | Collapse 10%<br>Syncope 9% | Uses the phase 1 and phase 2 patients |
| Thames et al.[27] | Syncope 13% | Angiographically proven series from Peter Bent Brigham Hospital |

**Table 10–6.** Frequency of Symptoms and Signs in 327 Patients of Phase I and Phase II Studies

| Symptoms and Signs | Total Series N = 327 (%) | Massive Emboli N = 197 (%) | Submassive Emboli N = 130 (%) |
|---|---|---|---|
| Symptoms | | | |
| Chest pain | 88 | 85 | 82 |
| Pleuritic | 74 | 64 | 85* |
| Nonpleuritic | 14 | 6 | 8 |
| Dyspnea | 84 | 85 | 82 |
| Apprehension | 59 | 65 | 50† |
| Cough | 53 | 53 | 52 |
| Hemoptysis | 30 | 23 | 40* |
| Sweats | 27 | 29 | 23 |
| Syncope | 13 | 20 | 4† |
| Signs | | | |
| Respirations > 16/min | 92 | 95 | 87 |
| Rales | 58 | 57 | 60 |
| ↑ $S_2P$ | 53 | 58 | 45‡ |
| Pulse > 100/min | 44 | 48 | 38 |
| Temperature > 37.8°C | 43 | 43 | 42 |
| Phlebitis | 32 | 36 | 26 |
| Gallop | 34 | 39 | 25‡ |
| Diaphoresis | 36 | 42 | 27* |
| Edema | 24 | 23 | 25 |
| Murmur | 23 | 27 | 16‡ |
| Cyanosis | 19 | 25 | 9† |
| Predisposing condition | | | |
| Current venous disease | 49 | 55 | 47 |
| Immobilization | 55 | 60 | 46‡ |
| Congestive heart failure and chronic lung disease | 38 | 36 | 40 |
| Malignant neoplasm | 6 | 8 | 5 |

NOTE: ↑ $S_2P$ = increase in the intensity of the pulmonic component of the second heart sound.
*Statistically significant ($p < 0.01$).
†Statistically significant ($p < 0.001$).
‡Statistically significant ($p < 0.05$).
Reproduced with permission from Bell, W. R., et al.: The clinical features of submassive and massive pulmonary emboli. Am. J. Med., *62*:355, 1977.

**Table 10–7.** Frequency of Coexisting Conditions in 167 Patients

| Condition | % Total | Condition | % Total |
|---|---|---|---|
| Thrombophlebitis | 39.5 | Angina | 5.4 |
| Venous varicosity and insufficiency | 15 | Congestive heart failure | 17.4 |
| | | Arrhythmia | 16.2 |
| Peripheral arterial disease | 4.8 | Rheumatic heart disease | 1.2 |
| Recent immobilization from fracture (casting) | 15 | Other heart disease | 9.0 |
| | | Primary pulmonary disease | 7.8 |
| Bed rest | 32.4 | Dehydration | 3.6 |
| Recent surgery | 31.2 | Diabetes mellitus | 8.4 |
| Recent termination of pregnancy | 1.2 | Malignancy | 7.2 |
| | | Hemoglobinopathy | 1.2 |
| Pelvic disease | 6.0 | Polycythemia | 0 |
| Obesity | 30 | No predisposing etiology | 6.0 |
| Cerebrovascular disease | 6.6 | | |
| Hypertension | 10.2 | | |
| Nephrotic syndrome | 0.6 | | |
| Myocardial infarction | 12.0 | | |

Reproduced with permission from Bell, W. R., et al.: The clinical features of submassive and massive pulmonary emboli. Am. J. Med., *62*:355, 1977.

**Table 10–8.** Unusual Clinical Circumstances for Massive Pulmonary Embolism

| |
|---|
| During open heart surgery[14] |
| Mycosis fungoides–reduced fibrinolytic activity[15] |
| Young wrestler, dehydration-increased viscosity[16] |
| SVC syndrome in polycythemia vera[17] |
| Right atrial myxoma[18] |
| Post CABG clot on right atrial suture line[19] |
| Tumor[20] |
| Hydatidiform mole[21] |
| Post-tourniquet anesthesia[22] |
| Right ventricular pacer electrode[23] |
| Fungus ball in pulmonary artery[24] |
| Thrombus at site of CVP line[25] |

SVC = superior vena caval; CABG = coronary artery bypass grafting; CVP = central venous pressure.

is electromechanical dissociation, that is, no palpable pulse but ventricular complexes on the cardiac monitor. Of course, this occurs in other settings such as extensive myocardial infarction, aortic stenosis, pericardial tamponade, pneumothorax, and extreme hypovolemia and is the final common pathway of most cardiac deaths. The inability to obtain a pulse with cardiac compression in this situation should further increase the suspicion of massive pulmonary embolism. Unless prevented by obesity, cardiac compression should result in a palpable pulse in extensive myocardial infarction, the most common cause of electromechanical dissociation.[26]

### Syncope or Shock

After cardiac arrest, the next most dramatic and ominous presentation of massive embolism is with syncope or acute shock. In the National Heart, Lung, and Blood Institute Trials, among 327 patients with angiographically documented pulmonary embolism, 26 (seven per cent) presented with shock. The majority of the 26 (23) had anatomically large (involvement of two or more pulmonary lobar arteries) pulmonary emboli.[1, 2] In a subset of 215 patients from the same trial judged free of prior cardiopulmonary disease, shock occurred in 10 per cent and syncope in nine per cent.[10] This paradoxically implies that the circulatory response to embolization was no worse among the patients with prior cardiopulmonary disease (shock in seven per cent) than those without (shock in 10 per cent). This finding is diametrically opposed to the conclusions of hemodynamic studies of pulmonary embolus (to be discussed later). In an analogous study of 132 angiographically documented cases, syncope (including cardiopulmonary arrest) was the mode of presentation in 13 per cent. Of this 13 per cent, 82 per cent had a 50 per cent or greater obstruction to pulmonary circulation.[27] Not all syncope in pulmonary embolus is related to obstruction to right ventricular output; vagal bradyarrhythmias may also play a role.[28]

### Cor Pulmonale

Acute cor pulmonale from pulmonary embolism, which is next in the spectrum of clinical presentation after cardiac arrest, syncope, and shock, was originally described by Sylvester McGinn and Paul Dudley White in 1935. Their observations were based on nine cases of massive postoperative embolism.[29] Little has been added to their clinical descriptions in the ensuing half century. The patient with acute cor pulmonale is tachycardic and tachypneic; cyanosis and evidence of peripheral hypoperfusion may be present. Anxiety is common, and occasionally dramatic alterations in mental status occur. The neck veins are distended. The pulmonary component of the second heart sound is prominent, perhaps even palpable. Depending on right ventricular compensation and subsequent right-sided ejection time, splitting may be prominent or absent. Extremely wide and fixed splitting should suggest the presence of right bundle branch block. Right-sided gallops, either an S3 or S4 or both, and RV lifts are possible. In an occasional patient, a localized pericardial rub is audible along the left sternal border. This sound, called the Means-Lerman scratch, was originally described in cases of thyrotoxicosis and is the result of a dilated pulmonary artery rubbing against the pericardium.[30] Pulsus paradoxus and Kussmaul's sign have been reported, both reflecting severe right ventricular decompensation.[31] In a small number of cases, new murmurs appear either as blood rushes past a large thrombus or because of tricuspid valve insufficiency. Extremely rarely, a right-sided intracardiac thrombus interferes with tricuspid or pulmonic valve function, leading to positional murmurs and even dramatic positional changes in circulatory status.[26] Though massive embolization of any material (blood clot, fat, tumor, bone marrow, air, amniotic fluid) can precipitate cor pulmonale, other potential causes include massive pneumothorax or atelectasis, mediastinal emphysema, or rupture of an aortic aneurysm into the pulmonary artery.[32]

Not all shocky patients with high right-sided pressures have acute cor pulmonale. Sepsis, superior vena caval syndrome, pericardial tamponade, right ventricular myocardial infarction, constrictive pericarditis, restrictive cardiomyopathy, hypertrophic cardiomyopathy, and severe cardiogenic shock also occasionally present with high right-sided pressures. Of course, in the emergency setting, acute and chronic cor pulmonale are clinically indistinguishable.

#### SYMPTOMS AND SIGNS

A study comparing the clinical presentation of anatomically massive (involvement of at least two lobar arteries, implying a minimum of 40 per cent obstruction) and nonmassive emboli in the 327 patients from the two National Heart, Lung and Blood Institute cooperative studies is summarized in Table 10–6. There was a great deal of common ground between the two groups. Two general conclusions may be drawn. First, patients with large emboli are more likely to present with the physical findings of acute cor pulmonale as previously described. This follows from the general correlation between the size of an embolus and the magnitude of hemodynamic response to it. This will be discussed in more detail in later sections of this chapter. Less expected is the finding that smaller emboli are more likely to present with a clinical syndrome of pulmonary infarction as defined by pleuritic chest pain and hemoptysis.[13] Physiologically, this occurs because with a large central embolus, collateral flow to distal pulmonary units preserves tissue integrity and prevents both pulmonary infarction and pulmonary hemorrhage. In a study of 41 angiographically proven cases, only 15 per cent of patients with emboli large enough to obstruct 50 per cent of pulmonary blood flow were associated with the clinical syndrome of pulmonary infarction.[33] Although pleuritic pain is considered classic for pulmonary embolism, in massive embolism, substernal chest pain that is virtually indistinguishable from coronary ischemia is observed in as many as 25 per cent of cases.[26] This pain may result from acute dilation of the pulmonary artery or because of right ventricular ischemia.[34]

### Laboratory Clues

Further clues to the possibility of a massive embolus may be found in the ECG, chest film, and arterial blood gases. With all three, there is at best a general trend toward more dramatic abnormalities with anatomically large emboli. Therefore, because anatomically larger emboli are also generally more likely to cause significant hemodynamic embarrassment and therefore be massive as pragmatically defined here, abnormalities of these laboratory tests are more likely to be found in massive than in nonmassive emboli.

#### ELECTROCARDIOGRAM

Electrocardiographic series are highly dependent on patient selection and electrocardiographic definitions. In three studies of ECG findings in anatomically large emboli, findings of RV strain are reported in 31 to 76 per cent of patients.[29, 35, 36] However, a perfectly normal electrocardiogram is unusual in anatomically large emboli and is reported in only six per cent of the emboli involving two or more lobar arteries in the two cooperative studies. Among these same patients, the development of new right bundle branch block was observed in 10 per cent.[37] The stratification in these studies has always been anatomic, never physiologic. Therefore, the incidence of ECG changes in the physiologically decompensated embolus, the massive embolus, is not known. It is frustrating to find patients with equal, dramatic hemodynamic disturbances, one with major ECG changes and another with no abnormalities beyond nonspecific ST and T wave changes.[38] Still, it is clear that when classic ECG findings occur, the probability of right ventricular pressure abnormalities and a reduction in cardiac output is very high. The relative insensitivity of the ECG in even anatomically massive embolism has been attributed to the fact that changes may be transient and that leads $V_1$ and $V_2$ are " 'multipurpose leads' reflecting left ventricular anteroseptal and posterobasal activity as well as right ventricular abnormalities."[39] One must be particularly wary of an electrocardiogram that suggests an anterior myocardial infarction, especially in the presence of evidence of inferior injury as well. One of Dr. Marriott's many aphorisms is that when one is tempted to diagnose both an anterior and an inferior infarction, one should think of a pulmonary embolism.[175] Such a "pseudoanterior infarction pattern" (for an example see Fig. 10–1) has been described in as many as 10 per cent of major emboli.[40]

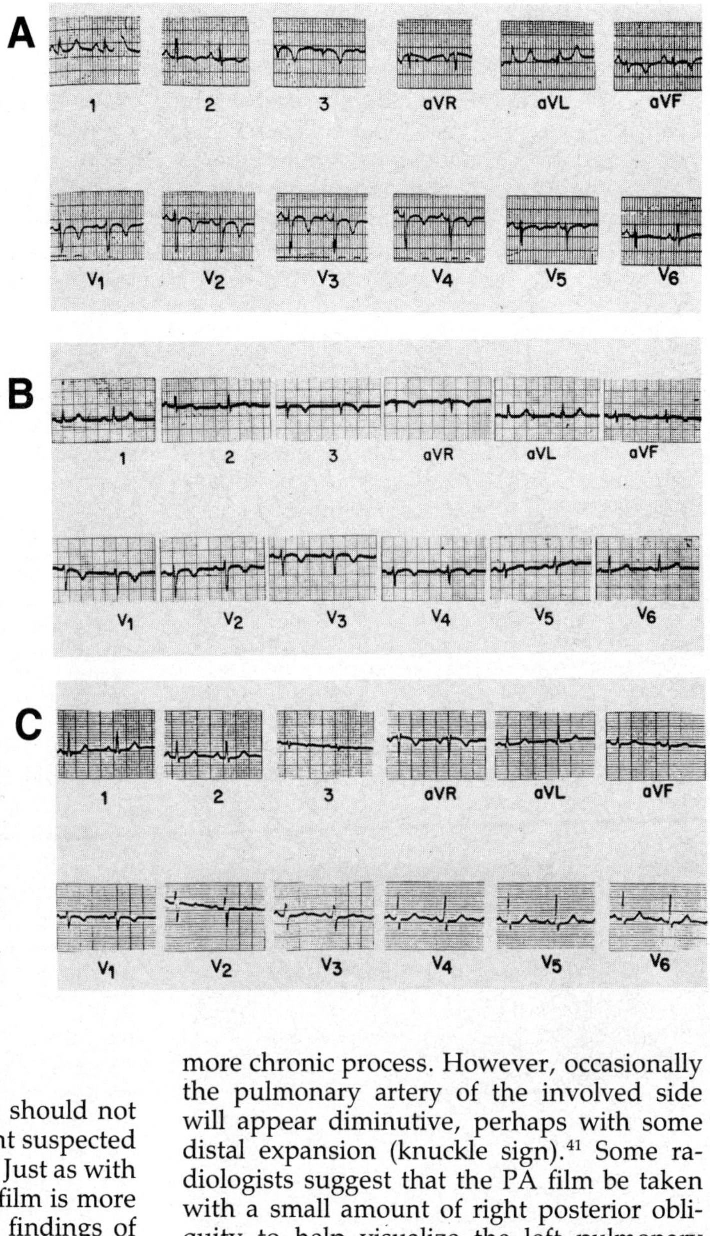


***Figure 10–1.*** Electrocardiographic evidence of acute massive pulmonary embolism. *A*, Deep T wave inversions in inferior and anterior leads on August 8; *B*, T wave abnormalities have become less marked on August 13; *C*, T wave abnormalities have resolved on November 22. (Reproduced with permission from McLarin, C. W., et al.: Pseudo-anterior myocardial infarction as a manifestation of severe pulmonary embolism. Journal of the Medical Association of Georgia, *70*:649, 1981.)

### Chest Roentgenogram

The PA and lateral chest films should not be ignored in the acutely ill patient suspected of massive pulmonary embolism. Just as with the electrocardiogram, the chest film is more likely to demonstrate the classic findings of embolization when emboli are anatomically large. A "normal" chest film is reported to occur in only nine per cent of major emboli.[8] Radiographic signs of major embolization include local atelectasis, a raised hemidiaphragm, and areas of focal oligemia (Westermark's sign [see Chapter 4, Fig. 4–2*A*]).[41] In an unblinded retrospective study of 100 chest films of patients with pulmonary embolism, all demonstrated this sign after close comparison with old films.[42] Contralateral hyperperfusion may simulate localized areas of pulmonary edema.[43] Alteration of the mediastinal silhouette is unusual in acute embolization, regardless of size, and implies a more chronic process. However, occasionally the pulmonary artery of the involved side will appear diminutive, perhaps with some distal expansion (knuckle sign).[41] Some radiologists suggest that the PA film be taken with a small amount of right posterior obliquity to help visualize the left pulmonary artery.[44]

### Arterial Blood Gases

Although larger emboli generally lead to greater increases in the alveolar-arterial oxygen gradient and subsequently to greater hypoxia, there are reported cases of anatomically massive emboli without hypoxia.[35] An unusual presentation of major embolism is that of hypoxia and paradoxic hypercarbia. This occurs because of extreme increases in the physiologic dead space: ventilated but nonperfused lung. This is the physiologic equivalent to placing a 20-foot section of additional tubing between the mouth and lungs. Under such circumstances, the effectiveness of ventilation declines dramatically. Haynes et al. reported a case of a previously healthy 40-year-old man who collapsed and was brought to an emergency room where, despite endotracheal intubation and a minute ventilation of 26 liters per minute (more than twice the normal value), the $P_{CO_2}$ remained 60 mm Hg. Pulmonary angiography demonstrated a 65 per cent obstructing embolus and the patient survived following treatment with pressors and streptokinase.[45]

If physical examination, ECG, chest film, and blood gases suggest a massive embolus, arrangements should quickly be made for a right heart catheterization and pulmonary angiogram (Fig. 10–2). This combined study not only provides the "gold standard" of diagnosis but is also very helpful in guiding further management.

### Lung Scan and Pulmonary Angiogram

One might have hoped, given the major alterations in pulmonary perfusion that result from a large embolus, that the nuclear scan might provide sufficient diagnostic information in many cases.[51] Rarely, such as when the perfusion scan demonstrates virtually no blood flow to a lung in the setting of a normal chest film and ventilation scan, the study is virtually diagnostic of a major embolus.[46] Furthermore, a scan demonstrating only minor abnormalities in the setting of an acutely ill, hemodynamically compromised patient, is against the diagnosis of massive embolism, provided that the patient is not already burdened by significant pulmonary or cardiac disease.[34] However, there are well-documented cases of large embolism with only minor abnormalities of the nuclear scan.[47] In a series of 106 patients who received a lung scan and pulmonary angiogram over a recent five-year period, angiography disproved a high- or low-probability lung scan in one-third of the patients.[48] In a recently published series, over 100 patients suspected of pulmonary embolus with abnormal perfusion scans underwent pulmonary angiography. Again, the nuclear scans were not always sufficiently specific to provide the only basis for important clinical therapeutic decisions.[49] Because patients suspected of massive embolization are acutely ill and in need of urgent, potentially hazardous therapy, the scan is usually bypassed in favor of the definitive right heart catheterization and pulmonary angiogram. Although the risks of such studies in hemodynamically compromised patients are not truly known (in a large series that included patients with diverse hemodynamic characteristics, angiographic mortality was under one per cent[50]), the benefits of rapid accurate diagnosis in such acutely ill patients tower above the risks. Further, in the rare patient with extreme hemodynamic compromise in whom surgical embolectomy is contemplated, partial cardiac bypass may be instituted using the femoral vein and artery to provide stability and support during the diagnostic procedure.[52, 53]

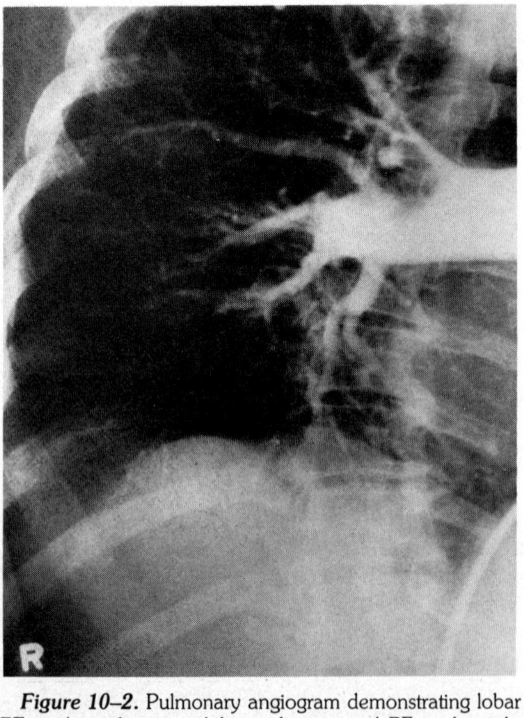


*Figure 10–2.* Pulmonary angiogram demonstrating lobar PE in the right upper lobe and segmental PE in the right middle and right lower lobes. (Figure kindly contributed by Dr. John A. Markisz, The New York Hospital and Cornell University Medical College.)

Not only will the angiogram demonstrate the size of the embolus, but simultaneously recorded hemodynamic information provides equally important prognostic information and guides to subsequent therapy. This is discussed in further detail in a later section of this chapter. Should embolism prove not to be the diagnosis, the hemodynamic study may help establish alternative diagnoses such as pericardial tamponade or right ventricular myocardial infarction.

In recent years, in an occasional case, the anatomic diagnosis of large, and therefore potentially massive, pulmonary embolism has been made in other ways. There is some experience with manual injection of contrast through a balloon-tipped pulmonary artery catheter at the bedside in an intensive care unit.[54–56] The balloon is inflated in a main pulmonary artery to occlude pulmonary blood flow, then 5 to 15 ml of contrast material, often mixed with lidocaine to suppress the cough response, is injected by hand. Plain films are then obtained. A major problem is that, in patients with emboli, diminished flow to the involved segment makes it less likely that the balloon catheter would float into that segment. With balloon injection, single-frame artifacts are possible, and examination of all lung fields is impossible.[56] At the present time, this technique must be considered experimental at best.

Inability to pass a pulmonary artery catheter beyond a point in a major pulmonary vessel, a damped "wedge-like" tracing in a main pulmonary vessel, and failure to obtain clinically plausible thermodilution cardiac outputs are further clues to embolization that may be obtained from a bedside right heart catheterization.[57]

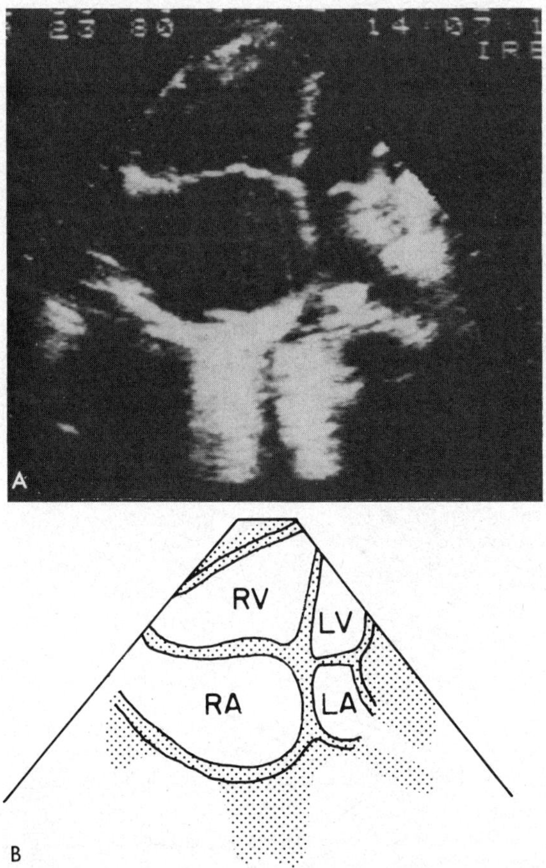


*Figure 10–3.* Apical four-chamber two-dimensional echocardiogram *(A)* and schematic drawing *(B)* from a patient with a massive pulmonary embolus. The apparent mass in the region of the left atrium is an imaging artifact.

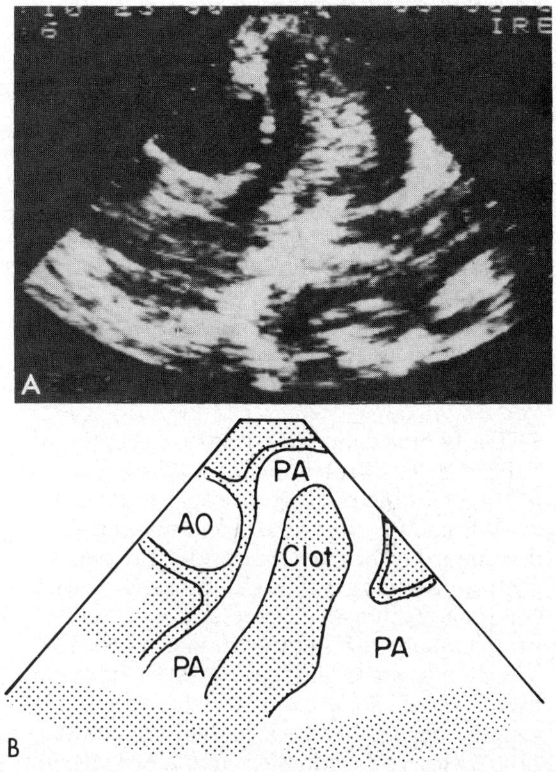


*Figure 10–4.* Two-dimensional echocardiogram in the short-axis parasternal view *(A)* and schematic drawing *(B)* demonstrating a thrombus in the pulmonary artery. This is the same patient as in Figure 10–3.

## Echocardiogram

An echocardiogram, especially a two-dimensional study, may occasionally be useful. Demonstration of an enlarged, volume-overloaded right ventricle in a hypoxic, shocky patient without right ventricular infarction is highly suggestive of massive embolization (Fig. 10–3).[58, 59] In rare cases, thrombus may be visualized inside the heart and/or a pulmonary artery[60, 61] (Fig. 10–4). Systolic fluttering from regurgitation as well as other abnormalities of tricuspid valve motion have been noted on M-mode study.[62, 63] There are a few reports of major embolization diagnosed with computed axial tomography and contrast.[61, 64] Some experience is beginning to accumulate with the use of intravenous digital subtraction angiography for the diagnosis of pulmonary embolism.[65–67] In an impressive recent series, 33 patients suspected of pulmonary embolism received both a digital subtraction study after a right atrial injection and a standard pulmonary angiogram. In 31 of the 33, an acceptable digital study was obtained that correctly identified pulmonary emboli in 12 cases and correctly excluded it in 18 cases. There was a single false-positive result. Emboli as peripheral as third-order pulmonary arteries were detected.[65] Finally, emboli may be directly visualized using transvenous angioscopy (see Chapter 14).[68, 69]

## HEMODYNAMICS

The hemodynamic response to acute embolization is a function not only of the size of the embolus but also of coexistent cardiac or pulmonary disease and the magnitude of the neurohumoral responses. In patients with underlying cardiopulmonary disease, especially congestive heart failure or multiple prior emboli, the hemodynamic response to a relatively small embolus may be devastating. This probably explains why at autopsy, only 50 per cent of fatal emboli are anatomically massive.[5] Dramatic circulatory decompensation as a response to a small embolus implies significant coexistent disease and a very poor prognosis. In the National Heart, Lung, and Blood Institute cooperative trials, only three patients with anatomically submassive emboli suffered shock, and all three failed to survive.[1]

To avoid this major impact of coexistent cardiopulmonary disease, formal hemodynamic study of the response to pulmonary embolus has focused on patients judged to be free of such disease prior to pulmonary embolus. In physiologic terms, a pulmonary embolus causes an increase in afterload, that is, an increase in forces resisting right ventricular ejection. On the right side of the circulation, this is measured roughly by the mean pulmonary arterial pressure or somewhat more accurately by calculating the pulmonary vascular resistance (PVR). Resistance, in Wood units, is the quotient of the mean pulmonary capillary wedge pressure ($\overline{PCW}$) subtracted from the mean pulmonary artery pressure ($\overline{PA}$) (i.e., the pressure drop across the circuit) divided by the cardiac output (CO) (i.e., the current across the circuit).

$$PVR = \frac{\overline{PA} - \overline{PCW}}{CO}$$

The value in Wood units, approximately one in normal patients, is often multiplied by 80 to obtain the results in metric units—dynes·sec·cm$^{-5}$. In these units the upper limit of normal at the Brigham and Women's Hospital is 100 dynes·sec·cm$^{-5}$.[70]

As demonstrated in Figure 10–5, the right ventricle is far less adept than the neighboring left at compensating for progressive increases in afterload analogous to a pulmonary embolism. Figure 10–5 demonstrates results obtained in dogs. Right ventricular failure occurs in two stages. First, as sug-

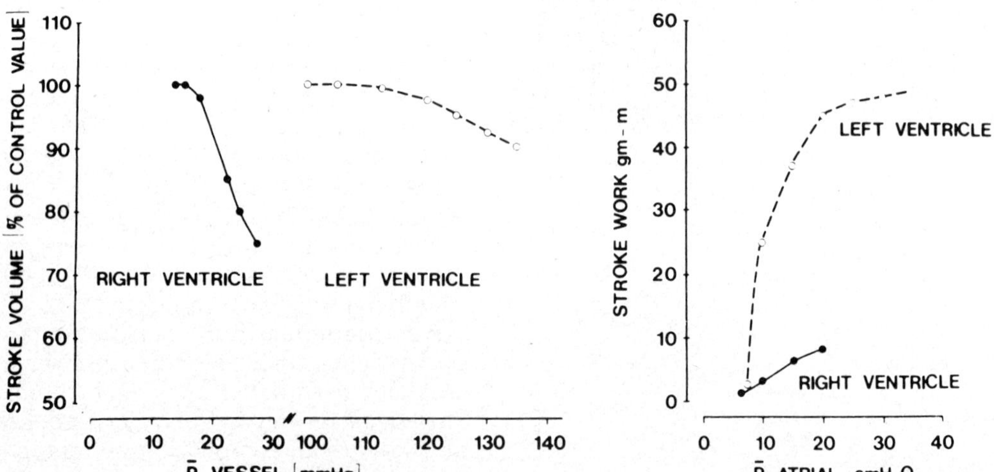


***Figure 10–5.*** Effects of increasing afterload ($\bar{P}$ vessel) and preload ($\bar{P}$ atrial) on right and left ventricular function. The data in the left panel were obtained by constricting the main pulmonary artery and aorta in dogs, thus increasing afterload. The right panel demonstrates the effect of increasing preload. (Reproduced with permission from McFadden, E. R., and Braunwald, E.: Cor pulmonale and pulmonary thromboembolism. *In* Braunwald, E. (ed.): Heart Disease. Philadelphia, W. B. Saunders, 1984, p. 1573.)

gested by the left panel of Figure 10–5, right ventricular stroke volume (volume of blood ejected with each beat) falls dramatically as afterload ($\bar{P}$ vessel) is increased. At this point, cardiac output is maintained primarily by tachycardia. If the right ventricle moves the same amount of blood across a circuit with a higher resistance, the right ventricle must do more work. For both the right and the left ventricle, a major mechanism for increasing cardiac work is to utilize the Frank-Starling relationship. If end-diastolic volume and pressure increase, then cardiac work increases (assuming a constant afterload or a constant resistance across the circuit). In other words, the heart is "better primed" before systole and is capable of doing more work. As the right ventricle calls on the Frank-Starling relationship, right ventricular end-diastolic pressure increases. This leads to an increase in mean right atrial and central venous pressure, the first phase of right ventricular failure. However, as demonstrated on the right panel of Figure 10–5, the ability of the right ventricle to increase cardiac work as preload increases ($\bar{P}$ atrial) is extremely limited. Eventually, forward output failure, a reduction in forward cardiac output, occurs. In dogs, with progressive constriction of the pulmonary artery, right ventricular and pulmonary artery pressures rise. When the pulmonary artery lumen is constricted 60 to 80 per cent of normal, right ventricular pressure reaches 80 mm Hg. Forward right ventricular failure occurs along with systemic hypoperfusion and shock.[32] Dog experiments reveal that at maximum right ventricular (RV) systolic pressure, right coronary flow reserve is exhausted, and oxygen supply is maximal. Further demands on the RV then lead to RV free wall ischemia and a deterioration in function. If coronary flow and oxygen supply are further augmented, for example by increasing central aortic pressure, this RV ischemia is alleviated and RV function improves.[71]

Figure 10–6 summarizes the results of three studies of the physiologic response to pulmonary embolism in patients without prior cardiopulmonary disease.[72–74] As demonstrated by the figure, there is a general relationship between the size of the embolus as measured by the percentage of obstructed pulmonary blood flow and increasing abnormalities of cardiac physiology. Mean pulmonary artery pressure starts to rise at about 25 per cent obstruction and rises with increasing degrees of obstruction until a maximum value of 40 mm Hg. Mean pulmonary artery pressure does not exceed this value unless acute embolization is superimposed on underlying cardiopulmonary disease, including previous embolization. Right atrial pressure rises at slightly higher degrees of anatomic obstruction and pulmonary artery pressure, because such a rise implies right ventricular congestive failure. Right atrial pressure is dependent on the underlying state of patient hydration, but in a patient with documented PE, an elevated jugular venous pressure often suggests an anatomically massive embolus. In one series, all patients with 50 per cent obstruction had a central venous pressure (CVP) of at least 10 mm Hg, whereas all those with obstruction of less than 25 per cent had a CVP of less than 10 mm Hg.[72] In

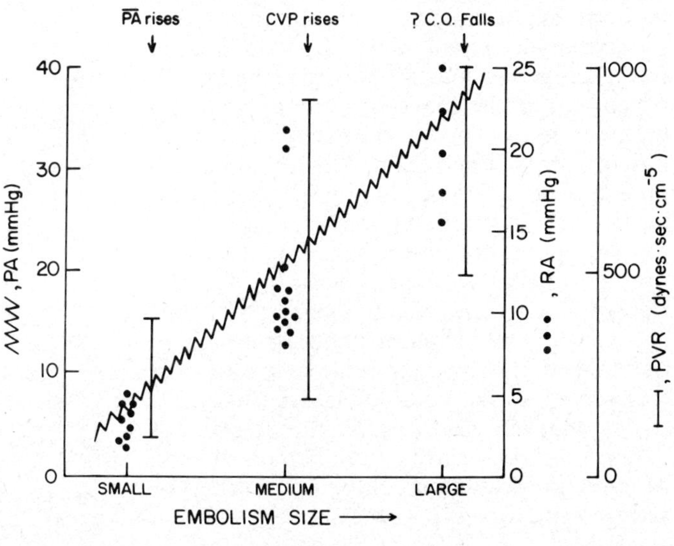


***Figure 10–6.*** Impact of embolus size on circulatory physiology. (See text for explanation.)

rare instances, acute dilation of the right ventricle inside a relatively rigid pericardium leads to a hemodynamic pattern mimicking constriction. This may lead to a situation in which filling of the left ventricle is also restricted, and left ventricular filling pressures may be elevated in the absence of left ventricular disease or systolic dysfunction.[75] There is a rough correlation between embolus size, pulse, and alveolar-arterial oxygen gradient.[8, 72–74]

In the absence of a quantifiable angiogram, measurement of the pulmonary vascular resistance (PVR) provides a crude guide to the size of an embolus. As implied by Figure 10–6, patients with a 25 per cent obstruction tend to have a PVR less than 500 dynes·sec·cm$^{-5}$, whereas patients with a 50 per cent or greater obstruction tend to have a PVR over 500 dynes·sec·cm$^{-5}$. Unfortunately, the high degree of overlap greatly reduces the predictive value of the PVR in the individual patient unless the measured value is extremely high or low.[74]

The larger the embolus, the greater the physiologic response, but, to state once again a major thesis of this chapter, the anatomically large embolus is not necessarily massive in terms of its consequences. In some patients, an anatomically large embolus is extremely well tolerated. For example, during phase 1 of the cooperative trials, only 12 of 107 patients with anatomically massive emboli suffered shock.[1] Clinical evidence of reduced cardiac output, not embolus size, correlates best with prognosis.

In McIntyre's series of 20 patients without previous cardiopulmonary disease,[73] cardiac output was often high, even in the face of anatomically large emboli. Among his five patients with at least a 50 per cent obstruction of pulmonary blood flow, two had normal filling pressures and high cardiac output. In other words, in his series, there were no patients who meet the criteria for a massive embolus as defined here. The anatomic degree of obstruction or pulmonary artery pressure is not a good predictor of cardiac output, although a reduced cardiac output is distinctly unusual without at least an obstruction of 50 per cent of pulmonary flow. This occurred in only three instances among 327 patients in the two cooperative trials.[1, 2] In this series, stroke volume was elevated, implying that elevated cardiac output was not a result of tachycardia (number of strokes/minute) but rather resulted from vasoconstriction, increased preload, and the Starling mechanism.[73] In Dalen's series of patients, most of whom had only moderate anatomically sized emboli, cardiac output again tended to be high. His study is one of the few to present cardiac output as a function of some other physiologic parameter, in this case right atrial pressure (Fig. 10–7). As this figure demonstrates, a reduced cardiac index (less than 2.0 liters/min/m$^2$) is rare without a right atrial pressure greater than 10, reflecting the physiologic fact that congestive right ventricular failure precedes forward failure.[72] In a contrasting series, McDonald found a greater tendency toward normal or low cardiac output. He noted a reduction in stroke volume and felt that tachycardia, probably mediated by hypoxia, was the mode of compensation.[8] The difference between the physiologic findings of the McDonald series and the Dalen and McIntyre series may lie in the size of the emboli involved. A greater percentage of McDonald's patients suffered an anatomically large embolus.

In summary, suspicion of massive embolism must be high when a patient in an appropriate clinical setting suffers a cardiac arrest, syncope, or the acute onset of shock, especially with a physical examination suggestive of acute cor pulmonale. The ECG, chest film, and blood gases may provide further evidence in support of the suspicion. If at pulmonary angiography the embolus is anatomically large and right ventricular pressures are abnormal, there is further support for the diagnosis. If clinical shock is present

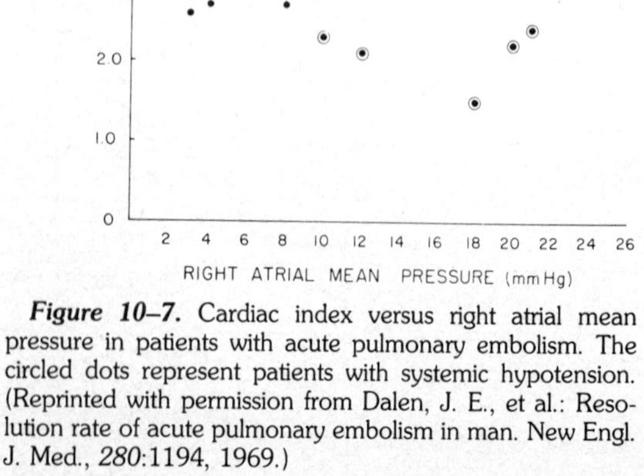


***Figure 10–7.*** Cardiac index versus right atrial mean pressure in patients with acute pulmonary embolism. The circled dots represent patients with systemic hypotension. (Reprinted with permission from Dalen, J. E., et al.: Resolution rate of acute pulmonary embolism in man. New Engl. J. Med., *280*:1194, 1969.)

at the time of angiography, confirmed by hemodynamic measurements at the time of right heart catheterization, and remains after optimization of both right and left heart filling pressures, then the diagnosis is clear: the patient is suffering from a massive pulmonary embolism and has a high likelihood of doing poorly with standard medical therapy. These are the patients who deserve the more individualized, more hazardous, and potentially more efficacious therapies that are the focus of the remainder of the chapter.

## THERAPIES FOR THE MASSIVE EMBOLUS

Faced with a patient with a pulmonary embolus and circulatory insufficiency, all avenues of traditional medical support should be fully explored. Steps in the fundamental medical support of a patient with a massive embolus are summarized in Table 10–9. Pain should be treated with intravenous opiates, usually morphine, because pain-mediated catecholamine release may contribute to elevated systemic and pulmonary vascular resistance, which reduces cardiac output. Opiates should not be used if the patient demonstrates an abnormal mental status or if there is evidence of pulmonary hypoventilation, usually best indicated by an inappropriately high $P_{CO_2}$.[32]

### Intensive General Medical Support

Oxygen should be administered to maintain the arterial $P_{O_2}$ over 60 mm Hg, not only to deliver oxygen to vital organs but also to counteract the pulmonary vasoconstrictor effects of hypoxia. If hypoxia persists despite high levels of inspired oxygen or if there is evidence of respiratory acidosis (or even perhaps inadequate pulmonary compensation for metabolic acidosis), intubation is necessary. Positive airway pressure, either in the form of continuous positive airway pressure (CPAP) or positive end-expiratory pressure (PEEP), is occasionally useful.[76] In many patients, the hypoxia of pulmonary embolism results partially from ventilation-perfusion mismatch, which is improved by positive pressure and augmentation of inspired oxygen concentration. Furthermore, there is experimental evidence, discussed in more detail later in this chapter, that PEEP may increase fibrinolysis and pulmonary production of vasodilatory prostaglandins. Unfortunately, in some patients, magnification of physiologic right-to-left shunting (rarely through a patent foramen ovale) from localized atelectasis, pulmonary edema, or intrapulmonary A-V anastomoses further contributes to hypoxia, and both increasing inspired oxygen concentrations and positive pressure are much less effective. Furthermore, positive pressure must be applied very cautiously in this clinical situation because of the high likelihood of detrimental effects on cardiac output. Still, in the common situation in which hypoxia is severe and cardiac output elevated, five to 10 cm of PEEP may be beneficial and well tolerated.[77–80]

In the hypotensive patient, in the absence of clinical evidence of pulmonary congestion, a major therapy should be a vigorous volume challenge. This increased fluid will augment the right ventricular end-diastolic pressure (preload) and will help to compensate for the afterload stress of a large embolus. Unfortunately, some patients who are free of prior cardiac disease develop cardiac rales at the time of embolization without true elevation of left heart filling pressures. In the cooperative trials, rales were extremely common, occurring in 58 per cent of all patients.[13] Nevertheless, until more accurate hemodynamic information is obtained invasively, it is reasonable to subject the patient without known cardiac disease to a cautious volume challenge. Evidence of elevated right-sided cardiac pressures on physical examination should not preclude a volume challenge. Because backward RV failure precedes forward failure, there will be some patients who are rescued from shock by pushing right-sided filling pressures far above the normal range. If cardiac output is increased by volume or by any other means, hypoxia may improve

***Table 10–9.*** Medical Support of the Massive Embolus with Conventional Modalities

| |
|---|
| Treat pain with intravenous morphine sulfate |
| Oxygen |
| Positive airway pressure (watch for detrimental effect on cardiac output) |
| Intubation if oxygenation or ventilation are unsatisfactory when unassisted |
| Hyperventilation may be necessary to compensate for metabolic acidosis |
| Positive end-expiratory pressure |
| Volume expansion |
| Sodium bicarbonate for metabolic acidosis |
| Isoproterenol |
| Other adrenergic stimulants |
| Maintain sinus rhythm |

as ventilated but underperfused areas of lung are perfused or "recruited." However, as discussed later, poorly ventilated areas may also be "recruited," and arterial oxygenation may subsequently deteriorate. One author suggests that dextran 40 might be an optimal form of volume challenge because of its anticoagulant and thrombolytic properties.[81] One should be aggressive with volume at this stage, but one should simultaneously be rushing the patient to right heart catheterization and pulmonary angiography. Right-sided pressures, wedge pressure, and cardiac output should be measured. Such measurements provide important guides for subsequent therapy and have greater prognostic significance than the angiographic anatomic information. Because many of these patients are old and at risk of left heart disease, measurement of pulmonary capillary wedge pressure and serial cardiac output is often essential to appropriate care. Further, there is evidence that pulmonary capillary permeability is increased in pulmonary embolization.[82] Therefore, left-sided filling pressures should be as low as possible to counteract the tendency of lung water to increase and contribute to hypoxia in this clinical setting.

If shock persists despite adequate filling pressures on both sides of the heart, isoproterenol should be used because of well-demonstrated pulmonary vasodilatory effects as well as the provision of inotropic and chronotropic support for the failing right ventricle. In animal models, isoproterenol lowers pulmonary vascular resistance as much as 50 per cent, usually by increasing cardiac output without a major change in pulmonary artery pressure.[83, 84] Isoproterenol dilates peripheral vascular beds, and adequate filling pressures (preload) are therefore essential to avoid a paradoxical drop in blood pressure during its administration. Generalized airway and vascular dilation from isoproterenol administration sometimes causes a fall in arterial oxygenation. It counteracts local pulmonary reflexes that restrict ventilation to poorly perfused alveoli and that reduce perfusion of underventilated ones. Similarly, underventilated areas of the lung may be "recruited" to receive increases in cardiac output.[85, 86] The major risk of isoproterenol is tachyarrhythmia. Isoproterenol greatly increases myocardial oxygen demands and should not be used in patients with coronary artery disease. Isoproterenol is not the best pressor in every patient, and others (e.g., dopamine) should be tried if the response to isoproterenol is not adequate.

Every effort should be made to maintain or achieve sinus rhythm in patients with a massive embolus. The pump-priming action of right atrial systole is vital to a stressed right ventricle. Acidosis is such a potent pulmonary vasoconstrictor that it should be aggressively treated with sodium bicarbonate. In the usual case, there is little risk of volume overload.

There is little controversy surrounding the basic medical support previously outlined. The addition of systemic anticoagulation with intravenous heparin completes the traditional medical care of the massive pulmonary embolus. However, clinical experience and the results of those few studies of pulmonary embolus that have been stratified by some index of disease severity (see Tables 10–1 and 10–3), either anatomic or hemodynamic, imply that some patients who receive only standard medical support will not do well. These are patients with evidence of circulatory insufficiency, e.g., shock. These patients are suffering a massive embolus and deserve more aggressive therapy. Two basic additional avenues of therapy are available, and they will be discussed in turn. First, the focus will be on more intensive medical therapies—thrombolytic agents, high-dose heparin, and vasodilators. Second, the focus will shift to surgical therapy, both by direct operative embolectomy and transvenous suction embolectomy. The chapter will conclude with a discussion of interruption of the inferior vena cava.

### Thrombolytic Agents

Unfortunately, efforts to define the proper role of thrombolytic therapy in the treatment of pulmonary embolism must rest on very little clinical research information. There are five published comparisons of heparin and thrombolytic agents, the results of which are summarized in Table 10–10. The total number of patients in these five studies combined is only 267. All studies demonstrated more dramatic anatomic or physiologic improvement in patients treated with thrombolytic agents. However, no study could translate these findings into an improvement in mortality or any other clinically useful parameter.[1, 87–90] In any event, limitations of sample size and the relatively low rate of mortality among control subjects greatly limit the power of these clin-

***Table 10–10.*** Summary of Comparative Trials of Heparin and Thrombolytic Agents

| Reference | N | Allocation | Findings | Mortality |
|---|---|---|---|---|
| Tibutt et al.[87] | 32 patients | Random<br>15 heparin<br>17 thrombolytic | Thrombolytic group improved by anatomy and right heart pressures | None |
| Hirsh et al.[88] | 27 patients | Nonrandom<br>10 heparin<br>17 streptokinase | Hemodynamic and anatomic improvement with streptokinase | None |
| Miller et al.[90] | 23 patients | Nonrandom<br>14 thrombolytic<br>9 heparin | Greater anatomic improvement with streptokinase | None |
| Ly et al.[89] | 25 patients | 20 random<br>5 nonrandom<br>14 thrombolytic<br>11 heparin | Statistically better anatomic improvement in thrombolytic group | 2—heparin therapy<br>1—thrombolytic therapy |
| Phase 1 Cooperative trials[1] | 160 patients | Random<br>78 heparin<br>82 urokinase | Improved hemodynamic and anatomic response in urokinase group | 6—urokinase<br>7—heparin |

ical studies. Survival rates may be considerably improved as a result of a specific therapy, but such benefit may not yet have been demonstrated, owing to the type II or beta error.[91]

The relatively large and randomized cooperative trials sponsored by the National Heart, Lung, and Blood Institute deserve further discussion. The first was a randomized comparison of heparin and urokinase in 160 patients with angiographically demonstrated pulmonary emboli. Patients received follow-up angiographic, nuclear, and hemodynamic studies. The urokinase patients had statistically greater anatomic improvement and comparatively more rapid resolution of hemodynamic abnormalities. The differences were most striking during the first few days of treatment and narrowed with time (Fig. 10–8) to the point where within five to seven days, benefit from thrombolytic therapy could not be demonstrated.[1, 34] A subsequent cooperative study, the Urokinase-Streptokinase Embolism Trial of identical design, compared 12 hours of urokinase with 12 and 24 hours of streptokinase among a total of 167 patients. These patients as a group further confirmed the anatomic and hemodynamic benefits of thrombolytic therapy in comparison with the heparin cohort from the first study. However, there was little difference detected among these three thrombolytic regimens. Urokinase appeared to act more quickly, especially in patients with anatomically large emboli, and streptokinase appeared to have greater favorable impact on hemodynamics. Mortality was equal in the three groups, reported as seven to nine per cent at two weeks and 10 to 15 per cent at six weeks (variation is among the three treatment groups).[2] The dramatic thrombolysis demonstrated in these studies stood in stark contrast to the natural history of pulmonary emboli treated with heparin alone. Prior to the cooperative trials, follow-up nuclear scan and angiographic studies had demonstrated that with anticoagulation therapy alone, resolution often did not begin for days and was frequently incomplete months after the acute event.[72, 92] A clear benefit of thrombolytic therapy in reducing mortality has never been demonstrated. In animal models, the anatomic and physiologic benefits of thrombolytic therapy have been confirmed.[93]

Other studies have refined our understanding of thrombolytic therapy in pulmo-

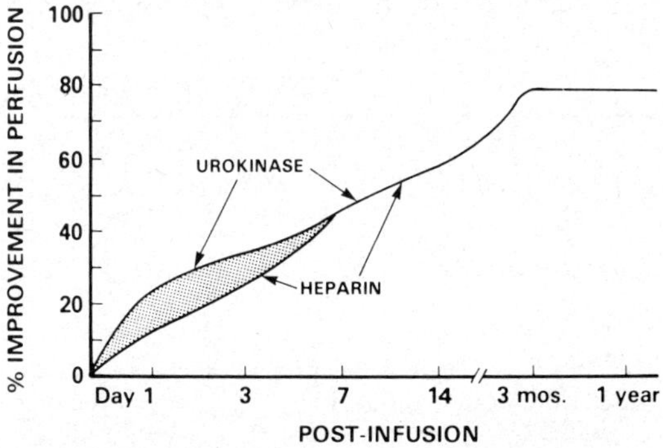


***Figure 10–8.*** Improvement in pulmonary perfusion after heparin treatment based on results of Urokinase Pulmonary Embolism Trial. There is a more rapid rate of lysis with urokinase in the first few days of treatment, but by one week, the extent of lysis is the same and thereafter the rate of lysis is identical. (Reprinted with permission from Hirsh, J., et al.: Venous Thromboembolism. Grune and Stratton, New York, 1981.)

nary emboli. Table 10–11 lists factors that appear to influence the efficacy of thrombolytic therapy. It appears that thrombolyis occurs more slowly in patients with underlying cardiopulmonary disease and that relatively older thrombi are more resistant to fibrinolysis. In the cooperative trials, patients with symptoms for longer than five days prior to angiography were excluded. In addition, emboli judged clinically to be less than 48 hours old appeared more vulnerable to thrombolysis.[1, 2, 94] Thrombolysis depends on the presence of plasminogen contained in a thrombus. Circulating human glutamyl-plasminogen does not remain fixed to a clot and may gradually leave, reducing the vulnerability of the clot to fibrinolysis. One investigator has proposed pretreatment of patients with placental plasminogen, which has a higher affinity for clot, when a thrombus proves resistant to standard thrombolytic regimens. This has proved effective in a small number of patients with pulmonary emboli.[95, 96] A new thrombolytic agent, human extrinsic plasminogen activator, which acts only at the site of a clot and does not induce a state of systemic fibrinolysis, may prove to be the optimal thrombolytic agent in the future.[97] No further benefit has been demonstrated from infusion of the thrombolytic agents directly into the pulmonary artery.[98] In some of the patients in the early trials of heparin versus thrombolytic agents, the latter were infused directly into the pulmonary artery without apparent ill effect or dramatic improvement in the degree of thrombolysis.[87] In a relevant experiment, peripheral and pulmonary artery infusions of streptokinase were compared in a canine autologous clot emboli preparation. Peripheral streptokinase proved more thrombolytic than pulmonary arterial administration.[99]

### High-Dose Heparin

Heparin has beneficial effects in the treatment of pulmonary emboli beyond its effects on the coagulation system. Specifically, heparin prevents some of the platelet-activating and degranulating effects of thrombin. In vitro experiments show that the antiplatelet effects of heparin require much higher concentrations of heparin than those required to achieve systemic anticoagulation. Therefore, very high doses of heparin have been recommended for large emboli, as much as 60,000 units per day, to try to take full advantage of this effect and to counteract the well-documented increase in heparin clearance in patients with pulmonary embolism.[42, 100] There is probably little clinical role for high-dose heparin today, because patients who are sick enough to need such therapy probably should receive thrombolytic therapy. Most of the contraindications to thrombolytic therapy apply equally to high-dose heparin.[42, 115, 116]

There has been some experimentation with the simultaneous administration of continuous infusion heparin and thrombolytic agents. In one series, 80 patients received urokinase (112,500 units per hour) and heparin (approximately 1500 units per hour) in an effort to achieve both heparin and thrombolytic benefits. Thrombolysis was achieved without an apparent increase in bleeding complications.[95] Unfortunately, this combination therapy, despite some hypothetical appeal, has never been tested in a controlled manner.

***Table 10–11.*** Factors Affecting the Degree of Thrombolysis

| Factor | Effect |
|---|---|
| Thrombus location | Thrombi in small or totally occluded vessels without blood flow are difficult to lyse |
| Thrombus duration | Lesions >7 days old usually do not resolve with thrombolytic therapy |
| Thrombus size | Complete thrombus dissolution is more difficult with massive, extensive clots |
| Activatibility of fibrinolytic system<br>Concentration of endogenous inhibitors<br>Dysproteinemia | If the endogenous inhibitors are abnormally elevated or the components of the fibrinolytic system dysfunctional, or abnormal proteins (myeloma, dysglobulinemia) present, it may not be possible to activate the fibrinolytic system adequately |
| Plasminogen concentration in thrombus | High intraclot plasminogen concentration will afford complete dissolution of thrombus |
| Body temperature | Extremes in body temperature reduce the efficiency of the fibrinolytic system |

Reproduced with permission from Bell, W. R., and Meek, A. G.: Guidelines for the use of thrombolytic agents. New Engl. J. Med., *301*:1266, 1979.

### Thrombolytic Agents vs. Heparin

The benefits of thrombolytic therapy are not without additional risks, the major risk being that of increased bleeding. During phase 1 of the cooperative trials, 45 per cent of the patients treated with urokinase, in contrast to only 27 per cent of the heparin-treated patients, suffered at least a moderate degree of blood loss. *Moderate* was defined as the loss of at least 500 ml of blood, a drop in hematocrit of at least five points, or the need for transfusion. The investigators point out that in phase 1, the rates of spontaneous bleeding (i.e., bleeding from a site other than where an invasive procedure had been performed) were equal (19 per cent), whether the patients received heparin or thrombolytic therapy. Most of the bleeding was from the sites of invasive procedures and was eventually controlled. Only one patient was withdrawn from the study because of bleeding, and bleeding never clearly contributed to mortality. Additionally, these patients were more heavily instrumented and manipulated than clinically necessary to meet the demands of the study protocol.[1] Unfortunately, complication rates between heparin and thrombolytic therapy have not been systematically compared. Contemporary clinical suspicion is that the risk of bleeding with either heparin or thrombolytic therapy is significantly less than that suffered in the cooperative trials but that heparin is still marginally safer than thrombolytic therapy. If systemic thrombolytic therapy for myocardial infarction becomes popular, more information on the relative safety of thrombolytic therapy in acutely ill patients will be generated.

As an example, Table 10–12 is a comparison of the bleeding experience in phase 2 of the cooperative trials in which all patients received thrombolytic therapy and a 1974 pilot study of peripheral streptokinase in myocardial infarction. Note that in the myocardial infarction trial, the percentage of patients with at least a five per cent drop in hematocrit was much less than in the phase 2 thrombolytic trial. Of even greater interest is the finding of an almost equal percentage of patients with a five per cent hematocrit drop among patients who received thrombolytic therapy for myocardial infarction and control patients who received no anticoagulation.[101] In a recent review of trials of intravenous thrombolytic therapy for myocardial infarction, only one to two per cent of patients were unable to tolerate intravenous streptokinase.[102] This complication rate is certainly comparable to what is experienced with continuous intravenous infusion of heparin. However, clinical suspicion remains that the incidence of serious, life-threatening bleeding is higher in patients who receive thrombolytic therapy. For example, it is estimated that the risk of an intracerebral hemorrhage with thrombolytic therapy is one per cent, compared with 0.5 per cent with intravenous heparin.[103]

In summary, there is evidence that thrombolytic therapy is more efficacious than heparin, but that thrombolytic therapy is associated with increased bleeding. The FDA approved thrombolytic agents for use in pulmonary embolism in 1977. Since then, the medical literature is replete with both anecdotal reports of extremely ill patients responding to thrombolytic therapy and semiofficial recommendations for its use. These recommendations attempt to define cohorts of patients with pulmonary emboli who are at sufficient risk of a poor outcome with traditional therapy to warrant the risks of thrombolytic therapy. The recommendations take two forms. Some recommend thrombolytic therapy for all eligible patients with emboli that involve at least two lobar arteries or 40 to 50 per cent of the pulmonary circulation—in other words, for all anatomically massive emboli regardless of hemodynamic consequences. Others require evidence of hemodynamic instability and downplay the anatomic size of emboli.[6, 11, 104–108] The Na-

***Table 10–12.*** Clinical Bleeding in Patients Undergoing Thrombolytic Therapy

| | | SMIT† | |
|---|---|---|---|
| | USPET* | *Strep-tokinase* | *Control* |
| Total patients | 167‡ | 53 | 54 |
| Type of bleeding | | | |
| Puncture site, cutdown, etc. | 92 (55)§ | 22 (41) | 4 (7) |
| Gastrointestinal | 8 (5) | 8 (15) | 3 (6) |
| Genitourinary | 12 (7) | 6 (11) | 0 (0) |
| Other | 7 (4) | 7 (13) | 3 (6) |
| Hematocrit decrease ≥5 points | 70 (42) | 14 (26) | 12 (22) |

*Urokinase-streptokinase Pulmonary Embolism Trial.
†Streptokinase myocardial infarction trial.
‡Includes 59 patients receiving urokinase for 12 hours, 54 receiving urokinase for 24 hours and 54 receiving streptokinase for 24 hours.
§Numbers in parentheses are percentages.
Reproduced with permission from Fratantoni, J. C., et al.: Thrombolytic therapy. Current status. New Engl. J. Med., *293*:1073, 1975.

tional Institutes of Health Consensus Development Conference (1980) deemed thrombolytic therapy appropriate for either an anatomically or physiologically defined massive embolus.

"the use of thrombolytic agents should be encouraged . . . for patients with pulmonary emboli with significant hemodynamic disturbances or in whom there has been obstruction of blood flow to a lobe or multiple segments. . . ."[103]

However, as discussed previously and as demonstrated in Tables 10–1 and 10–3, it is the hemodynamic response to embolization, not the anatomic size of an embolus, that best predicts prognosis. In fact, patients with an anatomically massive embolus and no evidence of circulatory insufficiency often do quite well with heparin alone (see Table 10–4). Most mortality and morbidity in this group is related not to pulmonary embolism but to comorbid medical conditions.[6] Therefore, thrombolytic therapy based on anatomy alone is a popular concept that rests on relatively little data. It is clear that another large-scale clinical trial of heparin and thrombolytic therapy is needed for this group of patients. The recommendation of thrombolytic therapy for patients with shock is on much firmer ground. The total numbers are small (see Table 10–3), but the mortality is impressive. Note again that in phase 1 of the cooperative trial, the mortality among patients with shock was 5/15 (33 per cent), or seven times the mortality of those without shock.[1] Unfortunately, a similar analysis for the phase 2 patients is not available. Among the six deaths in the urokinase-treated phase 1 cohort, only one died from shock, cardiac arrest, or congestive heart failure related directly to the embolus. In contrast, this was true of four of the seven deaths in the heparin-treated cohort.[108] In the only other hemodynamically stratified study, the mortality of patients in shock despite full therapy, including surgery when indicated, was 22 per cent, whereas the mortality without shock was seven per cent. In the same study, ten patients with a large embolus and shock received heparin therapy. Four of the 10 deteriorated on this therapy and required a change to either thrombolytic or surgical therapy.[9]

Overall, it is unfortunate that so much of this analysis must rest on the results of phase 1 of the cooperative study, which are now over a decade old. Contemporary methods of medical care might have an impact on these results. The phase 1 patients were relatively sick prior to embolization. For example, one third of them had clinical evidence of congestive heart failure prior to their admission into the study.[1] Because of the low mortality of patients with emboli and no hemodynamic embarrassment, it remains unresolved whether routine use of thrombolytic therapy in such cases is appropriate regardless of the anatomic size of the embolus. However, the high mortality of patients with shock implies that these are patients with enough to gain from thrombolytic therapy to justify the added risks, regardless of the anatomic size of the embolus.

There is a broad spectrum between patients with shock and those with no apparent embarrassment in circulatory function. For example, some patients are only transiently hypotensive, and it is uncertain whether this transient hypotension alters their prognosis sufficiently to justify thrombolytic therapy.[6, 27] In some patients, syncope represents vagally mediated bradyarrhythmia rather than overwhelming obstruction of right ventricular output.[28] Although clinical shock is the strongest predictor of poor prognosis, in the absence of shock, clinical or hemodynamic evidence of right ventricular failure has also in past experience been a predictor of relatively poor outcome. In Alpert's series of angiographically proven cases of massive PE, the mortality among patients with right ventricular failure was 14 per cent. Among 28 patients with right ventricular failure in this series, the frequency of shock was 57 per cent.[7] Some patients with large emboli and signs of right ventricular stress as reflected by elevated right atrial pressure but with preserved forward output are at increased risk of hemodynamic deterioration unless treated with thrombolytic therapy. As familiarity with thrombolytic therapy increases and estimates of its risk decline, it will become reasonable to recommend thrombolytic therapy for such patients, but further clinical trials in this area are needed.

### Approach to the Unstable Patient

The hemodynamically unstable patient suspected of massive embolization should be briefly medically stabilized and then rushed to right heart catheterization and angiography. A nuclear medicine scan is not worth the delay. Angiography should be performed from the arm to minimize the risk of dislodging a clot from the venous system in the legs or pelvis and because bleeding from the antecubital fossa is usually quickly recognized and controlled.[103] Once the diagnosis of massive embolism is confirmed by the presence of an embolus and persistent circulatory insufficiency, thrombolytic therapy should be instituted unless contraindicated. Invasive procedures should be avoided. Blood gases, if necessary, should be drawn from the radial artery with a 23- to 25-gauge needle and then the site should be compressed for a full 20 minutes. The optimum duration of thrombolytic therapy is not really known. The risk of a bleeding complication probably increases with each hour of therapy. Twenty-four to 72 hours is the current recommendation. In the patient who demonstrates dramatic hemodynamic improvement after a shorter period of time, a 24-hour infusion period should suffice before switching to heparin therapy. Twelve hours is the minimal time course of therapy that has undergone controlled study. In the phase 2 cooperative trial, 12- and 24-hour durations of therapy appeared to have equal efficacy.[2] There is no report of clinical deterioration or recurrent embolization at the time of crossover from thrombolytic to heparin therapy.

One nagging concern is the high rate of recurrent embolization reported in the cooperative thrombolytic trials. Though equal in both the heparin and thrombolytic groups, the reported recurrence rate was 20 per cent at one year.[1, 2] Limitations of sample size imply that considerable differences in the rate of recurrence could exist and have been missed by past studies. Furthermore, the high recurrence rate suggests that the practice of routinely discontinuing oral anticoagulation after six months should be critically reexamined (see page 127).

Finally, it has been argued that thrombolytic therapy should be used to reduce long-term mortality and morbidity from pulmonary embolism. In one study, using a subset of patients from the cooperative trials, 20 heparin-treated patients and 20 thrombolytic-treated patients had measurements of pulmonary capillary blood volume and carbon monoxide diffusing capacity at two weeks and one year after an acute embolus. The values for the heparin group were abnormal at both two weeks and one year. In contrast, among the thrombolytic-treated patients, values quickly returned to normal, sometimes as early as two weeks after embolism.[109] These differences in pulmonary physiology have never been shown to be of clinical significance. Complete resolution of large emboli without thrombolytic therapy has been well documented.[72, 104] In two similar studies of repeated right heart catheterization years after an acute embolus treated with heparin, no patient developed clinically significant pulmonary hypertension, including four patients whose embolus had been anatomically massive.[110, 111] The current impression is that if recurrent embolization is prevented, long-term morbidity from a single embolism, regardless of size, is usually minimal. The majority of such patients die from underlying cardiac or neoplastic disease.[112]

## Neurohumoral Factors

Another avenue for the medical therapy of the massive pulmonary embolus involves modification of the reflex-humoral responses to embolization. The relatively minor physiologic changes after surgical or balloon interruption of the pulmonary circulation imply that reflex and humoral forces must play a major role in pulmonary embolism. Smooth muscle cells in small distal pulmonary vessels can communicate with cells in major pulmonary vessels, because both are part of one large, spiral syncytium.[32] Compelling evidence is derived from cross-circulation experiments in which embolism in one animal leads to vascular and bronchial constriction in a second animal.[113] Humoral and reflex responses are not isolated, because in cats, humorally released serotonin causes vagally mediated reflex apnea and cardiac disturbances.[114]

Contemporary interest is focused on the role of prostaglandins and serotonin (see Chapter 16). In a dog model, intravenous prostacyclin ($PGI_2$), a vasodilator, improved fibrinolysis as well as cardiopulmonary physiology.[117] A subsequent dog experiment compared prostaglandin $E_1$, chosen because of greater in vivo stability than prostacyclin, and positive end-expiratory pressure (PEEP). As documented by clearance of radioactively labeled clot from dog lungs, PEEP augmented fibrinolysis and improved pulmonary physiology but had detrimental effects on cardiac function. Prostaglandin $E_1$ had no effect on thrombolysis and improved circulatory function slightly but was detrimental to pulmonary physiology, because generalized vasodilation exacerbated ventilation-perfusion mismatches. Measurements of prostaglandin metabolites suggested that embolism itself initiates the production of thromboxane $A_2$ and prostaglandins.[118] In a provocative experiment, plasma from embolized dogs reduced in vitro cat papillary muscle contractility and $Ca^{++}$-ATPase activity. The possibility that this cardiodepressive factor might be related to prostaglandins was supported by demonstrating that these responses could be blunted by pretreatment with indomethacin.[119] This experimental evidence is far too preliminary to support clinical recommendations but may pertain to the anecdotal successes reported with PEEP in human pulmonary emboli, which were discussed previously in this chapter.

Since 1953, when Comroe demonstrated that virtually all the physiology of pulmonary embolism can be duplicated by infusion of serotonin,[114] investigators have tried to modulate serotonin effects. Past successes with heparin, platelet depletion, clot aging, reserpine, cyproheptadine, and prostaglandins probably all derive at least partially from modulation of serotonin activity. A direct serotonin antagonist, ketanserin, is now available for investigational use. Ketanserin has significant physiologic benefit in animal experimental embolism. Treated animals demonstrate improved hemodynamics, pulmonary physiology, and pulmonary angiograms in comparison with control embolism animals. The only known major side effect is mild hypotension. The mechanism of this hypotension is currently not known. This drug is now undergoing a pilot experiment in human pulmonary emboli and may someday play a role in the routine medical treatment of pulmonary embolism (see Chapter 16).[122]

### Pulmonary Vasodilators

Because vasoconstriction is clearly present, pulmonary vasodilators other than isoproterenol may prove beneficial. There is a case report of a dramatic response to 100 mg of hydralazine in the setting of a massive embolism. However, the reported clinical recovery is not totally out of the bounds of what might be expected if a large embolus spontaneously broke into smaller pieces.[120] Among 13 patients with acute respiratory failure and $Po_2$ under 50, nifedipine led to a fall in mean PA pressure and pulmonary vascular resistance and an increase in cardiac output. However, when the experiment was repeated after the vasodilatory effect of an augmented concentration of inspired oxygen, nifedipine failed to demonstrate an additional vasodilatory action.[121] Unless a much greater response is demonstrated with other calcium antagonists, potential benefit does not warrant the risk of a detrimental influence on myocardial function.

### Pulmonary Embolectomy

One of the most difficult decisions in medicine is to attempt a pulmonary embolectomy for a critically ill patient, especially one so ill that even angiography to document the diagnosis is not feasible. Reported mortality rates for this procedure are exceedingly high but difficult to apply strictly to individual clinical situations, because they are so dependent on surgical skill, interval to surgical intervention, and degree of underlying cardiopulmonary disease.[7, 9, 53, 123–125] However, an emergency embolectomy is occasionally truly life-saving.

Trendelenburg's original operation, described in 1908 and first successfully employed by his student Kirschner in 1924, is a method of embolectomy without cardiopulmonary bypass. The operative mortality is reported between 87 and 95 per cent.[126] However, the operation is worth trying in the vanishingly rare situation of an otherwise healthy patient who would clearly be dead without surgery and who cannot be transported to a center where cardiopulmonary bypass is available.

Under cardiopulmonary bypass, first used for pulmonary embolectomy by Sharp in 1961, the operative mortality has steadily fallen.[126] A survey of 137 cases from 28 centers in the 1960s revealed an operative mortality of 57 per cent.[123] More recent estimates of mortality in otherwise healthy patients approach 25 per cent, a figure close to mortality with medical therapy in crudely comparable patients.[125] Obviously these patients are too rare and too ill for a randomized clinical trial.

For many patients, embolectomy is clinically inappropriate because of coexistent medical conditions. During nearly a decade at the Peter Bent Brigham Hospital, 45 patients with an anatomically massive pulmonary embolus were identified. There were six deaths among patients with a massive embolus and hypotension. Two died within an hour after angiography and therefore would not have survived long enough for mobilization of the surgical team. All four of the remaining patients had major comorbid illness, for example, metastatic carcinoma, which made an embolectomy "clinically inappropriate."[7] Similarly, in a review of 101 patients who died of pulmonary embolus at the Cleveland Clinic, only five were retrospectively deemed candidates for embolectomy.[127]

In the thrombolytic era, surgical therapy should be reserved for the "supermassive" embolus.[128] This is the patient with refractory or recurrent cardiac arrest who cannot be stabilized long enough to receive aggressive medical management or the patient who is clearly failing on medical management, hopefully including thrombolytic therapy. In the arrest situation, one should not forget that vigorous cardiopulmonary resuscitation has been shown to break up emboli.[126] In rare cases, the chest could be opened for more direct massage. An exceedingly difficult clinical situation occurs when a patient who is obviously extremely ill is briefly stabilized but in a state that if allowed to continue for hours will jeopardize vital organ function. An example is the patient with persistent shock and hypoxia despite maximal medical management. Some of these patients will improve dramatically within hours on thrombolytic therapy, but others will not and may suffer irreversible damage such that recovery, even with successful embolectomy, is impossible.

In reviews of surgical experience, a major source of morbidity and mortality has been severe, prolonged, preoperative hypoxia, acidosis, and shock as well as sudden cardiopulmonary arrest, either during angiography or at the time of induction of anesthesia for embolectomy. It has been suggested that appropriate patients receive partial cardiopulmonary bypass using the femoral vein and artery prior to angiography or the induction of anesthesia.[52, 53, 124, 126, 127] Contemporary techniques of "crashing onto bypass" may make such suggestions obsolete. A few patients have been saved with prolonged extracorporeal membrane oxygenator support with or without embolectomy.[85, 130, 131] Occasionally, patients undergo embolectomy but have sustained such severe right ventricular injury that they cannot be weaned off bypass. Such patients can be maintained with the aid of a right ventricular assist device, which consists of the roller pump from the heart-lung machine and cannulae in the superior and inferior vena cavae.[132]

Operative technique is good enough today that embolectomy should be considered in otherwise healthy patients with large emboli and shock who cannot receive thrombolytic therapy, for example, a young patient who suffers a massive embolism in the immediate postoperative period. In addition, thrombolytic therapy may be reversed and a patient readied for embolectomy within one hour.[133]

Most surgeons believe that all patients who undergo embolectomy should receive a prophylactic interruption of the inferior vena cava. This is easily done by extending the midline sternotomy incision to allow abdominal exploration and exposure of the inferior vena cava.[134] Some have reported intraoperative placement of transvenous devices through the right atrium. However, this requires radiographic equipment and can be cumbersome in a surgical suite.[135] Although the utility of such prophylactic maneuvers makes intuitive sense and probably does not contribute to surgical morbidity, surgeons who do not routinely interrupt the inferior vena cava report comparable long-term morbidity and mortality for embolectomy.[9]

In a small number of patients, success has been reported using transvenous suction techniques to remove emboli in the angiographic suite.[136, 137] Greenfield and coworkers report results with this technique in 15 patients. Despite the fact that all 15 were hypoxic and in shock, embolic material was removed in 13 (87 per cent). In one case, the pulmonary artery was perforated, and in two cases, cardiac arrest occurred at the time of injection of contrast material into the pulmonary artery. Four of the 15 patients died.

## INTERRUPTION OF THE INFERIOR VENA CAVA

### Ligation

In 1868, 12 years after Virchow identified the legs as the major source of pulmonary emboli, Trousseau first suggested that recurrent embolization could be prevented by ligation of the inferior vena cava.[138] However, because surgical exposure of the cava is relatively difficult, the first operation to prevent embolization was ligation of the femoral veins. Unfortunately, the rate of recurrent embolization was exceeding high, 26 per cent according to one report. Often the clot had propagated past the accessible femoral vein by the time the patient reached the operating table.[139] Currently, femoral vein ligation is

***Table 10–14.*** Reported Indications for Interruption of the Inferior Vena Cava

| Indication | N | % |
|---|---|---|
| Complication or failure of AC | 502 | 44 |
| Heparin contraindicated | 257 | 23 |
| Caval/iliofemoral vein thrombosis | 152 | 13 |
| Prophylactic | 92 | 8 |
| Severe PE initial therapy | 87 | 8 |
| PE requiring embolectomy | 25 | 2 |
| Recurrent PE | 24 | 2 |
| Septic thrombophlebitis or PE | 19 | 2 |
| Total | 1133 | 102 |

AC = anticoagulants; N = number of patients; % = percentage of total patients reported receiving vena caval interruption; total percentage is greater than 100 per cent owing to multiple indications in some patients.

Reproduced with permission from Bomalaski, J. S., et al.: Inferior vena caval interruption in the management of pulmonary embolism. Chest, *82*:767, 1982.

ple, in a series of 180 patients undergoing aortic surgery, 112 received a clip and did well without embolization. However, in 68 without a prophylactic clip, seven suffered an embolism, two of which resulted in death.[173] There have been efforts to identify patients at high risk of postoperative embolization and provide them with prophylactic clips. However, such risk factor analysis has failed to identify all of the patients who go on to suffer a postoperative embolism.[173, 174]

### Complications

Reported rates of surgical mortality and morbidity for IVC interruption are overwhelmingly dependent on the preoperative condition of the patients included.

#### Leg Swelling

The rate of venous complications is greatly dependent on the preexisting extent of venous disease as well as on definitions of venous sequelae.[139, 141, 144, 147] Most postoperative swelling is controlled with elevation and support stockings. Edema improves with time and may reflect the successful trapping of a large embolus by the device.[155] There is disagreement about whether postoperative anticoagulation significantly influences the rate of venous sequelae.[144, 152] This has never been studied with any rigor. However, in eligible patients, anticoagulation is strongly recommended because of the possibility of recurrent embolization through the venous anastomoses and collaterals that inevitably develop.[141, 155]

#### Recurrent Embolization

Accurate information on rates of recurrent embolization is difficult to gather. Some patients clearly develop recurrent symptoms suggestive of embolization when large central emboli break up and move distally. With either anticoagulation or interruption, the rate of recurrent fatal pulmonary emboli is relatively low.[1, 138, 139, 141, 144, 145, 148–152, 159–163]

### Transvenous Devices

Most patients who are candidates for clipping of the inferior vena cava are relatively poor surgical risks and must pass through the angiography area where the diagnosis of pulmonary embolism or deep vein thrombosis is confirmed. In recent years, there has been a great deal of enthusiasm for transvenous umbrellas or filters, which can be placed through a venotomy under radiographic control without general anesthesia.

Three major transvenous devices exist. One is the Hunter detachable balloon occluder. This device may be used in the rare situation in which a patient requires total interruption of the inferior vena cava from the transvenous route. A significant clinical experience with this device does not exist. The first clinically popular transvenous filter was the Mobin-Uddin filter system introduced in 1967 (Fig. 10–10).[163] Although still occasionally preferred because of prior experience or more facile maneuverability under certain situations, most contemporary angiographers prefer the Kimray-Greenfield filter, which was introduced in 1973. The Kimray-Greenfield device (Fig. 10–11) is cone-shaped so that it may be 80 per cent filled with clot and lead to only a 64 per cent reduction in effective cross-sectional area.[141] Table 10–15 summarizes available information comparing these two filters. Both are probably equally effective at preventing recurrent embolization, but the Kimray-Greenfield device has a higher patency rate and, probably as a consequence, a lower rate of venous sequelae. This high patency rate allows placement of the Kimray-Greenfield filter above the renal veins when necessary. Also, the Kimray-Greenfield device can be placed from either the femoral or internal jugular vein, whereas the Mobin-Uddin filter must be inserted through the internal jugular vein.

Although these devices do not require general anesthesia, great care is required for

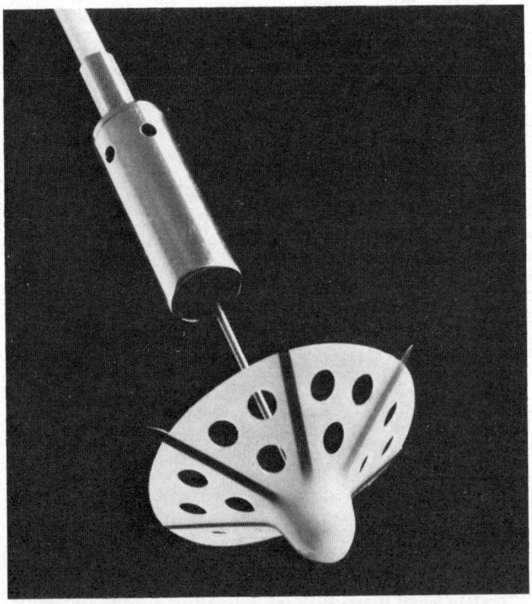

***Figure 10–10.*** Mobin-Uddin umbrella. American Edwards Laboratories, P.O. Box 11150, Santa Ana, California 92711.

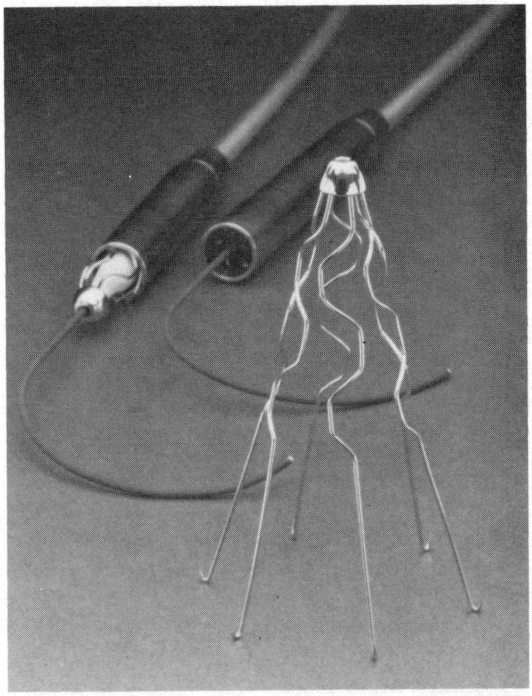

***Figure 10–11.*** Kimray-Greenfield vena cava filter. Medi-Tech, Inc., 150 Coolidge Ave., Watertown, Massachusetts 02172.

appropriate placement. Even in expert hands, placement is impossible or anatomically incorrect in a small percentage of patients.[164] Inferior vena caval angiography should precede placement. This procedure is best performed from the left femoral vein to detect venous anomalies. Both devices may migrate after placement or erode the inferior vena caval wall. A potential problem with these devices is that they preclude the use of thrombolytic therapy because of fear of excessive bleeding retroperitoneally or from the large venotomy site.[145]

In hospitals with angiographers and surgeons skilled in the transvenous technique, most patients at increased risk of complication from anesthesia should receive the transvenous umbrella. However, in the absence of a controlled clinical trial, no recommen-

***Table 10–15.*** Comparison of Transvenous Devices

**Mobin-Uddin Device**

| *Reference* | *Number of Patients* | *Mortality* | *Venous Problems* | *Recurrent Emboli* | *Patency Rate* |
|---|---|---|---|---|---|
| MGH[141] | 41 | 5% | 56% | 10% | — |
| Wingerd[158] | 38 | 0% | 75% | 3 fatal | 45% |
| Bomalaski[146] | 2,966 | 0.6% | 9% | 3.4% | 40% |
| Cimochowski[140] | 65 | 4% | — | — | 27% |
| Edwards Labs. | 4,700 | — | 5% | 2.2% | — |
| Mobin-Uddin[165] | 100 | 15% | — | 45 | — |
| Fullen[166] | 80 | 15% | — | 2% | — |
| Lawrence[167] | 28 | 1% | — | 11% | — |
| Senties[168] | 51 | 0% | — | 0% | — |
| Menzoian[169] | 128 | 7% | — | 0% | — |
| Schlosser[170] | 125 | — | — | 2% | — |

**Kimray-Greenfield Device**

| *Reference* | *Number of Patients* | *Mortality* | *Venous Problems* | *Recurrent Emboli* | *Patency Rate* |
|---|---|---|---|---|---|
| MGH[141] | 56 | 5% | 13% | 3.6% | — |
| Wingerd[158] | 33 | 0% | 38% | none fatal | 95% |
| Bomalaski[146] | 141 | 3.5% | 15% | — | — |
| Cimochowski[140] | 32 | 4% | — | — | 95% |
| Greenfield[164] | 152 | 0% | 17% | 2% (none fatal) | 95% |

dation between a surgical clip and a transvenous filter is possible in patients who are at relatively low risk of a poor response to anesthesia.[171] The transvenous technique is particularly popular for the large number of patients with advanced malignancy who need interruption. For such patients, the relative simplicity of the transvenous technique clearly outweighs concern about long-term efficacy.

## SUMMARY

To summarize briefly, although pulmonary embolism is most destructive when the diagnosis is missed repeatedly or when it leads to sudden death, some patients do poorly despite prompt diagnosis and adequate medical care. These are patients suffering a massive pulmonary embolism.

Although anatomically large emboli pose a greater threat than smaller ones, the hemodynamic response to embolization proves to be a more powerful predictor of prognosis. When a small embolus causes a great deal of hemodynamic distress, underlying cardiopulmonary disease must be present, and the prognosis is poor. When a large embolus causes little hemodynamic embarrassment, the outlook is good with traditional "prophylactic" heparinization.

There is a spectrum of hemodynamic response to pulmonary embolism. At one end, patients experience tachycardia and a high cardiac output. At the opposite end, some develop shock or cardiac arrest. In between are patients who demonstrate signs of right ventricular congestive failure, although forward output is maintained. The more dramatic the hemodynamic abnormalities, the greater the risk of a poor outcome with standard care. These are the patients who deserve the potentially more efficacious but uniformly more hazardous therapies, which have been described previously. Diagnosis by pulmonary angiography should be prompt and should be combined with a complete right heart catheterization. Hemodynamic information should guide the general medical management of these critically ill patients, which may influence outcome as much as any more efficacious antiembolism therapy that is employed.

Thrombolytic therapy may be indicated when cardiac output is reduced and may also be recommended for patients who demonstrate dramatic signs of right ventricular distress. Embolectomy is reserved for appropriate patients who cannot be stabilized medically. Vasodilators are the object of much clinical investigation and may play a role in the treatment of these patients in the future. Unfortunately, the controlled clinical experience with patients with massive embolization and with the therapies discussed here is too limited for more specific recommendations. Therefore, the treatment of the patient with a massive embolism must rest to a great degree on individualized clinical judgment.

## REFERENCES


1. Urokinase pulmonary embolism trial. Phase 1 results. JAMA, *214*:2163, 1970.
2. Urokinase-streptokinase embolism trial. Phase 2 results. JAMA, *229*:1606, 1972.
3. Alpert, J. S., Smith, R., Carlson, J., et al.: Mortality in patients treated for pulmonary embolism. JAMA, *236*:1477, 1976.
4. Hall, R. J. C., Sutton, G. C., and Kerr, I. H.: Long-term prognosis of treated acute massive pulmonary embolism. Br. Heart J., *39*:1128, 1977.
5. Dalen, J. E., and Alpert, J. S.: Natural History of Pulmonary Embolism. *In* Sasahara, A. A., Sonnenblick, E. H., and Lesch, M., (Eds.): Pulmonary Emboli. Grune & Stratton, New York, 1974, p. 77.
6. Dalen, J. E.: Controversy. The case against fibrinolytic therapy. J. Cardiovasc. Med., *5*:799, 1980.
7. Alpert, J. S., Smith, R. E., Ockene, I. S., et al.: Treatment of massive pulmonary embolism: The role of pulmonary embolectomy. Am. Heart J., *89*:413, 1975.
8. McDonald, I. G., Hirsh, J., Hale, G. S., et al.: Major pulmonary embolism, a correlation of clinical findings, haemodynamics, pulmonary angiography, and pathological physiology. Br. Heart J., *34*:356, 1972.
9. Miller, G. A. H., Hall, R. J. C., and Paneth, M.: Pulmonary embolectomy, heparin, and streptokinase: Their place in the treatment of acute massive pulmonary embolism. Am. Heart J., *93*:568, 1977.
10. Stein, P. D., Willis, P. W. III, and DeMets, D. L.: History and physical examination in acute pulmonary embolism in patients without preexisting cardiac or pulmonary disease. Am. J. Cardiol., *47*:218, 1981.
11. Fishman, W. P. (Ed.): Pulmonary Disease and Disorders. McGraw-Hill, New York, 1979, p. 816.
12. Samkoff, J. S., and Comstock, G. W.: Epidemiology of pulmonary embolism mortality in a general population. Am. J. Epidemiol., *114*:488, 1981.
13. Bell, W. R., Simon, T. L., and DeMets, D. L.: The clinical features of submassive and massive pulmonary emboli. Am. J. Med., *62*:355, 1977.
14. Cleveland, J. C., Lebenson, I. M., and Friedman, J. W.: Successful management of pulmonary embolism occurring during cardiopulmonary by-pass for mitral valve replacement. Chest, *73*:236, 1978.
15. Kounis, N. G.: Pulmonary embolism with neurological and abdominal manifestations. Practitioner, *223*:115, 1979.
16. Croyle, P. H., Place, R. A., and Hilgenberg, A. D.:

Massive pulmonary embolism in a high school wrestler. JAMA, *241*:827, 1979.
17. Lesser, L., Walter P. F., and Hardison, J. E.: Ligation of the superior vena cava for recurrent pulmonary emboli. South. Med. J., *72*:940, 1979.
18. Gonzalez, A., Altieri, P. I., Marquez, E., et al.: Massive pulmonary embolism associated with a right ventricular myxoma. Am. J. Med., *69*:795, 1980.
19. Formolo, J. M., Giraldo, A., and Shors, C. M.: Fatal pulmonary embolism from massive right atrial thrombus postcoronary artery bypass surgery. Am. Heart J., *101*:510, 1981.
20. Milne, B., Cervenko, F. W., Morales, A., et al.: Massive intraoperative pulmonary tumor embolus from renal cell carcinoma. Anesthesiology, *54*:253, 1981.
21. Natonson, R., Shapiro, B. A., Harrison, R. A., et al.: Massive trophoblastic embolization and PEEP therapy. Anesthesiology *51*:469, 1979.
22. Estrera, A. S., King, R. P., and Platt, M. R.: Massive pulmonary embolism: A complication of the technique of tourniquet ischemia. J. Trauma, *22*:60, 1982.
23. Kinney, E. L., Allen, R. P., Weidner, W. A., et al.: Recurrent pulmonary emboli secondary to right atrial thrombus around a permanent pacing catheter: A case report and review of the literature. Pace, *2*:196, 1979.
24. Noble, J., and Cohen, R.: Case records of the Massachusetts General Hospital. New Engl. J. Med., *286*:1309, 1972.
25. Bradway, W., Biondi, R. J., Kaufman, J. L., et al.: Internal jugular thrombosis and pulmonary embolism. Chest, *80*:335, 1981.
26. Case records of the Massachusetts General Hospital. New Engl. J. Med., *296*:33, 1977.
27. Thames, M. D., Alpert, J., and Dalen, J. E.: Syncope in patients with pulmonary embolism. JAMA, *238*:2509, 1977.
28. Simpson, R. J., Podolak, R. P., Mangano, C. A., et al.: Vagal syncope during recurrent pulmonary embolism. JAMA, *249*:390, 1983.
29. McGinn, S., and White P. D.: Acute cor pulmonale resulting from pulmonary embolism. JAMA, *104*:1473, 1935.
30. Lerman, J., and Means, J. H.: Cardiovascular symptomatology in exophthalmic goiter. Am. Heart J., *8*:55, 1932.
31. Cohen, S. I., Kupersmith, J., Aroesty, J., et al.: Pulsus paradoxus and Kussmaul's sign in acute pulmonary embolism. Am. J. Cardiol., *32*:271, 1973.
32. McFadden, E. R., and Braunwald, E.: Cor Pulmonale and Pulmonary Thromboembolism. *In* Braunwald, E., (Ed.): Heart Disease. W. B. Saunders, 1980, p. 1643.
33. Dalen, J. E., Haffajee, C. I., Alpert, J. S., et al.: Pulmonary embolism, pulmonary hemorrhage, and pulmonary infarction. New Engl. J. Med., *296*:1431, 1977.
34. Hirsh, J., Genton, E., and Hull, R.: Venous Thromboembolism. Grune & Stratton, New York, 1981.
35. Wenger, W. K., Stein, P. D., and Willis, P. W. III: Massive acute pulmonary embolism. JAMA, *220*:843, 1972.
36. Miller, G. A. H., and Sutton, G. C.: Acute massive pulmonary embolism. Br. Heart J., *32*:518, 1970.
37. Stein, P. D., Dalen, J. E., McIntyre, K., et al.: The Electrocardiogram in Acute Pulmonary Embolism. *In* Sasahara, A. A., Sonnenblick, E. H., and Lesch, M., (Eds.): Pulmonary Embolism. Grune & Stratton, New York, 1974, p. 65.
38. McIntyre, K. M., Sasahara, A. A., and Littmen, D.: Relation of the electrocardiogram to hemodynamic alterations in pulmonary embolism. Am. J. Cardiol., *30*:205, 1972.
39. Spodick, D. H.: Electrocardiographic response to pulmonary embolism. Mechanisms and sources of variability. Am. J. Cardiol., *30*:695, 1972.
40. McLarin C. W., Latting, C. A., Walter, P. F., et al.: Pseudo-anterior myocardial infarction as a manifestation of severe pulmonary embolism. Journal of the Medical Association of Georgia, *70*:649, 1981.
41. Torrance, D. J.: The Chest Film in Massive Pulmonary Embolism. Charles C Thomas, Springfield, Illinois, 1963.
42. Rosenow, E. C. III, Osmundon, P. J., and Brown, M. L.: Pulmonary embolism. Mayo Clin. Proc., *56*:161, 1981.
43. Hyers, T. M., Fowler, A. A., and Wicks, A. B.: Focal pulmonary edema after massive pulmonary embolism. Am. Rev. Respir. Dis., *123*:232, 1981.
44. Viamonte, M., Jr., Koolpe, H., Janowitz, W., et al.: Pulmonary thromboembolism—update. JAMA, *243*:2229, 1980.
45. Haynes, J. B., and Iseman, M. D.: Massive pulmonary embolism presenting with hypercapnia and minimal intrapulmonary shunting. Rocky Mountain Med. J. *76*:135, 1979.
46. Klein, E. W., McCarten, K., Dimcheff, D. G., et al.: Massive pulmonary emboli diagnosed and followed by lung imaging and radionuclide pulmonary angiography. Circulation, *50*:1260, 1974.
47. Bell, W. R., and Simon T. L.: Current status of pulmonary thromboembolic disease: Pathophysiology, diagnosis, prevention, and treatment. Am. Heart J., *103*:239, 1982.
48. Marsh, J. D., Glynn, M., and Torman, H. A.: Pulmonary angiography: Application in a new spectrum of patients. Am. J. Med., *75*:763, 1983.
49. Hull, R. D., Hirsh, J., Carter, C. J., et al.: Pulmonary angiography, ventilation lung scanning, and venography for clinically suspected pulmonary embolism and abnormal perfusion lung scan. Ann. Inter. Med., *98*:891, 1983.
50. Cheely, R., McCartney, W. H., Perry, J. R., et al.: The role of noninvasive tests versus pulmonary angiography in the diagnosis of pulmonary embolism. Am. J. Med., *70*:17, 1981.
51. Robin, E. D.: Overdiagnosis and overtreatment of pulmonary embolism; The emperor may have no clothes. Ann. Intern. Med., *87*:775, 1977.
52. Berger, R. L.: Pulmonary embolectomy with preoperative circulatory support. Ann. Thorac. Surg., *16*:217, 1973.
53. Mattox, K. L., Feldtman, R. W., Beall, A. C., et al.: Pulmonary embolectomy for acute massive pulmonary embolism. Ann. Surg., *195*:726, 1982.
54. Bynum, L. J., Wilson, J. E. III, Christensen, E. E., et al.: Radiographic techniques for balloon-occlusion pulmonary angiography. Radiology, *133*:518, 1979.
55. Dougherty, J. E., LaSala, A. F., and Fieldman, A.: Bedside pulmonary angiography utilizing an existing Swan-Ganz catheter. Chest *77*:43, 1980.
56. LePage, J. R., and Gracia, R. M.: The value of bedside wedge angiography in the detection of pulmonary emboli; a predictive and prospective evaluation. Radiology, *144*:67, 1982.
57. Lewis, J. E., Anderson, T. W., Fennell, W. H. et

al.: A clue to pulmonary embolism obtained during Swan-Ganz catheterization. Chest, *81*:527, 1982.
58. Steckley, R., Smith, C. W., and Robertson, R. M.: Acute right ventricular overload: An echocardiographic clue to pulmonary embolism. Johns Hopkins Med. J. *143*:122, 1978.
59. Shiina, A., Kunio, K., Kawai, N., et al.: Echocardiographic manifestation of acute pulmonary thromboembolism. Jpn. Heart J., *22*:853, 1981.
60. Starkley, I. R., and DeBono, D. P.: Echocardiographic identification of right-sided cardiac intracavity thromboembolus in massive pulmonary embolism. Circulation, *66*:1322, 1982.
61. DiCarlo, L. A., Jr., Schiller, W. B., Herfkens, R. L., et al.: Noninvasive detection of proximal pulmonary thrombosis by two-dimensional echocardiography and computerized tomography. Am. Heart J., *103*:879, 1982.
62. Tadaakiiwasaki, M. T., Yamamoto, T., Makihata, S., et al.: Echocardiographic abnormalities of tricuspid valve motion in pulmonary embolism. Br. Heart J., *47*:454, 1982.
63. Dianzumba, S. B., Montello, N. J., and Joyner, C. R.: Systolic flutter of the tricuspid valve associated with massive pulmonary embolism. South. Med. J., *76*:83, 1983.
64. Godwin, J. D., Webb, W. R., Gamsu, G., et al.: Computed tomography of pulmonary embolism. Am. J. Roentgenol., *135*:691, 1980.
65. Pond, G. D., Ovitt, T. W., and Capp, P. M.: Comparison of conventional pulmonary angiography with intravenous digital subtraction angiography for pulmonary embolic disease. Radiology, *147*:345, 1983.
66. Ludwig, J. W. Verhoeven, L. A., Kersbergen, J. J., et al.: Digital subtraction angiography of the pulmonary arteries for the diagnosis of pulmonary embolism. Radiology, *147*:639, 1983.
67. Goodman, P. C., and Brant-Zawadzki, M.: Digital subtraction pulmonary angiography. Am. J. Radiology *139*:305, 1982.
68. Moser, K. M., Shure D., Harrell, J. H., et al.: Angioscopic visualization of pulmonary emboli. Chest, *77*:198, 1980.
69. Shure, D., Moser, K. M., Harrell, J. H., et al.: Identification of pulmonary emboli in the dog: Comparison of angioscopy and perfusion scanning. Circulation, *64*:618, 1981.
70. Grossman, William (Ed.): Cardiac Catheterization and Angiography. Lea and Febiger, Philadelphia, 1980, p. 118.
71. Vlahakes, G. J., Turley, K., and Hoffman, J. I. E.: The pathophysiology of failure in acute right ventricular hypertension: Hemodynamic and biochemical correlations. Circulation, *63*:87, 1981.
72. Dalen, J. E., Banas, J. S., Brooks, H. C., et al.: Resolution rate of acute pulmonary embolism in man. New Engl. J. Med., *280*:1194, 1969.
73. McIntyre, K. M., and Sasahara, A. A.: The hemodynamic response to pulmonary embolism in patients without prior cardiopulmonary disease. Am. J. Cardiol., *28*:288, 1971.
74. Dalen, J. E., and Grossman, W.: Profiles in Pulmonary Embolism. *In* Grossman, W. (Ed.): Cardiac Catheterization and Angiography. Lea and Febiger, Philadelphia, 1980, pp. 336, 345.
75. Myers, M. L., Calvin, J. E., Driedger, A. A., et al: Myocardial dysfunction associated with massive pulmonary embolus as evaluated by radionuclide angiography. Crit. Care Med. *10*:417, 1982.
76. Suter, P. M., Fairley, H. B., and Isenberg, M. D.: Optimum end-expiratory airway pressure in patients with acute pulmonary failure. New Engl. J. Med., *292*:284, 1975.
77. Orta, D. A., Tucker, N. H., Green, L. E., et al.: Severe hypoxemia secondary to pulmonary embolization treated successfully with the use of a CPAP (continuous positive airway pressure) mask. Chest, *74*:588, 1978.
78. Dantzger, D. R., and Bower, J. S.: Alterations in gas exchange following pulmonary embolism. Chest, *81*:495, 1982.
79. Vegas, A. M., Grindlinger, G. A., McLoughlin G. A., et al.: Control of pulmonary fibrinolytic activity by prostaglandins. Surgical Forum, *30*:180, 1979.
80. Poe, R. H., Sahler, C. P., Betts, L. W., et al.: Right to left shunt measurement in patients suspect for pulmonary embolism. Respiration, *46*:174, 1981.
81. Hauser, C. J., and Shoemaker, W. C.: Volume loading in massive acute pulmonary embolus. Crit. Care Med., *7*:304, 1979.
82. Malik, A. B., Lee, D. C., Zee, H. V., et al.: The role of fibrin in the genesis of pulmonary edema after embolization in dogs. Cir. Res., *45*:120, 1979.
83. Shepard, J. W., Hauer, D., Sgrori, V., et al.: Effects of isoproterenol on distribution of perfusion in embolized dog lungs. J. Nucl. Med., *20*:950, 1979.
84. McDonald, I. G., Hirsh, J., Hale, G. S., et al.: Isoproterenol in massive pulmonary embolism: Hemodynamic and clinical effects. Med. J. Aust., *2*:201, 1968.
85. Jardin, F., Gurdjian, P., Desfonds, P., et al.: Hemodynamic factors influencing arterial hypoxemia in massive pulmonary embolism with circulatory failure. Circulation, *59*:909, 1979.
86. Moser, K. M.: Pulmonary embolism. Am. Rev. Respir. Dis., *115*:829, 1977.
87. Tibutt, D. A., Davies, J. A., Anderson, J. A., et al.: Comparison by controlled clinical trial of streptokinase and heparin in the treatment of life-threatening pulmonary embolism. Br. Med. J., *2*:343, 1974.
88. Hirsh, J., McDonald, I. G., Hale, G. A., et al.: Comparison of the effects of streptokinase and heparin in the early rate of resolution of major pulmonary embolism. Can. Med. Assoc. J., *104*:485, 1971.
89. Ly, B., Arnesen, H., Hol, E., et al.: A controlled clinical trial of streptokinase and heparin in the treatment of major pulmonary embolism. Acta Med. Scand., *203*:456, 1978.
90. Miller, G. A. H., Sutton, G. C., Kerr, I. H., et al.: Comparison of streptokinase and heparin in the treatment of isolated acute massive pulmonary embolism. Br. Med. J., *2*:681, 1971.
91. Freiman, J. A., Chalmers, T. C., Smith, H., et al.: The importance of beta, the type II error and sample size in the design and interpretation of the randomized control trial. Survey of 71 "negative" trials. New Engl. J. Med., *299*:690, 1978.
92. Tow, D. E., and Wagner, N. H., Jr.: Recovery of pulmonary artery flow in patients with pulmonary embolism. New Engl. J. Med., *276*:1053, 1967.
93. Mazuch, J., Pavlik, V., Kukura, A., et al.: Acute massive pulmonary thromboembolism in experiment. Comparison of the effect of fibrinolytic and anticoagulant treatment. Acta Med. Acad. Sci. Hung., *35*:317, 1978.
94. Bell, W. R., and Meek, A. G.: Guidelines for the use of thrombolytic agents. New Engl. J. Med., *301*:1266, 1979.
95. Griguer, P., Charbonnier, B., Latour, F., et al.:

Plasminogen and moderate doses of urokinase in the treatment of acute pulmonary embolism. Angiology *30*:1, 1979.
96. Kwaan, H. C.: The Status of Thrombolytic Therapy. *In* Bergan, J. J., and Yao, J. S. T. (Eds.): Venous Problems. Year Book Medical Publisher, Chicago, 1976, p. 281.
97. Bergman, S. R., Keith, A. A., Fox, M. B., et al.: Coronary thrombolysis achieved with human extrinsic plasminogen activator, a clot selective activator, administered intravenously. J. Am. Coll. Cardiol. *1*:615, 1983 (abstract).
98. Edwards, I. R., MacLean, K. S., and Dow, J. D.,: Low-dose urokinase in major pulmonary embolism. Lancet, *2*:409, 1973.
99. Johnson, W. C., Widrich, W. C., Patten, D. H., et al.: Effects of streptokinase on canine pulmonary emboli: Local vs. peripheral infusion. J. Surg. Res., *24*:366, 1978.
100. Simon, T. L., Hyers, T. M., Gaston, J. P., et al.: Heparin pharmacokinetics: Increased requirements in pulmonary embolism. Br. J. Haematol., *39*:111, 1978.
101. Fratantoni, J. C., Ness, P., and Simon, T. L.: Thrombolytic therapy. Current status. New Engl. J. Med., *293*:1073, 1975.
102. Stampfer, M. J., Goldhaber, S. Z., Yusuf, S., et al.: Effect of intravenous streptokinase in acute myocardial infarction. Pooled results from randomized trials. New Engl. J. Med., *307*:1180, 1982.
103. Thrombolytic therapy in thrombosis: A National Institutes of Health consensus development conference. Ann. Intern Med., *93*:141, 1980.
104. Porter, J. M., and Goodnight, S. H., Jr.: The clinical use of fibrinolytic agents. Am. J. Surg., *134*:217, 1977.
105. Genton, E.: Thrombolytic therapy of pulmonary thromboembolism. Prog. Cardiovasc. Dis., *21*:333, 1979.
106. Porter, J. M.: Thrombolysis as an alternative to pulmonary embolectomy. Vasc. Surg., *11*:373, 1977.
107. Hinshaw, H. C., and Murray, J. F.: Disease of the Chest. W. B. Saunders, Philadelphia, 1980, p. 670.
108. Sasahara, A. A.: Controversy. The case for fibrinolytic therapy. J. Cardiovasc. Med., *5*:793, 1980.
109. Sharma, G. V. R. K., Burleson, V. A., and Sasahara, A. A.: Effect of thrombolytic therapy of pulmonary-capillary blood volume in patients with pulmonary embolism. New Engl. J. Med., *303*:842, 1980.
110. De Soyza, N. D. B., and Murphy, M. L.: Persistent post-embolic pulmonary hypertension. Chest, *62*:665, 1972.
111. Riedel, M., Stanek, V., Widimsky, J., et al.: Long term follow-up of patients with pulmonary thromboembolism. Chest, *81*:151, 1982.
112. Paraskos, J. A., and Adelstein, S. J.: Late prognosis of acute pulmonary embolism. New Engl. J. Med., *289*:55, 1973.
113. Halmagyi, D. F. J., Starzecki, B., and Horner, G. J.: Humoral transmission of cardiorespiratory changes in experimental pulmonary embolism. Circ. Res., *14*:546, 1964.
114. Comroe, J. H., Jr., Lingen, B. V., Stroud, R. C., et al.: Reflex and direct cardiopulmonary effects of 5-OH tryptamine (serotonin). Am. J. Physiol., *173*:379, 1953.
115. Thomas, D. P.: Heparin in the prophylaxis and treatment of venous thromboembolism. Semin. Hematol. *15*:1, 1978.
116. Gurewich, V., Cohen, M. L., and Thomas D. P.: Humoral factors in massive pulmonary embolism. An experimental study. Am. Heart J., *76*:784, 1968.
117. Utsunomiya, T., Krausz, M. M., Valeri, C. R., et al.: Treatment of pulmonary embolism with prostacyclin. Surgery, *88*:25, 1980.
118. Utsunomiya, T., Krausz, M. M., Dunham, B., et al.: Treatment of pulmonary embolism with positive end-expiratory pressure and prostaglandin E1. Surg. Gynecol. Obstet., 153:161, 1981.
119. Utsunomiya, T., Krausz, M. M., Dunham, B., et al.: Circulating negative inotropic agent(s) following pulmonary embolism. Surgery, *91*:402, 1982.
120. Bates, E. R., Crevey, B. J., Sprague, F. R., et al.: Oral hydralazine therapy for acute pulmonary embolism and low output state. Arch. Intern. Med., *141*:1537, 1981.
121. Simonneau, G., Escourrou, P., Duroux, P., et al.: Inhibition of hypoxic pulmonary vasoconstriction by nifedipine. New Engl. J. Med., *304*:1582, 1981.
122. Huval, W. V., Mathieson, M. A., Stemp, L. I., et al.: Therapeutic benefits of 5 hydroxy-tryptamine inhibition following pulmonary embolism. Ann. Surg., *197*:220, 1983.
123. Cross, F. S., and Mowlem, A.: A survey of current status of pulmonary embolectomy for massive pulmonary embolism. Circulation, (Suppl. I):86, 1967.
124. Reul, G. J., and Beall, A. C.: Emergency pulmonary embolectomy for massive pulmonary embolism. Circulation, *50*:(Supp. II):236, 1974.
125. Tschirkov, A., Kraus, E., Elert, O., et al.: Surgical management of massive pulmonary embolism. J. Thorac. Cardiovasc. Surg., *75*:730, 1978.
126. Sautter, R., Myers, W. O., Ray, J. F. III, et al.: Pulmonary Embolectomy: Review and Current Status. *In* Sasahara, A. A., Sonnenblick, E. H., and Lesch, M. L., (Eds.): Pulmonary Emboli. Grune and Stratton, New York, 1974, p. 143.
127. Meyerowitz, B. R.: Pulmonary embolism in surgical patients: Is embolectomy superior to prophylaxis? Surgery, *60*:521, 535, 1966.
128. Alpert, J. S., and Dalen, J. E.: Reply. Am. Heart J., *91*:134, 1976.
129. Estrera, A. S., Platt, M. R., and Mills, L. J.: Pulmonary embolectomy for massive pulmonary embolism. Tex. Med., *77*:46, 1981.
130. Krellenstein, D. J., Bryan-Brown, C. W., Fayena, A. O., et al.: Extracorporeal membrane oxygenattion for massive pulmonary thromboembolism. Ann. Thorac. Surg., *23*:421, 1977.
131. Cooper, J. D., Teasdale, S., Nelems, J. M., et al.: Cardiorespiratory failure secondary to peripheral pulmonary emboli. Survival following a combination of prolonged extra corporeal membrane oxygenator support and pulmonary embolectomy. J. Thorac. Cardiovasc. Surg., *761*:872, 1976.
132. Pennington, D. G.: Clinical Experience with a Centrifugal Pump Ventricular Assist Device. *In* Pierce, W. S. (Ed.): Circulatory Assistance and the Artificial Heart. USA-USSR Joint Symposium. U.S. Department of Health and Human Services, Washington, DC, 1980. (NIH publication No. 80-2082)
133. Sasahara, A. A., Sharma, G. U. R. K., Tow, D. E., et al.: Clinical use of thrombolytic agents in venous thromboembolism. Arch. Intern. Med. *142*:684, 1982.
134. Moran, J. M.: Vena cava interruption after pulmonary embolectomy. Ann. Thorac. Surg., *25*:248, 1978.
135. Pellegrini, R.: Pulmonary embolectomy. Ann. Thorac. Surg., *27*:96, 1979.
136. Scoggins, W. G., and Greenfield, L. J.: Transven-

ous pulmonary embolectomy for acute massive pulmonary embolism. Chest, *71*:213, 1977.
137. Greenfield, L. J., and Zocco, J. J.: Intraluminal management of acute massive pulmonary thromboembolism. J. Thorac. Cardiovasc. Surg., *77*:402, 1979.
138. Anonymous. The role of partial caval occlusion in the prevention of fatal pulmonary emboli. (Editorial) Med. J. Aust., 516, 1980.
139. Donaldson, M. C., Wirthlin, L. S., and Donaldson, G. A.: Thirty-year experience with surgical interruption of the inferior vena cava for prevention of pulmonary embolism. Ann. Surg., *191*:367, 1980.
140. Cimochowski, G. E., Evans, R. H., Zarins, C. K., et al.: Greenfield filter versus Mobbin-Uddin umbrella. J. Thorac. Cardiovasc. Surg., 79:358, 1980.
141. McNamara, M. F., Creasy, J. K., Takaki, H., et al.: Vena Caval Surgery to Prevent Recurrent Pulmonary Embolism. *In* Bergan, J. J., and Yao, J. S. T. (Eds.): Venous Problems. Year Book Medical Publishers, Chicago, 1976, p. 319.
142. Josey, W. E., and Staggers, S. R.: Heparin therapy in septic pelvic thrombophlebitis. A study of 46 cases. Am. J. Obstet. Gynecol., *120*:228, 1974.
143. Toole, A. L., Lowman, R., and Stern, H.: Pulmonary embolism and intracardiac shunt. A unique indication for operation. Ann. Thorac. Surg., *22*:296, 1976.
144. Couch, N. P., Baldwin, S. S., and Crane, C.: Mortality and morbidity rates after inferior vena caval clipping. Surgery, *77*:106, 1975.
145. Novelline, R. A.: Transvenous Devices for Interruption of the Inferior Vena Cava. *In* Wilkins, R. A., and Viamonte, M. (Eds.): Interventional Radiology. Blackwell Scientific Publications, Oxford, 1982, p. 243.
146. Bomalaski, J. S., Martin, G. J., Hughes, R. L., et al.: Inferior vena cava interruption in the management of pulmonary embolism. Chest, *82*:767, 1982.
147. AbuRahma, A. F., Boland, J., Lawton, W. E., Jr., et al.: Long term follow up of prophylactic caval clipping. J. Cardiovasc. Surg., *22*:550, 1981.
148. Coon, W. W.: Operative therapy of venous thromboembolism. Mod. Concepts Cardiovasc. Dis., *43*:71, 1974.
149. Moretz, W. H., Still, J. M., Jr., Griffin, L. H., et al.: Partial occlusion of the inferior vena cava with a smooth Teflon clip: Analysis of long-term results. Surgery, *71*:710, 1972.
150. DeWeese, M. S., Kraft, R. O., Nichols, W. K., et al.: Fifteen-year clinical experience with the vena cava filter. Ann. Surg., *178*:247, 1973.
151. Moran, J. M., Kahn, P. C., and Callow, A. D.: Partial versus complete caval interruption for venous thromboembolism. Am. J. Surg., *117*:471, 1969.
152. Blumenberg, R. M., and Gelfand, M. L.: Long-term follow-up of vena caval clips and umbrellas. Am. J. Surg., *134*:205, 1977.
153. Pollack, E. W., Sparks, F. C., and Barker, W. F.: Pulmonary embolism. An appraisal of therapy in 516 cases. Arch. Surg., *107*:66, 1973.
154. Gardner, A. M. N.: Inferior vena caval interruption in the prevention of fatal pulmonary embolism. Am. Heart J., *95*:679, 1978.
155. Askew, A. R., and Gardner, A. M. N.: Long term follow-up of partial caval occlusion by clip. Am. J. Surg., *140*:441, 1980.
156. Crane, C.: Venous interruption for pulmonary embolism: Present status. Prog. Cardiovasc. Dis., *17*:329, 1975.
157. Ebert, P. A.: The role of surgery in the treatment of pulmonary thromboembolism. Surg. Clin. North Am., *54*:1107, 1974.
158. Wingerd, M., Bernhard, V. M., Maddison, F., et al.: Comparison of caval filters in the management of venous thromboembolism. Arch. Surg., *113*: 1264, 1978.
159. Basu, D., Gallus, A., Hirsh, J., et al.: A prospective study of the value of monitoring heparin treatment with the activated partial thromboplastin time. New Engl. J. Med., *287*:324, 1972.
160. Salzman, E. W., Deykin, D., Shapiro, R. M., et al.: Management of heparin therapy. Controlled prospective trial. New Engl. J. Med., *292*:1046, 1975.
161. Wilson, J. E. III, Bynum, L. J., and Parkey, R. W.: Heparin therapy in venous thromboembolism. Am. J. Med., *70*:808, 1981.
162. Glazier, R. R., and Crowell, E. B.: Randomized prospective trial of continuous vs. intermittent heparin therapy. JAMA, *236*:1365, 1976.
163. Mobin-Uddin, K., Utley, J. R., and Bryant, L. R.: The inferior vena cava umbrella filter. Prog. Cardiovasc. Dis., *17*:391, 1975.
164. Greenfield, L. J., Peyton, R. P., Caute, S., et al.: Greenfield vena cava filter experience. Late results in 150 patients. Arch. Surg., *116*:1451, 1981.
165. Mobin-Uddin, K., Calland, G. M., Bolooki, H., et al.: Transvenous caval interruption with umbrella filter. New Engl. J. Med., *286*:55, 1972.
166. Fullen, W. D., McDonough, J. J., and Altmeier, W. A.: Clinical experience with vena cava filters. Arch. Surg., *106*:582, 1973.
167. Lawrence, G. H., and Beebe, H. G.: An evaluation of the Mobin-Uddin umbrella in the prevention of pulmonary thromboembolism. Am. J. Surg., *132*:204, 1976.
168. Senties, A. C., Carrera, W. F., and Gordillo, O. C.: Inferior vena cava ligation versus the Mobin-Uddin filter for the prevention of recurrent pulmonary embolism. Int. Surg., *62*:420, 1977.
169. Menzoian, J. O., LoGerfo, F. W., Witzman, A. F., et al.: Clinical experience with the Mobin-Uddin vena cava umbrella filter. Arch. Surg., *115*:1179, 1980.
170. Schlosser, V.: Late Results of the Transvenous Cava Block Operation. *In* May, R., and Weber, J. (Eds.): Pelvic and Abdominal Veins. Progress in Diagnosis and Therapy. Excerpta Medica, Amsterdam, 1981, p. 327.
171. Goldhaber, S. Z., Buring, J. E., Lipnick, R. J., et al.: Interruption of the inferior vena cava by clip or filter. Am. J. Med., *76*:512, 1984.
172. Rosenthal, D., Cossman, D., Matsumoto, G., et al.: Prophylactic interruption of the inferior vena cava. A retrospective evaluation. Am. J. Surg., *137*:388, 1979.
173. Korwin, S. M., Callow, A. D., Rosenthal, D., et al.: Prophylactic interruption of the inferior vena cava. Immediate and long-term hemodynamic effects. Arch. Surg., *114*:1037, 1979.
174. Kusminsky, R. E., Medina, S., AbuRahma, A. F., et al.: Prophylactic inferior vena cava clipping in colonic surgery. Dis. Colon Rectum, *25*:108, 1982.
175. Marriott, H. J. L.: Practical Electrocardiography. The Williams and Wilkins Co., Baltimore, 1972, p. 288.

CHAPTER 11

# NONTHROMBOTIC PULMONARY EMBOLISM

DALE S. ADLER, M.D.

The clinical features of nonthrombotic pulmonary embolism differ from the clinical features of thrombotic pulmonary embolism in several ways.

First, some types of nonthrombotic pulmonary emboli are uncommon. Many physicians never see a single case of venous air embolism or amniotic fluid pulmonary embolism. Second, in nonthrombotic pulmonary emboli, the embolizing substance can consist of almost any material. It can be derived from the body's organ systems, such as fat or bile emboli; it can be derived from pathologic processes invading the body, such as tumors or infectious microorganisms; and it can be foreign material introduced into the body, such as polyethylene catheters or talc. Third, the factors that predispose patients to nonthrombotic pulmonary embolism are usually circumscribed. Fat embolism, for example, occurs almost exclusively in the setting of trauma. Tumor emboli obviously cannot occur unless the patient has cancer. Fourth, the clinical presentations of nonthrombotic pulmonary emboli, with the exception of tumor pulmonary emboli, are quite predictable.

This chapter reviews the most common types of nonthrombotic pulmonary emboli. The order of discussion is based on clinical presentation. Tumor and septic pulmonary emboli are discussed first, because both can mimic thrombotic pulmonary embolism. Air, amniotic fluid, and fat emboli are then reviewed. Each of these can present with features of the adult respiratory distress syndrome. Next discussed are foreign particle pulmonary emboli, which, except for oil emboli, present as chronic lung disease. Last, there is a miscellaneous section that discusses rare types of nonthrombotic pulmonary emboli that cannot be readily classified by clinical presentation.

Emphasis has been placed on the pathophysiology and clinical presentations of each of the different types of emboli. When appropriate, treatment and prophylaxis are also considered.

## TUMOR

Since 1897, multiple case reports have shown that hepatocellular carcinoma and nearly every other type of carcinoma and sarcoma can embolize to the lungs. In the lungs, tumor emboli cause most of their damage by mechanically obstructing the pulmonary arterial circulation. Unlike metastases, tumor emboli initially do not affect the pulmonary parenchyma. Unlike thrombotic pulmonary emboli, tumor emboli may trigger little in the way of vasoactive mediators.[1]

The mechanism whereby tumor fragments gain access to the pulmonary circulation and the pulmonary pathology associated with tumor embolism are well described. Tumor emboli arrive in the lungs both directly, by invading capillary and venous networks, and indirectly, by invading the lymphatic system and traveling to the thoracic duct and venous circulation.[2] In the lungs, tumor emboli appear as intravascular tumor fragments, usually engulfed by thrombus. Over a period of weeks or months, the tumor emboli either necrose and are obliterated or they establish themselves as metastases.[3, 4] Some authors feel that the formation of thrombus around

***Table 11–1.*** Winterbauer Grading System for Quantitating Tumor Pulmonary Embolism

| Grade | Definition |
|---|---|
| 0 | 0 to 1 small arterial or arteriolar tumor embolus |
| I | 2 to 15 small arterial tumor emboli |
| II | ≥16 small arterial tumor emboli and no more than 10% of all small arteries occluded<br>or<br>Occlusion of one or more subsegmental arteries |
| III | Occlusion of 15–30% of all small arteries<br>or<br>Occlusion of one or more segmental arteries |
| IV | Occlusion of more than one-third of all small arteries<br>or<br>Occlusion of a main or lobar pulmonary artery |

From the methodology described by Winterbauer, R. H., Elfenbein, I. B., and Ball, W. C.: Incidence and clinical significance of tumor embolization to the lungs. Am. J. Med., *45*:271, 1968.

a tumor embolus kills the tumor cells.[1, 2] Others feel that platelets and clotting factors promote tumor invasion.[5]

The clinical significance and frequency of pulmonary tumor embolism were best delineated in a 1968 report by Winterbauer and coworkers.[2] In their classic report, they first devised a grading system for quantitating tumor embolization to the lungs (Table 11–1). Next, they classified the clinical significance of the pulmonary tumor emboli into three groups. Emboli were considered "incidental" findings if the patient had no respiratory symptoms and if death was due to a non-pulmonary cause. Emboli were considered "primary" causes of the patient's morbidity or mortality if their grade was III or IV and if the patient had respiratory distress without other substantial cardiac or pulmonary processes. Emboli were labeled "contributory" to the patient's morbidity and mortality if their grade was II, III, or IV and if the patient had respiratory distress in the setting of significant parenchymal pulmonary diseases (metastases, lymphatic spread, and so forth) or cardiac impairment.[2]

Case reports had suggested that five types of tumor frequently embolized to lung: hepatocellular carcinoma, renal cell carcinoma, breast carcinoma, gastric carcinoma, and choriocarcinoma. Therefore, Winterbauer and coworkers reviewed 366 autopsies of patients with these five types of tumor (Table 11–2). They determined that the overall frequency of tumor pulmonary embolism in these five tumors was 26 per cent. The overall frequency of grade III or grade IV tumor pulmonary embolism was 6 per cent. With one exception, all cases of clinically significant pulmonary tumor emboli (emboli considered the "primary" cause of respiratory symptoms) occurred in patients with grade III or grade IV emboli.[2]

Frequency figures for the five tumors were as follows: hepatoma (79 patients), 51 per cent grade I or higher, 8 per cent grade III or IV; hypernephroma, metastatic or > 4 cm (78 patients), 31 per cent grade I or higher, 2 per cent grade III or IV; breast carcinoma (100 consecutive cases), 17 per cent grade I or higher, 9 per cent grade III or IV; gastric carcinoma (100 consecutive cases), 12 per

***Table 11–2.*** Frequency of Pulmonary Tumor Embolism in Five Selected Tumors

| Tumor | Number of Autopsies | Per Cent of Cases with Grade I or Higher Pulmonary Tumor Embolism | Per Cent of Cases with Grade III or Grade IV Pulmonary Tumor Embolism |
|---|---|---|---|
| Hepatoma* | 79 | 51 | 8 |
| Hypernephroma** (metastatic or >4 cm) | 78 | 31 | 2 |
| Breast carcinoma | 100 | 17 | 9 |
| Gastric carcinoma | 100 | 12 | 4 |
| Choriocarcinoma | 9 | 2/9 cases | 0 |
| Total | 366 | 26 | 6 |

Adapted from Winterbauer, R. H., Elfenbein, I. B.,, and Ball, W. C.: Incidence and clinical significance of tumor embolization to the lungs. Am. J. Med., *45*:271, 1968.

*Synonymous with hepatocellular carcinoma.

**Synonymous with renal cell carcinoma.

cent grade I or higher, 4 per cent grade III or IV; choriocarcinoma (9 cases), 2 cases grade I and higher, no cases grade III or IV[2] (see Table 11–2).

The frequency of pulmonary tumor embolism in other types of neoplasia is unknown. The overall frequency of pulmonary tumor embolism, based on 1085 autopsies of patients with all types of solid tumors, is 2.4 per cent.[1] Not surprisingly, this figure is far lower than Winterbauer's figure of 26 per cent, because he selected five types of solid tumors which frequently embolized to the lungs.

With rare exceptions, only grade III and grade IV tumor pulmonary emboli are clinically significant.[2] In an autopsy review of 32 cases of clinically significant tumor pulmonary embolism, 13 patients presented with respiratory distress of unknown etiology.[2] Although pulmonary symptoms may be absent in a few cases of grade III or grade IV tumor embolism, they are usually quite prominent. They are not related to tumor type. Of the 32 cases just mentioned, dyspnea was present in 24; pleuritic pain was present in seven.[2] Hemoptysis has been reported, but in patients with underlying malignancy, its significance is unclear.[1]

The time course of symptoms varies widely in patients with tumor pulmonary embolism. Acute presenting symptoms occur, including sudden collapse, that are indistinguishable from acute, thrombotic pulmonary embolism.[6] At times, patients present with gradually increasing dyspnea, that mimics recurrent "silent" thrombotic pulmonary embolism.[7, 8]

Heart and lung examination of patients with grade III or grade IV tumor pulmonary embolism is similar to that of patients with thrombotic pulmonary embolism. In chronic cases, pulmonary hypertension and cor pulmonale may be present.[8, 9]

As in thrombotic pulmonary embolism, the chest roentgenogram in tumor pulmonary embolism can be normal or can show an infarction pattern. (In Winterbauer's review of the literature on clinically significant tumor pulmonary emboli, eight of 28 patients had normal chest x-rays, and 15 had infarction patterns only.[2]) At presentation, blood gases may reveal hypoxemia and hypocarbia, just like thrombotic pulmonary embolism. Similarly, electrocardiograms may show right heart strain or right ventricular hypertrophy. These abnormalities rarely revert to normal as they might in thrombotic pulmonary embolism. At times, even after all the routine laboratory work has been reviewed, there is still no hint of malignancy.[1]

A negative lung scan is unhelpful in pulmonary tumor emboli. Too often, the emboli occlude arterioles that are <2 mm in diameter.[10, 11] However, a positive scan that does not evolve over several weeks can sometimes distinguish tumor from thrombotic pulmonary embolism. Peripheral perfusion defects rather than central perfusion defects may also be a characteristic of tumor embolism to the lungs. A case of osteogenic sarcoma pulmonary embolism was diagnosed by combining routine $^{99m}$Tc MDP bone scanning with additional scintigraphic views of the lungs.[12] $^{99m}$Tc MDP, which is taken up by osteoid, accumulated at the base of a nonperfused segment. Chest CT was negative, thus suggesting tumor embolus, not metastasis.

As expected, pulmonary angiography may sometimes document the presence of obstruction. However, no study evaluating its sensitivity has been performed. One would expect that, because of the peripheral location of tumor emboli, pulmonary angiography might sometimes miss the diagnosis. Right heart catheterization frequently discloses elevated pulmonary artery pressures.

Because pulmonary tumor embolism can present so variably, it should be part of the differential diagnosis almost every time thrombotic pulmonary embolism is under consideration in a patient with suspected or known malignancy. Even lower extremity swelling does not exclude tumor pulmonary embolism, because lymphatic and venous obstruction by tumor could cause this. When patients with pulmonary infarction, pulmonary hypertension, or respiratory symptoms have constitutional signs or organomegaly, pulmonary tumor embolism should be considered strongly.[2, 10]

At least four factors are postulated to predispose a cancer patient to tumor pulmonary embolism: (1) Pulmonary embolization of tumors, like metastatic behavior of tumors, probably varies according to ill-defined, type-specific tumor "tropism" and "stickiness." Just as some breast cancers have a tendency to metastasize to liver and bone, some tumors are more likely to embolize to the lungs.[2] (2) Advanced tumor stage, particularly advanced hepatic metastases, may correlate with higher grades of pulmonary tumor embolism. This is true in breast and gastric carcinoma.[1, 2] (3) A tumor's tendency to invade vascular structures might make it more likely to embolize to the lungs. For example, gastric and breast carcinomas, tumors which rarely invade the inferior vena cava, have a lower frequency of pulmonary tumor embolization than do hepatoma and hypernephroma.[2] (4) Chemotherapy, radiation therapy, and especially surgical manipulation have all been correlated with the rapid onset of pulmonary tumor embolism. Within two days of irradiation, parotid and hepatic tumors have been reported to have embolized to the lung.[2] Intraoperative pulmonary embolization of hypernephroma, lung carcinoma, Wilms' tumor, retroperitoneal sarcoma, teratoma, and myxoma have been reported.[4, 5, 13–15] Not surprisingly, insertion of a LeVeen shunt to drain ascitic fluid into the superior vena cava can cause large-scale tumor pulmonary embolism.[3]

### Therapy

There is no specific treatment for tumor pulmonary embolism. The underlying neoplastic process must be addressed. Acute, massive tumor embolism has been treated with embolectomy.[6] Heparinization, in scattered cases, has not been helpful and can be deleterious if there is bleeding into the underlying neoplasms. During surgery, special care should be taken to prevent tumor embolization. In Wilms' tumor and renal cell carcinoma resections, the renal vein should be ligated early.[5, 14]

The prognosis for patients with grade III or IV tumor pulmonary embolism is grim. In Winterbauer's review, they died within 12 weeks of diagnosis, death frequently being caused by the tumor emboli.[2] All of these patients had advanced stages of tumor, however, and whether pulmonary tumor embolism significantly changed their survival is unclear. No data exist comparing survival among patients with and without grade I and grade II pulmonary tumor emboli.

However, on the bright side, pulmonary tumor emboli do not always result in pulmonary parenchymal metastases. Daughtry[6] reported on a patient with renal cell carcinoma who presented with massive tumor pulmonary embolism. Following embolectomy and surgical resection of a large primary tumor, the patient survived for several years. Tumor did not escape the pulmonary arterial circulation. Metastases were not created. Hence, pulmonary tumor emboli should not be equated with pulmonary metastases, and the presence of pulmonary tumor emboli should not discourage vigorous treatment of the primary tumor.

## SEPTIC PULMONARY EMBOLI

Septic pulmonary emboli were first described by Hussey in 1945. He carefully distinguished septic emboli from bacteremia that caused abscesses.

> "In any case of septicemia caused by a pyogenic organism, abscesses may occur in the lungs as well as elsewhere. In a sense, these are embolic abscesses, but we have not included cases of this type in this discussion. Rather, we have been interested in the situation in which a septic thrombus in the peripheral veins or the right side of the heart becomes dislodged, enters the pulmonary circulation, and causes infarction."[16]

Other authors have relied on this original definition of septic emboli. MacMillan and coworkers[17] pointed out that a bland pulmonary embolus that becomes secondarily infected is not a true septic embolus. McHenry,[18] and later Soave,[19] stated that the necrotizing pneumonia that may occur after *Pseudomonas* bacteremia is not secondary to septic emboli but rather to on-site bacterial colonization. In other words, septic embolism can be diagnosed only in the presence of septic thrombosis.

In three series, infected tricuspid valve thrombi (tricuspid endocarditis), seen almost exclusively in intravenous drug abusers, led to at least half the cases of septic pulmonary emboli. The remaining cases of septic pulmonary emboli resulted equally from endogenously and exogenously induced septic peripheral thrombi[17, 20, 21] (Table 11–3).

Common causes of endogenous peripheral thrombi are: (1) jugular venous system thrombophlebitis secondary to facial, dental, sinus, and pharyngeal infections; (2) pelvic thrombophlebitis in the setting of abortion or delivery; and (3) deep vein thrombophlebitis related to cellulitis, arthritis, and subcutaneous abscesses. Septic thrombi can also form in bone secondary to osteomyelitis or in the inferior vena cava or hemorrhoidal veins when abdominal or perirectal infections occur. Infected tips of transvenous pacemakers, intravenous catheters, and artificial dialysis shunts are the sites where most peripheral, exogenous septic thrombi form. At times, drug addicts inject large boluses of

***Table 11–3.*** Sources of Septic Pulmonary Emboli: Three Series of Septic Pulmonary Embolism

| Location of Septic Thrombus | MacMillan[17] 60 patients | Jaffe[21] 17 patients* | Fred[20] 7 patients |
|---|---|---|---|
| Tricuspid endocarditis | 32/60 | 13/17 | 3/7 |
| Peripheral endogenous septic thrombi (e.g., peripheral venous, inferior vena caval, pelvic, pharyngeal, hemorrhoidal, or bone thrombophlebitis) | 13/60 | 6/17 | 4/7 |
| Exogenous septic thrombi<br>catheters<br>pacemakers<br>shunts<br>foreign particles | 15/60 | 0/17 | 0/7 |

*Two patients had both septic thrombophlebitis and tricuspid endocarditis.

infected material that either form peripheral septic thrombi or embolize to the lungs directly.[16, 17, 22–25]

The pathophysiology of septic pulmonary embolism is uncomplicated. In typical thromboembolic (i.e., "bland") pulmonary processes, collateral vessels often prevent infarction. In septic embolic events, however, the already infected embolus rapidly infects the pulmonary tissues. Inflammation ensues, and the collateral circulation is quickly compromised. Infarction and abscesses appear within days. When an infected embolus contacts pleura, empyema readily results.[17]

The bronchioles are also distorted by inflammation. They form one-way check valves that trap air. The trapped air, under pressure, flattens ruined alveolar septa, and thus, thin-walled cysts are formed. When a piece of necrotic consolidated parenchyma is in the midst of one of these cysts, the radiologic "target sign" is seen.[26, 27]

Hemoptysis results not only from ischemia-induced hemorrhagic infarction but from actual invasion of blood vessels by colonies of microorganisms. Mycotic aneurysms and bronchioloarterial fistulas can be formed and cause massive, fatal hemoptysis.[28, 29]

The overall frequency of true septic embolism is far less than the frequency of bland thromboembolic pulmonary embolism. In a 1969 series, only .25 per cent of autopsies showed evidence of septic emboli, whereas 20 per cent of the autopsies had bland pulmonary embolism.[20] Among populations predisposed to septic thrombus formation, however, the frequency of septic pulmonary emboli is quite high, and septic emboli must be considered even before bland emboli. In a group of 28 intravenous drug abusers with pulmonary, vascular, and cardiac complications, 11 patients had septic pulmonary emboli.[28] In a group of 46 postpartum women with signs of septic pelvic thrombophlebitis, 15 had infiltrative chest processes that may have represented septic pulmonary embolism and infarction.[30] In patients with osteomyelitis, serious pharyngeal infection, or dialysis shunts, septic pulmonary embolism must at least be considered whenever respiratory symptoms develop.[24, 31]

The presenting signs of septic pulmonary embolism are rarely masked by the underlying septic process. Patient complaints are similar whether the embolus originates on the tricuspid valve or from a peripheral endogenous or exogenous source. Shaking chills, pleuritic pain, and cough are common. Hemoptysis occurs and can be massive, but it is rare. Dyspnea is also rare. Unlike bland pulmonary emboli, spontaneous remission of symptoms does not occur among patients with septic pulmonary embolism.[17, 20, 23]

Physical examination nearly always reveals fever. Pleural rubs occur at times but probably no more frequently than they do with bland emboli. On a thorough examination, the site of thrombosis will very frequently be apparent.

White blood cell counts reflect the underlying septic picture, not the presence of pulmonary infarction, and thus range from decreased to elevated.[17, 23] The chest roentgenogram is central to the suspicion and diagnosis of septic pulmonary embolism. It is found to be abnormal early in almost all cases.[31] It usually has multiple nodular densities ranging in size from a few millimeters to greater than seven centimeters, involving both lobes[20, 23] (Fig. 11–1). Over a period of days, the roentgenogram rapidly changes. Sequentially, new individual nodules or groups of nodules appear, predominantly in the lower lobes. The older nodules extend, coalesce into abscesses, and become wedge-shaped or cavitate.[21] The lesions that cavitate

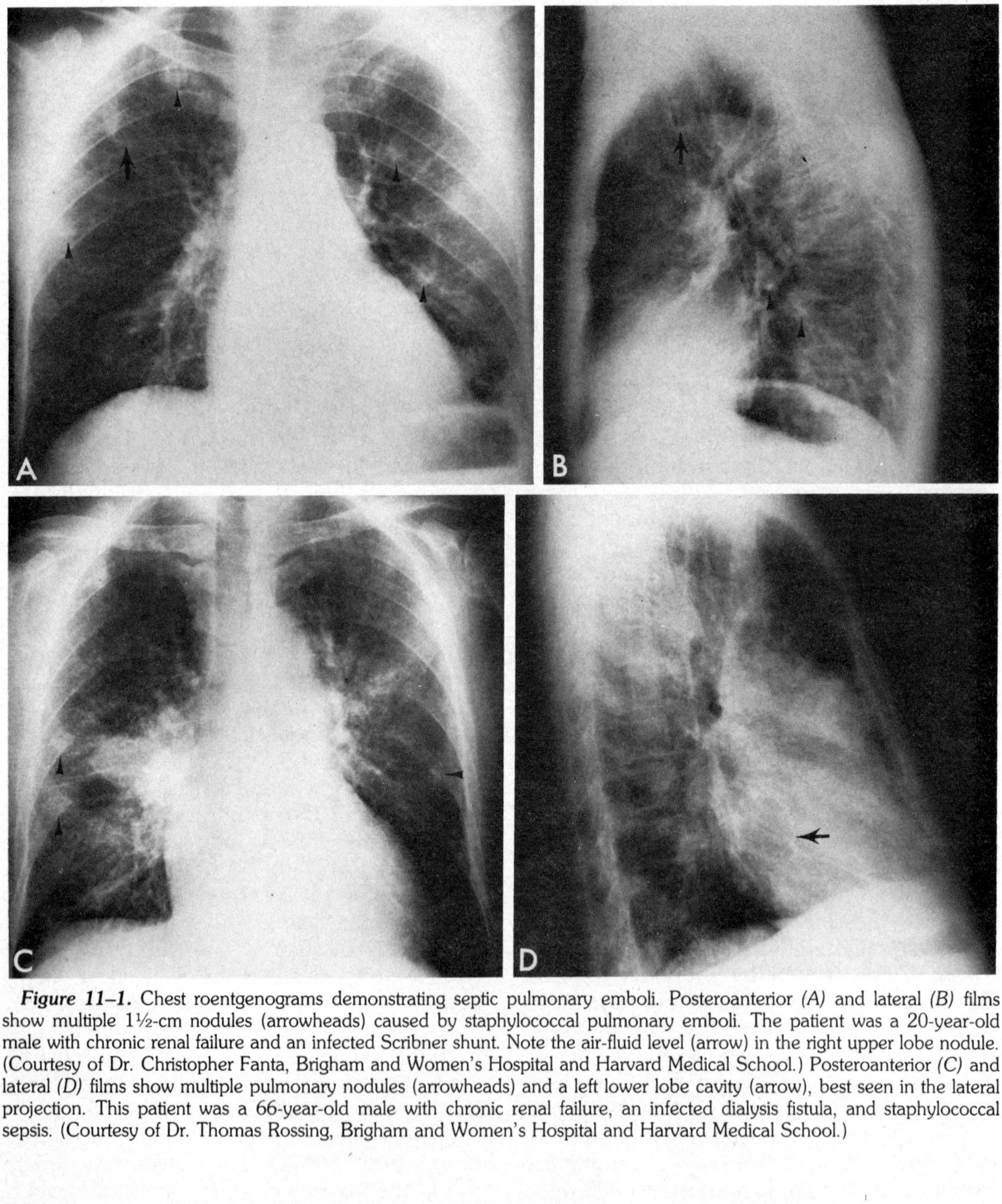


***Figure 11–1.*** Chest roentgenograms demonstrating septic pulmonary emboli. Posteroanterior *(A)* and lateral *(B)* films show multiple 1½-cm nodules (arrowheads) caused by staphylococcal pulmonary emboli. The patient was a 20-year-old male with chronic renal failure and an infected Scribner shunt. Note the air-fluid level (arrow) in the right upper lobe nodule. (Courtesy of Dr. Christopher Fanta, Brigham and Women's Hospital and Harvard Medical School.) Posteroanterior *(C)* and lateral *(D)* films show multiple pulmonary nodules (arrowheads) and a left lower lobe cavity (arrow), best seen in the lateral projection. This patient was a 66-year-old male with chronic renal failure, an infected dialysis fistula, and staphylococcal sepsis. (Courtesy of Dr. Thomas Rossing, Brigham and Women's Hospital and Harvard Medical School.)

in communication with a bronchus form the "target sign," defined as an "area of pulmonary density suspended within an air-filled, thin-walled pseudocystic formation."[27] Pleural effusions and empyema are frequently present.[23] Hilar and mediastinal adenopathy can also occur.[32] X-rays obtained from neutropenic patients have been reported to undergo similar changes.[27]

Sputum can be purulent, but in one series of 11 patients with septic pulmonary emboli, no patients had positive sputum cultures.[23] However, blood cultures tend to be positive, because the lungs are poor filters of microorganisms. Cultures reflect the underlying septic pathology. Fungal, staphylococcal, and gram-negative organisms predominate in cases of tricuspid endocarditis and vary in different geographic regions. Alpha hemolytic streptococcal, anaerobic, enterococcal, gram-negative, and staphylococcal organisms frequently grow in the setting of peripheral septic thrombosis.[17, 23]

Because the chest roentgenogram is almost always abnormal, lung scans are of little value in the diagnosis of septic pulmonary embolism.[20] Angiography is generally avoided in patients who appear septic to avoid seeding the cardiac valves. When performed, however, it is usually helpful. In one report, it demonstrated large lobar obstructive defects that turned out to be Candida.[33] In a group of seven septic patients with chest infiltrates and surgically proven septic pulmonary emboli, angiography was positive in six.[17] In other scattered reports, angiography has demonstrated subsegmental occlusions and aided in the diagnosis of septic embolism.[21] However, because septic embolism can involve small vessels (<2 mm in diameter), angiography is not a very sensitive diagnostic test.[20]

When a patient presents with chills, pleuritic pain, and multiple, sequentially developing cavitary pulmonary densities, the diagnosis of septic pulmonary embolism must be considered, but it is by no means certain unless a source of infected thrombi is detected. Aside from the myriad causes of necrotizing pneumonia,[32] two entities that can closely mimic the clinical presentation of septic pulmonary embolism are Pseudomonas bacteremia[18, 19] and aseptic necrosis of bland pulmonary emboli.[34] In the former, angiography, although risky, could be helpful. In the latter, the absence of both a fever and an elevated white count might steer the diagnostician away from septic pulmonary emboli.

### Therapy

Therapy for endogenously formed septic pulmonary emboli consists of initial medical treatment of the underlying septic process, followed by surgical treatment if the patient fails to respond to conservative management. The pulmonary process should be treated similarly.[17] Therapy for exogenously formed septic emboli from tips of transvenous pacemakers and dialysis shunts requires foreign body extirpation as well as medical treatment.[24]

Frequently, tricuspid endocarditis, like left-sided endocarditis, requires surgery. The presence of septic pulmonary emboli prior to antibiotic treatment does not portend a poor prognosis. Continued septic pulmonary emboli during antibiotic treatment would be one of several reasons for surgery, however. Heparin is of doubtful benefit in tricuspid endocarditis.

Septic pelvic thrombophlebitis and other forms of septic phlebitis will most often respond to a combination of antibiotics and aggressive systemic heparinization. Heparinization can be a diagnostic aid; if a postpartum patient has spiking fevers unresponsive to antibiotics but rapidly defervesces once heparin therapy is initiated, the diagnosis of septic pelvic thrombophlebitis is virtually assured[35] (Fig. 11–2). Even patients

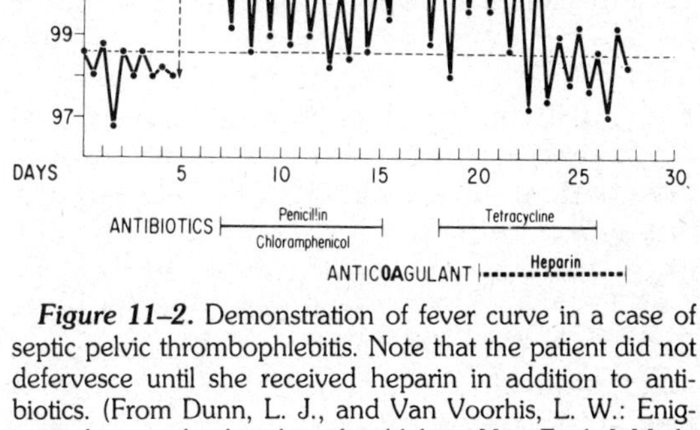


***Figure 11–2.*** Demonstration of fever curve in a case of septic pelvic thrombophlebitis. Note that the patient did not defervesce until she received heparin in addition to antibiotics. (From Dunn, L. J., and Van Voorhis, L. W.: Enigmatic fever and pelvic thrombophlebitis. New Engl. J. Med., *276*:265, 1967.)

with massive ovarian vein thrombosis usually respond quickly to medical management.[30] Some authors, in cases of septic pelvic thrombophlebitis with septic pulmonary infarction, keep patients anticoagulated for three months,[36] but there are few data to support this. When septic pelvic and deep vein thrombi do not respond to medical management and the patient has ongoing episodes of septic pulmonary infarction or fever, surgery is required. Drainage and vein ligation are then performed.[20]

Pulmonary lesions, such as empyema, abscesses, and bronchopleural fistulae require treatment in their standard fashion, as if they did not arise from septic emboli. Reasonable indications for surgery include loculated empyema that fails drainage, persistent large abscess and ongoing sepsis, and bronchopleural fistulae with empyema. Massive hemoptysis, defined as "a single expectoration of greater than 50 cc" requires, as it always does, prompt attention including bronchoscopy and angiography.[29] Bronchioloarterial fistulae and ruptured mycotic aneurysms can result in fatal aspiration. Intubation equipment should be on hand, and surgery should be performed promptly.

Prognosis in cases of septic pulmonary emboli is determined mostly by the underlying septic process. In patients who respond to medical or surgical management, the chest roentgenogram improves remarkably, often leaving only mild fibrosis, pneumatoceles, or pleural thickening.[31]

## AMNIOTIC FLUID EMBOLISM

In 1941, Steiner and Lushbaugh[37] described eight pregnant women who, during labor, suddenly developed tachypnea and pulmonary edema followed by shock, hemorrhage, and death. Postmortem findings in all eight patients were the same: particles of amniotic fluid were showered throughout the pulmonary arterioles. In the same report, Steiner and Lushbaugh noted that pulmonary amniotic fluid particles were not present in the postmortem examinations of 34 women dying from other delivery complications such as eclampsia, rheumatic heart disease, or hemorrhage. They concluded that amniotic fluid embolism was a distinct clinicopathologic entity and not simply a by-product of other birth complications.

Amniotic fluid emboli are made up of variable combinations of vernix caseosa and meconium mucin. (Vernix caseosa refers to the greasy, cheesy substance that coats the fetal skin. It is composed of dead epidermal cells and the fatty secretions of fetal sebaceous glands.[38]) The amniotic fluid components gain access to the placental sinuses and thus the venous circulation when the fetal membranes tear or leak at the placental margin[39] (Fig. 11–3). In the lungs, the amniotic fluid emboli plug arterioles and capillaries. Usually, a dense inflammatory reaction surrounds the embolus, and nodules form that may involve the alveolar septa. Diffuse pulmonary edema and hemorrhage are usually present.[40] Amniotic fluid embolization does not occur during normal deliveries.[41, 42]

The overall frequency of amniotic fluid embolism is low. Steiner estimated that the syndrome complicated one in 8000 births.[37] Later authors suggested that the frequency is even lower: between one in 20,000 and one in 37,000 births.[41, 43] Although the overall frequency of amniotic fluid embolism is low, the frequency of the syndrome among mothers who die during delivery is quite high. Steiner and Lushbaugh said that it was the most common cause of death during labor and the first nine hours after labor. Among 30 consecutive patients dying during this interval, eight of the deaths were attributed to amniotic fluid embolism. (The second leading cause of death during this interval was rheumatic heart disease complications.[37]) As the death rates from infection, hemorrhage,

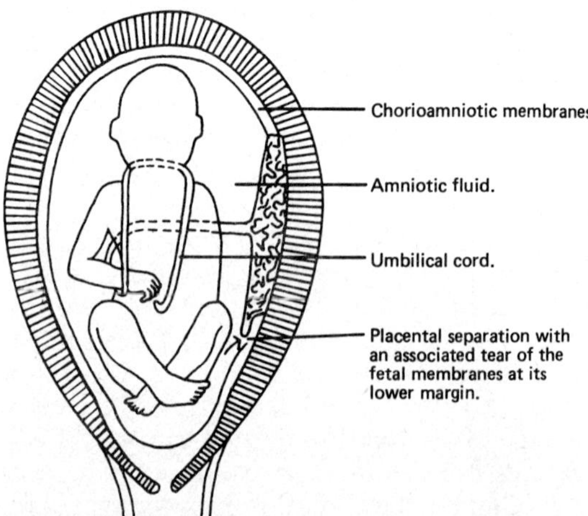


*Figure 11–3.* Pathogenesis of amniotic fluid embolism. The arrow indicates the portal of entry of amniotic fluid into the placental sinuses and thence into the maternal circulation. (From Corridan, M., Kendall, E. D., and Begg, J. D.: Cord entanglement causing premature placental separation and amniotic fluid embolism. Br. J. Obstet. Gynecol., 87:935, 1980.)

and eclampsia have fallen, the proportion of maternal deaths due to amniotic fluid embolism has risen.[44]

Not all cases of amniotic fluid embolism are fatal, as will be discussed later. As of 1979, 26 cases of nonfatal amniotic fluid embolism had been reported.[40] The proportion of maternal cases of respiratory distress syndrome caused by amniotic fluid embolism may be quite high, but it is unknown.

The clinical syndrome associated with amniotic fluid embolism begins during labor or within 24 hours after delivery.[37, 45] The main symptoms are dyspnea, shock, and hemorrhage. Though Steiner and Lushbaugh reported that six of their eight patients first noted chills, others have reported that chills occur only five to 20 per cent of the time[37, 46] (Table 11–4).

The sudden onset of dyspnea and restlessness was noted early in seven of eight patients in Steiner's series, but in only 40 per cent of Aguillon's 60 cases compiled from the literature.[46]

The most common feature of amniotic fluid embolization is shock. In all of Steiner's patients and all of Aguillon's own patients, marked hypotension occurred as the presenting symptom or within hours of the onset of dyspnea. Shock or dyspnea or both were present in 53 of the 60 cases from the literature.[37, 46]

Hemorrhage, defined as blood loss greater than 500 ml, occurred in half of Steiner's patients, 40 per cent of Aguillon's own patients, 47 per cent of the patients in Aguillon's literature review, and 27 per cent of Barno's series. Of note, in both Barno's and Aguillon's series, hemorrhage occurred in almost every patient who survived for more than one hour.[37, 45, 46]

Physical examination of the patient with amniotic fluid embolism almost always reveals tachypnea, hypotension, and tachycardia. Rales are frequently heard and, within hours, nearly all patients will develop pulmonary edema.[43]

The white blood cell count can be greater than 30,000 and frequently displays a left shift.[40] In the patients who are hemorrhaging, coagulation studies disclose disseminated intravascular coagulation with hypofibrinogenemia, thrombocytopenia, and elevated fibrin degradation products and clotting parameters. The chest roentgenogram reveals alveolar infiltration in nearly all cases. The electrocardiogram can show right heart strain. Blood gas determinations disclose profound hypoxemia. Right heart catheterization reveals low pulmonary capillary wedge pressures and elevated pulmonary artery pressures even when the patient is in shock. In the setting of floridly abnormal chest roentgenograms, lung scanning is not helpful in diagnosing amniotic fluid embolism. Angiography experience is limited. A recent case report mentioned an erroneously negative pulmonary angiogram.[47]

Short of lung biopsy, there is no guaranteed accurate diagnostic test for amniotic fluid embolism. Tests that appear useful involve examination of maternal sputum for fetal squamous cells[48] and examination of buffy coat smears.[40, 47] The buffy coat smears are prepared from blood aspirated from a CVP line or preferably from a pulmonary artery catheter. After centrifugation and washing, smears can be viewed with both Wright stains and polarized lenses. Clusters of fetal squamous cells will be birefringent. No study has compared the accuracy of this relatively noninvasive test with open lung biopsy. The time course for buffy coat positivity is unknown. In one report, a sample drawn 30 hours after the onset of symptoms was positive for fetal squamous cells. Forty-eight hours later, a second sample was negative.[47]

A case taken from Steiner and Lushbaugh's original report exemplifies the rapid, fulminant course that can be associated with amniotic fluid embolism. A 30-year-old woman had an uneventful pregnancy until two weeks before term when fetal heart sounds

***Table 11–4.*** Symptoms Associated with Amniotic Fluid Embolism

| Author | Type of Series | Number of Cases | Chills | Dyspnea or Restlessness | Shock | Hemorrhage (>500 cc Blood Loss) |
|---|---|---|---|---|---|---|
| Steiner[37] | Autopsy | 8 | 6/8 | 7/8 | 8/8 | 4/8 |
| Aguillon[46] | Literature; autopsy | 60 | 3/60 | 24/60 | 42/60 | 27/60 |
| Aguillon[46] | Autopsy and clinical | 5 | 1/5 | 2/5 | 5/5 | 2/5 |
| Barno[45] | Autopsy and clinical | 15 | Not given | Not given | 15/15 | 4/15 |

ceased. She had mild labor pains. "Suddenly . . . the patient was awakened by an attack of . . . air hunger and profuse perspiration. She was in shock with cyanosis of the lips . . ." After delivering a macerated fetus, the patient quickly died from amniotic fluid embolism, three hours and 45 minutes after her shock began.[2]

A case report by Wasser and coworkers in 1979 illustrates a slightly less fulminant pattern.[40] A 23-year-old woman underwent a normal cesarean section. "Two hours after delivery, the patient became dyspneic and cyanotic. The blood pressure was 80/60 mm Hg, the pulse 124 per minute . . . respiratory rate 40 per minute, and the temperature was 36.2° C rectally. Physical examination revealed diffuse rhonchi, bibasilar rates, and an accentuated pulmonic second sound. Arterial blood gases showed a pH of 7.47, a $PaO_2$ of 32 torr, and $PaCO_2$ of 31 torr. Chest x-ray revealed bilateral alveolar infiltrates. The white blood cell count was 31,600 per $mm^3$." Clotting parameters were normal.

During the peripartum period, the rapid onset of hypotension, pulmonary edema, and hemorrhage in the absence of chest pain is virtually diagnostic of amniotic fluid embolism. Other processes that can mimic aspects of the early phase of amniotic fluid embolism are improperly diagnosed or mismanaged rheumatic heart disease, peripartum cardiomyopathy, eclampsia, aspiration, air and thrombotic pulmonary embolism, drug reactions, and sepsis.

Multiple conditions predispose to the development of amniotic fluid embolism. All of these conditions enhance the entry of amniotic fluid into the venous circulation by a two-part process: They promote tearing or leaking of the fetal membrane, and they cause disruption of the uterine and placental venous systems.

Tumultuous labor, induced labor, and cesarean section can cause membrane tearing as well as venous laceration and placental loosening that widens the placental sinusoids.[37, 43] As expected, these processes are associated with amniotic fluid embolism (Table 11–5). In Aguillon's review, 15 of 19 patients had "difficult" labor. In his own series, two of five patients had difficult labor.[46] In Barno's series, 14 of 15 patients had what he calls "hard" labor. The 15th had a cesarean section.[45] In Steiner and Lushbaugh's series, all eight patients had strong labor.[37]

Other processes that cause placental separation, membrane tearing, and the onset of especially forceful uterine contractions include placenta previa, premature separation, and abruptio placentae. These also are associated with amniotic fluid embolism.[43]

The status of the fetus is also a factor in amniotic fluid embolization. A dead or distressed fetus, particularly one that has caused meconium staining of the amniotic fluid, predisposes to membrane permeability and tearing as well as placental separation. Over half the cases reported by Steiner and Lushbaugh, Barno, and Aguillon had either dead fetuses or meconium staining.[37, 45, 46]

Maternal age and parity are not related to the development of amniotic fluid emboli in many series. Fetal size, fetal age, and duration of labor do not seem to correlate with amniotic fluid embolism.[46]

The pathophysiology of amniotic fluid embolism involves three phases (Table 11–6). Initially, the pulmonary emboli cause mechanical obstruction to pulmonary arterial flow. During this phase, some patients experience dyspnea. Early dyspnea may depend on the quantity of emboli showered.

The next phase is characterized by an anaphylaxis-like reaction involving systemic

***Table 11–5.*** Factors that Predispose to Amniotic Fluid Embolism

| Author | Type of Series | Number of Cases | Difficult Labor | Dead Fetus or Distressed Fetus (Meconium Staining) |
|---|---|---|---|---|
| Steiner[37] | Autopsy | 8 | 8/8 | 4/8 |
| Aguillon[46] | Literature; autopsy | 60 | 15/19* | 36/60 |
| Aguillon[46] | Autopsy and clinical | 5 | 2/5 | 3/5 |
| Barno[45] | Autopsy and clinical | 15 | 14/15 | 4/14** |

*Only 19/60 cases mentioned quality of labor.
**Only 14/15 cases mentioned status of fetus.

***Table 11–6.*** Pathophysiology of Amniotic Fluid Embolism: Three Overlapping Phases

| Phase | Clinical Manifestation |
|---|---|
| 1. Mechanical obstruction | Dyspnea and hypoxia |
| 2. Anaphylaxis | Pulmonary edema<br>nonelevated PCW* pressure<br>elevated PA* pressure<br>Hypotension<br>decreased SVR* |
| 3. Disseminated intravascular coagulation (DIC) | Hemorrhage<br>decreased platelets, fibrinogen; increased clotting time and fibrin split products |

*PCW = pulmonary capillary wedge; PA = pulmonary artery; SVR = systemic vascular resistance.

vasodilation, pulmonary vasoconstriction, and capillary leak.[43] During this phase, which may completely overshadow the first phase, the patient develops hypotension and pulmonary edema. In a pregnant ewe model, Reis and coworkers[49] demonstrated that seconds following intravenous injection of autologous amniotic fluid, central aortic pressure and systemic vascular resistance fell, whereas pulmonary artery pressure and pulmonary vascular resistance rose. The left atrial pressure did not change (Fig. 11–4).

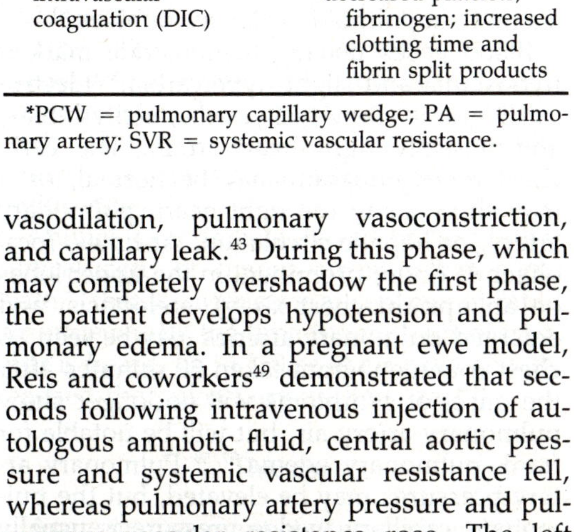


***Figure 11–4.*** Experimental amniotic fluid injection into a ewe. Pressure tracings depict the hemodynamics noted before and after the intravenous injection of 150 cc of amniotic fluid. The solid black bar indicates the time of injection. Following injection, mean aortic pressure decreased, pulmonary arterial pressure and right atrial pressure increased, and cardiac output (pulmonary arterial flow) decreased. (From Reis, R. L., Pierce, W. S., and Benrendt, D. M.: Hemodynamic effects of amniotic fluid embolism. Surg. Gynecol. Obstet., *129*:45, 1969.)

The third phase of the amniotic fluid embolism syndrome involves the onset of disseminated intravascular coagulation (DIC). It is initiated by the release of thromboplastic amniotic materials into the circulation. The patient's hypotension and diminished hepatic circulation probably serve to potentiate the DIC.[50] As discussed earlier, hemorrhage is seen in only about 40 per cent of amniotic fluid embolism cases but is seen in nearly all cases that survive longer than one hour.[46]

### Therapy

Treatment for amniotic fluid embolism consists of rapidly removing the fetus and amniotic fluid and then vigorously supporting the patient. The hypotension, adult respiratory distress syndrome, and DIC are treated conventionally.

Amniotic fluid embolism carries a grave prognosis. In a series compiled before 1960, it was 80 per cent fatal.[46] Although many cases of nonfatal amniotic fluid embolism have recently been reported, there are no recent data on overall survival.[40, 41, 51, 52] Hopefully, sophisticated hemodynamic monitoring and vigorous treatment of DIC will improve the outlook in this fulminant disease. Some authors feel that they can prevent amniotic fluid embolism by avoiding rigorous labor induction, particularly in the setting of distressed or dead fetuses.[45]

## VENOUS AIR EMBOLISM

Venous air embolism does not lend itself to epidemiologic study, because it is difficult to document and frequently inapparent. Even when the syndrome of venous air embolism is full blown, replete with the adult respiratory distress syndrome, it is often misdiagnosed. Not surprisingly, the overall frequency of venous air embolism is unknown.[53]

The cause of venous air embolism, however, is known. Whenever air that is at a higher pressure than the venous circulation comes into communication with the venous circulation, venous air embolism occurs. Communication between air and the venous circulation can exist via an unconnected or improperly connected intravenous catheter, via a surgically or traumatically exposed vein, or via a bronchopulmonary arterial fistula. Positive air–venous pressure gradients occur in a number of settings. Elevated or pressur-

## FAT EMBOLISM SYNDROME

### Diagnosis

The relationship between fat emboli (an anatomic finding) and fat embolism syndrome (a clinicopathologic entity) is far more complex than the relationship between other types of emboli and the syndromes that they produce. Unlike the simple connection, for example, between septic embolism and septic embolism syndrome, there is no simple connection between fat embolism and the fat embolism syndrome.

Fat embolism as an anatomic entity was first described by Zenker in 1862. He noted fat emboli in the lungs of a patient who died from a massive crush injury to the chest and abdomen.[67] In 1876, Holm found pulmonary fat emboli in 21 patients who died following fractures. He concluded that fat embolism was a common anatomic finding that was not clinically significant.[67] Over the past 100 years, most authors have agreed with Holm's conclusion. Several groups have demonstrated that nonclinically significant pulmonary fat emboli are present in 67 to 97 per cent of patients dying with fractures.[67–70] Herndon and coworkers suggested that inconsequential pulmonary fat emboli are present in the lungs of 94 per cent of patients who undergo uncomplicated hip surgery.[71]

The pathology associated with clinically insignificant fat embolism has been well described. Variable numbers of pulmonary arterioles and capillaries are "plugged with large fat globules, which frequently coalesce." At times, the tissue distal to the plugs shows changes of ischemic necrosis and slight hemorrhage.[69]

Unlike fat embolism, which is defined anatomically and is usually clinically insignificant, fat embolism syndrome is defined clinically and, by definition, is clinically significant. The fat embolism syndrome is a diagnosis of exclusion in trauma patients who have a constellation of abnormal pulmonary, neurologic, cutaneous, and laboratory findings. Regrettably, there are no agreed-upon criteria for what constitutes a "constellation" of findings, and nearly every investigator has used a different definition to

***Table 11–8.*** Representative Definitions of the Fat Embolism Syndrome

| Author | Year | Institution | Definition of Fat Embolism Syndrome* |
|---|---|---|---|
| Linscheid[72]<br>Dines[73]<br>Burgher[74]<br>Dines[68] | 1969<br>1972<br>1974<br>1975 | Mayo Clinic<br>Mayo Clinic<br>Mayo Clinic<br>Mayo Clinic | Pulmonary and cerebral dysfunction, long bone fracture, fever, hypoxia and one of the following: abnormal CXR, petechiae, retinal fat, fat in clotted blood, lipuria |
| Stoltenberg[75] | 1979 | Hennepin County Medical Center | Hypoxemic and central nervous system symptoms |
| Gurd[76] | 1974 | Royal Victoria Hospital Northern Ireland | One major: respiratory insufficiency, cerebral involvement, petechial rash<br>Four minor: fever, tachycardia, retinal fat, jaundice, renal changes, and fat macroglobulinemia |
| Curtis[77] | 1979 | Yale–New Haven Hospital | Neurologic dysfunction, respiratory insufficiency, petechiae |
| Moore[78] | 1981 | Royal Newcastle Hospital, Australia | Cerebral and respiratory disorders |
| Guentner[79] | 1981 | University of Calgary, Canada | Two of the following: fever (>38° C), change in sensorium, hypoxemia, petechiae, diffuse pulmonary infiltrates |
| Schonfeld[80] | 1983 | University of Cincinnati | ≥5 points: Petechiae 5 point(s); Diffuse alveolar infiltrate 4 "; Hypoxemia 3 "; Confusion 1 "; Fever ≥38° C 1 "; Pulse ≥120/min 1 "; R.R.** ≥30/min 1 " |

*All authors specified that listed criteria were not explainable on the basis of other processes, such as aspiration pneumonia or heart failure and so forth.

**R.R. = respiratory rate.

diagnose the fat embolism syndrome. Table 11–8 lists representative definitions from 10 recent series on the fat embolism syndrome.

Fortunately, there is a great deal of overlap among the definitions; therefore, studies can be at least roughly compared. Several authors considered both respiratory and neurologic dysfunction as major criteria, whereas one author required only respiratory dysfunction or neurologic dysfunction to make the diagnosis. Only two authors required neither. The list of other criteria included petechiae (representative of both cutaneous fat emboli and thrombocytopenia), fever, retinal emboli, hypoxia, and pulmonary infiltrates. Authors required anywhere from one to four of these, in addition to the major criteria of respiratory and/or neurologic dysfunction, to diagnose fat embolism syndrome.

The use of major and minor criteria to diagnose the fat embolism syndrome was nicely exemplified by Dines and coworkers of the Mayo Clinic. According to these authors, fat embolism syndrome is a clinical syndrome characterized by the major findings of cerebral dysfunction, hypoxemia, and fever, and at least one minor finding, such as an abnormal chest x-ray, petechiae, or retinal fat.[73]

The frequency of fat embolism syndrome among trauma patients varies according to its definition. Using a rigorous definition that required both pulmonary and neurologic impairment, several groups of investigators[68, 70, 78, 81] estimated that 0.5 to 6 per cent of fracture patients develop fat embolism syndrome. Using a less rigorous definition that did not require both pulmonary and neurologic impairment, Gurd and coworkers estimated that 19 per cent of fracture patients developed the fat embolism syndrome.[76] All of these figures are far lower than the estimated frequency of simple fat embolism among trauma patients (67 to 97 per cent).[67–70]

The pathology associated with fat embolism syndrome differs from the pathology associated with simple fat embolism. Fat embolism syndrome patients have fat emboli in multiple organs, and in each of these organs, the fat emboli cause extensive damage.[68] Pulmonary capillaries are occluded by combinations of fat globules, fibrin, and platelet clumps. Often, there is a diffuse chemical pneumonitis, pulmonary capillary hemorrhage, and interstitial and alveolar edema. Hyaline membranes and adult respiratory distress syndrome pathology are also seen.[68, 77] Cerebral arterioles and capillaries are also plugged by fat globules, fibrin, and platelets. Perivascular edema and hemorrhage are present. Ischemic necrosis is seen in areas distal to the plugs. Similar pathology is seen in the liver and kidney.[69] Biopsies of petechiae reveal cutaneous, capillary fat emboli, surrounded by hemorrhage.[81]

Because the pathology and clinical significance of fat embolism syndrome vary so greatly from mere fat embolism, many investigators have attempted to determine whether certain types of trauma particularly predispose fat emboli patients to the development of the fat embolism syndrome. They have found a gradation among fractures: patients with single, upper extremity fractures have a low risk for developing fat embolism syndrome; patients with lower extremity long bone fractures have a moderate risk of developing the fat embolism syndrome;[72, 74, 76] and patients with multiple lower extremity long bone fractures have the highest risk for the development of the fat embolism syndrome—27 per cent (5 of 18 patients) in one series.[82] Patients who were transferred from one hospital to another shortly after trauma also had an increased risk for developing fat embolism syndrome.[83]

Avikainen performed stress, metabolic, and coagulation studies on 10 patients one year after they sustained fat embolism syndrome and on 10 controls one year after they sustained trauma without fat embolism syndrome.[84] He concluded that the fat embolism syndrome group had higher stress-induced blood sugar and beta lipoprotein levels. He wondered whether these stress responses had contributed to the development of fat embolism syndrome in these people.

Although many authors include fracture in their definitions of the fat embolism syndrome, there are rare reports of a similar clinicopathologic entity occurring in nonfracture patients. The conditions that seem to predispose to this rare form of fat embolism syndrome include: (1) bone disease, e.g., osteoporosis, myelodysplasia, and osteomyelitis; (2) diseases associated with fatty liver formation, e.g., pancreatitis, diabetes mellitus, prolonged steroid usage, and alcoholism; (3) sickle cell disease; and (4) severe burns.[68, 81, 85, 86]

Children below the age of 10 seem to have a very low frequency of fat embolism syndrome.[81, 87] All other age groups are probably equally predisposed.[74, 78, 79] Whether methylmethacrylate, the cement used frequently in hip arthroplasty, contributes to the risk of developing fat embolism syndrome is not clear.[71, 88]

Fat embolism syndrome can present as early as two hours after trauma or orthopedic surgery. Approximately 20 per cent of the time, it presents within the first 12 hours, 60 per cent of the time within the first 24 hours, and 85 per cent of the time within 48 hours. Some cases have occurred seven days after injury[76, 78, 84] (Table 11–9). There is no correlation between the syndrome's delay in onset and its severity.[79] The possible mechanisms for the delay will be discussed in the section on pathophysiology.

As assured by the definitions of fat embolism syndrome, the most important symptoms are respiratory and cerebral. The first sign of the fat embolism syndrome is often dyspnea or tachypnea and restlessness. Nearly all patients develop respiratory symptoms within the first day of the onset of the syndrome. Chest pain and hemoptysis are reported in about 20 per cent of patients, but both are partly related to patients' underlying injuries.[76]

Cerebral symptoms occur, by definition, as often as respiratory symptoms. In the Gurd series, of 69 fat embolism syndrome patients who were oriented on admission, nine became confused, 35 became drowsy, and 25 became comatose.[76] In Avikainen's series, four of 10 patients became unconscious, and three others became confused.[84] Often, the neurologic symptoms precede the respiratory symptoms; hence they are not entirely attributable to hypoxemia.

On physical examination, nearly all patients are febrile (see Table 11–10). Temperatures can be greater than 103°F (39.4°C). Examination of the skin and mucous membranes discloses petechiae of the bucca, anterior axillary fold, and root of the neck in about one-third to two-thirds of the patients.

***Table 11–9.*** Time Interval Between Trauma and the Onset of the Fat Embolism Syndrome

| Author | Average Interval | Range |
|---|---|---|
| Linscheid[72] | Not given | 4 hrs to 7 days |
| Burgher[74] | 40 hrs | 6 hrs to 3 days |
| Dines[68] | Not given | Immediate to 3 days |
| Gurd[76] | 46 hrs | 4 hrs to 15 days |
| Curtis[77] | 40 hrs | 2 hrs to 5 days |
| Moore[78] | Not given | Within 2 days |

The petechiae, representative of both fat emboli and thrombocytopenia, can be an early, first sign of the syndrome, or they can develop over the first few days.[74, 76, 79] Funduscopic exam reveals "multiple white fluffy exudates, fine streaks of hemorrhage, and macular edema" in up to one-third of patients.[74, 76] Patients may have scotomata that can sometimes outlast the syndrome.[89] Rarely, the chest examination can be normal very early, but nearly all patients go on to develop diffuse rales within 24 hours of the onset of the syndrome.

Laboratory data (see Table 11–10) are almost always abnormal in patients with the fat embolism syndrome. Hematocrits frequently drop more than 10 points, but the significance of the drop is unclear in trauma patients who are being hydrated intravenously. White blood cell counts are either slightly elevated or normal. Platelets drop in the majority of patients and in the setting of disseminated intravascular coagulation fall below 100,000. Prothrombin times increase, and fibrinogen decreases in the DIC patients. The percentage of patients who actually develop DIC is not known. Many authors do not report serum calcium. Others report that it decreases in nearly 80 per cent of patients. Some, if not all, of the decrease may be secondary to multiple transfusions rather than fat embolism syndrome. Erythrocyte sedimentation rate was elevated in 87 per cent of patients in Gurd's series. Values above 70 were common.[76]

Blood gases reveal $PaO_2$ less than 60 mm Hg and as low as 26 mm Hg in well over 80 per cent of the reported cases. Usually, $PaCO_2$ is diminished as well. At times hypoxia precedes the development of an abnormal chest roentgenogram. The converse is almost never true.[75] Chest roentgenograms are abnormal within 24 hours of onset of the fat embolism syndrome in over 80 per cent of patients in most series.[74, 79] Typical chest films disclose diffuse bilateral interstitial and alveolar infiltrates; patchy, predominantly lower lobe infiltrates; or diffuse pulmonary edema with a normal-sized heart (adult respiratory distress syndrome). Rarely, patients have pleural effusions.[76–78] Electrocardiograms often disclose right heart strain. In a few cases, paradoxical fat embolism to the coronary arteries has occurred, causing acute infarction.[77]

Because the chest roentgenograms are ordinarily so abnormal, there is little experience with lung scanning or angiography. Special-

***Table 11–10.*** Frequency of Abnormal Signs and Laboratory Values: Five Representative Series of Fat Embolism Syndrome*

| Author | Cases | | Age (Years) | | Fever >38° | Petechiae | Retinal Abnormality** | Platelet Count | $PaCO_2$ | Chest X-ray |
|---|---|---|---|---|---|---|---|---|---|---|
| | *Number* | *Type* | *Mean* | *Range* | | | | | | |
| Burgher[74] | 36 | Clinical Autopsy | 41 | 18–88 | Required for inclusion | 21/36 | 13/36 | Not given | <60 mm Hg 21/25 | 29/36 alveolar infiltrates |
| Gurd[76] | 100 | Clinical | 34 | 14–91 | 83/100 | 57/100 | 9/63 | 12/38 <90,000 per $mm^3$ | <50 mm Hg 24/50 | 43/52 alveolar infiltrates |
| Curtis[77] | 30 | Clinical Autopsy | 50 | 17–81 | 30/30 | Required for inclusion | Not given | 10/30 <100,000 per $mm^3$ | <50 mm Hg 18/20 | 25/30 abnormal |
| Moore[78] | 17 | Clinical | 23 | 17–41 | 17/17 | 9/17 | Not given | 4/14 "below normal" | <60 mm Hg 17/17 | 17/17 abnormal |
| Guentner[79] | 54 | Clinical | 27 | 15–74 | 54/54 | 39/54 | Not given | Not given | Range 23–72 mm Hg | 44/54 diffuse infiltrates |

*Cerebral and respiratory symptoms not included in this table, because they are part of definitions used by most authors.
**Fat or hemorrhage.

ized tests looking for fat macroglobulinemia (Gurd test) and urine fat globules are of no benefit in the diagnosis of fat embolism syndrome.[90–93]

The course and outcome in the fat embolism syndrome series depended partly on the definitions the authors used to enroll patients and partly on whether patients developed the adult respiratory distress syndrome. In the studies that required both respiratory and cerebral symptoms, patients often developed the adult respiratory distress syndrome. Mortality was often as high as 60 per cent in those series.[68, 77] In the series that required a less rigorous definition, far fewer patients developed the adult respiratory distress syndrome, and the mortality rate was less than 20 per cent.[97, 94] Deaths occurred from one day to months after the onset of the syndrome.

Patients who survived rarely had residual neurologic defects. Roentgenograms become normal over days to weeks. Pulmonary function tests reportedly become normal over a period of a few months. Survivors who undergo repeated orthopedic procedures are not at an increased risk for developing the fat embolism syndrome.[70, 78]

The following case, reported by Naver and coworkers, nicely demonstrates many features of the fat embolism syndrome.[95] A 25-year-old male sustained a left femoral shaft fracture. He was admitted to the hospital and placed in traction. Thirty-nine hours after admission, he became dyspneic. Physical examination disclosed a temperature of 100.4°F (38°C), tachypnea, and a petechial rash on the abdomen and chest. The $PaO_2$ was 47 mm Hg and the $PaCO_2$ was normal. The initial chest radiograph was normal. Twenty-four hours later, his blood gases had deteriorated further, and the chest film showed diffuse, bilateral infiltrates. The patient was treated with continuous positive airway pressure and oxygen. Over a two-day period, he began to improve. After seven days, all treatment was stopped. On day 10, he underwent internal fixation of his fracture without complications.

## Pathophysiology

It is important to emphasize that the diagnosis of the fat embolism syndrome is a diagnosis of exclusion. Other causes of diffuse pulmonary, cerebral, and febrile processes must be eliminated (Table 11–11). The fat embolism syndrome tends to present more slowly than air embolism or amniotic fluid embolism, but both of these should be considered in the appropriate circumstances. Additionally, the adult respiratory distress syndrome can be produced by hypovolemic or septic shock, pancreatitis, and severe head and thoracic crush injuries. Aspiration pneumonia and cardiogenic shock should also be considered.

***Table 11–11.*** Illnesses that Can Mimic the Fat Embolism Syndrome

| |
|---|
| Embolic processes, e.g., thrombotic pulmonary embolism, air embolism, amniotic fluid embolism |
| Other causes of the adult respiratory distress syndrome, e.g., hypovolemic or septic shock, pancreatitis, CNS trauma |
| Aspiration pneumonia |
| Cardiogenic shock |
| Anaphylaxis or narcotic lung syndrome |
| Thoracic crush injuries |
| Pulmonary hemorrhage |

The pulmonary, cerebral, and cutaneous pathology associated with fat embolism syndrome was discussed previously. Five important pathophysiologic questions remain, although question five is not answerable:

1. Where do fat emboli originate?
2. What causes the development of the adult respiratory distress syndrome?
3. What is the role of the coagulation system?
4. Why is there a delay in the onset of symptoms?
5. What turns commonplace, clinically insignificant fat embolism into the fat embolism syndrome?

Two theories have long been used to explain where the fat globules originate. The physicochemical theory proposes that the fat emboli arise from circulating lipoproteins and albumin-complexed free fatty acids. Stress-induced catecholamine release and some poorly defined process cause an increased production of free fatty acids. Proponents of this theory argue that it can explain the rare nontraumatic cases of fat embolism syndrome in addition to the standard trauma-induced cases of fat embolism syndrome.[76, 81] The mechanical theory proposes that the fat emboli originate in the marrow cavity. In the setting of fractures and stress, marrow fat somehow enters the venous circulation. Evidence for the bone marrow–mechanical theory comes from three lines of reasoning: (1) animal experiments have shown that $^{14}C$-labeled marrow fat fills the lungs after experimentally-induced fractures; (2) clinically, fat embolism occurs more frequently in patients with multiple long bone fractures; and (3) diseases that are associated with an increased marrow space, such as myelodysplasia, are also associated with an increased risk of fat embolism.[70, 81, 96]

Presently, the mechanical theory is more popular than the physicochemical theory. The mechanical theory makes no attempt to explain nontraumatic fat embolism syndrome, in which the liver might give rise to fat emboli.

The pulmonary damage associated with the fat embolism syndrome occurs in three overlapping stages (Fig. 11–5). In the first stage, fat emboli obstruct arterioles and then gradually break up and occlude capillaries. Mechanical obstruction causes pulmonary hypertension. This first stage, the obstructive effect, can be produced by infusing free fatty acids into animals. Of note, hypovolemic animals often are unable to survive this first phase, but euvolemic animals tend to survive this first phase.[81, 97] In the second stage, which occurs with some delay, fat globules are hydrolyzed by lipoprotein lipase to free fatty acids. The free fatty acids are toxic to the lungs and cause pericapillary inflammation and edema. Additionally, the free fatty acids destroy surfactant and make the lungs stiff.[81] During this second, delayed stage, hypoxemia occurs in experimental animals.[97] In the third stage, which partly overlaps the first two stages, the thromboplastin released during the initial traumatic tissue injury, acting perhaps in concert with the thromboplastin-like activity of fat, causes platelet aggregation and fibrin thrombi formation in the pulmonary capillaries. The platelet aggregates not only cause additional mechanical obstruction, but they lead to a release of vasoactive mediators that cause pulmonary vasoconstriction.[70, 81, 98] Hence, the pulmonary damage seen in the fat embolism syndrome is caused by mechanical obstruction, free fatty acid toxicity, and vasoactive mediators.

The role of the coagulation system in fat embolism syndrome has been alluded to previously. The combination of tissue-released and fat-associated thromboplastin enhances clotting. Trauma and shock often disrupt fibrinolysis. The result can be the disseminated intravascular coagulation that is often seen in the fat embolism syndrome.[70, 76]

The delay in the onset of respiratory symptoms probably represents the time it takes for neutral fat hydrolysis and for the initiation of the coagulation cascade. Neurologic symptoms do not occur until the fat emboli cross either the pulmonary capillary bed or right-to-left shunts.[96, 99]

### Therapy

Treatment of fat embolism syndrome is largely supportive. Oxygenation and fluid balance should be monitored carefully. High-dose steroids have been recommended for the patients who develop signs of the adult respiratory distress syndrome. In theory, steroids might decrease the inflammation associated with free fatty acid toxicity and might stimulate Type II pneumocyte proliferation, enhancing surfactant synthesis.[81] In several uncontrolled series, steroids were frequently used, but the results are not easily interpretable.[73, 74, 81] No controlled steroid treatment studies have been carried out. Heparin therapy, thought to be valuable for inhibiting the thromboplastin-induced clotting, has not shown promise in several uncontrolled trials. Several authors argue that heparin's stimulatory effect on lipolysis might be detrimental, because it enhances the production of free fatty acids[81] toxic to the lungs. Hypertonic glucose or glucose and insulin treatments that might inhibit lipolysis have not proved beneficial in uncontrolled treatment trials.[81] Alcohol is a lipoprotein inhibitor, but it has not been shown to be effective in uncontrolled trials.[70]

### Prophylaxis

Stoltenberg has argued that treating fat embolism syndrome is difficult, because the fat, free fatty acids, and platelet aggregates have already been in the lungs for several hours or days by the time the syndrome presents.[75] He and others suggest that measures to prevent the fat embolism syndrome might be more beneficial than measures that attempt to treat the syndrome.

No randomized controlled studies of heparin prophylaxis have been performed. Al-

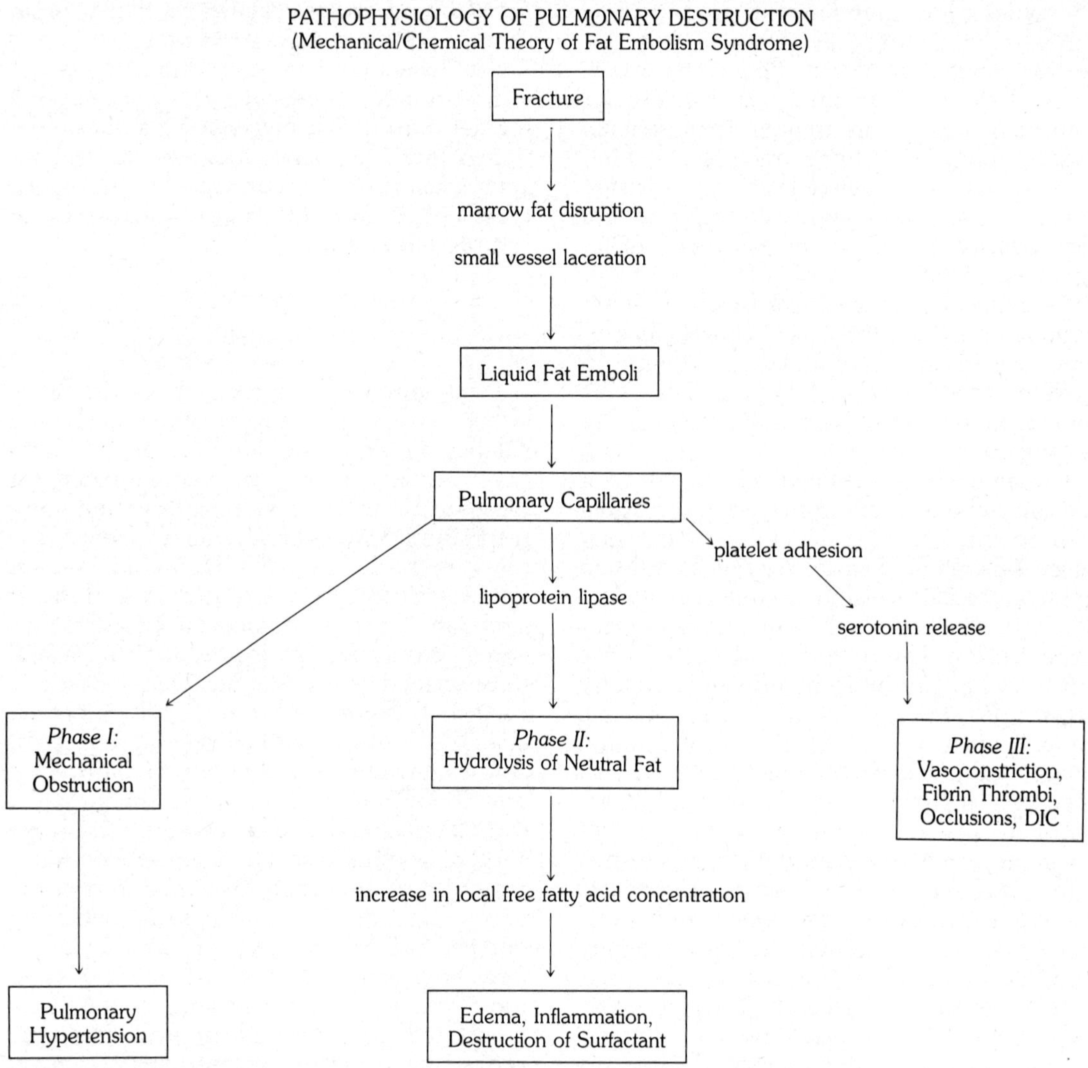


***Figure 11–5.*** The three overlapping phases of pulmonary fat embolism syndrome: (1) mechanical obstruction; (2) hydrolysis of neutral fat, resulting in free fatty acids that are toxic to the lungs; (3) activation of the coagulation system, resulting in the release of vasoconstrictive mediators and localized disseminated intravascular coagulation (DIC). (Modified from Stoltenberg, J. J., and Gustilo, R. B.: The use of methylprednisolone and hypertonic glucose in the prophylaxis of fat embolism syndrome. Clin. Orthop., *143*:211, 1979.)

cohol "prophylaxis" was retrospectively reviewed by Myers in 1977. He found that 16 cases of fat embolism syndrome developed in 74 trauma patients who had alcohol levels on admission of less than 0.02 gm per 100 ml. Only one case of fat embolism syndrome developed in the 26 trauma patients who had alcohol levels on admission of greater than 0.02 gm per 100 ml. The two groups had equal percentages of multiple fracture patients.[100] Hypertonic glucose and fluids have been shown to be of no prophylactic benefit in two small controlled studies.[75, 101] Small studies by Stoltenberg[75] and Rokkanen[102] (Table 11–12) have suggested that three large doses of steroids during the first 24 hours after admission may prevent the development of the fat embolism syndrome. Schonfeld and coworkers[80] conducted a prospective randomized, double-blind study comparing placebo with 12 doses of methylprednisolone, 7.5 mg per kg per dose. The groups were well matched in terms of fracture index. Nine of 41 placebo patients developed fat embolism syndrome. There were no cases of fat embolism syndrome among 21 steroid-treated patients ($p<0.05$). The steroid-treated group did not have excess wound infection or problems with delayed healing. The authors suggest that certain, as yet undefined, classes of high-risk patients might benefit from steroid prophylaxis.[80] Other authors suggest that patients who have two lower extremity long bone fractures should receive steroid prophylaxis.[75] Clearly, further prospective randomized, controlled studies are needed to assess the value of fat embolism syndrome prophylaxis and treatment measures.

### Summary

The fat embolism syndrome is not rare. It should be suspected any time a trauma patient develops unexplained respiratory or cerebral symptoms. Careful funduscopic and cutaneous examinations might reveal diagnostic lipemia retinalis or petechiae, respectively. Steroid prophylaxis should be considered in patients who have multiple long bone fractures. Early diagnosis allows the physician to initiate important supportive measures and to avoid extraneous antibiotic, cardiotonic, or anticoagulation regimens. Specific treatment for patients with fat embolism syndrome has not yet been established.

## FOREIGN PARTICLE EMBOLISM

When an intravenous drug abuser injects insoluble substances into his or her veins, or when a lymphangiographer injects oil into a patient's lymphatic system, the injected particles, by definition, embolize to the lungs. Some types of injected foreign particles, such as starch, cause little damage. Other injected material, such as talc or cotton, can cause pulmonary hypertension and interstitial fibrosis. This section reviews pulmonary emboli that are composed of commonly injected foreign particles. The first part discusses the foreign particle emboli associated with drug addiction. The second part discusses foreign particle emboli associated with diagnostic radiographic procedures.

### Foreign Particle Emboli Associated with Drug Addiction

In this country, heroin is the most commonly abused intravenous drug. Undiluted, pure heroin is usually smuggled into the United States. Here it is diluted with soluble materials such as quinine, lactose, or maltose that do not embolize to the lungs. Before injection, however, heroin is mixed with water, heated, and drawn into an eyedropper or syringe through a cotton filter (perhaps an item of clothing, like a sock). Cotton fibers enter the solution, and on injection, these fibers embolize to the lungs.[22]

***Table 11–12.*** Steroid Prophylaxis Against Fat Embolism Syndrome

| Author | Number of Patients | Trauma to Randomization Interval | Steroid Dose Methylprednisolone (IV) | Fat Embolism Syndrome *Placebo Therapy* | Fat Embolism Syndrome *Steroid Therapy* |
|---|---|---|---|---|---|
| Rokkanen[102] | 29 | Not given | 10 mg/kg × 3 doses | 6/15 | 1/14 |
| Stoltenberg[75] | 64* | Not given | 1 gm × 3 doses | 2/23 | 0/21 |
| Schonfeld[80] | 62 | <12 hrs | 7.5 mg/kg × 12 doses | 9/41 | 0/21 |

*20 patients were treated with 50 ml $D_{50}W$ q 4 hr × 4 days. In this group, 3/20 developed fat embolism syndrome.

Heroin is not always available, and so some abusers intravenously inject amphetamine-like substances (mephentermine sulfate) that they squeeze off the cotton pledgets found in nasal inhalers. Many more abusers intravenously inject oral opiates (oral methadone, oral meperidine), oral "uppers" (methamphetamine—speed, methylphenidate hydrochloride—Ritalin), oral antihistamines (tripelennamine hydrochloride—Pyribenzamine), and oral "downers" (secobarbital—Seconal).[103] Two oral preparations that are frequently injected are nicknamed for the colors that result when the tablets are crushed into solution. "Blue velvet" is made by crushing 50-mg tablets of tripelennamine into 30 ml of paregoric. "Red devil" is made by crushing secobarbital tablets into water.[104]

All of the oral medications have insoluble fillers. Methadone, meperidine, methylphenidate, tripelennamine, and methamphetamine contain talc (magnesium silicate) (see Fig. 2–13*A*). Secobarbital contains starch. When these preparations are injected, the talc and starch embolize to the lungs.[105] When normally inhaled substances such as mephentermine sulfate (Wyamine sulfate) are injected, cotton pledget contaminants embolize to the lungs. Other injected contaminants, such as hair, also embolize to the lungs (see Fig. 2–13*B*).

Talc crystals and cotton fibers, alone or in combination, lodge in the pulmonary arterioles. Thrombus forms around the foreign material. Endothelial cells proliferate, and vessel sclerosis occurs. If a large number of arterioles are involved in this process, termed angiothrombosis, pulmonary hypertension results. Starch granules, on the other hand, simply lodge in the pulmonary circulation. Although they produce mechanical obstruction, they cause no pathologic damage.[28, 104, 105]

Cotton fibers and talc crystals can also pass between damaged endothelial cells into the pulmonary interstitium. There, they trigger a granulomatous reaction that can ultimately lead to interstitial fibrosis and restrictive lung disease. In some cases, parenchymal destruction is so severe that lung elasticity is ruined and obstructive lung disease occurs. At times, interstitial foreign particles are picked up by the lymphatic system, where they also incite a granulomatous response.[103, 105] In some patients, angiothrombosis is the major lesion. In others, interstitial fibrosis and angiothrombosis are equally important.

It is important to emphasize that the arteriolar sclerosis and interstitial fibrosis seen in the lungs of drug abusers are caused by fillers, not by the "pleasure" drugs. In animal experiments, Puro and coworkers could produce the entire range of pulmonary pathology simply by injecting talc or starch.[104] The addition of the full "blue velvet" or "red devil" ingredients did not alter the pathology. In humans, the quantity of filler needed to produce significant pulmonary disease is unknown. In one study, patients had injected from 10 to 40 crushed tablets per day for several years.[105]

Intravenous drug abusers are at risk for the development of several types of acute pulmonary disease. For unclear reasons, but perhaps related to drug overdose, hypoxia, or gastric aspiration, they commonly develop an acute noncardiogenic pulmonary edema known as heroin lung. When groggy, they are predisposed to aspiration and to the development of aspiration pneumonia. They frequently inject infected materials, and they often develop peripheral septic thrombophlebitis and right-sided endocarditis. Thus, they frequently generate septic thrombi that can embolize to the lungs and cause necrotizing pneumonia.[22, 103]

Foreign particle embolization, with its attendant angiothrombosis and pulmonary granulomatosis, is not as common a clinical problem as heroin lung aspiration, pneumonia, or septic pulmonary embolism. In a 1967 clinical study, Louria and coworkers found that pulmonary complications of intravenous drug abuse accounted for 21 per cent of the total complications caused by intravenous drug abuse. However, they did not find a single clinical case of foreign particle pulmonary embolization.[22] In a 1970 clinical study of 28 intravenous narcotic addicts with major cardiopulmonary and vascular complications, Jaffe and Koschmann[28] found only one case of foreign particle emboli–induced angiothrombosis.

In autopsy series, the frequency of foreign body–induced angiothrombosis and pulmonary granulomatosis varies, depending on regional drug abuse patterns. Hopkins found angiothrombosis in 12 of 100 consecutive autopsies performed on patients in either Seattle or San Diego whose deaths were due to narcotics.[106] Siegel, looking at a similar population in New York City, found only a four per cent frequency of foreign particle embolization and secondary angiothrombosis and granulomatosis.[107]

Foreign particle embolization to the lungs,

***Table 11–13.*** Foreign Particle Embolization: Frequency of Presenting Complaints and Chest Abnormalities

| Author and Number of Patients | Chronic Resting or Exertional Dyspnea | Cough | Hemoptysis | Chest Pain | Rhonchi or Rales |
|---|---|---|---|---|---|
| Douglas[105] 7 patients | 5/7 | 5/7 | 1/7 | 0/7 | 2/7 |
| Paré[103] 17 patients | 10/17 | 4/17 | 0/17 | 0/17 | 2/17 |
| Robertson[108] 4 patients | 4/4 | 0/4 | 0/4 | 0/4 | 1/4 |

then, occurs rarely. It is not a major cause of acute pulmonary disease in drug addicts. It is, however, an important entity, because among young intravenous drug abusers it is the major cause of potentially severe chronic lung disease.

Chronic dyspnea is the major presenting symptom of talc and cotton fiber pulmonary embolization. As shown in Table 11–13, the majority of patients in three different clinical series presented with either chronic resting or chronic exertional dyspnea. In this group of smokers, cough may not carry as much predictive value. Chest pain was not noted by any patients, and hemoptysis was rare. One patient with pulmonary hypertension presented with syncope.[103, 105, 108]

Physical examination of patients with talc and cotton fiber pulmonary embolization can be helpful but is never diagnostic. Vital signs are often normal. The skin frequently has multiple "track marks," representing sclerosed veins, and multiple venous puncture sites. Fundi sometimes show yellow-white particles in the retinal capillaries, thought to represent left-sided talc embolism. In one series, nine of 15 patients had abnormal retinal particles.[103] Visual acuity is rarely impaired, although Lederer reported on an intravenous methylphenidate (Ritalin) abuser who suffered loss of vision due to talc-induced neovascularization.[109] The chest examination reveals rhonchi or rales in only a few patients (see Table 11–13). In severe cases, signs of pulmonary hypertension and even cor pulmonale are present.[108]

Important laboratory results are summarized in Table 11–14. Chest roentgenograms reveal infiltrates in less than half of the patients. The infiltrates are usually bilateral but are otherwise quite variable. They can be diffuse or localized; apical, mid-zone, or basal; reticular or nodular. The nodules are usually 1 mm or less. Lung volumes may be diminished. Rarely, patients will have bilateral adenopathy. Electrocardiograms may reveal right heart strain. Restrictive lung disease is common. In Paré's series of 17 abusers, who were selected for their sustained, long-term intravenous use of oral drugs, nearly all had restrictive lung disease based on pulmonary function tests.[103] Over half the patients had decreased carbon monoxide diffusion capacity.[103, 105, 108]

There are few data on the role of lung scanning. Because the chest roentgenograms are often abnormal, scans may be of little help. In cases in which the roentgenogram is normal, one would expect to find peripheral patchy defects. Because foreign particle emboli often involve 2-mm pulmonary vessels, the scans may show nothing at all.

Right heart catheterization may be notable for pulmonary hypertension with normal

***Table 11–14.*** Foreign Particle Embolization: Frequency of Abnormal Cardiopulmonary Laboratory Data

| Author and Number of Patients | Infiltrate on CXR | Right Heart Strain on ECG | Restrictive Lung Disease** | $D_LCO$* Below Normal |
|---|---|---|---|---|
| Douglas[105] 7 patients | 3/7 | 2/7 | 1/7 | 6/7 |
| Paré[103] 17 patients | 7/17 | 2/17 | 15/17 | 10/17 |
| Robertson[108] 4 patients | 2/4 | 3/4 | 2/4 | 3/4 |

*Carbon monoxide diffusion capacity.
**Diagnosed by pulmonary function tests.

pulmonary embolism is usually mild. Most patients develop cough, slight dyspnea, or mild pleuritic pain during the radiographic procedure. Subsequently, they have fever that can be greater than 39° C. Chest examination often reveals diffuse moist rales. Clinical diagnosis rests on an abnormal chest roentgenogram within 12 hours following the contrast procedure. Diffuse, bilateral, fine nodular stippling is the hallmark of the disease.[111, 112] Blood gases demonstrate slight hypoxia.

Patients with preexisting pulmonary disease, particularly patients with right heart strain, can have difficulty tolerating oil embolism–induced pulmonary capillary obstruction and hypoxia. Bron and coworkers[111] described two patients, both with preexisting lung disease, who developed acute hypotension, cyanosis, and right heart strain during lymphangiography.

The vast majority of patients who suffer pulmonary oil embolism improve over one to two days. Thus fever, cough, and dyspnea subside. The chest roentgenogram may have residual "fluffiness," but this resolves over several days.[111, 112]

#### THERAPY

Treatment for oil embolism is supportive. Prophylaxis against clinically important pulmonary oil embolism includes (1) avoiding lymphangiography in patients with significant pulmonary disease, (2) stopping injection of contrast material when lymphatic obstruction is detected, and (3) avoiding myelography for one week following routine, but especially traumatic, lumbar puncture. The use of more water-soluble contrast agents could potentially eliminate clinical pulmonary oil embolism.[111, 112]

## MISCELLANEOUS CAUSES OF PULMONARY EMBOLISM

An endless list of thus far undiscussed substances has been known to embolize to the lungs. These substances can be classified into three groups (Table 11–16): (1) Endogenous body fluids or organs, which include trophoblasts, bile, bone marrow, and cerebrum; (2) parasitic life cycle constituents, which include echinococcal cysts and dirofilarial worms; and (3) nonbiologic, exogenous materials, which include polyethylene catheters, bullets, prosthetic valve coating, and silicone. This section will briefly review the clinical syndromes that occur when each of these substances embolizes to the lungs.

### Endogenous Body Fluids or Organs

#### TROPHOBLASTS FROM MOLAR PREGNANCY

Although placental trophoblasts embolize to the lungs during normal pregnancies, large numbers of trophoblastic emboli and the clinical syndrome of trophoblastic pulmonary embolism, with rare exceptions, occur only in association with molar pregnancies.[114] A 1971 to 1976 study reported that the frequency of clinical trophoblastic embolism among molar pregnancies was 2.4 per cent (nine cases in 376 molar pregnancies).[115]

Trophoblastic pulmonary embolism can occur at any time during or shortly following molar pregnancy. The patient may be asymptomatic but can also have acute or chronic dyspnea. Physical examination is usually notable only for tachypnea, perhaps some rales, an enlarged-for-dates uterus, and chocolate-colored staining. Blood gases disclose hypoxemia. The chest roentgenogram can be normal or show localized haziness. Lung scanning or angiography can often make the diagnosis of pulmonary embolism. Pelvic ultrasound and elevated human chorionic gonadotropin levels can make the diagnosis of molar pregnancy.

Treatment includes evacuation of the mole and supportive measures. Some authors suggest several days of high-dose steroid treatment, although the efficacy of this is unproven.[115]

Patients usually improve over 72 hours. It is unclear whether trophoblastic embolism increases a patient's risk for metastatic trophoblastic disease, or choriocarcinoma. Therefore, the chest roentgenogram and human chorionic gonadotropin levels should be followed closely. If either test remains abnormal, chemotherapy should be considered.[115]

#### BILE

A clinical syndrome of bile pulmonary embolism has been reported in a patient following attempted percutaneous transhepatic drainage for biliary obstruction. According to Armellin and coworkers,[116] a 69-year-old male became acutely disoriented and tachypneic several hours after insertion of a per-

***Table 11–16.*** Miscellaneous Etiologies of Nonthrombotic Pulmonary Embolism

| Embolizing Material | Predisposing Factors | Clinically Significant | Clinical Presentation | Chest X-ray | Treatment |
|---|---|---|---|---|---|
| ***Endogenous Fluids or Organs*** | | | | | |
| Trophoblasts | Molar pregnancy | Yes | Acute or gradual onset of dyspnea | Diffuse haze or normal | Remove mole, ? steroids, follow HCG,* chemoprophylaxis |
| Bile | Liver disease, biliary obstruction, percutaneous biliary drainage | Sometimes | Asymptomatic or acute dyspnea | ? | ? |
| Bone marrow | Trauma<br>CPR** | Pulmonary—no<br>Paradoxical—yes | Pulmonary—asymptomatic<br>Paradoxical—stroke or MI | ? | ? |
| Cerebral | Massive head trauma | No | None | ? | ? |
| ***Parasitic Life Cycle Constituents*** | | | | | |
| Hydatid | Preexisting cardiac or hepatic cysts | Yes | Can mimic all presentations of pulmonary embolism | May show cysts | Remove surgically |
| Dirofilaria | Preexisting dirofilaria infection of the right ventricle or pulmonary artery | Yes | Acute: wheezing, like pulmonary embolism<br>Chronic: asymptomatic | Pulmonary infarct or solitary nodule | Surgical (for diagnosis and treatment) |
| ***Nonbiologic, Exogenous Materials*** | | | | | |
| Catheters/introducers | Withdrawing catheter through needle, patient flexion at catheter site, catheter poorly secured to skin | Yes | Arrhythmia, cardiac/pulmonary thrombosis, cardiac perforation, pulmonary infarction, sepsis | Shows catheter | Remove if new (see text) |
| Bullet | Bullet entry into venous circulation | Yes | Acute pulmonary embolism | Shows bullet | Remove (see text) |
| Valve particles | Aged right-sided prosthetic valve | ? | ? | ? Fibrosis | Valve probably needs replacement |
| Silicone | Silicone injections, intramuscularly | Yes | Fever, chest pain, dyspnea | Pulmonary infiltrates | Supportive |

*Human chorionic gonadotropin.
**Cardiopulmonary resuscitation.

cutaneous transhepatic drain established external, but not internal, biliary drainage. The patient rapidly died. At autopsy, numerous pulmonary arterioles contained bile plugs. The authors suggested that during placement of the hepatic catheter into the biliary tree, small hepatic veins were nicked. In the midst of distal biliary obstruction, bile duct pressure was greater than hepatic vein pressure, and so bile entered the venous circulation.

Bile emboli do not always cause symptoms. Brozinsky and coworkers[117] noted incidental pulmonary bile emboli when they autopsied a patient who had previously undergone external percutaneous hepatic drainage. Others have also described incidental bile pulmonary emboli at autopsy in patients with liver disease in the absence of percutaneous drainage. How bile plugs gain spontaneous access to the hepatic venous system is unclear.[116]

### Bone Marrow

Bone marrow spicules, in the setting of trauma or cardiopulmonary resuscitation, are often forced into the venous system. If pulmonary arterial pressures are elevated and a right-to-left communication exists, paradoxical bone marrow embolism to the cerebral and coronary arteries can occur.[118] This process has been implicated as the cause of death in a patient who underwent successful cardiopulmonary resuscitation.[119] Unlike paradoxical bone marrow embolism, pulmonary bone marrow embolism rarely causes symptoms and is usually an incidental postmortem finding.[83]

### Cerebral Tissue

Cerebral tissue, following severe head trauma, can enter the superior sagittal sinus and embolize to the lungs. In the single case report of cerebral pulmonary embolism, not surprisingly, the pulmonary lesions were incidental findings compared with the patient's fatal head wounds.[120]

## Parasitic Life Cycle Constituents

### Hydatid

Many cases of hydatid pulmonary embolism have been reported. Hydatid cyst products, consisting of liquid, daughter cysts, brood capsules, and protoscolices, enter the circulation when hepatic cysts rupture into the inferior vena cava or when cardiac cysts rupture into the heart. The cyst products embolize to the lungs, where they can immediately cause an acute allergic reaction or mimic an acute thrombotic pulmonary embolism. Alternatively, the cyst products, such as the daughter cysts and protoscolices, can slowly grow into large mature cysts that obstruct the pulmonary arteries, creating pulmonary hypertension and cor pulmonale.[121]

Hydatid pulmonary embolism should be suspected in echinococcus-infested areas when patients have symptoms of acute, recurrent, or chronic pulmonary embolism. Eosinophilia and calcified hepatic, cardiac, or pulmonary cysts on roentgenography can help make the diagnosis. Lung scans and pulmonary angiograms can establish the presence of intravascular obstruction. Treatment requires operative removal not only of the pulmonary artery cysts but of cardiac and hepatic cysts as well.[121]

### Dirofilaria

*Dirofilaria imitis* (dog heartworm) commonly infects domesticated dogs and rarely infects human beings. The adult parasite

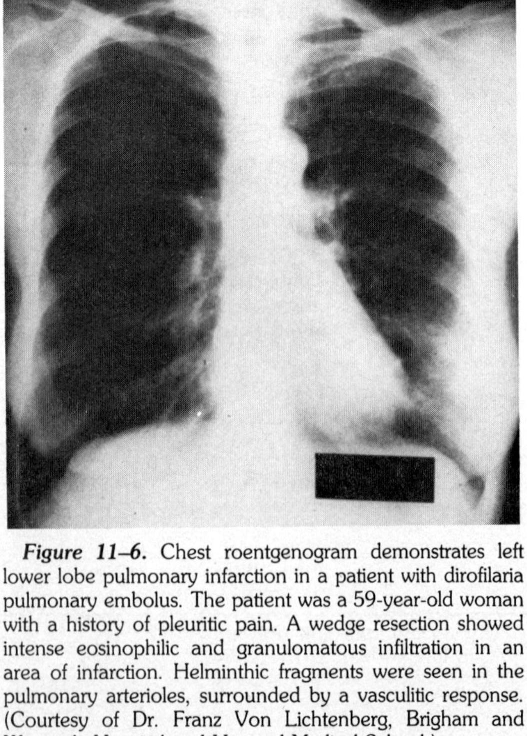

***Figure 11–6.*** Chest roentgenogram demonstrates left lower lobe pulmonary infarction in a patient with dirofilaria pulmonary embolus. The patient was a 59-year-old woman with a history of pleuritic pain. A wedge resection showed intense eosinophilic and granulomatous infiltration in an area of infarction. Helminthic fragments were seen in the pulmonary arterioles, surrounded by a vasculitic response. (Courtesy of Dr. Franz Von Lichtenberg, Brigham and Women's Hospital and Harvard Medical School.)

lodges in the right ventricle and produces circulating microfilaria. There are rare case reports that suggest that, in people, the microfilaria can plug pulmonary capillaries and cause arteritis and pulmonary infarction. Acutely, patients can present with wheezing, shortness of breath, pulmonary infarction on chest roentgenogram, and eosinophilia. Chronically, symptoms disappear, but patients can develop a solitary pulmonary nodule in an area of infarcted lung (Fig. 11–6).

Early lung biopsy might show intravascular dead microfilaria and infarcted distal lung tissue. Late biopsy of a pulmonary nodule can reveal intravascular dead microfilaria amidst nonspecific coagulative necrosis and inflammation.

#### THERAPY

Dirofilaria pulmonary embolism is rarely diagnosed in its acute stages, and treatment of its early, wheezing phase has not been addressed. In chronic disease, when the patient has developed a solitary pulmonary nodule, diagnosis and treatment consist of careful surgical excision of the nodule. The role of antinematodal agents is unclear, because the worms are usually dead by the time a radiographically apparent nodule is seen.[122, 123]

### Nonbiologic, Exogenous Materials

#### CATHETER

Polyethylene catheter and catheter introducer pulmonary embolism occurs frequently. Usually, the polyethylene tubing is severed when a catheter is drawn through a sharp introducing needle. At times, the catheter or introducer breaks apart from its connecting piece during dressing changes or when the patient vigorously moves around.[124–126]

Antecubital, femoral, internal jugular, and subclavian vein catheters have all been reported to embolize to the great veins, right heart, main pulmonary arteries, and distal pulmonary arteries. Paradoxical catheter embolization can also occur.[127]

Reported complications from unremoved catheter emboli include sepsis and endocarditis, intracardiac and intrapulmonary thrombosis, cardiac arrhythmias and perforation, septic and thrombotic pulmonary embolism, and pulmonary infarction.[126] Estimated rates of complications in cases of unremoved catheters vary between 12 and 55 per cent. Fatal complications of unremoved catheter emboli have been reported to be as high as 24 per cent in a series of 76 patients.[127] Right ventricular and pulmonary artery catheter emboli have the highest rates of associated complications. Great vein, atrial, and peripheral lung catheter emboli have slightly lower associated complication rates.[127]

Some authors argue that ideally, all catheter emboli, no matter how long they have been present, should be removed.[124, 125, 128] Percutaneous snare techniques, which have very low complication rates, can be attempted first.[127] If these methods fail and the patient is well enough to withstand thoracotomy, open chest removal of catheter emboli can be carried out.

Other authors caution wisely that the high complication rates in nonoperative cases can be attributed, in part, to the underlying debilitated condition of the patients who were denied surgery. These authors suggest that new catheter emboli and right heart and main pulmonary artery catheter emboli of any age should be removed, whereas old, incidentally noted great vein or peripheral pulmonary catheter emboli can be left alone.[127, 129] This latter approach is more reasonable and practical than the aggressive approach in which all catheter emboli must be removed, whatever their age or location.

Catheter embolism can often be prevented by (1) avoiding withdrawal of the catheter through a needle, (2) firmly securing the catheter to the skin, and (3) preventing elbow or hip flexion when an antecubital or femoral catheter is present, respectively.[124, 127]

#### BULLET

Bullet pulmonary embolism is rare. In 1976, only 17 cases had been reported.[130] Bullets migrate to the pulmonary circulation after entering peripheral veins, the right heart, or the superior sagittal vein.[131, 132] Usually, bullets migrate to the pulmonary circulation shortly after the initial injury. Rarely, a bullet dislodges from the peripheral circulation and embolizes to the lungs a few weeks after injury.[131]

Bullet embolization to the lungs should be suspected whenever an exit wound cannot be found and roentgenography of the injured area does not show a bullet.[131] Patients are usually asymptomatic; however, they may complain of sudden, pleuritic chest pain, dyspnea, and hemoptysis. In one reported case, fatal bullet pulmonary embolization presented with signs of massive thrombotic pulmonary embolism.[133] Chest roentgenography discloses a pulmonary bullet and, occasionally, pulmonary infarction. Lung scans and angiography are ordinarily helpful because the bullets, depending on their size, tend to lodge in the major pulmonary artery or in the segmental pulmonary arteries.[131]

Unremoved bullet pulmonary emboli, like unremoved catheter emboli, can cause sepsis, pulmonary thrombosis, erosion of the involved vessel (even years later), and cardiac neurosis.[131] In a review of 17 patients, Stephenson and coworkers[130] noted that in the nine patients who did not undergo embolectomy, seven died from factors that may have been related to the bullet pulmonary embolus. In the eight patients who underwent embolectomy, no deaths occurred.

Most authors feel that new bullet pulmonary emboli, like new catheter emboli, should be surgically removed. What to do with incidentally discovered, long-term bullet pulmonary emboli is less clear.[132]

### Prosthetic Valve

Right heart prosthetic valve fragments can embolize to the lungs. Robinson and coworkers[134] found pulmonary intravascular Teflon particles and granulomas in a patient who was undergoing replacement of a seven-year-old, stenotic, teflon-coated Beall tricuspid valve. The patient had no specific pulmonary complaints. As more patients receive prosthetic valves, pulmonary embolization of valve coating may become more common. It is not known whether prosthetic valve materials can produce pulmonary hypertension and restrictive lung disease.

### Silicone

Injectable silicone fluid (polydimethylsiloxane) ordinarily remains pooled at its injection site. Thus, females and male transsexuals use silicone fluid to augment breast and gluteal size. Chastre and coworkers[135] reported three cases of silicone particle pulmonary embolism following intramuscular injection of silicone fluid. All three patients presented with high fever, chest pain, dyspnea, and cough within 24 hours of the injection. Physical examination disclosed rales. Chest roentgenograms showed bilateral alveolar infiltrates. Patients were hypoxemic. In one patient, pulmonary artery pressures were elevated despite a normal pulmonary capillary wedge pressure. All sputum and blood cultures were negative. Bronchoalveolar washings revealed silicone particle–laden macrophages. All the patients improved spontaneously over one week. This syndrome should be considered whenever a patient develops dyspnea shortly after silicone injection.

Multiple endogenous and exogenous substances have been reported to embolize to the lungs. Although many substances silently embolize, embolic trophoblasts, parasites, catheters, and bullets can cause significant morbidity and mortality. In the appropriate clinical settings, they must be considered whenever the question of thrombotic pulmonary embolism is raised.

## CONCLUSION

Nonthrombotic pulmonary emboli are rare. Amniotic fluid emboli, air emboli, and foreign particle emboli are almost never documented. Fat, septic, and tumor emboli are more common, but they too are infrequent compared with thrombotic pulmonary emboli.

However, infrequency does not connote clinical insignificance. Patients with tachypnea or acute pulmonary edema from nonthrombotic pulmonary emboli require unique diagnostic tests and treatment strategies: air and amniotic fluid emboli, for example, are diagnosed via right heart aspiration, not via angiography. Anticoagulants, the mainstay in the treatment of thrombotic pulmonary emboli, have virtually no role in the treatment of tumor and fat emboli. Therefore, all physicians should be aware of the nonthrombotic pulmonary embolism syndromes. When certain subsets of patients, such as peripartum females, develop respiratory symptoms, nonthrombotic pulmonary embolism should not only be considered but should lead the list of differential diagnoses.

## REFERENCES

1. Kane, R. D., Hawkins, H. K., Miller, J. A., et al.: Microscopic pulmonary tumor emboli associated with dyspnea. Cancer, 36:1473, 1975.

2. Winterbauer, R. H., Elfenbein, I. B., and Ball, W. C., Jr.: Incidence and clinical significance of tumor embolization of the lungs. Am. J. Med., *45*:271, 1968.
3. Smith, R. R. L., Sternberg, S. S., Paglia, M. A., et al.: Fatal pulmonary tumor embolization following peritoneovenous shunting for malignant ascites. J. Surg. Oncol., *16*:27, 1981.
4. Arbeit, J. M., Flye, M. W., Mundinger, G. H., et al.: Latent pulmonary embolus from a retroperitoneal sarcoma. Cancer, *46*:1492, 1980.
5. Shurin, S. B., Gauderer, M. W. L., Dahms, B. B., et al.: Fatal intraoperative pulmonary embolization of Wilms tumor. J. Pediatr., *101*:559, 1982.
6. Daughtry, J. D., Stewart, B. H., Golding, L. A. R., et al.: Pulmonary embolus presenting as the initial manifestation of renal cell carcinoma. Ann. Thorac. Surg., *24*:178, 1977.
7. Graham, J. P., Rotman, H. H., and Weg, J. G.: Tumor emboli presenting as pulmonary hypertension. Chest, *69*:229, 1976.
8. Brisbane, J. U., Howell, D. A., and Bonkowsky, H. L.: Pulmonary hypertension as a presentation of hepatocarcinoma. Am. J. Med., *68*:466, 1980.
9. Gonzalez, A., Altieri, P. I., Marquez, E., et al.: Massive pulmonary embolism associated with a right ventricular myxoma. Am. J. Med., *69*:795, 1980.
10. Varma, J. S.: Subacute pulmonary hypertension and systemic tumour embolism from cervical cancer. Scott. Med. J., *27*:336, 1982.
11. Meyers, J. D.: Letter to the Editor. New Engl. J. Med., *304*:610, 1981.
12. Hoefnagel, C. A., Marcuse, H. R., and Somers, R.: Pulmonary tumor-embolism from intravascular osteosarcoma demonstrated by bone scintigraphy. Clin. Nucl. Med., *12*:574, 1982.
13. Yue, W. Y.: Fatal neoplastic pulmonary embolism during general anesthesia. Minn. Med., *55*:540, 1972.
14. Milne, B., Cervenko, F. W., Morales, A., et al.: Massive intraoperative tumor embolus from renal cell carcinoma. Anesthesiology, *54*:253, 1981.
15. Kennan, D. J. M., Morton, P., and O'Kane, H. O.: Right atrial myxoma and pulmonary embolism. Rational basis for investigation and treatment. Br. Heart J., *48*:510, 1982.
16. Hussey, H. H., and Katz, S.: Septic pulmonary infarction; Report of 8 cases. Ann. Intern. Med., *22*:526, 1945.
17. MacMillan, J. C., Milstein, S. H., and Samson, P. C.: Clinical spectrum of septic pulmonary embolism and infarction. J. Thorac. Cardiovasc. Surg., *75*:670, 1978.
18. McHenry, M. C., Baggenstoss, A. H., and Martin, W. J.: Bacteremia due to gram-negative bacilli. Am. J. Clin. Pathol., *50*:160, 1968.
19. Soave, R., Murray, H. W., and Litrenta, M. M.: Bacterial invasion of pulmonary vessels. Pseudomonas bacteremia mimicking pulmonary thromboembolism with infarction. Am. J. Med., *65*:864, 1978.
20. Fred, H. L., and Harle, T. S.: Septic pulmonary embolism. Chest, *55*:483, 1969.
21. Jaffe, R. B., and Koschmann, E. B.: Septic pulmonary emboli. Radiology, *96*:527, 1970.
22. Louria, D. B., Hensle, T., and Rose, J.: The major medical complications of heroin addiction. Ann. Intern. Med., *67*:1, 1967.
23. Osei, C., Berger, H. W., and Nicholas, P.: Septic pulmonary infarction: Clinical and radiographic manifestations in 11 patients. Mt. Sinai J. Med., *46*:145, 1979.
24. Goodwin, N. J., Castronuovo, J. J., and Friedman, E. A.: Recurrent septic pulmonary embolization complicating maintenance hemodialysis. Ann. Intern. Med., *71*:29, 1969.
25. Waisser, E., Kuo, C. S., and Kabins, S. A.: Septic pulmonary emboli arising from a permanent transvenous cardiac pacemaker. Chest, *61*:503, 1972.
26. Zelefsky, M. N., and Lutzker, L. G.: The target sign: A new radiologic sign of septic pulmonary emboli. Am. J. Roentgenol., *129*:453, 1977.
27. Silingardi, V., Canossi, G. C., Torelli, G., et al.: The radiologic "target sign" of septic pulmonary embolis in a case of acute myelogenous leukemia. Respiration, *42*:61, 1981.
28. Jaffe, R. B., and Koschmann, E. B.: Intravenous drug abuse. Pulmonary, cardiac, and vascular complications. Am. J. Roentgenol. Radium. Ther. Nucl. Med., *109*:107, 1970.
29. Webb, D. W., and Thadepalli, H.: Hemoptysis in patients with septic pulmonary infarcts from tricuspid endocarditis. Chest, *76*:99, 1979.
30. Josey, W. E., and Staggers, S. R.: Heparin therapy in septic pelvic thrombophlebitis: A study of 46 cases. Am. J. Obstet. Gynecol., *120*:228, 1974.
31. Felman, A. H., and Shulman, S. T.: Staphylococcal osteomyelitis, sepsis, and pulmonary disease. Radiology, *117*:649, 1975.
32. Gumbs, R. V., and McCauley, D. I.: Hilar and mediastinal adenopathy in septic pulmonary embolic disease. Radiology, *142*:313, 1982.
33. Noble, J., and Cohen, R. B.: Case 24–1972. New Engl. J. Med., *286*:1309, 1972.
34. Scharf, J., Nahir, A. M., Munk, J., et al.: Aseptic cavitation in pulmonary infarction. Chest, *59*:456, 1971.
35. Dunn, L. J., and Van Voorhis, L. W.: Enigmatic fever and pelvic thrombophlebitis. New Engl. J. Med., *276*:265, 1967.
36. Ledger, W. J., and Peterson, E. P.: The use of heparin in the management of pelvic thrombophlebitis. Surg. Gynecol. Obstet., *113*:1115, 1970.
37. Steiner, P. E., and Lushbaugh, C. C.: Maternal pulmonary embolism by amniotic fluid. JAMA, *117*:1245, 1340, 1941.
38. Moore, K. L.: The Developing Human, 3rd ed. W. B. Saunders, Philadelphia, 1982, p. 97.
39. Corridan, M., Kendall, E. D., and Begg, J. D.: Cord entanglement causing premature placental separation and amniotic fluid embolism. Br. J. Obstet. Gynecol., *87*:935, 1980.
40. Wasser, W. G., Tessler, S., Kamath, C. P., et al.: Nonfatal amniotic fluid embolism: A case report of post-partum respiratory distress with histopathologic studies. Mt. Sinai J. Med., *46*:388, 1979.
41. Masson, R. G., Ruggieri, J., and Siddiqui, M. M.: Amniotic fluid embolism: Definitive diagnosis in a survivor. Am. Rev. Resp. Disp., *120*:187, 1979.
42. Roche, W. D., and Norris, H. J.: Detection and significance of maternal pulmonary amniotic fluid embolism. Obstet. Gynecol., *43*:729, 1974.
43. Courtney, L. D.: Amniotic fluid embolism. Obstet. Gynecol. Survey, *29*:169, 1974.
44. Guha-Ray, D. K.: Maternal mortality in an urban hospital. Obstet. Gynecol., *47*:430, 1976.
45. Barno, A., and Freeman, D. W.: Amniotic fluid embolism. Am. J. Obstet. Gynecol., *77*:1199, 1959.
46. Aguillon, A., Andjus, T., Grayson, A., et al.:

Amniotic fluid embolism: A review. Obstet. Gynecol. Survey, *17*:619, 1962.
47. Dolyniuk, M., Orfei, E., Vania, H., et al.: Rapid diagnosis of amniotic fluid embolism. Obstet. Gynecol., *61*:28s, 1983.
48. Chung, A. F., and Merkatz, I. M.: Survival following amniotic fluid embolism with early heparinization. Obstet. Gynecol., *42*:809, 1973.
49. Reis, R. L., Pierce, W. S., and Benrendt, D. M.: Hemodynamic effects of amniotic fluid embolism. Surg. Gynecol. Obstet., *129*:45, 1969.
50. Taenaka, N., Shimada, Y., Kawai, M., et al.: Survival from DIC following amniotic fluid embolism. Successful treatment with a serine proteinase inhibitor; FOY. Anesthesia, *36*:389, 1981.
51. Scott, M. M.: Cardiopulmonary considerations in nonfatal amniotic fluid embolism. JAMA, *183*:989, 1963.
52. Meier, P. R., and Bowes, W. A.: Amniotic fluid embolus-like syndrome presenting in the second trimester of pregnancy. Obstet. Gynecol., *61*:31s, 1983.
53. O'Quin, R. J., and Lakshminarayan, S.: Venous air embolism. Arch. Intern. Med., *142*:2173, 1982.
54. Campkin, T. V., and Perks, J. S.: Venous air embolism. Lancet, *1*:235, 1973.
55. Cholankeril, J. V., Joshi, R. R., Cenizal, J. S., et al.: Massive air embolism from the pulmonary artery. Radiology, *142*:33, 1982.
56. Doblar, C. C., Jinkle, J. C., Fay, M. L., et al.: Air embolism associated with pulmonary artery catheter introducer kit. Anesthesiology, *56*:307, 1982.
57. Tuddenham, W. J., and Paskin, D. L.: Radiographic demonstration of air embolism. Med. Radiogr. Photogr., *50*:16, 1974.
58. Ordway, C. B.: Air embolus via CVP catheter without positive pressure: Presentation of case and review. Ann. Surg., *179*:479, 1974.
59. Kizer, K. W., and Goodman, P. C.: Radiographic manifestations of venous air embolism. Radiology, *144*:35, 1982.
60. Warren, B. A., Philp, R. B., and Inwood, M. J.: The ultrastructural morphology of air embolism: Platelet adhesion to the interface and endothelial damage. Br. J. Exp. Path., *54*:163, 1973.
61. Moosavi, H., Utell, M. J., Hyde, R. W., et al.: Lung ultrasructure in noncardiogenic pulmonary edema induced by air embolization in dogs. Lab. Invest., *45*:456, 1981.
62. Ericsson, J. A., Gottlieb, J. D., and Sweet, R. B.: Closed-chest cardiac massage in the treatment of venous air embolism. New Engl. J. Med., *270*:1353, 1964.
63. Ence, T. J., and Gong, H.: Adult respiratory distress syndrome after venous air embolism. Am. Rev. Resp. Dis., *119*:1033, 1979.
64. Kogutt, M. S.: Systemic air embolism secondary to respiratory therapy in the neonate: Six cases including one survivor. Am. J. Roentgenol., *131*:425, 1978.
65. Fowler, A. A., Hamman, R. F., Good, J. T., et al.: Adult respiratory distress syndrome: Risk with common predispositions. Ann. Intern. Med., *98*:593, 1983.
66. Furuya, H., Suzuki, T., Okumua, F., et al.: Detection of air embolism by transesophageal echocardiography. Anesthesiology, *58*:124, 1983.
67. Sevitt, S.: Fat Embolism. Butterworth and Company, London, 1962.
68. Dines, D. E., Burgher, L. W., and Okazaki, H.: The clinical and pathologic correlation of fat embolism syndrome. Mayo Clin. Proc., *50*:407, 1975.
69. Tedeschi, C. G., Walter, C. E., and Tedeschi, L. G.: Shock and fat embolism: An appraisal. Surg. Clin. North Am., *48*:431, 1968.
70. Benatar, S. R., Ferguson, A. D., and Goldschmidt, R. B.: Fat embolism—some clinical observations and a review of controversial aspects. Q. J. Med., *41*:85, 1972.
71. Herndon, J. H., Bechtol, C. O., and Crickenberger, D. P.: Fat embolism during total hip replacement. J. Bone Joint Surg., *56A*:1350, 1974.
72. Linscheid, R. L., and Dines, D. E.: The fat-embolism syndrome. Surg. Clin. North Am., *49*:1137, 1969.
73. Dines, D. E., Linscheid, R. L., and Didier, E. P.: Fat embolism sndrome. Mayo Clin. Proc., *47*:237, 1972.
74. Burgher, L. W., Dines, D. E., Linscheid, R. L., et al.: Fat embolism and the adult respiratory distress syndrome. Mayo Clin. Proc., *49*:107, 1974.
75. Stoltenberg, J. J., and Gustilo, R. B.: The use of methylprednisolone and hypertonic glucose in the prophylaxis of fat embolism syndrome. Clin. Orthop., *143*:211, 1979.
76. Gurd, A. R., and Wilson, R. I.: The fat embolism syndrome. J. Bone Joint Surg., *56B*:408, 1974.
77. Curtis, A. McB., Knowles, G. D., Putnam, C. E., et al.: The three syndromes of fat embolism: Pulmonary manifestations. Yale J. Biol. Med., *52*:149, 1979.
78. Moore, P., James, O., Saltos, N.: Fat embolism syndrome: Incidence, significance and early features. Aust. N. Z. J. Surg., *51*:546, 1981.
79. Guentner, C. A., and Braun, T. E.: Fat embolism syndrome. Chest, *79*:143, 1981.
80. Schonfeld, S. A., Ploysongsang, Y., DiLisio, R., et al.: Fat embolism prophylaxis with corticosteroids. Ann. Intern. Med., *99*:438, 1983.
81. Gossling, H. R., and Pellegrini, V. D.: Fat embolism syndrome. A review of the pathophysiological basis of treatment. Clin. Orthop., *165*:68, 1982.
82. Rokkanen, P., Lahdensuu, M., Kataja, J., et al.: The syndrome of fat embolism: Analysis of thirty consecutive cases compared to trauma patients with similar injuries. J. Trauma, *10*:299, 1970.
83. Buchanan, D., and Jason, D. K.: Occurrence of pulmonary fat and bone marrow embolism. Am. J. Forensic Med. Path., *3*:73, 1982.
84. Avikainen, V., Willman, K., and Rokkanen, P.: Stress hormones, lipids, and factors of hemostasis in trauma patients with and without fat embolism syndrome: A comparative study at least one year after severe trauma. J. Trauma, *20*:148, 1980.
85. Pastore, L., and Kessler, S.: Pulmonary fat embolization in the immunocompromised patient. Its relationship to steroid medication. Am. J. Surg. Pathol., *6*:315, 1982.
86. Hill, R. B.: Fatal fat embolism from steroid-induced fatty liver. New Engl. J. Med., *265*:318, 1961.
87. Limbird, T. J., and Ruderman, R. J.: Fat embolism in children. Clin. Orthop., *136*:267, 1978.
88. Gittman, J. E., Buchanan, T. A., Fisher, B. J., et al.: Fatal fat embolism after spinal fusion for scoliosis. JAMA, *249*:779, 1983.
89. Adams, C. B. T.: The retinal manifestations of fat embolism. Injury, 2:221, 1971.
90. Tedeschi, C. G., Castelli, W., Kropp, G., et al.: Fat macroglobulinemia and fat embolism. Surg. Gynecol. Obstet., *126*:83, 1968.

91. Gurd, A. R.: Fat embolism: An aid to diagnosis. J. Bone Joint Surg., *52B*:732, 1970.
92. Nolte, W. J., Olofsson, T., Schersten, T., et al.: Evaluation of the Gurd test for fat embolism. J. Bone Joint Surg., *56B*:417, 1974.
93. Cole, W. G.: Urinary fat and fat embolism. Med. J. Aust., *1*:1187, 1973.
94. Burgher, L. W.: Fat embolism syndrome. Chest, *79*:131, 1981.
95. Naver, L., Walter, S., and Glowinski, J.: Pulmonary fat embolism treated by intermittent continuous positive airway pressure given by face mask. Br. Med. J., *1*:1413, 1980.
96. Alho, A.: Fat embolism syndrome: Etiology, pathogenesis and treatment. Acta Chir. Scand. (Suppl.) *499*:75, 1980.
97. Bruecke, P., Burke, J. F., Lam, K. W., et al.: The pathophysiology of pulmonary at embolism. J. Thorac. Cardiovasc. Surg., *61*:949, 1971.
98. Saldeen, T.: The importance of intravascular coagulation and inhibition of the fibrinolytic system in experimental fat embolism. J. Trauma, *10*:287, 1970.
99. Peltier, L. F., and Sevitt, S.: Trauma workshop report: Fat embolism. J. Trauma, *10*:1074, 1970.
100. Myers, R., and Taljaard, J. J. F.: Blood alcohol and fat embolism syndrome. J. Bone Joint Surg., *59A*:878, 1977.
101. Shier, M. R., Wilson, R. F., James, R. E., et al.: Fat embolism prophylaxis: A study of four treatment modalities. J. Trauma, *17*:621, 1977.
102. Rokkanen, P., Alho, A., Avikainen, V., et al.: The efficacy of corticosteroids in severe trauma. Surg. Gynecol. Obstet., *138*:69, 1974.
103. Paré, J. A. P., Fraser, R. G., Hogg, J. C., et al.: Pulmonary "mainline" granulomatosis: Talcosis of intravenous methadone abuse. Medicine, *58*:229, 1979.
104. Puro, H. E., Wolf, P. L., Skirgaudas, J., et al.: Experimental production of human "blue velvet" and "red devil" lesions. JAMA, *187*:1100, 1966.
105. Douglas, F. G., Kafilmout, K. J., and Patt, N. L.: Foreign particle embolism in drug addicts: Respiratory pathophysiology. Ann. Intern. Med., *75*:865, 1971.
106. Hopkins, G. B.: Pulmonary angiothrombotic granulomatosis in drug offenders. JAMA, *221*:909, 1972.
107. Siegel, H.: Human pulmonary pathology associated with narcotic and other addictive drugs. Hum. Pathol., *3*:55, 1972.
108. Robertson, C. H., Reynolds, R. C., and Wilson, J. E.: Pulmonary hypertension and foreign body granulomas in intravenous drug abusers. Am. J. Med., *61*:657, 1976.
109. Lederer, C. M., and Sabates, F. N.: Ocular findings in the intravenous drug abuser. Ann. Ophthalmol., *14*:436, 1982.
110. Peach, M. J.: Anions: Phosphate, Iodine, Fluoride, and Other Anions. *In* Goodman, L. S., and Gilman, A. (eds.): Other Anions. The Pharmacological Basis of Therapeutics. MacMillan Publishing Co., New York, 1975, pp. 798.
111. Bron, K. M., Baum, S., and Abrams, H. L.: Oil embolism in lymphangiography. Incidence, manifestations, and mechanism. Radiology, *80*:194, 1963.
112. Yousef, M. M. A., and Mudarris, M. F.: Non-water soluble contrast intravasation and pulmonary embolization in myelography. J. Neuroradiol., *80*:426, 1979.
113. Hallgrimsson, J., and Clouse, M. E.,: Pulmonary oil emboli after lymphography. Arch. Pathol., *80*:426, 1965.
114. Marcuse, P. M.: Pulmonary syncytial giant cell embolism. Obstet. Gynecol., *3*:210, 1954.
115. Kohorn, E. I., McGinn, R. C., Gee, B. L., et al.: Pulmonary embolization of trophoblastic tissue in molar pregnancy. Obstet. Gynecol., *51*:16s, 1978.
116. Armellin, G. M., Smith, R. C., and Faithfull, G. R.: Pulmonary bile emboli following percutaneous cholangiography and biliary drainage. Pathol., *13*:615, 1981.
117. Brozinsky, S., DeSoto-Lapaix, F., Jimenez, F., et al.: Bile emboli: A complication of PTC. J. Clin. Gastroenterol., *3*:135, 1981.
118. Ghatak, N. R., and Zimmerman, H. M.: Cerebral bone marrow embolism. Arch. Pathol., *92*:112, 1971.
119. Lin, C.-S., and Zar, F. G.: Paradoxical bone marrow coronary embolism following cardiopulmonary resuscitation. JAMA, *248*:33, 1982.
120. Hatfield, S., and Challa, V.: Embolism of cerebral tissue to lungs following gunshot wound to head. J. Trauma, *20*:353, 1980.
121. Palant, A., Deutsch, V., Kishon, Y., et al.: Pulmonary hydatid embolization. Report on 2 operated cases and review of published reports. Br. Heart J., *38*:1086, 1976.
122. Brown, H. W.: Basic Clinical Parasitology. Appleton-Century-Crofts, New York, 1975.
123. Goodman, M. L., and Gore, I.: Pulmonary infarct secondary to dirofilaria larvae. Arch. Intern. Med., *113*:702, 1964.
124. Bernhardt, L. C., Wegner, G. P., and Mendenhall, J. T.: Intravenous catheter embolization to the pulmonary artery. Chest, *57*:329, 1970.
125. Wellmann, K. F., Reinhard, A., and Salazar, E. P.: Polyethylene catheter embolism. Circulation, *37*:380, 1968.
126. Weinsaft, M. H., Khan, R. G., and Piccone, V.: Teflon pacemaker introducer embolization. NY State J. Med., *79*:925, 1979.
127. Richardson, J. D., Grover, F. L., and Trinkle, J. K.: Intravenous catheter emboli. Experience with twenty cases and collective review. Am. J. Surg., *128*:722, 1974.
128. Edwards, A. C., and Sowton, E.: Management of Embolized Central Venous Catheters. Br. Med. J., *2*:669, 1978.
129. Wajsbort, F., Monies-Chass, I., Peleg, A., et al.: Embolization of detached fragments of intravenous plastic catheter. Anaesthesist, *27*:492, 1978.
130. Stephenson, L. W., Workman, R. B., Aldrete, J. S., et al.: Bullet emboli to the pulmonary artery: A report of 2 patients and review of the literature. Ann. Thorac. Surg., *31*:333, 1976.
131. Symbas, P. N.: Bullet emboli in the pulmonary and systemic arteries. Ann. Surg., *185*:318, 1977.
132. Nehme, A. E.: Intracranial bullet migrating to pulmonary artery. J. Trauma, *20*:344, 1980.
133. Saltzstein, E. C., and Freeark, R. J.: Bullet embolism to the right axillary artery following gunshot wound of the heart. Ann. Surg., *158*:65, 1963.
134. Robinson, M. J., Nestor, M., and Rywlen, A. M.: Pulmonary granulomas secondary to embolic prosthetic valve material. Hum. Pathol., *12*:759, 1981.
135. Chastre, J., Basset, F., Viau, F., et al.: Acute pneumonitis after subcutaneous injections of silicone in transsexual men. New Engl. J. Med., *308*:764, 1983.

CHAPTER **12**

# VENOUS THROMBOEMBOLISM IN CHILDREN

*DAVID R. FULTON, M.D.*

Pulmonary embolism (PE) and deep vein thrombosis (DVT) are well-recognized, common entities in the adult but in general are considered unusual among children. As a result, when present, they are usually not diagnosed ante mortem. In part, failure to recognize these entities may be the result of concurrent severe underlying illness, which may mask the presenting features. The purpose of this chapter is to provide current information about the frequency, pathogenesis, and clinical presentation of thromboembolic disease in the pediatric patient as well as diagnostic modalities and therapeutic interventions. Outlining the present status of these disorders will serve to heighten clinical recognition and thereby expand the experience in diagnostic and therapeutic intervention, which, to date, has been limited.

## FREQUENCY

The first case of pulmonary embolism in a child was reported in 1861 by Löeschner, who described a fatal illness lasting three days following a tibial fracture. The illness was characterized by pain and edema of the left leg and was associated with delirium. At postmortem examination, in addition to pulmonary embolus, thrombosis of the left femoral, popliteal, and anterior tibial veins was found and was presumed secondary to the phlebitis resulting from trauma.[1] Since this report, many additional case reports of pulmonary embolism have originated; however, even small case series among children are rare, and nearly all have been the result of retrospective analysis.[2–8]

In the larger series, the frequency of pulmonary embolus found at autopsy ranged from 0.73 to 3.1 per cent.[2, 5–7] When available, the data indicated that the majority of children found to have pulmonary embolus were under one year of age. No series presented data that enabled estimation of the frequency of pulmonary embolus in surviving children. Several authors attributed the inability to derive this figure to the difficulty of diagnosing pulmonary embolism ante mortem, because severe underlying disease processes are thought to mask the presenting features of embolism. In an autopsy review of 500 children from our institution over a 10-year period, we have identified 26 patients with pulmonary emboli (thrombotic and nonthrombotic) involving vessels of all dimensions (Table 12–1). In 50 per cent of the cases, the finding occurred in children less than 1 year of age. In all instances, the patients had significant underlying medical illness or conditions that predisposed to pulmonary embolus. In 50 per cent of our cases, severe congenital heart disease was present, and overwhelming infection was identified in 21 per cent. Only once was the diagnosis considered ante mortem, but the patient died of a massive pulmonary embolus before therapy could be initiated.

***Table 12–1.*** Age Distribution of Children with Pulmonary Embolism Diagnosed at Autopsy at the New England Medical Center, 1974–1983

| Age Category | Mean Age | Number of Patients |
|---|---|---|
| Less than 1 yr | 1.5 months | 13 |
| 1–10 yrs | 2.7 years | 7 |
| 10–19 yrs | 13.2 years | 6 |

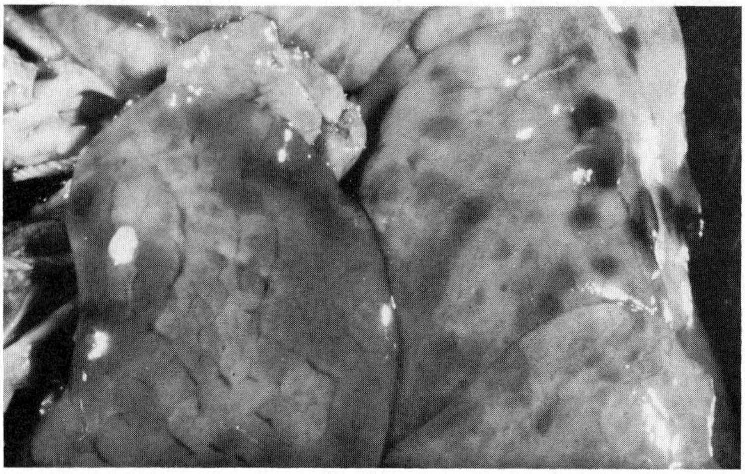

***Figure 12–1.*** Bilateral infarcts of the lung (darker areas) resulting from multiple pulmonary thromboemboli in a 20-day-old infant who had undergone surgical repair of coarctation of the aorta. Thrombus was found in association with venous catheters located in the inferior and superior vena cava. (The bright areas represent artifacts related to photographic technique.)

## PATHOGENESIS

The pathophysiologic consequences of pulmonary emboli are similar to those found in adults. Pulmonary emboli obstruct pulmonary artery vessels of varying size and, depending on the degree of flow limitation, may lead to pulmonary parenchymal infarction (Fig. 12–1). The composition of thrombus is often a fibrin-protein collection, but other components, including fat,[9–11] tumor,[12] septic debris,[7, 12–16] and cerebral tissue[17–22] have been described in children. For the purpose of categorization, the etiology of venous thromboembolic disease in children may be separated into intrinsic and extrinsic disorders (Table 12–2). Intrinsic abnormalities of both vessel walls and the coagulation system or low flow through the venous system may lead to stasis and thrombus formation. Damage to the vessel wall from extrinsic sources such as indwelling catheters may cause thrombi to form in areas of trauma. Predicting the probability of pulmonary embolism from a source of thrombosis is difficult, because few prospective studies have described the natural history of deep vein thrombosis in the younger individual.

***Table 12–2.*** Causes of Pulmonary Embolism in Children

| |
|---|
| **Intrinsic** |
| Deep leg vein thrombosis |
| Renal vein thrombosis |
| Infection |
| Primary pulmonary artery thrombosis |
| Genetic |
| Hughes-Stovin syndrome |
| Antithrombin III deficiency |
| Klinefelter's syndrome |
| Malignancy |
| **Extrinsic** |
| Ventriculoatrial shunts |
| Cardiac catheterization |
| Indwelling venous catheters (e.g., TPN lines, central venous pressure lines, etc.) |
| Cerebral birth trauma |
| Pharmacologic agents |
| Fat embolism |

TPN = total parenteral nutrition.

### Intrinsic Disorders

#### Deep Leg Vein Thrombosis

Deep leg vein thrombosis, the most common cause of pulmonary embolus in adults,[23] occurs less frequently in children, although its actual incidence is unknown. In fact, children with pulmonary emboli often have identifiable sources of thrombus other than the leg, including the renal vein, the vena cava, the cerebral venous system, or nonthrombotic etiologies. In addition, spontaneous pulmonary artery thrombosis in childhood can occur, particularly in association with underlying congenital heart disease. Predisposing factors to deep leg vein thrombosis are superficial skin infections,[16] osteomyelitis,[24] subperiosteal abscess,[25] trauma,[26] and pre- or postoperative settings associated with immobilization.[8, 16, 27, 28] In the last case, diminished muscular activity of the lower extremities results in stasis near valves of deep veins, predisposing to thrombosis, not unlike that occurring in adults. Halo-femoral traction, used in the preoperative management of scoliosis, involves wire cable connection of a cranial halo to pins placed bilaterally in the supracondylar area of the femur. Successive weights are added, creating traction and correcting scoliotic deformities prior to insertion of Harrington rods.[29] Deep leg vein thrombosis occurring during halo-femoral traction in children has prompted one of the few prospective evaluations of deep vein thrombosis in childhood.[29] In this study, 54 children in halo-femoral traction from eight to 53 days (mean of 28 days) underwent venography two days prior to corrective surgery. Only two patients (4 per cent) had demonstrable deep vein thrombosis, both of whom had already developed clinical signs consistent with the diagnosis, whereas none of the venogram-negative individuals had symptoms.

### Renal Vein Thrombosis

Renal vein thrombosis, which may cause pulmonary embolism if sufficiently extensive, most often presents as an acute event in the young infant with intravascular depletion and hemoconcentration following a diarrheal illness. An association has also been shown between renal vein thrombosis and maternal diabetes,[30–32] nephrotic syndrome,[33] cytomegalovirus,[34] maternal use of thiazides,[35] and trauma.[30] Current theory suggests that diminished renal blood flow or hemoconcentration promotes stasis and thrombosis in the smaller veins of the renal system, which may then propagate to include the main renal vein and extend to involve the inferior vena cava. Pulmonary embolism found concurrently with renal vein thrombosis has been reported at autopsy and is thought to play a major role in the demise of the patient.[6, 7, 36] However, data regarding the frequency of pulmonary embolism in patients surviving with renal vein thrombosis are incomplete. It has been suggested that pulmonary embolism occurs only when renal vein thrombosis is accompanied by extension to the inferior vena cava.[36]

### Infection

The role of infection in causing pulmonary embolism has changed over the past 50 years. In children, the first report of pulmonary embolism related to infection occurred in a six-year-old boy with otitis media and mastoiditis with extension to the right lateral and occipital sinuses. The thrombophlebitis proliferated further to the internal jugular vein, from which septic emboli seeded the pulmonary bed.[37] Local infection and venous thrombosis have been associated with subsequent pulmonary embolism in children in many case reports and include such diverse etiologies as measles,[37] diphtheria,[38] suppurative otitis media and mastoiditis,[5, 7, 37, 39–41] meningitis,[5] peritonitis,[5, 6, 12, 13] bacterial endocarditis,[15, 41] septicemia,[6, 7] and osteomyelitis.[24] The frequency of reported thrombophlebitis associated with these processes has decreased since the introduction of antibiotics and immunization, although overwhelming infection, particularly in the immunocompromised host, continues to predispose to septic pulmonary emboli.

### Primary Pulmonary Artery Thrombosis

The presence of congenital heart disease has occasionally been correlated with primary thrombosis of a pulmonary artery. Diminished pulmonary blood flow with increased blood viscosity from polycythemia in cyanotic heart disease appears to be the major predisposing factor.[42–44] In addition, some children with cyanotic heart disease but without polycythemia have evidence for low-grade chronic disseminated intravascular coagulation, rendering these individuals relatively hypercoagulable.[45] The most common lesions associated with primary pulmonary artery thrombosis include tetralogy of Fallot,[42, 46–49] pulmonary atresia,[7, 50] and, less frequently, ventricular septal defect with and without pulmonic stenosis.[51, 52]

Persistent fetal circulation or primary pulmonary hypertension of the newborn is a disorder of heterogeneous etiologies uniformly characterized by systemic or suprasystemic pulmonary artery pressure resulting in right-to-left shunting at the level of the ductus arteriosus or interatrial septum. The resulting cyanosis and metabolic acidosis aggravate pulmonary vasoconstriction and pulmonary hypertension, frequently leading to death.[52–56] In a number of these newborn infants, the presence of pulmonary microthrombi is demonstrated at autopsy.[56] One theory postulates that these thrombi may be initiated by intrapulmonary platelet aggregation caused by newborns' inhalation of amniotic fluid, a known thrombogenic agent.[57] The resulting effect is a decrease in the cross-sectional area of the pulmonary bed due to mechanical obstruction combined with a vasoconstrictive effect of vasoactive substances.[58–60] The presence of mechanical obstruction may explain the frequent failure of tolazoline, $PGE_1$, and $PGI_2$ to reverse the pulmonary hypertension or reduce arterial hypoxemia.[56]

### Genetic

**Hughes-Stovin Syndrome.** The Hughes-Stovin syndrome is a rare anatomic disorder that is marked by the presence of peripheral venous thrombosis and multiple pulmonary artery aneurysms.[61–66] The clinical expression is usually one of peripheral vein thrombophlebitis, cough, hemoptysis, and fever. Death usually results from aneurysm rupture into a bronchus. Postmortem examination shows aneurysm formation of the pulmonary arteries and in some cases pulmonary thromboemboli, presumably initiated from the sites of venous thrombosis.[66] The etiology of the anatomic abnormalities is unknown. Administration of anticoagulants has failed to prevent the venous thromboses.[66]

**Antithrombin III Deficiency.** Although its presentation is often later in life,[67–69] antithrombin III deficiency has been described in children as well (see Chapter 9).[70–72] The inheritance of the disorder in a recently studied family has suggested an autosomal dominant pattern.[70]

**Klinefelter's Syndrome.** A genetic predisposition to thromboembolic events is also supported by the reports of a fivefold increase in frequency of deep vein thrombosis and pulmonary embolism in adult males with Klinefelter's syndrome.[71] Although not reported in children with Klinefelter's syndrome, the discrepancy in frequency may result from the failure to consider the diagnosis.

### Malignancy

Neoplastic processes, in children as in adults, have been associated with pulmonary embolism. Solid tumors rather than lymphoproliferative disorders predominate. Wilms' tumor, the most common intra-abdominal malignancy of childhood, originates from renal parenchyma and is characterized by mesenchymal and epithelial components in varying stages of maturity. This neoplasm is known to invade the inferior vena cava, leading to obstruction and calcification,[72–75, 76] and may travel from the vessel into the right atrium, producing symptoms and signs of right heart failure.[77]

## Extrinsic Sources

Advances in therapy for childhood illness have led to the use of catheters and other devices that can predispose to venous thrombosis and subsequent pulmonary embolism. Extrinsic causes of pulmonary embolism include ventriculoatrial catheters, indwelling venous catheters and their infusates, cerebral birth trauma, and certain drugs (see Table 12–2).

### Ventriculoatrial Shunts

A recent predominant therapy for decompression of hydrocephalus was placement of a shunt that linked the lateral ventricle of the central nervous system with the right atrium. The early experience included findings of thrombosis at the distal catheter site and, in some cases, involvement of the superior vena cava and right atrium.[78] One series estimated that 25 per cent of patients with ventriculoatrial catheters had thrombus formation in the right atrium,[79] and the risk of pulmonary embolism in this setting was high, approaching 55 per cent at autopsy.[79–81] In some, the embolic episodes were catastrophic, directly contributing to the patients' demise,[2] whereas in others, embolization was low grade and continuous, leading to progressive pulmonary hypertension and cor pulmonale.[79, 82] Because of these complications, ventriculoatrial shunts have generally been replaced with ventriculoperitoneal catheters. However, some ventriculoatrial shunts are still patent, and in these individuals, complications must be considered (Fig. 12–2).

### Cardiac Catheterization

Cardiac catheterization in children is accomplished most often by access from the lower extremities either by femoral venous cutdown or by percutaneous technique.[83, 84] These procedures have been complicated by the thrombosis of the deep venous system, including the femoral and iliac veins as well as the inferior vena cava (Fig. 12–3).[85–91] In two recent reports, the frequency of thrombosis at repeat catheterization was 4 per cent among those initially undergoing study at under six months of age.[90, 91] Various factors have been suggested as the cause of obstruction, including percutaneous technique,[93] arterial hypoxemia,[87, 88, 90] use of balloon cathe-

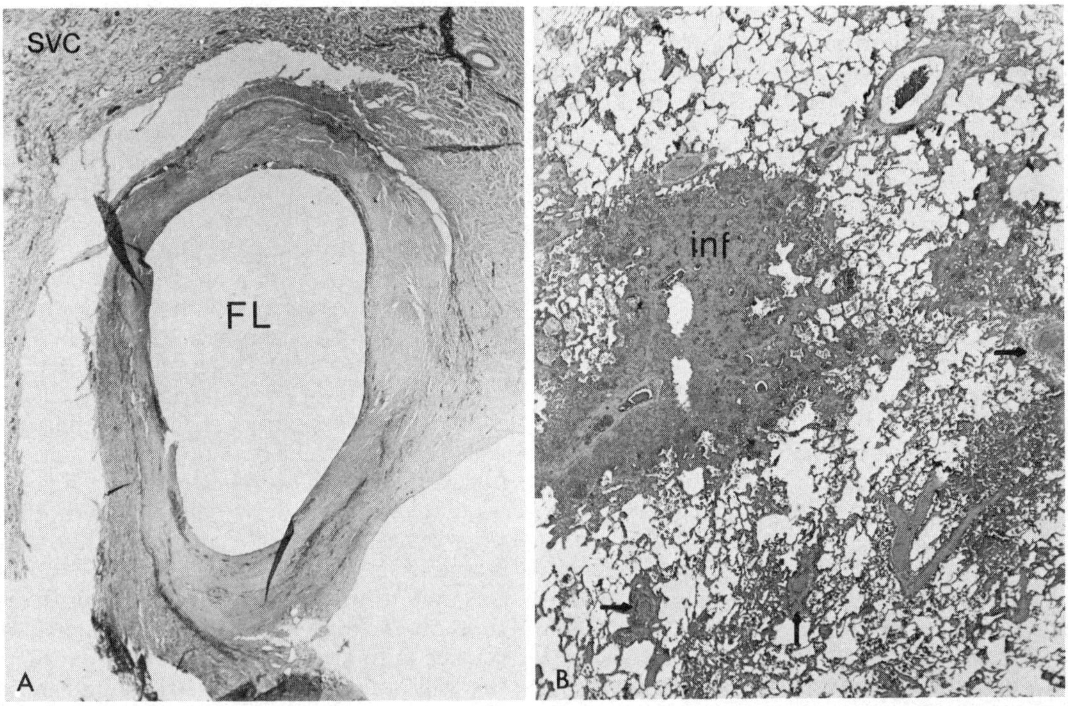


***Figure 12–2.*** *A,* Microscopic section from the superior vena cava (SVC) of a 17-year-old male with a ventriculoatrial shunt who died following a massive pulmonary embolus. A well-organized thrombus is present with a false lumen (FL) formed by the catheter tip.

*B,* Microscopic section of the lung in the same patient showing infarction (inf) and pulmonary emboli (arrows) of varying vessel sizes.

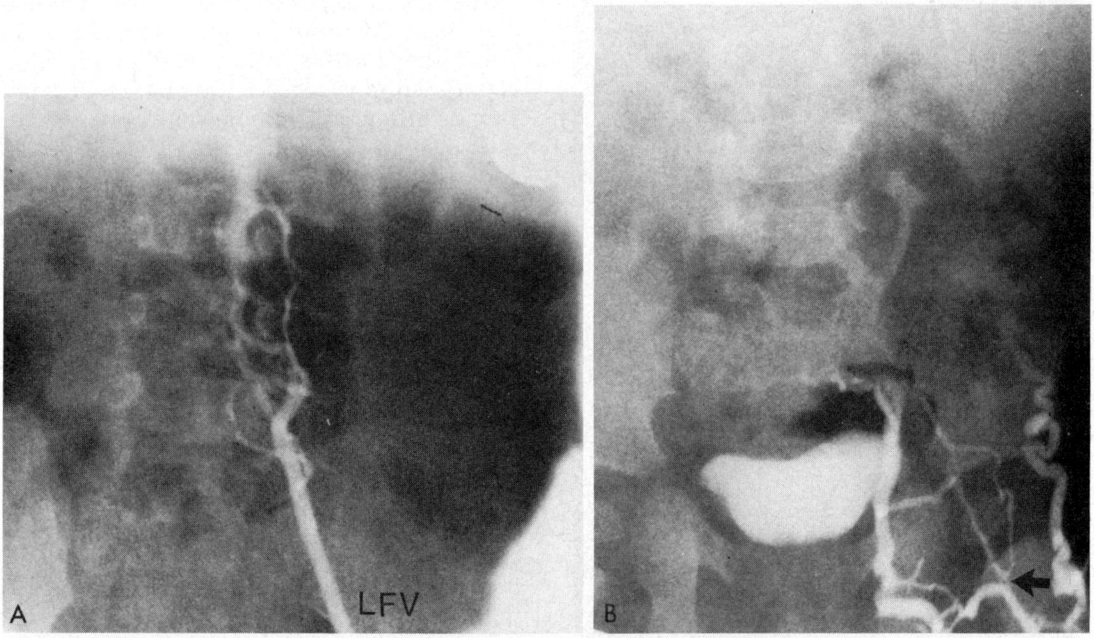


***Figure 12–3.*** *A,* Injection of dye into the left femoral vein (LFV) of an eight-month-old infant with D-transposition of the great arteries during repeat cardiac catheterization; initial catheterization was via the right femoral vein. The left femoral vein is visualized; however, no contrast agent crosses the midline, thus indicating inferior vena caval obstruction resulting from the initial catheterization.

*B,* Left femoral vein injection in a 10-month-old infant during a repeat cardiac catheterization showing obstruction of the femoral vein (arrow). Venous drainage occurs via superficial and paravertebral collateral vessels.

ters,[85, 88] or duration of the procedure;[86, 88, 92] however, despite the presence of extensive venous thrombosis, evidence is lacking for subsequent pulmonary embolism from these sources.

INDWELLING CENTRAL VENOUS CATHETERS

The use of indwelling central venous catheters for administering total parenteral nutrition in the form of amino acid solution, elevated glucose concentration, and fat emulsion has gained widespread acceptance in the chronically debilitated infant or child with gastrointestinal anomalies or disease (Fig. 12–4), prolonged ventilatory requirements, or oncologic disease. The propensity for venous thrombosis of the indwelling catheter was first noted in a six-month-old infant with aganglionosis of the colon. This infant required ileostomy and subsequent hyperalimentation for failure to thrive on oral feedings. Several catheters were removed because of Candida sepsis, and four weeks following reparative surgery, the infant died after the sudden onset of respiratory distress and cyanosis. Bilateral pulmonary embolism was confirmed at autopsy.[43] Others have reported similar findings,[94–96] and in one well-documented case, the diagnosis was made ante mortem using a $^{99m}$Tc lung perfusion scan following the onset of respiratory distress.[97] The use of bilateral jugular venous catheters for hyperalimentation in premature infants has resulted in superior vena cava and bilateral innominate thrombosis, which can interfere with pulmonary lymphatic and thoracic duct drainage, with subsequent development of chylothoraces.[98] Thrombus formation from a central venous catheter can propagate in the right atrium (Fig. 12–5), causing a ball-valve phenomenon that may cause superior vena cava obstruction or acute cyanosis from right-to-left shunting through a patent foramen ovale.[99] Intensive care settings have also employed indwelling catheters in the pulmonary arteries of neonates for monitoring pulmonary artery pressure, pulmonary capillary wedge pressure, and cardiac output without hyperalimentation infusion,[100] and fatal pulmonary embolism has been known to occur in this setting as it has in adults.[101]

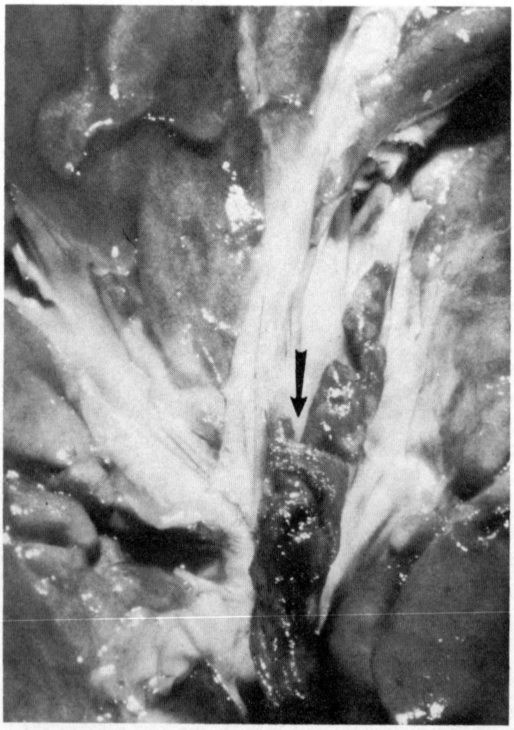

*Figure 12–4.* Thrombus occluding the superior vena cava in a four-year-old boy with severe inflammatory bowel disease necessitating a central venous catheter. Multiple large and small vessel pulmonary emboli were found at autopsy.

These observations raise the question of the mechanism of thrombus formation and its relationship to the type of intravenous fluid infusion. A group of 27 infants with indwelling peripheral vein catheters had phlebography prior to and every 12 to 24 hours after the onset of the study until intravenous support was no longer required.[102] Saline, Intralipid, Vamine, glucose 5.5%, or invertose was infused, most without heparin added to the solution. Mild edema without vessel damage occurred in those receiving saline. With the other solutions, all infants exhibited mural irregularities and variation in the width of the vessel lumen on phlebography and in some cases occlusion of the vessels. Edema of the surrounding soft tissue was noted in 50 per cent of the infants after 12 hours of infusion and in 100 per cent by 24 hours, whereas only two infants of five receiving heparin-containing solutions had mild edema at 24 hours. Some infants had leakage of contrast material when early vessel changes were noted. A parallel study using the cheek pouch of the hamster indicated that these various solutions exhibit different degrees of toxicity. Vamine retarded flow velocity immediately in small vessels, followed by complete cessation of flow within one to five minutes after the onset of infusion. Glucose 5.5% and invertose 10% retarded flow, with full arrest of flow occurring

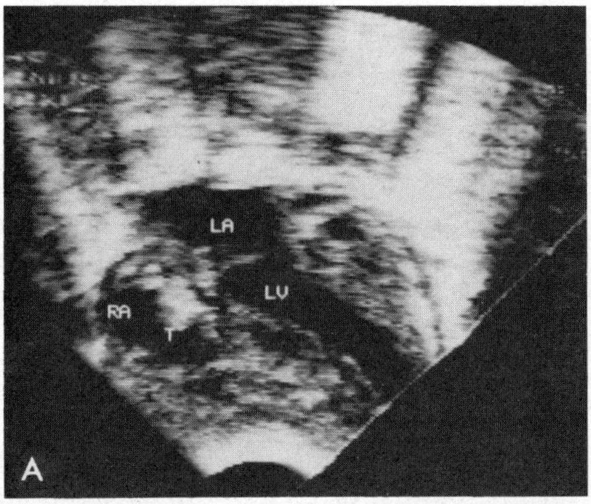


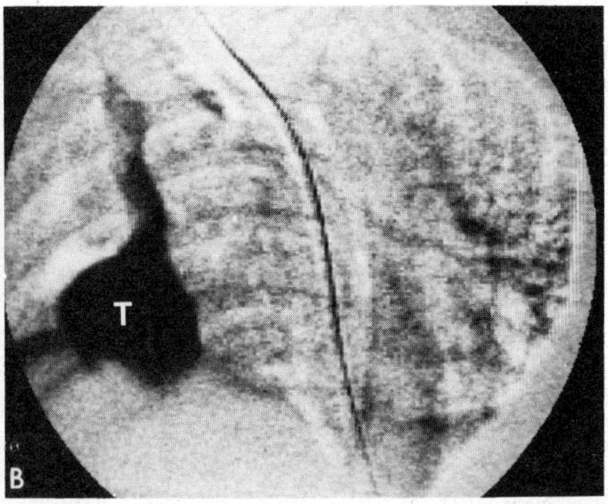


***Figure 12–5.*** *A,* A two-dimensional echocardiogram from the subxiphoid position in a nine-month-old male patient with *Staph. epidermidis* septicemia and a central hyperalimentation line. A large thrombus (T) can be seen in the lower portion of the right atrium (RA), just above the tricuspid valve. Right ventricular inflow was obstructed by the mass, which acted as a partial ball-valve thrombus. LA = left atrium; LV = left ventricle.

*B,* Digital subtraction pulmonary angiography was attempted in the same patient, with contrast material injected through the hyperalimentation catheter. The catheter tip is situated in the superior aspect of the right atrium. Contrast material enters a large cavitary right atrial thrombus (T), which acts as a cul-de-sac. Therefore, we do not visualize contrast agent in the right atrium or in the right ventricle. This thrombus is an ominous nidus for potential pulmonary embolization.

in 50 per cent. Intralipid and saline produced no measurable changes. Thus, although direct vessel trauma plays a role in thrombus formation, the type of infused fluid may accentuate vessel damage, leading to accelerated vessel occlusion.

### Cerebral Tissue

Fatal embolism of cerebral tissue to the pulmonary bed in neonates has been reported from several postmortem studies.[17–22] The pathogenesis of this often catastrophic event is uncertain; however, one theory is that elevated intracranial pressure from severe birth trauma reverses blood flow in the cerebral circulation, with forced entry of brain tissue into the circulation and subsequent embolization.[21] Another theory implicates tentorial tears from pressure changes as the mode of entry of cerebral tissue to the venous system.[20] Brain tissue has been found in the branches of pulmonary arteries and is thought to occur from trauma at a point in early gestation. In these rare situations, the brain is generally severely maldeveloped, supporting the concept of a traumatic episode in early pregnancy leading to embolization of cerebral tissue.[103–106]

### Pharmacologic Agents

Oral contraceptives affect hemostasis through an effect on platelets, coagulation factors, and fibrinolysis.[107, 108] They are widely used by adolescents and, therefore, those individuals taking these drugs should be considered at increased risk for development of thromboembolism. The use of steroids has also been associated with the development of pulmonary thromboembolism.[109, 110] In addition, an increased propensity for pulmonary artery thrombosis has been reported in children with nephrotic syndrome being treated with prednisone and a thiazide diuretic,[111] but the degree to which these drugs contribute is unclear.

### Fat Embolism

Fat embolism in children probably differs little in mechanism from that in adults (see Chapter 11). Although initially thought not to occur following trauma in children under 14 years of age because of the relative paucity and difference in composition of bone marrow fat,[112] later reports indicated that young age did not appear to reduce the frequency of fat embolism.[113–115] Fat is apparently extruded into the venous system from the marrow of traumatized bone and embolizes to the lungs, where free fatty acids are liberated, inducing an inflammatory pneumonitis.[116, 117] Coexisting pathologic conditions, including myelodysplasia,[115] collagen vascular disease,[113] and steroid therapy[113] are thought to predispose to fat embolism by causing osteoporosis with relative enlargement of the marrow cavity.[118] Fat embolism has also been found in infants at autopsy who were treated with infusion of liquid emulsions. These infants received Intralipid in quantities (3 gm/kg/day)[119] or rates (0.17 gm/kg/hr)[120, 121] in excess of the daily recommendations.

## CLINICAL PRESENTATION

The presence of venous thromboembolic disease in infants and children is often unsuspected because the process is frequently superimposed on an underlying systemic disease that may mimic or mask the clinical presentation. In addition, because little emphasis has been placed on the risk for developing this disorder in childhood, the physician may fail to consider this possibility. Therefore, our understanding of the clinical aspects leans heavily on retrospective analysis of autopsy series.

### Symptoms

Pulmonary embolism presents as an acute, life-threatening crisis or as a chronic process with development of cor pulmonale. In many children presenting acutely, the signs are often preceded by a history of upper respiratory tract infection, otitis media, or gastroenteritis with vomiting, diarrhea, and dehydration. Then, most commonly, there is an abrupt change in the child's condition with agitation, cyanosis, and tachypnea. The older individual may complain of chest pain, occasionally marked by a pleuritic component or suprascapular pain. In some, the progression may be so rapid toward cardiovascular collapse that gasping or agonal breathing may predominate. These symptoms may be accompanied by diaphoresis or cough with hemoptysis. More chronic symptoms include onset of dyspnea and cough with blood-tinged sputum. These features may continue for months without significant change but then may accelerate in severity. The source of emboli in older children may be suggested by complaints of leg pain, tenderness, or swelling, indicating deep vein thrombosis, although silent presentation is not uncommon. Similarly, tenderness over intravenous catheter sites should raise suspicion of venous inflammation with thrombosis. The complaint of fever often accompanies the onset of thrombosis; in fact, in some cases, fever without a source has been the only presenting feature of a deep vein thrombosis confirmed subsequently.

### Signs

The signs associated with pulmonary embolus are striking in the absence of concomitant disease. Significant respiratory distress and cyanosis are almost always present; the rate of respiration usually varies with the age of the child. Hypotension and tachycardia are found in 30 to 50 per cent. Auscultatory findings include wheezing, bronchovesicular breath sounds, or pleural rub over the lung fields. The pulmonic component of the second heart sound is accentuated. A new systolic murmur may be heard along the left sternal border or right chest, or over the back.[122, 123] The pulses may be thready, reflecting systemic hypotension. Neck vein distention, a frequent finding in adults with cor pulmonale, is difficult to assess in younger children and infants, even in the presence of significant right ventricular hypertension. Other signs of right-sided congestive heart failure have been described, including hepatomegaly and, in more chronic situations, ascites and edema of the lower extremities. Such signs are not generally observed in the younger patient. Peripheral sources for pulmonary emboli are suggested by typical findings of deep vein thrombosis with edema, tenderness, and erythema of the lower extremities, especially in sites of previous trauma or indwelling venous cannulae.

In infants with renal vein thrombosis, a palpable flank mass is present on the side of involvement. Systemic hypertension, sometimes severe, is often found. Obstruction of superficial abdominal veins and prominent edema of the sacrum and lower extremities may prevail. Oliguria or even anuria is indicative of compromised renal function. Dehydration, a frequent concurrent condition with renal vein thrombosis, is indicated in infants by decreased skin turgor, dry mucous membranes, absent lacrimation, weight loss, oliguria, and, in more severe cases, hypotension and tachycardia resulting from depletion of the intravascular space, diminished peripheral perfusion, and metabolic acidosis.

When central catheter thrombosis occurs in the major venous systems of the thorax, edema of the neck with periorbital and facial edema is a nearly constant sign. Focal neurologic signs indicate infection and thrombosis of the cerebral veins and sinuses. The presence of a ventriculoatrial shunt should suggest a cerebral source for those presenting with typical signs of pulmonary embolus. Rapid, progressive cyanosis in a child with cyanotic heart disease and the finding of a new murmur or loss of a continuous shunt murmur indicate a probable pulmonary artery thrombosis. Children with fat embolism related to trauma will show the minor signs of fever, tachycardia, petechiae, and cyanosis as well as major neurologic involvement with coma or paresis; the diagnosis of fat embolism can be strongly supported by the findings of retinal embolism.[11, 114, 124]

## Laboratory Findings

### CHEST X-RAY

Findings on chest x-ray are frequently related to an underlying pulmonary process or the presence of congenital heart disease. In the absence of these disorders, the chest x-ray in children with pulmonary embolus may indicate cardiac enlargement,[140] selective pulmonary hypoperfusion,[97] parenchymal densities,[15, 41, 52, 125, 126] or central pulmonary artery engorgement[125] with diminished peripheral perfusion in more chronic states[4] and globally decreased flow in persistent fetal circulation of the newborn. Pleural effusions are present in many with embolism and infarction, including those with superior vena cava thrombosis resulting from central venous catheters.[98, 127] Calcification on x-ray has been described with a right atrial ball-valve thrombus, confirmed by echocardiography and cardiac catheterization, in an infant receiving hyperalimentation.[99] The chest x-ray in fat embolism often demonstrates interstitial infiltrates in a characteristic "snowstorm" pattern.[113, 115]

### ELECTROCARDIOGRAM

Descriptions of electrocardiographic changes following pulmonary embolism in infants and children are infrequent and derived entirely from isolated case reports. In the normal newborn, right ventricular forces predominate and gradually diminish over the course of the first year. Therefore, assessing right ventricular hypertrophy resulting from pulmonary emboli may be difficult, particularly without an earlier tracing for comparison. Nonetheless, abnormal electrocardiographic findings have been noted, including right axis deviation,[123, 128] right bundle branch block,[125] right atrial enlargement,[128, 129] and right ventricular hypertrophy.[128, 129] In addition, ST segment elevation[122, 123] or depression[111] has been observed. However, normal electrocardiograms have been noted in cases of significant pulmonary emboli,[97, 126] indicating the lack of sensitivity of this test.

### ARTERIAL BLOOD GASES

As with other laboratory tests associated with pulmonary embolus in children, arterial blood gas data are relatively scant. Most reports indicate the presence of arterial hypoxemia ranging from a $PO_2$ of 24 to 73 mm Hg.[11, 97, 101, 114, 115, 123, 126, 130] The $PCO_2$ decreases to 24 to 34 mm Hg, reflecting hyperventilation in some[123, 126] and respiratory compensation for metabolic acidosis[42, 97] in others.

## Cardiac Catheterization

A small number of children have undergone cardiac catheterization for confirmation of presumptive pulmonary embolus. Hemodynamic data have shown elevated pulmonary artery pressure ranging from one-half systemic to suprasystemic levels.[82, 123, 125, 129] Pulmonary angiography has disclosed obstruction of large pulmonary arteries[123, 125, 126] as well as loss of visualization of smaller peripheral vessels[82, 129] and, in some instances, has demonstrated pulmonary artery aneurysms with thrombus formation.[64] In several other studies of patients with intracardiac thrombus, the right atrial mean pressures were increased but no evidence of pulmonary embolus was found on angiography.[77, 99] Cardiac catheterization in infants with persistent fetal circulation has been performed frequently and demonstrates near-systemic or suprasystemic pulmonary artery pressure with right-to-left shunting at the ductal level, atrial level, or both, resulting in arterial desaturation.[55] Lesions consistent with pulmonary emboli are generally not appreciated, although they are demonstrated in some at postmortem examination.[56]

Cardiac catheterization with angiography is more accurate than other methods for confirming the diagnosis of pulmonary embolism in adults.[131, 132] Its limited use in pediatrics probably results most often from failure to consider the diagnosis ante mortem. In those individuals in whom the differential diagnosis includes pulmonary embolism, some die before reaching the catheterization laboratory, whereas in others, catheterization and angiography have been considered too risky and of little potential benefit in an unstable patient.

Use of digital subtraction angiography may represent the best alternative, because small amounts of contrast material may be injected through peripheral venous access sites, thereby minimizing the invasiveness and risks of the procedure, while still providing high-resolution images of the pulmonary arterial bed. Use of a 9-inch image intensifier, although suboptimal in adults, provides an excellent field size in younger children and infants (Fig. 12–6). In addition, use of cardiac cycle–gated techniques may decrease the difficulty posed by motion artifact.[133] Further evaluation of this technique in children seems warranted and requires comparison with lung scanning and conventional pulmonary angiography to determine its utility.

### Contrast Venography

Injections of contrast material in peripheral vessels have helped to determine the presence of deep leg vein thrombosis as well as obstruction from thrombus in thoracic venous structures or the right heart.[77, 98, 99, 127, 134] Technically, deep leg vein phlebograms in children are relatively easy to obtain and involve minimal risk in the several large series reported.[29, 145, 147] The studies have confirmed the presence of deep venous thrombosis following prolonged immobilization,[29] infection,[145, 147] surgery,[136] and trauma,[26] thus permitting the judicious institution of anticoagulant therapy.

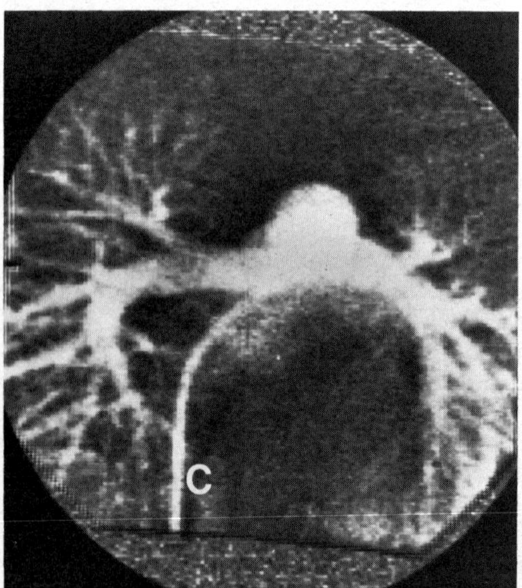


*Figure 12–6.* Normal digital subtraction pulmonary angiogram in a six-month-old infant. The catheter (C) was advanced from the right femoral vein. A 9-inch image intensifier was utilized.

### Radionuclide Scanning

Perfusion scans of the pulmonary bed are widely used in adults to assess the involvement of the vascular compartment in disease states. The technique is sensitive for highlighting abnormalities but lacks specificity. In children with possible pulmonary embolus, the lack of prospective studies comparing the scan with angiography makes it impossible to assess the utility of scanning. Isolated case reports exist in which the scan successfully predicted a pulmonary embolus that was confirmed subsequently by arteriogram or postmortem examination.[123, 126] The technique has also been applied in a case of suspected fat embolism in which a diffuse, nonsegmental pattern of abnormal perfusion was demonstrated, supporting the diagnosis.[115] In addition, a normal lung scan in the presence of massive right atrial ball-valve thrombus diagnosed by venography made the presence of distal embolization highly unlikely.

Radionuclide venography utilizing $^{99m}Tc$ macroaggregated albumin (see Chapter 4) was successful in diagnosing deep vein thrombosis in an infant who concurrently showed a small perfusion defect of the right lung consistent with a pulmonary embolus.[135] Although resolution does not compare with that of contrast venography (see Chapter 4), the radionuclide method is able to provide simultaneous information regarding two separate vascular beds (deep leg veins and pulmonary arteries) with minimal risk.

More widespread use of the radionuclide scanning technique in pulmonary embolism will help to assess its usefulness. Doppler ultrasound, impedance plethysmography,[125] and radioiodinated fibrinogen uptake have not been used enough to assess their utility in the pediatric patient.

## TREATMENT

Following diagnosis of venous thromboembolic disease in children, therapy is directed toward maintenance of adequate ventilation and circulatory support. Underlying infections are treated with antibiotics; indwelling catheters serving as possible sources of thrombus are removed whenever possible. Intralipid therapy and other infused vessel irritants should be at least temporarily withheld, and polycythemic patients should undergo phlebotomy to decrease blood hyperviscosity. In addition to these maneuvers, potential therapy includes anticoagulants, thrombolytic agents, embolectomy, or interruption of the venous embolic pathway. The experience with these modes of therapy in children with venous thromboemboli is limited.

### Anticoagulation

Despite the frequent use of heparin for treatment of deep vein thrombosis and pulmonary embolism in children,[8, 26, 27, 97, 123, 125, 126, 135, 136] no large case series has been reported that provides dosage recommendations or assessment of heparin's clinical efficacy. Newborn infants often demonstrate accelerated whole blood clotting time,[137] despite a prolonged activated partial thromboplastin time (PTT).[137, 138] However, in a comparison study of pharmacokinetics following single-bolus infusions of heparin in normal newborn infants and adults, a larger volume of distribution, faster clearance, and shorter plasma half-life were found for heparin in the infants.[139] A follow-up evaluation in which heparin was administered continuously to a group of infants with predominantly arterial thrombosis confirmed the existence of increased heparin clearance in younger individuals.[140] To achieve satisfactory steady state levels, we suggest heparin administration by continuous infusion.

Despite the presence of low levels of serum antithrombin III in infants, which might be expected to interfere with effective heparin anticoagulation, adequate clinical response has been obtained using doses of 16 to 35 U/kg/hr (mean = 27 U/kg/hr).[140] Further study is warranted utilizing a seven- to 10-day protocol to determine the applicability of these results to children with deep vein thrombosis or pulmonary embolism.

Prophylactic use of low doses of heparin administered subcutaneously prior to surgery in adults has been shown to decrease the frequency of deep vein thrombosis and pulmonary embolism in certain types of surgery[142–144] (see Chapter 8), but no data are available regarding the efficacy of venous thromboembolism prophylaxis in children. Warfarin therapy for prolonged anticoagulation in chronic disease states has not undergone extensive evaluation in children, but it is widely used clinically for prophylaxis in younger children after valve replacement with nontissue mechanical prostheses. Prothrombin time adjusted to 150 to 200 per cent of control values is a reasonable target for clinical effect. Thrombolytic therapy for venous thromboembolism in children should be assessed in clinical trials.

### Surgical Procedures

The surgical approach has been used in children both for interruption of the inferior vena cava and for thrombus removal.[64, 123, 125] Thrombectomy for deep vein thrombosis has been employed successfully but rarely in younger individuals.[8, 145] However, most have improved without surgery by using heparin and warfarin anticoagulation. A relative indication for thrombectomy exists in renal vein thrombosis with bilateral renal vein involvement and caval extension.[36, 146] However, utilization of thrombolytic agents in the future may establish medical therapy as the preferred approach in infants with the disorder. Surgical closure of a ventricular septal defect for recurrent septic pulmonary emboli has been reported[15] and probably represents the therapy of choice.

## SUMMARY

Advances in pediatric pulmonary thromboembolism are limited by underdiagnosis of the disorder ante mortem, even though it is not infrequently found at postmortem examination. Failure to consider the diagnosis generally occurs because serious concurrent medical illness may obscure the presence of pulmonary embolism. In turn, because the diagnosis is rarely postulated, assessment of those diagnostic modalities well described in adult patients has not been possible in children. Even in the rare instances in which venous thromboembolism is detected in children ante mortem, standard pediatric therapeutic regimens have not been established, emphasizing the need for well-controlled clinical trials to determine dosage, efficacy, and safety of anticoagulants and thrombolytic agents. Future improvements in diagnosis and therapy will be possible only after recognition of pulmonary embolism as an important disease entity in children.

## REFERENCES


1. Löeschner, J. W.: Phlebitis venae cruralis sinistrae, peri- et myocarditis, embolia et oedema pulmonum. Jahrb. Kinderh. Phys. Erziehung, *4*:66, 1861.
2. Buck, J. R., Connors, R. H., Coon, W. W., et al.: Pulmonary embolism in children. J. Ped. Surg., *16*:385, 1981.
3. Zuschlag, E.: Infarction of the lung in children. Am. J. Dis. Child., *74*:399, 1947.
4. Stevenson, G. F., and Stevenson, F. L.: Pulmonary embolism in childhood. J. Pediatr., *34*:62, 1949.
5. DeCamp, P. T., and Ochsner, A.: Thrombo-embolism in children. Analysis of 35 cases. Ann. Surg., *133*:611, 1951.
6. Emery, J. L.: Pulmonary embolism in children. Arch. Dis. Child., *37*:591, 1962.
7. Jones, R. H., and Sabiston, D. C.: Pulmonary embolism in childhood. Monog. Surg. Sci., *3*:35, 1966.
8. Jones, D. R. B., and MacIntyre, I. M. C.: Venous thromboembolism in infancy and childhood. Arch. Dis. Child., *50*:153, 1975.
9. Hill, R. B.: Fatal fat embolism from steroid-induced fatty liver. New Engl. J. Med., *265*:318, 1961.
10. Barson, A. J., Chiswick, M. L.,and Doig, C. M.: Fat embolism in children after intravenous fat infusions. Arch. Dis. Child., *53*:218, 1978.
11. Weisz, G. M., Schramek, A., Abrahamson, J., et al.: Fat embolism in children: Tests for its early detection. J. Ped. Surg., *9*:163, 1974.
12. Haber, S. L., and Bennington, J. I.: Pulmonary embolism in an infant. J. Pediatr., *61*:759, 1962.
13. Hosoi, K.: Pulmonary embolism and infarction. Ann. Surg., *95*:67, 1932.
14. Crutcher, R. R., and Daniel, R. A.: Pulmonary embolism. Surgery, *23*:47, 1948.
15. Windsor, H. M., Noble, N., and Chang, V. P.: Infected ventricular septal defect. Aust. N.Z. J. Surg., *51*:271, 1981.
16. Wise, R. C., and Todd, J. K.: Spontaneous, lower-extremity venous thrombosis in children. Am. J. Dis. Child., *126*:766, 1973.
17. Krakower, C.: Pulmonary embolus containing cerebral tissue. Arch. Path., *22*:113, 1936.
18. Gardiner, W. R.: Massive pulmonary embolization of cerebral cortical tissue: An unusual fetal birth injury. Stanford Med. Bull., *14*:226, 1956.
19. Tryfus, H.: Massive pulmonary embolism of cerebellar tissue in a newborn. Arch. Dis. Child., *38*:292, 1963.
20. Valdes-Dapena, M. A., and Arey, J. B.: Pulmonary emboli of cerebral origin in the newborn. A report of two cases. Arch. Path., *84*:643, 1967.
21. Tan, K. L., and Hwang, W. S.: Neonatal brain tissue embolism in the lung. Aust. N.Z. J. Med., *6*:146, 1976.
22. Pillay, S. V.: Pulmonary embolism of cerebral tissue in a neonate. A case report. S. Afr. Med. J., *58*:498, 1980.
23. Bell, W. R., and Simon, T. L.: Current status of pulmonary thromboembolic disease: Pathophysiology, diagnosis, prevention, and treatment. Am. Heart J., *103*:239, 1982.
24. Horvath, F. L., Brodeur, A. E., and Cherry, J. D.: Deep thrombophlebitis associated with acute osteomyelitis. J. Pediatr., *79*:815, 1971.
25. Jupiter, J. B., Ehrlich, M. G., Novelline, R. A., et al.: The association of septic thrombophlebitis with subperiosteal abscesses in children. J. Pediatr., *101*:690, 1982.
26. Zionts, L. E., McCampbell, E. J., Szentfulopi, T., et al.: Deep vein thrombosis in children following trauma. A report of two cases. J. Bone Joint Surg., *65A*:839, 1983.
27. Leslie, I. J., Dorgan, J. C., and Bentley, G.: Deep-venous thrombosis in child during halofemoral traction. Lancet, *2*:847, 1979.
28. Hodgson, D. C.: Venous stasis during surgery. Anaesthesia, *19*:96, 1964.
29. Leslie, I. J., Dorgan, J. C., Bentley, G., et al.: A prospective study of deep vein thrombosis of the leg in children on halo-femoral traction. J. Bone Joint Surg., *63B*:168, 1981.
30. Oppenheimer, E. H., and Esterly, J. R.: Thrombosis in the newborn: Comparison between infants of diabetic and nondiabetic mothers. J. Pediatr., *67*:549, 1965.
31. Takeuchi, A., and Benirschke, K.: Renal vein thrombosis of the newborn and its relation to maternal diabetes. Biol. Neonat., *3*:257, 1961.
32. Ward, T. F.: Multiple thromboses in an infant of a diabetic mother. J. Pediatr., *90*:982, 1977.
33. Lewy, P. R., and Wellington, J.: Nephrotic syndrome in association with renal vein thrombosis in infancy. J. Pediatr., *85*:359, 1974.
34. Vorlicky, L. N., and Balfour, H. H.: Cytomegalovirus and renal vein thrombosis in a newborn infant. Am. J. Dis. Child., *127*:742, 1974.
35. Seeler, R. A.: Renal vein thrombosis in the newborn. JAMA, *213*:1906, 1970.
36. Duncan, R. E., Evans, A. T., and Martin, L. W.: Natural history and treatment of renal vein thrombosis in children. J. Ped. Surg., *12*:639, 1977.
37. Péhu, M. M., and Horand, R.: Gangrene pulmonaire embolique otogène chez un enfant de six ans. Lyon Med., *104*:1307, 1905.
38. Prettin, F.: Thrombose und tödliche Lungenembolie. Virchows Arch. f. Path. Anat., *297*:535, 1936.
39. Guillemot, L.: Gangrène pulmonaire otogène chez un nourrisson de 7 mois. Bull. Soc. de Pédiat. de Paris, *8*:229, 1906.
40. Jones, J. A.: Pulmonary embolism in an infant following aural infection. Lancet, *2*:1070, 1930.
41. Aziz, K. U., Newfeld, E. A., and Paul, M. H.: Echocardiographic detection of bacterial vegetations in a child with a ventricular septal defect. Chest, *70*:780, 1976.
42. Svane, S.: Primary thrombosis of a pulmonary artery in a child with tetralogy of Fallot. Br. Heart J., *39*:815, 1977.
43. Dormandy, J. A., and Edelman, J. B.: High blood viscosity: An aetiological factor in venous thrombosis. Br. J. Surg., *60*:187, 1973.
44. Kontras, S. B., Bodenbender, J., Craenen, J., et al.: Hyperviscosity in congenital heart disease. J. Pediatr., *76*:214, 1970.
45. Komp, D. M., and Sparrow, A. W.: Polycythemia in cyanotic heart disease—a study of altered coagulation. J. Pediatr., *76*:231, 1970.

46. Best, P. V., and Heath, D.: Pulmonary thrombosis in cyanotic congenital heart disease without pulmonary hypertension. J. Path. Bact., *75*:281, 1958.
47. Ferencz, C.: The pulmonary vascular bed in tetralogy of Fallot. Bull. Johns Hopkins Hosp., *106*:81, 100, 1960.
48. Ferencz, C.: Pulmonary vascular changes in tetralogy of Fallot. Dis. Chest, *46*:664, 1964.
49. Ring, A., and Bakke, J. R.: Chronic massive pulmonary artery thrombosis. Ann. Intern. Med., *43*:781, 1955.
50. Ball, K., Goodwin, J. F., and Harrison, C. V.: Massive thrombotic occlusion of the large pulmonary arteries. Circulation, *14*:766, 1956.
51. Dickinson, L.: Thrombosis of the pulmonary artery in a case of congenital stenosis of the orifice. Trans. Path. Soc. London, *48*:57, 1897.
52. Harvey, E. B., and Hogg, P.: Thrombosis of the pulmonary artery in children. Am. J. Dis. Child., *71*:67, 1946.
53. Gersony, W. M., Duc, G. V., and Sinclair, J. C.: "PFC" syndrome (persistence of the fetal circulation). Circulation, *40*(Suppl. 3):87, 1969.
54. Levin, D. L., Heymann, M. A., Kitterman, J. A., et al.: Persistent pulmonary hypertension of the newborn infant. J. Pediatr., *89*:626, 1976.
55. Peckham, G. J., and Fox, W. W.: Physiologic factors affecting pulmonary artery pressure in infants with persistent pulmonary artery hypertension. J. Pediatr., *93*:1005, 1978.
56. Levin, D. L., Weinberg, A. E., and Perkin, R. M.: Pulmonary microthrombi syndrome in newborn infants with unresponsive persistent pulmonary artery hypertension. J. Pediatr., *102*:299, 1983.
57. Suzuki, S., Wake, N., and Yoshiaki, K.: New neonatal problems of blood coagulation and fibrinolysis. II. Thromboplastic effect of amniotic fluid and its relation to lung maturity. J. Perinat. Med., *4*:221, 1976.
58. Segall, M. L., Goetzman, B. W., and Schick, J. B.: Thrombocytopenia and pulmonary hypertension in the perinatal aspiration syndromes. J. Pediatr., *96*:727, 1980.
59. Morrow, W. R., Haas, J. E., and Benjamin, D. R.: Nonbacterial endocardial thrombosis in neonates: Relationship to persistent fetal circulation. J. Pediatr., *100*:117, 1982.
60. Stenmark, K. R., James, S. L., Voelkel, N. F., et al.: Leukotriene $C_4$ and $D_4$ in neonates with hypoxemia and pulmonary hypertension. New Engl. J. Med., *309*:77, 1983.
61. Hughes, J. P., and Stovin, P. G. I.: Segmental pulmonary artery aneurysms with peripheral venous thrombosis. Br. J. Dis. Chest, *53*:19, 1959.
62. Beattie, J. M., and Hall, A. J.: Multiple embolic aneurysms of the pulmonary arteries from veins of leg. Death from rupture of the aneurysm into the lung. Proc. Roy. Soc. Med., *5*:147, 1911–1912.
63. Frater, R. W. M., Beck, W., and Schrire, V.: The syndrome of pulmonary artery aneurysms, pulmonary artery thrombi and peripheral venous thrombi. J. Thorac. Cardiovasc. Surg., *49*:330, 1965.
64. Roberts, D. H., Jiminez, J. F., and Golladay, E. S.: Multiple pulmonary artery aneurysms and peripheral venous thromboses—the Hughes-Stovin syndrome. Pediatr. Radiol., *12*:214, 1982.
65. Egeberg, O.: Inherited deficiency causing thrombophilia. Thromb. Diath. Haemorrh., *13*:516, 1965.
66. Marciniak, E., Farley, C. H., and De Simone, P. A.: Familial thrombosis due to antithrombin III deficiency. Blood, *43*:219, 1974.
67. Mackie, M., Bennet, B., Ogston, D., et al.: Familial thrombosis: Inherited deficiency of antithrombin III. Br. Med. J., *1*:136, 1978.
68. Mendelsohn, G., Gomperts, E. D., and Gurwitz, D.: Severe antithrombin III deficiency in an infant associated with multiple arterial and venous thromboses. Thromb. Haemost. (Stuttg.), *36*:495, 1976.
69. Leone, G., Volari, V. M., Shorti, S., and Myers, T. J.: Inferior vena cava thrombosis in a child with familial antithrombin III deficiency. Thromb. Haemost., *43*:74, 1980.
70. Haas, H. A., Scully, M. F., and Clark, S. E.: A case of familial antithrombin III deficiency in an English family. Thromb. Haemost., *42*:185, 1979.
71. Campbell, W. A., and Price, W. H.: Venous thromboembolic disease in Klinefelter's syndrome. Clin. Genet., *19*:275, 1981.
72. Singleton, E. B., and Rosenberg, H. S.: Intraluminal calcification of the inferior vena cava. AJR, *86*:556, 1961.
73. Kassner, E. G., Baumstark, A., Kinkhabwala, M. N., et al.: Calcified thrombosis in the inferior vena cava in infants and children. Pediatr. Radiol., *4*:167, 1976.
74. Schullinger, T. N., Santulli, T. V., Berdon, W. E., et al.: Calcific thrombi of the inferior vena cava in infants and children. J. Pediatr. Surg., *13*:429, 1978.
75. Kirks, D. R., Ponzi, J. W., and Korobkin, M.: Computed tomographic diagnosis of calcified inferior vena cava thrombus in a child with Wilms' tumor. Pediatr. Radiol., *10*:110, 1980.
76. Noonan, J. A.: Pulmonary thromboembolism in children. *In* Mobin-Uddin, K. (Ed.): Pulmonary Thromboembolism. Charles C Thomas, Springfield, Ill., 1975, p. 137.
77. Anselmi, G., Suarez, J. A., Machado, I., et al.: Wilms' tumor propagated through the inferior vena cava into the right heart cavities. Br. Heart J., *32*:575, 1970.
78. Shurtleff, D. B., and Foltz, E. L.: Clinical observations on 20 hydrocephalic children subjected to ventriculo-atrial shunt: A preliminary report (abstr.). Am. J. Dis. Child., *98*:467, 1959.
79. Anderson, F. M.: Ventriculo-cardiac shunts. J. Pediatr., *82*:222, 1973.
80. Emery, J. L., and Hilton, H. B.: Lung and heart complications of treatment of hydrocephalus with ventriculo-atrial shunt. Surgery, *50*:309, 1961.
81. Friedman, S., Zita Gozum, C., and Chaten, J.: Pulmonary vascular change complicating ventriculo-vascular shunting for hydrocephalus. J. Pediatr., *64*:305, 1964.
82. Sperling, D. R., Patrick, J. R., Anderson, F. M., et al.: Cor pulmonale secondary to ventriculo-auriculostomy. Am. J. Dis. Child., *107*:308, 1964.
83. Boizsen, E., and Lundstrom, N. R.: Percutaneous cardiac catheterization and angiocardiography in infants and children. Am. J. Cardiol., *22*:572, 1968.
84. Simovitch, H., Hohn, A. R., Wagner, H. R., et al.: Percutaneous right and left heart catheterization in children: Experience with 1000 patients. Circulation, *41*:513, 1970.
85. Hawker, R. E., Celermajer, J. M., Cartmill, J. B., et al.: Thrombosis of the inferior vena cava following balloon septostomy in transposition of the great arteries. Am. Heart J., *82*:593, 1971.
86. Kirkpatrick, S. E., Takahashi, M., Petry, E. L., et al.: Percutaneous heart catheterization in infants and children: II. Prospective study of results and complications in 127 consecutive cases. Circulation, *42*:1049, 1970.

87. Kuehl, K. S., Perry, L. W., and Scott, L. P.: Thrombosis of the inferior vena cava in patients with cyanotic congenital heart disease. J. Pediatr., *79*:430, 1971.
88. Wigger, H. J., Bransilver, B. R., and Blanc, W. A.: Thromboses due to catheterization in infants and children. J. Pediatr., *76*:1. 1970.
89. Porter, C. J., Gillette, P. C., Mullins, C. E., et al.: Cardiac catheterization in the neonate: A comparison of three techniques. J. Pediatr., *93*:97, 1978.
90. Matthews, R. A., Park, S. C., Neches, W. H., et al.: Iliac venous thrombosis in infants and children after cardiac catheterization. Cathet. Cardiovasc. Diagn., *5*:67, 1979.
91. Keane, J. F., Lang, P., Newburger, J., et al.: Iliac vein-inferior caval thrombosis after cardiac catheterization in infancy. Pediatr. Cardiol., *1*:257, 1980.
92. Carter, G. A., Girod, D. A., and Hurwitz, R. A.: Percutaneous catheterization of the neonate. Pediatrics, *55*:662, 1975.
93. Firor, H. S.: Pulmonary embolization complicating total intravenous alimentation. J. Ped. Surg., *7*:81, 1972.
94. Ryan, J. A., Abel, R. M., Abbott, W. M., et al.: Catheter complications in total parenteral nutrition. New Engl. J. Med., *290*:757, 1974.
95. Muller, K. M., and Blaeser, B.: Fatal thromboembolism after central-vein catheterisation. Dtsch. Med. Wochenschr., *101*:411, 1976.
96. Nichols, M. M., and Tyson, K. R. T.: Saddle embolus occluding pulmonary arteries. Am. J. Dis. Child., *132*:926, 1978.
97. Wesley, J. R., Keens, T. G., Miller, S. W., et al.: Pulmonary embolism in the neonate: Occurrence during the course of total parenteral nutrition. J. Pediatr., *93*:113, 1978.
98. Kramer, S. S., Taylor, G. A., Garfinkel, D. J., et al.: Lethal chylothoraces due to superior vena caval thrombosis in infants. AJR, *137*:559, 1981.
99. Pliam, M. B., McGough, E. C., Nixon, G. W., et al.: Right atrial ball-valve thrombus: A complication of central venous alimentation in an infant. Diagnosis and surgical management of a case. J. Thorac. Cardiovasc. Surg., *78*:579, 1979.
100. Todres, I. D., Crone, R. K., Rogers, M. C., et al.: Swan-Ganz catheterization in the critically ill newborn. Crit. Care Med., *7*:330, 1979.
101. Pokora, T. J., Boros, S. J., Brennom, W. S., et al.: Fatal neonatal thrombosis associated with a pulmonary arterial catheter. Crit. Care Med., *9*:618, 1981.
102. Enger, E., Jacobson, B., and Sorenson, S. F.: Tissue toxicity of intravenous solutions. A phlebographic and experimental study. Acta Paediatr. Scand., *65*:248, 1976.
103. Askanazy, M.: Contribution to the relationship between malformation and tumor based on an observation of a unique encephalocele with gliomas in the lung. Arch. Geb. Path. Anat. Inst. zu Tübingen *6*:433, 1908.
104. Hückel, R.: On ectopic glial tissue in the lung of a newborn with frontal encephalocele. Verhandl. Deutsch Path. Gesellsch., *24*:272, 1919.
105. Gruenwald, P.: Emboli of brain tissue on fetal lungs. Am. J. Path., *17*:879, 1914.
106. Potter, E. L., and Young, R. L.: Heterotopic brain tissue in the lungs of two anencephalic monsters. Arch. Path., *34*:1009, 1942.
107. Ygge, J.: Changes in blood coagulation and fibrinolysis during the puerperium. Am. J. Obstet. Gynecol., *104*:2, 1969.
108. Bell, W. R., Simon, T. L., and De Mets, D. L.: The clinical features of submassive and massive pulmonary emboli. Am. J. Med., *62*:355, 1977.
109. Cosgriff, S. W., Diefenbach, A. F., and Vogt, W.: Hypercoagulability of the blood associated with ACTH and cortisone therapy. Am. J. Med., *9*:752, 1950.
110. Cosgriff, S. W.: Thromboembolic complications associated with ACTH and cortisone therapy. JAMA, *147*:924, 1951.
111. Gootman, N., Gross, J., and Mensch, A.: Pulmonary artery thrombosis. A complication occurring with prednisone and chlorothiazide therapy in two nephrotic patients. Pediatrics, *34*:861, 1964.
112. James, E. S.: Fat embolism. Can. Med. Assoc. J., *62*:548, 1950.
113. Drummond, D. S., Salter, R. B., and Boone, J.: Fat embolism in children: Its frequency and relationships to collagen disease. Can. Med. Assoc. J., *101*:200, 1969.
114. Weisz, G. M., Rang, M., and Salter, R. B.: Posttraumatic fat embolism in children: Review of the literature and of experience in the Hospital for Sick Children, Toronto. J. Trauma, *13*:529, 1973.
115. Limbird, T. J., and Ruderman, R. J.: Fat embolism in children. Clin. Orthop., *136*:267, 1978.
116. Peltier, L. F.: An appraisal of the problem of fat embolism. Int. Abst. Surg., *104*:313, 1957.
117. Gauss, H.: The pathology of fat embolism. Arch. Surg. (Chicago), *9*:593, 1924.
118. Shulman, S. T., and Grossman, B. J.: Fat embolism in children. Am. J. Dis. Child., *120*:480, 1970.
119. Barness, L. A., Dallman, P. R., and Anderson, H.: Use of intravenous fat emulsions in pediatric patients. Pediatrics, *68*:738, 1981.
120. Wretlind, A.: Complete intravenous nutrition. Theoretical and experimental background. Nutr. Metab., *14*(Suppl.):1, 1972.
121. Gustafson, A., Kjellmer, I., and Oligard, R.: Nutrition in low birth weight infants. II. Repeat injections of fat emulsion. Acta Ped. Scand., *63*:177, 1974.
122. Cohen, S. I., Hecht, H., Cantor, J., et al.: Flow murmur associated with partial occlusion of the right pulmonary artery. Am. Heart J., *90*:376, 1975.
123. Croyle, P. H., Place, R. A., and Hilgenberg, A. D.: Massive pulmonary embolism in a high school wrestler. JAMA, *241*:827, 1979.
124. Adams, C. B. T.: The retinal manifestations of fat embolism. Injury, *2*:221, 1971.
125. Banks, D. C., Raftery, E. B., and Oram, S.: Thromboembolic pulmonary hypertension of unusual cause in a teenager. Br. Med. J., *3*:563, 1970.
126. Nudelman, R., Best, L., and Tharp, S.: Pulmonary embolism in a 14 year old following an elective abortion. Pediatrics, *68*:584, 1981.
127. Dhande, V., Kattwinkel, J., and Alford, B.: Recurrent bilateral pleural effusions secondary to superior vena cava obstruction as a complication of central venous catheterization. Pediatrics, *72*:109, 1983.
128. McMahon, D. P., and Aterman, K.: Pulmonary hypertension due to multiple emboli. J. Pediatr., *92*:841, 1978.
129. Talner, N. S., Liu, H., Oberman, H. A., et al.: Thromboembolism complicating Holter valve shunt. Am. J. Dis. Child., *101*:602, 1961.

130. Krous, H. F.: Neonatal nonbacterial thrombotic endocarditis. Arch. Path. Lab. Med., *103*:76, 1979.
131. Dalen, J. E., Brooks, H. L., Johnson, L. W., et al.: Pulmonary angiography in acute pulmonary embolism: Indications, techniques, and results in 367 patients. Am. Heart J., *81*:175, 1971.
132. Gilday, D. L., Poulose, K. P., and Deland, F. H.: Accuracy of detection of pulmonary embolism by lung scanning correlated with pulmonary angiography. AJR, *115*:732, 1972.
133. Goldhaber, S. Z., and Markisz, J.: Digital subtraction angiography: An internist's and radiologist's view. Cardiovasc. Intervent. Radiol., *6*:239, 1983.
134. Rocchini, A. P., Cho, K. J., and Byrum, C.: Transluminal angioplasty of superior vena cava obstruction in a 15 month old child. Chest, *82*:506, 1982.
135. DeLong, S. R., Gober, A. E., Fernandez-Ulloa, M., et al.: Iliofemoral venous thrombosis in an infant: Diagnosis by radionuclide venography. J. Pediatr., *94*:91, 1979.
136. Joffe, S.: Postoperative deep vein thrombosis in children. J. Ped. Surg., *10*:539, 1975.
137. Barnard, D. R., and Hathaway, W. E.: Neonatal thrombosis. Am. J. Pediatr. Hematol. Oncol., *1*:235, 1979.
138. Barnard, D. R., Simmons, M. A., and Hathaway, W. E.: Coagulation studies in extremely young premature infants. Pediatr. Res., *13*:1330, 1979.
139. McDonald, M. M., Jacobson, L. J., Hay, W. W., et al.: Heparin clearance in the newborn. Pediatr. Res., *15*:1015, 1981.
140. McDonald, M. M., and Hathaway, W. E.: Anticoagulant therapy by continuous heparization in newborn and older infants. J. Pediatr., *101*:451, 1982.
141. Negus, D., Freidgood, A., Cox, S. J., et al.: Ultra-low dose intravenous heparin in the prevention of postoperative deep vein thrombosis. Lancet, *1*:891, 1980.
142. Kakkar, V. V., Corrigan, T., Spindler, J., et al.: Efficacy of low doses of heparin in prevention of deep vein thrombosis after major surgery. Lancet, *2*:101, 1972.
143. Gallus, A. S., Hirsh, J., Tuttle, R. J., et al.: Small subcutaneous doses of heparin in prevention of venous thrombosis. New Engl. J. Med., *288*:545, 1973.
144. Nachbur, B., Baumgartner, G., and Huser, J. J.: Deep thrombophlebitis of the lower extremities in children. Vasa, *8*:53, 1979.
145. Thompson, I. M., Schneider, R., and Lababidi, Z.: Thrombectomy for neonatal renal vein thrombosis. J. Urol., *113*:396, 1975.
146. Gorenstein, A., Gordon, R. L., Schiffrin, E., et al.: Phlebography of the deep venous system of the leg in children. Radiology, *144*:519, 1982.

PART IV

# FUTURE PROSPECTS

5. Alteration in the anticoagulant—ACD: saline ratio[30, 33]

We have found that the best platelet preparation is achieved by using a modification of Heaton's method.[8] The platelet suspension is incubated at room temperature (22° C) for 20 minutes using the desired activity of indium-111 chloride in dilute HCl, complexed to 50 μl of 8-OH quinoline (oxine) in absolute alcohol (1 mg/ml) diluted in 4 ml of a solution of ACD:saline (1:7), the pH of which is adjusted to 6.5 to 7.0. Centrifugation forces of 200 G × 15 minutes for platelet harvesting and 2000 G × 5 minutes for washings are used.[14]

Of interest is a method developed by Hawker[11] that demands only 26 ml of blood for platelet harvesting and requires only 45 minutes from the initial drawing of blood to reinjection of the labeled platelet suspension. This halves both the volume of blood required and the procedural time of the more established methods while apparently preserving physiologic function. It therefore may be adopted as the preferred method for widespread use.

## ANIMAL STUDIES (Table 13–2)

Using experimentally induced venous thrombi in a dog model, workers have attempted to define the following:

1. The diagnostic accuracy of the technique
2. The optimal time delay from injection of the platelet suspension to imaging of the area of interest
3. The effect of antiplatelet and anticoagulant therapy as well as thrombus age on the sensitivity of the thrombus visualization by platelet scintigraphy

These studies have demonstrated that imaging of fresh venous thrombi and pulmonary emboli is possible within an hour of injection of labeled platelets. Thrombi older than six hours may be imaged with lower sensitivity. Heparin administered intravenously by continuous infusion inhibits platelet uptake on established thrombi, provided the activated partial thromboplastin time is maintained at 2.5 times baseline values. This effect is reversed by protamine and heparin's biologic decay.

Sostman and coworkers[21] have shown that Renografin-76 injected intraarterially immediately before platelet injection does not affect venous thrombus visualization in dogs, whereas others have shown that platelet aggregation is inhibited by contrast agents both in vivo and in vitro.[34, 35] Inhibition of aggregation may only apply to certain types of contrast media and needs further study.

This work in animals has provided a firm basis for potentially rewarding studies in humans.

## STUDIES IN HUMANS (Table 13–3; Figures 13–1 and 13–2)

Since 1978, several studies have been performed in humans. All demonstrate the feasibility of platelet scintigraphy with respect to the diagnosis of deep vein thrombosis and pulmonary embolism.

In the first systematic study performed, Fenech and coworkers[24] found a sensitivity of 95 per cent and a specificity of 100 per cent for a diagnosis of deep vein thrombosis (see Table 13–3). Successful imaging was possible within one hour after injection of the platelet suspension. We studied 76 consecutive patients following a major orthopedic procedure. In 64, venograms were obtained within eight days following surgery. For analysis, the limb was divided into two segments (above and below the knee). The overall sensitivity and specificity rates were 90 and 95 per cent, respectively. Potential sources of false-positive studies included hematoma, wounds, platelet accumulation around freshly implanted orthopedic prostheses, infection, and platelet uptake by prosthetic arterial grafts—both Dacron grafts and saphenous bypass grafts. With experience, however, these entities were in most cases easily differentiated from true venous thrombi. This study nevertheless emphasizes the need to identify nonvenous hematoma or wounds as well as orthopedic and vascular prostheses prior to the interpretation of the platelet images. Sources of infection tend to produce a diffuse area of uptake that does not conform to any well-defined vascular channel. Uptake by surgical wounds can be minimized by the injection of platelets 24 to 48 hours following surgery.

Although controversy exists concerning the optimum therapy for patients with deep venous thrombosis, the consensus favors intravenous heparin as an effective agent in preventing platelet accumulation on established thrombi, provided the activated partial thromboplastin time is maintained at 2.5 times control values.

***Table 13–2.*** Studies in Animals for Diagnosis of Deep Vein Thrombosis and Pulmonary Emboli

| Author | Labeling Medium | Harvesting Forces | Washing Forces | Reference Standard DVT | Reference Standard PE | Conclusion |
|---|---|---|---|---|---|---|
| Thakur[1] | NS | 180 G × 15 min | 1500 G × 15 min | Venography + surgery | ND | 1. Possible to identify DVT within 50 minutes of injection of platelet suspension<br>2. 100% accurate |
| McIlmoyle[4] | NS | 480 G × 15 min | 1500 G × 15 min | ND | Autopsy | 1. 70% autopsy proved PE identified by PS |
| Knight[9] | ACD/NS | 180 G × 15 min | 1700 G × 15 min | Autopsy | ND | 1. Possible to identify DVT within 2 hours of injection of platelet suspension<br>2. Optimal time for imaging 12–15 hrs after injection of platelets. Up to 6-hr-old DVT visualized; older thrombus not visualized |
| Moser[19] | NS | 7000 G × 45 sec<br>or<br>200 G × 15 min | 700 G × 20 sec<br>200 G × 15 min<br>or<br>1400 G × 10 min | Autopsy | Autopsy | 1. Heparin inhibits platelet accumulation on thrombi. This effect is reversed by protamine |
| Fedullo[20] | NS | 200 G × 15 min | 1400 G × 10 min | None | None | 1. Labeled platelet accumulation on DVT inhibited by IV heparin at APTT 2.5 times control. Reversed by biologic decay of heparin and protamine |
| Sostman[21] | NS | 180 G × 15 min | 1500 G × 15 min | None | Autopsy | 1. PE identified up to 72 hours after formation<br>2. IV heparin prevented platelet accumulation; protamine and biologic decay of heparin reversed this |

Abbreviations: ACD = acid citrate dextrose, G = gravitational force, NS = normal saline, DVT = deep vein thrombosis, PS = platelet scintigraphy, PE = pulmonary emboli, ND = not done, min = minutes, sec = seconds, APTT = activated partial thromboplastin time.

***Table 13–3.*** Studies in Humans Using Platelet Scintigraphy to Diagnose Deep Venous Thrombosis and Pulmonary Embolism

| Author | n | Patient Population | Labeling Medium | Harvesting Forces | Washing Forces | μCi Injected | Conclusion |
|---|---|---|---|---|---|---|---|
| Goodwin[7] | 6 | 3 venogram + 1 PA − 2 VQ + IPG + | Plasma | 200 G × 5 min | 1000 G × 5–15 min | 200–500 | 1. 5/5 positive by venography or VQ scan were positive by PS 2. 1 patient negative by PS and PA |
| Davis[22] | 2 | 2 venogram + | Modified Tyrodes | 180 G × 15 min or | 1500 G × 15 min or | 500 | 1. Both positive by PS |
| Davis[23] | 20 | 3 venogram + 2 PA and VQ + 4 IPG + | Modified Tyrodes or ACD/saline | 200 G × 15 min | 2000 G × 10–15 min | 100–550 | 1. 6/7 positive by IPG or venography were positive by PS 2. 1/11 with positive VQ scan or PA was positive by PS; all 10 negative by PS on IV heparin 3. 6/6 with positive PS and IPG or venography on IV heparin APTT between 2.0 and 2.5 |
| Fenech[24] | 48 | 33 fractured femurs, 15 clin. susp. DVT; all had venography | Tyrodes Calcium free and $PGE_1$ | 200 G × 10 min | 640 G × 10 min | 180–220 | 1. Sensitivity 95%, specificity 100% |
| Grimley[25] | 27 | All had venography | | (See Fenech[24]) | | 150 | 1. Correlation between venography and PS 84%. 2 FP with thigh thrombosis; 1 FP in the calf |
| Ezekowitz[26] | 1 | Case report PE | ACD/saline | 200 G × 15 min | 2000 G × 5 min | 622 | 1. Identification of PE surgically proven in spite of 25,000 IU heparin IV for 5 weeks |
| Sostman[27] | 1 | Case report PE | | (See Thakur[16]) | | | 1. Identification of PE off heparin |
| Ezekowitz[28] | 108 | 1. Clinically suspected DVT (n = 30) 2. Postop. orthop. procedure (n = 76) | ACD/saline | 200 G × 15 min | 2000 G × 5 min | 300–500 | 1. DVT may be identified within 1 hr of injection of labeled platelets 2. Technique 100% sensitive in patients off IV heparin |

Abbreviations: n = number, + = positive, − = negative, VQ scan = ventilation perfusion scan, PS = pulmonary scintigraphy, PA = pulmonary angiography, IPG = impedance plethysmography, min = minutes, PE = pulmonary embolism, postop = postoperative, $PGE_1$ = prostaglandin $E_1$, APTT = activated partial thromboplastin time, FP = false-positive.

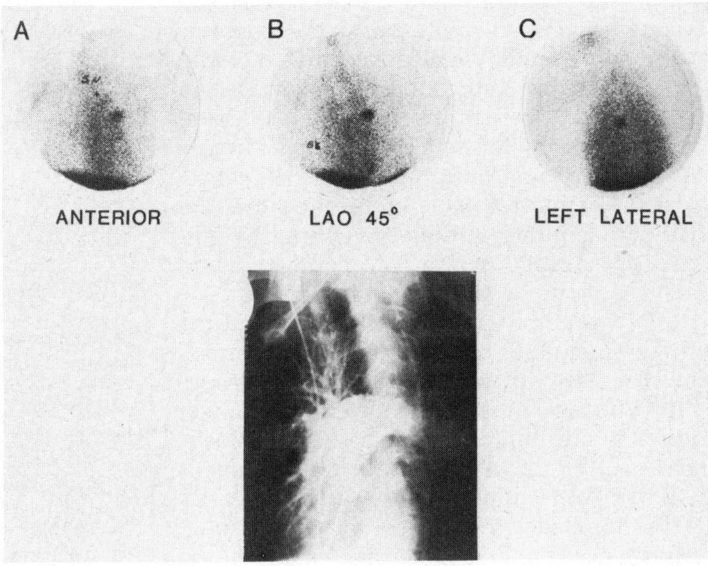


***Figure 13–1.*** Upper panels: *A, B,* and *C* represent scintiphotos obtained 96 hours after injection of the platelet suspension. Lower panel: Pulmonary angiogram in left anterior oblique view. All images are oriented with the top cephalad. In the upper panels *A, B,* and *C,* the increased activity represents a pulmonary artery embolus. The corresponding pulmonary angiogram demonstrates complete obstruction of the left pulmonary artery. (From Ezekowitz, M. D., et al.: Diagnosis of a persistent pulmonary embolus by Indium-111 platelet scintigraphy with angiographic and tissue confirmation. Am. J. Med., *72*:839–842, 1982.)

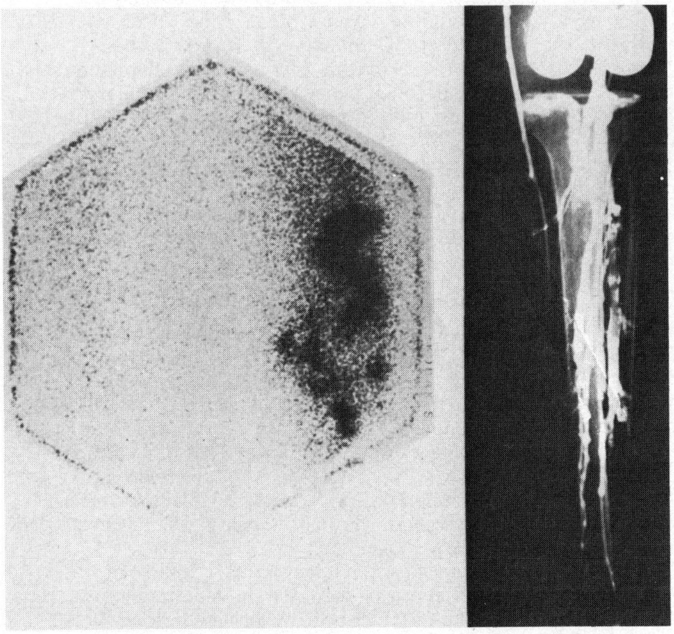

***Figure 13–2.*** The image on the left is a scintiphoto of both lower limbs obtained 48 hours after injection of the platelet suspension. The area of increased activity in the left lower limb reflects an extensive deep venous thrombosis that corresponds to the venogram on the adjacent panel. These images were obtained four days after a total knee replacement.

To determine the effects of intravenous heparin on the incorporation of platelets into acute venous thrombi, we studied 30 patients with clinically suspected deep vein thrombosis. All patients had a clinically indicated venogram. Patients with positive venograms were all treated with intravenous heparin unless a contraindication to anticoagulant therapy was present. The sensitivity of platelet scintigraphy for detecting venous thrombi fell from 90 to 39 per cent. This difference was directly attributable to the effect of intravenous heparin. Studies evaluating the efficacy of aspirin, dipyridamole, coumadin, and subcutaneous heparin are under way.

Only three reports have demonstrated the successful identification of pulmonary emboli in man.[7, 26, 27] It appears that intravenous heparin effectively prevents platelet accumulation at sites of embolism. The diagnostic accuracy of the technique in this setting is yet to be determined.

In summary, indium-111 platelet scintigraphy has exciting potential value in the diagnosis and management of patients with deep vein thrombosis. The method is accurate, noninvasive, and may be used for diagnosis as well as a direct means of monitoring thrombus propagation and response to therapy for as long as seven days following the injection of the platelet suspension. Evaluation of its role in the diagnosis of pulmonary embolism needs further investigation.

## REFERENCES


1. Thakur, M. L., Welch, M. J., Joist, J. H., et al.: Indium-111 labeled platelets: Studies on preparation and evaluation of in vitro and in vivo functions. Thromb. Res., *9*:345, 1976.
2. Baker, J. R. J., Butler, K. D., Eakins, M. N., et al.: Subcellular localization of $^{111}$In in human and rabbit platelets. Blood, *59(2)*:351, 1982.
3. Scheffel, U., McIntyre, P. A., Evatt, B., et al.: Evaluation of Indium-111 as a new high photon yield gamma-emitting "physiological" platelet label. Johns Hopkins Med. J., *140(6)*:285, 1977.
4. McIlmoyle, G., Davis, H. H., Welch, M. J., et al.: Scintigraphic diagnosis of experimental pulmonary embolism with In-111–labelled platelets. J. Nucl. Med., *18(9)*:910, 1977.
5. Wistow, B. W., Grossman, Z. D., McAfee, J. G., et al.: Labelling of platelets with oxine complexes of Tc-99m and In-111. Part I. In vitro studies and survival in the rabbit. J. Nucl. Med., *19(5)*:483, 1978.
6. Dewanjee, M. K., Fuster, V., Kaye, M. P., et al.: Imaging platelet deposition with 111-In-labelled platelets in coronary artery bypass grafts in dogs. Mayo Clin. Proc., *53(5)*:327, 1978.
7. Goodwin, D. A., Bushberg, J. T., Doherty, P. W., et al.: Indium-111–labelled autologous platelets for location of vascular thrombi in humans. J. Nucl. Med., *19(6)*:626, 1978.
8. Heaton, W. A., Davis, H. H., Welch, M. J., et al.: Indium-111: A new radionuclide label for studying human platelet kinetics. Br. J. Haematol., *42(4)*:613, 1979.
9. Knight, L. C., Primeau, J. L., Siegel, B. A., et al.: Comparison of In-111–labeled platelets and iodinated fibrinogen for the detection of deep vein thrombosis. J. Nucl. Med., *19(8)*:891, 1978.
10. Joist, J. H., Baker, R. K., Thakur, M. L., et al.: Indium-111–labelled human platelets: Uptake and loss of label and in vitro function of labelled platelets. J. Lab. Clin. Med., *92(5)*:829, 1978.
11. Hawker, R. J., Hawker, L. M., and Wilkinson, A. R.: Indium (111-In)–labelled human platelets: Optimal method. Clin. Sci., *58(3)*:243, 1980.
12. Heyns, A. DuP., Badenhorst, P. N., Pieters, H., et al.: Preparation of a viable population of indium-111–labelled human blood platelets. Thromb. Haemost., *42(5)*:1473, 1980.
13. Klonizakis, I., Peters, A. M., Fitzpatrick, M. L., et al.: Radionuclide distribution following injection of 111-Indium–labelled platelets. Br. J. Haematol., *46(4)*:595, 1980.
14. Ezekowitz, M. D., Leonard, J. C., Smith, E. O., et al.: Identification of left ventricular thrombi in man using Indium-111–labelled autologous platelets. Circulation, *63(4)*:803, 1981.
15. Mathias, C. J., and Welch, M. J.: Labelling mechanism and localization of Indium-111 in human platelets. J. Nucl. Med., *20*:659, 1979 (Abstract).
16. Thakur, M. L., Walsh, L., Malech, H. L., et al.: Indium-111–labelled human platelets: Improved method, efficacy and evaluation. J. Nucl. Med., *22*:381, 1981.
17. Joist, J. H., and Baker, R. K.: Loss of $^{111}$Indium as indicator of platelet injury. Blood, *58(2)*:350, 1981.
18. Scheffel, U., Tsan, M.-F., Mitchell, T. G., et al.: Human platelets labelled with In-111 8-hydroxyquinoline: Kinetics, distribution and estimates of radiation dose. J. Nucl. Med., *23*:149, 1982.
19. Moser, K. M., Spragg, R. G., Bender, F., et al.: Study of factors that may condition scintigraphic detection of venous thrombi and pulmonary emboli with Indium-111 labelled platelets. J. Nucl. Med., *21*:1051, 1980.
20. Fedullo, P. F., Moser, K. M., Moser, K. S., et al.: Indium-111–labelled platelets: Effect of heparin on uptake by venous thrombi and relationship to the activated partial thromboplastin time. Circulation, *66(3)*:632, 1982.
21. Sostman, H. D., Neumann, R. D., Zoghbi, S. S., et al.: Experimental studies with $^{111}$Indium-labelled platelets in pulmonary embolism. Invest. Radiol., *17*:367, 1982.
22. Davis, H. H., Heaton, W. A., Siegel, B. A., et al.: Scintigraphic detection of atherosclerotic lesions and venous thrombi in man by indium-111–labelled autologous platelets. Lancet, June 3, p. 1185, 1978.
23. Davis, H. H., Siegel, B. A., Sherman, L. A., et al.: Scintigraphy with $^{111}$In-labelled autologous platelets in venous thromboembolism. Radiology, *136*:203, 1980.
24. Fenech, A., Hussey, J. K., Smith, F. W., et al.: Diagnosis of deep vein thrombosis using autologous indium-111–labelled platelets. Br. Med. J., *282*:1020, 1981.
25. Grimley, R. P., Rafiqi, E., Hawker, R. J., et al.: Imaging of $^{111}$In-labelled platelets—a new method for the diagnosis of deep vein thrombosis. Br. J. Surg., *68*:714, 1981.
26. Ezekowitz, M. D., Eichner, E. R., Scatterday, R., et

al.: Diagnosis of a persistent pulmonary embolus by Indium-111 platelet scintigraphy with angiographic and tissue confirmation. Am. J. Med., *72*:839, 1982.

27. Sostman, H. D., Neumann, R. D., Loke, J., et al.: Detection of pulmonary embolism in man with $^{111}$In-labelled autologous platelets. Am. J. Radiol., *138*:945, 1982.
28. Ezekowitz, M. D., Pope, C. F., Smith, E. O., et al.: Unpublished data, 1983.
29. Dewanjee, M. K., Rao, S. A., Rosemark, J. A., et al.: Indium-111 tropolone, a new tracer for platelet labelling. Radiology, *145*:149, 1982.
30. Scheffel, U., Tsan, M. F., McIntyre, P. A.: Labelling of human platelets with $^{111}$In-8-hydroxyquinoline. J. Nucl. Med., *20*:524, 1979.
31. Bunting, R. W., Callahan, R. J., Finkelstein, S., et al.: A modified method for labelling human platelets with Indium-111 oxine using albumin density-gradient separation. Radiology, *145*:219, 1982.
32. Danpure, H. J., Osman, S., and Brady, F.: The labelling of blood cells in plasma with $^{111}$In-tropolonate. Br. J. Radiol., *55*:247, 1982.
33. Danpure, H. J., and Osman, S.: Cell labelling and cell damage with $^{111}$In-acetylacetone—an alternative to indium-111-oxine. Br. J. Radiol., *54*:597, 1981.
34. Zir, L. M., Carvalho, A. C., Harthorne, J. W., et al.: Effect of contrast agents on platelet aggregation and $^{14}$C-serotonin release. New Engl. J. Med., *291(3)*:134, 1974.
35. Gafter, U. Creter, D., Zevin, D., et al.: Inhibition of platelet aggregation by contrast media. Radiology, *132*:341, 1979.

CHAPTER 14

# PULMONARY ANGIOSCOPY

DEBORAH SHURE, M.D.

## INTRODUCTION

There are a number of clinical and investigational situations in which a direct look at the interior of the heart or the pulmonary arteries in vivo would be useful. In particular, thrombus within the heart, valvular vegetations, intracardiac tumor, and chronic pulmonary emboli are anatomic problems that often evade our currently available diagnostic instruments, but that could be accessible by a direct visualization technique. For several years we have been developing an instrument and a technique for this purpose. We call the instrument an angioscope and the procedure angioscopy.

## HISTORY

There has actually been a long-standing interest in viewing the interior of the heart and great vessels in vivo. The first recorded attempt to view the heart, cardioscopy, was made by Rhea and Walker in 1913 and described in a paper by Cutler.[1] Their device was a tube with an inset lens, which was inserted into the heart at the time of thoracotomy. They never achieved good visualization and had additional problems with hemodynamic instability and sepsis.

Over the next 70 years a number of investigators have developed a variety of devices to achieve the goal of visualization of the interior of the vasculature and to allow some degree of surgical manipulation. The major problem posed by vascular endoscopy is visualization of structures through the opaque medium of blood. This problem has been dealt with by all the devices in one of two basic ways. Blood has either been flushed transiently from the field of view, or blood has been mechanically displaced by the lens itself or by an optically transparent device creating a chamber in front of the lens. The method of flushing the field of view has usually been complicated by circulatory overload in order to achieve an adequate view.

In 1922, Allen and Graham[2] reported on the use of a cardioscope with a convex lens, which displaced blood by direct contact. It was inserted through the left atrial appendage and was capable of visualizing and, by way of an attached knife, cutting a stenosed mitral valve. The postoperative mortality of this procedure (done only in animals) was high, mainly due to sepsis.

In 1943, Harken and Glidden[3] described the experimental use of a cardioscope in which the lens was covered by a saline-filled plastic balloon. This instrument was also inserted through the atrial appendage (left or right). Its insertion was tolerated for prolonged periods in animals, and the visualization was reported to be good.

In 1948, Brock[4] described the clinical use of an instrument similar to that of Allen and Graham for use in pulmonary valvulotomy. The instrument was inserted through the left pulmonary artery. It was successful at visualizing a subvalvular stenosis in one of the two cases in which the procedure was performed. In the other case, the cardioscope could not be passed into the main pulmonary artery.

Two years later, Bloomberg described his experience with a cardioscope in the discussion of a paper presented by Bailey.[5] The instrument was used in dogs to visualize the aortic valve. Good visualization was achieved by flushing the field of view with short, high-pressure bursts of saline, but blood had to be withdrawn during the procedure to prevent circulatory fluid overload. That same year, Murray[6] described another cardioscope for intraoperative use that displaced blood by direct contact of the lens with the structure to be viewed and allowed for insertion of surgical cutting devices. It is not clear what use was made of this instrument.

One year later, in 1951, Butterworth[7] described a simple cardioscope fashioned from one piece of Lucite (methyl methacrylate). It was narrower (½ inch in diameter) and could carry more light to the interior of the heart than previous instruments. It was inserted through the atrial appendage and was used experimentally in animals to visualize and cut stenotic mitral valves. In 1954, Boulton[8] described the clinical and experimental use of a similar instrument.

In 1958, Sakakibara[9] described two cardioscopes for intraoperative use. In one instrument the lens was covered by an inflatable balloon; in the other, it was covered by a transparent, solid polyvinyl cap that became pliable at body temperature. In both instruments blood displacement was also aided by an irrigation channel. The instruments were inserted through the ventricular wall. Aortic valvulotomy was performed in seven cases using a serrated edge built into the cardioscope equipped with the polyvinyl cap. In some cases, adequate visualization was only achieved by clamping the vena cava and pulmonary vein and filling the left heart with saline.

A major improvement in cardioscopy was made by Carlens and Silander.[10] In 1961, they described the first cardioscope that did not require intraoperative insertion through the heart wall. Their cardioscope was a long metal tube with a side viewing lens covered by an inflatable latex balloon. The instrument was inserted through the right jugular vein (in animals) and passed into the right atrium and right ventricle. Visualization was obtained by inflating the balloon and touching it to the structure to be viewed to displace blood. Two years later, they reported the successful use of this instrument in six patients to diagnose atrial septal defects and anomalous venous return. Although the procedure was carried out under general anesthesia, they believed that such anesthesia was not essential.[11]

The next major improvement was made by Gamble and Innis[12] in 1967. They described the first experimental use of a fiberoptic cardioscope in animals. The instrument had a diameter of 4.1 mm, and the lens was covered by an inflatable latex balloon. The instrument was used in three dogs and could be inserted from the femoral artery, the carotid artery, or the jugular vein. The right heart and main pulmonary artery could be visualized from the jugular approach. The femoral artery approach was found to be inadequate for visualization of the aortic valve, but this could be well seen from the carotid approach, and the left ventricle could be entered. The instrument could not, however, be turned in the left ventricle or passed into the left atrium. No adverse effects of the procedure were noted. Ten years later, Dee and Crosby[13] used a fiberoptic instrument inserted through the carotid artery to visualize aortic valves in animals. Their procedure required the production of transient asystole (produced by raising intrabronchial pressure) to decrease venous return and the rapid infusion of saline to flush blood from the aortic valves.

## CURRENT WORK

We first reported the use of a fiberoptic instrument to visualize the interior of the right side of the heart and the pulmonary arteries in 1980.[14] We called our technique "angioscopy" rather than cardioscopy because of our interest in the extension of the procedure to include the pulmonary arterial vascular tree. Our instrument was a pediatric bronchoscope modified by an inflatable latex balloon. We demonstrated the ability of the apparatus to visualize acute pulmonary emboli.

In 1981, we reported further studies with a modified instrument, the one currently in use.[15] The angioscope is longer and narrower than the previous version (80 cm long, 4 mm diameter) and it differs from that of Gamble and Innis in the addition of a directional control (Fig. 14–1). The distal tip can be flexed 90° by a control lever on the proximal handle. The tip is covered by a transparent polyurethane balloon, which is secured to the angioscope with 6/0 Teflon-coated nylon suture (Fig. 14–2). The polyurethane balloon is optically superior to the latex balloon. The balloon can be inflated or deflated through an 0.8-mm channel within the angioscope. Carbon dioxide is used for balloon inflation to prevent air embolism if a balloon should break. A conventional cold xenon light source is used for illumination.

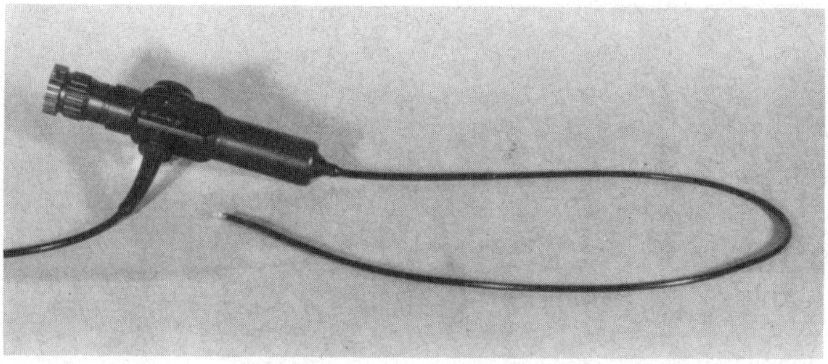

*Figure 14–1.* The angioscope. (Courtesy of Machida America).

### Technique

The angioscope is inserted through a jugular venotomy (internal or external jugular). The procedure requires only local anesthesia for the venotomy. To maintain sterility, the procedure should be performed by two people. One person manipulates the distal end and the other person holds the proximal end with the eye piece and flexion controls, which of necessity must be held near the face. After inserting the distal tip into the venous system, the balloon can be inflated during passage through the veins to the right atrium, which can be recognized with the angioscope, or the angioscope can be passed into the heart with the balloon deflated using fluoroscopic guidance. Once in the right atrium, visualization can be obtained by rotating the angioscope or using its flexion control to gently touch the inflated balloon to the structures to be viewed. The angioscope can then be passed through the tricuspid valve and into the right ventricle and main pulmonary artery. With experience, one can recognize the structures seen through the angioscope, but intermittent fluoroscopy can be useful to confirm the location of the angioscope. Fluoroscopy is particularly useful when the angioscope is in the pulmonary vasculature, since, unlike a bronchoscopic examination in which one can see some distance ahead in the bronchial tree, angioscopy provides only a view of the region immediately adjacent to the inflated balloon. Using this technique, the angioscope can be guided through the pulmonary arteries (left and right), and lobar and sublobar arteries can be visualized. The examination can be carried out to arteries of a 4-mm diameter. The procedure lasts approximately 20 minutes.

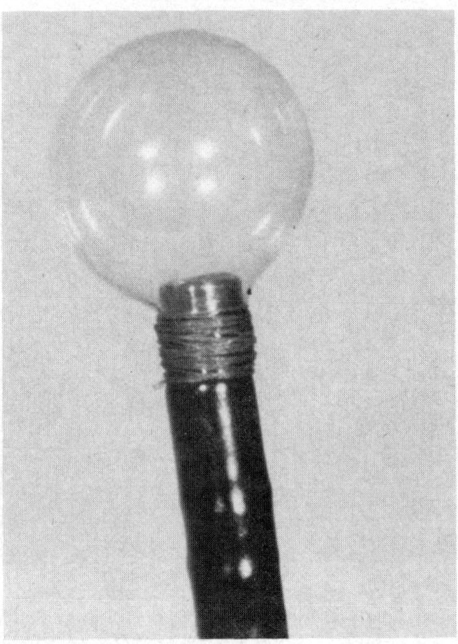

*Figure 14–2.* Distal end of the angioscope with polyurethane balloon inflated.

### Capability

Internal structures within the range of the angioscope can be visualized with remarkable clarity. The tricuspid valve with its chordal attachments (Fig. 14–3) and papillary muscle (Fig. 14–4) can be seen in the right heart. The pulmonic valve itself is a thin structure and difficult to visualize, but the right ventricular outflow tract and the pulmonary artery can be clearly seen. Pulmonary arterial branches can also be identified (Fig. 14–5). The entire pulmonary arterial intima normally has a smooth, pale appearance as seen in Figure 14–5. The blood seen directly in front of the angioscope normally appears bright red. An acute pulmonary embolus, in contrast, appears as a dark blue mass in front of the angioscope (Fig. 14–6). Although the view is quite clear, photographic documentation (still or ciné) is useful to review anatomic abnormalities that may not have been fully appreciated during the procedure.

Anatomic accuracy is the major advantage of the angioscope. In a study comparing

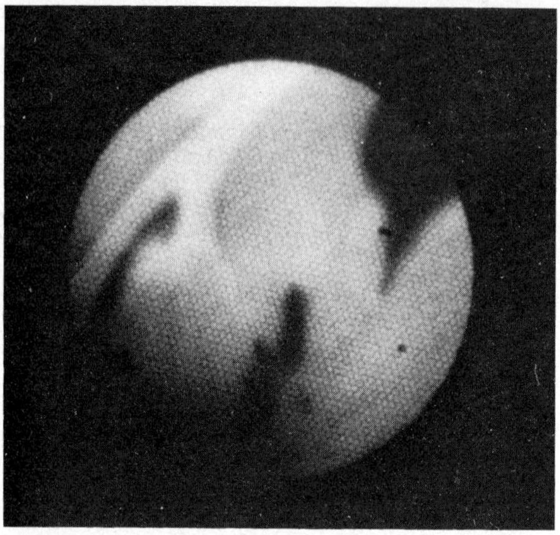

***Figure 14–3.*** Tricuspid valve with chorda tendineae. (From Shure, D., et al.: Identification of pulmonary emboli in the dog: Comparison of angioscopy and perfusion scanning. Circulation, *64*:618, 1981. By permission of the American Heart Association, Inc.)

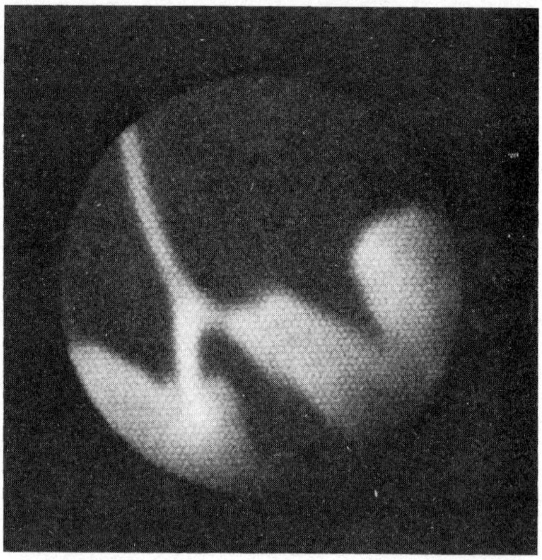

***Figure 14–4.*** Papillary muscle with chordae tendineae. (From Shure, D., et al.: Identification of pulmonary emboli in the dog: Comparison of angioscopy and perfusion scanning. Circulation, *64*:618, 1981. By permission of the American Heart Association, Inc.)

identification and localization of acute pulmonary emboli by lung perfusion scanning and angioscopy,[15] we found that angioscopy could detect all emboli within its range (vessels 4 mm or larger in diameter) and was more anatomically accurate than perfusion scanning, which reflected the functional distribution of blood flow. This distinction was seen in three cases in which the angioscopic and autopsy findings were identical and differed from those seen on the perfusion scans. In two experimental animals, a single branching central embolus produced two lobar defects on scan. In the third animal, three sublobar emboli produced one lobar defect on the scan. This degree of anatomic accuracy with angioscopy should be useful in clinical applications of the procedure.

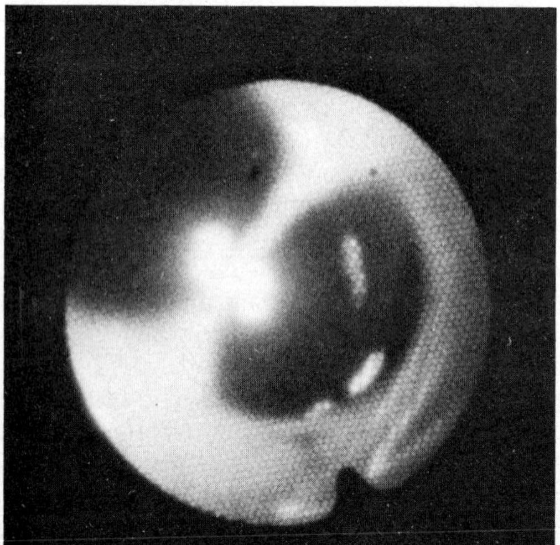

***Figure 14–5.*** Normal pulmonary arteries showing pale intima, smooth vessel wall contour, and bright red blood. (From Shure, D., et al.: Identification of pulmonary emboli in the dog: Comparison of angioscopy and perfusion scanning. Circulation, *64*:618, 1981. By permission of the American Heart Association, Inc.)

### Safety

We have examined the physiologic effects of angioscopy on animals before and after

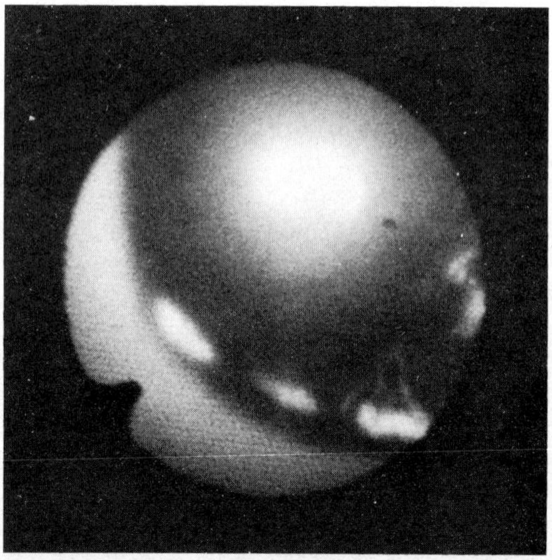

***Figure 14–6.*** Acute pulmonary thromboembolus in a pulmonary artery. (From Shure, D., et al.: Identification of pulmonary emboli in the dog: Comparison of angioscopy and perfusion scanning. Circulation, *64*:618, 1981. By permission of the American Heart Association, Inc.)

pulmonary embolization.[16] No effects on arterial blood gases, heart rate, cardiac output, systemic blood pressure, or pulmonary arterial pressure are seen during angioscopy in animals without pulmonary emboli. After substantial pulmonary embolization, clinically small increases were seen in cardiac output, systemic pressure, and heart rate during angioscopy. The effects were not related to the angioscopic balloon inflation. There was no effect on arterial blood gases. Both before and after pulmonary embolization, angioscopy produced minor arrhythmias (atrial and ventricular premature contractions) that were not hemodynamically significant and that were comparable to those seen during right heart catheterization. The right ventricular outflow tract appears to be the most sensitive area during passage of the angioscope. This absence of significant physiologic effects is to be expected based on the previous benign experiences with right heart catheterization[7] and with temporary occlusion of the pulmonary artery.[8, 9]

## THE ROLE OF ANGIOSCOPY

Experimentally, angioscopy is a potentially useful tool in the investigation of pulmonary emboli, clot lysis, vasculitis, and possibly in the development of endocarditis. It also has great clinical potential, the extent of which remains to be defined. The technique is clearly feasible as shown from animal studies,[12, 14, 15] and Tanabe and his associates[20] have already used a fiberoptic instrument similar to ours in humans to diagnose atrial and ventricular septal defects. The questions at this time are: When is angioscopy indicated, and when are conventional studies adequate?

We are currently engaged in a study of these questions. Our study focuses on the usefulness of angioscopy in the detection of chronic, central organized pulmonary emboli and right ventricular lesions such as thrombus, tumor, and endocarditis. These areas were chosen because their diagnosis is often in doubt after conventional diagnostic imaging procedures such as echocardiography, angiography, and perfusion scanning. Our particular interest has been in chronic pulmonary emboli, in which the angiogram can be difficult to interpret and lung perfusion scans can underestimate the degree of vascular obstruction.[21] These difficulties may arise, in part, from the tendency of chronic emboli to partially recanalize over time, producing a variety of unusual and often misleading images. Because chronic embolic obstruction is surgically correctable if the obstruction is relatively central (see Chapter 15), its diagnosis is of particular clinical significance. Conventional procedures are performed first in our study. If the diagnosis is still in doubt, angioscopy is performed as described previously. During the procedure, the electrocardiogram, systemic pressure, and pulmonary arterial pressure are continuously monitored, and arterial blood gases are measured intermittently. In most cases, a final diagnosis should be established by surgery or, in some cases, at autopsy. By this systematic approach we hope to establish the indications, contraindications, benefits, and problems of human applications of angioscopy.

Our initial experiences with human application of angioscopy for identification and localization of chronic embolic obstruction have been encouraging.[22] We have been able to visualize subtle irregularities in the pulmonary arterial intima, which probably represent the residua of old emboli that have resolved. Perhaps more importantly, we have been able to clearly see both central,

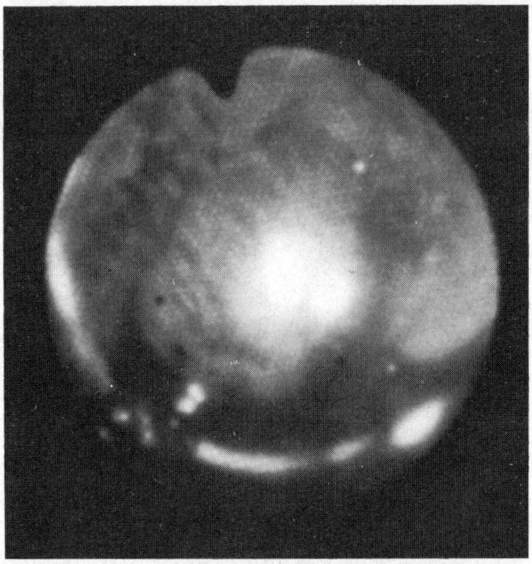

***Figure 14–7.*** Organized chronic pulmonary embolus showing the white, pitted surface. The embolus is totally obstructing a pulmonary artery. (From Shure, D., et al.: Identification of pulmonary emboli in the dog: Comparison of angioscopy and perfusion scanning. Circulation, *64*:618, 1981. By permission of the American Heart Association, Inc.)

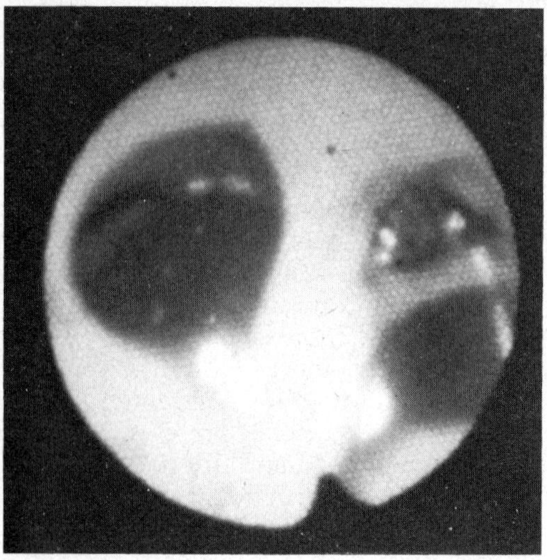

***Figure 14–8.*** Partial recanalization of a chronic pulmonary embolus in a sublobar pulmonary artery. Webbing and irregularities of the arterial wall can be seen. (From Shure, D., et al.: Identification of pulmonary emboli in the dog: Comparison of angioscopy and perfusion scanning. Circulation, *64*:618, 1981. By permission of the American Heart Association, Inc.)

obstructing, organized thrombus (Fig. 14–7) as well as more peripheral abnormalities associated with partially obstructing organized emboli (Fig. 14–8). The obstructing organized embolus, in contrast to the smooth, dark blue appearance of a fresh embolus, presents as a white mass with a pitted surface (Fig. 14–7). On the other hand, emboli that have partially recanalized present as narrowing of the vessel (which can be appreciated from the feel of the angioscope) with webbing and irregularities of the contour of the vessel wall (Fig. 14–8). These changes can be appreciated even more by contrast to the normal pulmonary artery appearance of a perfectly smooth contour (see Fig. 14–5).

This clarity of anatomic detail seen with angioscopy indicates the potential diagnostic advantages of the procedure. It is our hope that fiberoptic angioscopy, like fiberoptic bronchoscopy, may provide us with new insights into diseases that were relatively inaccessible to direct visualization. As the visualization capabilities of the instrument become defined, future modifications of the angioscope could permit biopsy, injection, or suctioning to expand its diagnostic and possibly therapeutic capabilities.

## REFERENCES


1. Cutler, E. C., Levine, S. A., and Beck, C. S.: The surgical treatment of mitral stenosis. Arch. Surg., *9*:689, 1924.
2. Allen, D. S., and Graham, E. A.: Intracardiac surgery—a new method. JAMA, *79*:1028, 1922.
3. Harken, D. E., and Glidden, E. M.: Experiments in intracardiac surgery. J. Thorac. Surg., *12*:566, 1943.
4. Brock, R. C.: Pulmonary valvulotomy for the relief of congenital pulmonary stenosis. Br. Med. J., *1*:1121, 1948.
5. Bailey, C. P., Glover, R. P., O'Neill, T. J. E., et al.: Experiences with the experimental surgical relief of aortic stenosis. J. Thorac. Surg., *20*:516, 1950.
6. Murray, G.: A cardioscope. Angiology, *1*:334, 1950.
7. Butterworth, R. F.: A new operating cardioscope. J. Thorac. Surg., *22*:319, 1951.
8. Boulton, H. E., Bailey, C. P., Costas-Durieux, J., et al.: Cardioscopy—simple and practical. J. Thorac. Surg., *27*:323, 1954.
9. Sakakibara, S., Iikawa, T., Hattori, J., et al.: Direct visual operation for aortic stenosis: Cardioscopic studies. J. Internat. Coll. Surg., *29*:548, 1958.
10. Carlens, E., and Silander, T.: Method for direct inspection of the right atrium: Experimental investigation in the dog. Surgery, *49*:622, 1961.
11. Carlens, E., and Silander, T.: Cardioscopy. J. Cardiovasc. Surg., *4*:512, 1963.
12. Gamble, W. J., and Innis, R. E.: Experimental intracardiac visualization. New Engl. J. Med., *276*:1397, 1967.
13. Dee, P., and Crosby, I.: Fiberoptic studies of the aortic valve in dogs. Br. Heart J., *39*:459, 1979.
14. Moser, K. M., Shure, D., Harrell, J. H., et al.: Angioscopic visualization of pulmonary emboli. Chest, *77*:198, 1980.
15. Shure, D., Moser, K. M., Harrell, J. H. II, et al.: Identification of pulmonary emboli in the dog: Comparison of angioscopy and perfusion scanning. Circulation, *64*:618, 1981.
16. Shure, D., Moser, K. M., and Konopka, R. G.: Hemodynamics, and gas exchange during angioscopy in the dog. Angiology, *35*:97, 1984.
17. Swan, H. J. C., Ganz, W., Forrester, J., et al.: Catheterization of the heart in man with use of a flow-directed balloon-tipped catheter. New Engl. J. Med., *283*:447, 1970.
18. Swenson, E. W., Finley, T. N., and Guzman, S. V.: Unilateral hypoventilation in man during temporary occlusion of one pulmonary artery. J. Clin. Invest., *40*:828, 1961.
19. Carlens, E, Hanson, H. E., and Nordenstrom, B.: Temporary unilateral occlusion of the pulmonary artery. A new method of determining separate lung function and of radiographic examination. J. Thorac. Surg., *22*:527, 1951.
20. Tanabe, T., Yokota, A., and Sugie, S.: Cardiovascular fiberoptic endoscopy: Development and clinical application. Surgery, *87*:375, 1980.
21. Moser, K. M., Spragg, R. G., Long, W. B., et al.: Chronic thrombotic obstruction of major pulmonary arteries: Results of thromboendarterectomy in 15 patients. (Abstract) Am. Rev. Respir. Dis., *4*:87, 1982.
22. Shure, D., Moser, K. M., Gregoratos, G., et al.: The role of angioscopy in the diagnosis of chronic pulmonary emboli. Chest, *84*:341, 1983.

CHAPTER 15

# PULMONARY THROMBOENDARTERECTOMY

*JOE R. UTLEY, M.D.*

Chronic symptoms are relatively unusual in patients with pulmonary emboli. Most patients have acute syndromes, and the most common clinical decisions are related to the management of acute emboli and the prevention of their recurrence. In a few patients, the pulmonary emboli do not lyse but rather progress to chronic pulmonary vascular obstruction. This progression may produce no symptoms in patients with chronic obstruction of a small portion of the pulmonary vascular bed. Some patients develop vascular obstruction of a major degree in both lungs and become chronically symptomatic due to pulmonary hypertension and decreased cardiac output. We have performed bilateral pulmonary thromboendarterectomy in a highly selected group of these patients with debilitating symptoms.[2, 4-7, 11, 12]

## PATHOGENESIS

Our concepts regarding pathogenesis of this condition have developed from the patients' clinical history, progression of their symptoms, progression of evidence of vascular obstruction, the operative findings, and the pathology of the material removed surgically. Most of the patients we have evaluated for chronic pulmonary vascular obstruction have had a history of cardiopulmonary symptoms for many years. Frequently, the symptoms were of an episodic nature in the beginning and became constant later in the patient's course. In several patients, the early episodes were not recognized as pulmonary emboli, and many patients did not receive anticoagulants after their initial episode. The history in some patients suggested only a single episode of embolization. However, most patients had a history of multiple episodes. In a few patients, nothing in the history suggested acute pulmonary emboli, and the possibility of chronic pulmonary emboli was only considered late in the course of the patient's disease. It is possible that one of the risk factors in the progression to chronic vascular obstruction due to recurrent emboli is atypical early manifestations, failure to diagnose the acute episode, or failure to begin anticoagulant therapy. Other factors that might influence the lysis of emboli are the age of the thrombotic material at the time of embolization and abnormalities or variations in the local and systemic factors that promote either thrombosis or fibrinolysis.

The gross appearance of the thrombotic material at operation suggests great variation in the age of the emboli. We have found recent red clots that have embolized to areas of incomplete fibrous obstruction. Large emboli may show fibrosis at the periphery and degenerated blood clot at their centers. The organized material within the pulmonary artery may peel away in layers between portions of emboli of different ages. The cohesion of the obstructive material is a function of the age of the emboli. Emboli that are recent may crumble as they are extracted. As the emboli become older, the material becomes more fibrotic, and the extraction of fibrous cores from segmental arteries is facilitated by the ability to apply traction on the fibrous material. The ideal situation is thrombus material that has become strong and cohesive owing to fibrosis but has not become densely adherent to the arterial wall. After many years, the dense fibrosis obliterates the plane of cleavage between the embolic material and the arterial wall, making extraction difficult. Thus, in some areas the material may be too young to remove satisfactorily and in other areas too old. Different pathology may be seen in different areas in the same patient.

One patient with complete obstruction of the right pulmonary artery had developed a hypoplastic pulmonary artery distal to the obstruction. This patient had the most severe reperfusion pulmonary edema we have seen. Biopsy of the lung distal to areas of pulmonary artery obstruction showed diffuse thickening of the walls of the arterioles and venules. The degree of small vessel disease has not been a predictor of benefit of the operation. Organized thrombus in the walls of pulmonary veins may be a contributing factor in reperfusion pulmonary edema.

Although variations in the pathology of the embolic material are important determinants of the results of the operation, excellent results can be achieved many years after the first episode of embolization.

A factor that may contribute to the progression of the patient's symptoms late in the course of the disease is the development of arteriolar thickening and a form of reactive vascular obstruction in areas of perfused lung. The evidence that muscular/arteriolar obstruction is a significant factor in patients is twofold. First, the pulmonary vascular obstruction will frequently respond transiently to vasodilators in patients with recurrent emboli. Second, perfusion scans obtained soon after thromboendarterectomy show diminished flow in previously perfused areas and increased flow in areas opened by thromboendarterectomy.

## PREOPERATIVE EVALUATION

All patients had severe exercise intolerance, fatigability, and dyspnea. One patient had recurrent massive hemoptysis as well. Five patients were in New York Heart Association functional class III and five were in functional class IV. All patients were evaluated by right heart catheterization, pulmonary angiography, and ventilation/perfusion scanning. All patients had elevated pulmonary vascular resistance. Pulmonary hypertension was severe at rest or exercise in all patients. All patients had angiographic obstruction in both lungs, with occlusion at the level of lobar arteries or proximal to them. One patient had severe tricuspid valve insufficiency, and one patient had right-to-left shunting across an atrial septal defect. Five patients had complete obstruction of a pulmonary artery, three on the right and two on the left.

In one patient there was no history suggestive of pulmonary emboli, but the angiogram suggested bilateral vascular obstruction. The scan showed segmental perfusion defects. Two patients had peripheral pulmonary artery angiograms and were found to have partial obstruction in the main pulmonary artery at operation, which the angiogram did not demonstrate. At present, we employ central as well as peripheral angiography in evaluating these patients. Although the bronchial circulation is increased in these patients and is an important consideration in their operative management, we have not performed bronchial angiography routinely. When we have obtained bronchial angiograms, we have found that bronchial circulation is increased. In our experience, failure to demonstrate patent peripheral pulmonary vessels has not been a predictor of failure to benefit from the operation or of inoperability.

## OPERATIVE MANAGEMENT

Coumadin therapy is discontinued, and heparin anticoagulation is instituted preoperatively. Arterial pressure, central venous pressure, and left atrial pressure of all patients are monitored postoperatively. We have chosen not to use Swan-Ganz catheters or indwelling pulmonary artery lines because of the risk of their contributing to postoperative pulmonary artery thrombosis.

We have operated on all patients through a median sternotomy incision with complete cardiopulmonary bypass, deep hypothermia, and circulatory arrest. Unilateral thromboendarterectomy through a lateral thoracotomy employing unilateral pulmonary artery occlusion is not an appropriate approach in these patients for several reasons.[1] First, all patients have bilateral obstructions. Second, half of the patients have complete obstruction of one pulmonary artery at its origin, making occlusion for thromboendarterectomy difficult without compromising the flow to the opposite lung. The view of the segmental branches of the pulmonary artery through central arteriotomies is facilitated by a sternotomy approach. Because respiratory insufficiency is the most common problem in these patients postoperatively, the sternotomy incision contributes to lung dysfunction less than the lateral thoracotomy incision.

Through a median sternotomy incision, the patient is prepared for cannulation of the ascending aorta and superior and inferior vena cava. The pericardium is incised on both right and left to expose the proximal extrapericardial portion of the right and left pulmonary artery. Both phrenic nerves are mobilized from the pericardium for 5 to 6 cm. The right pulmonary artery is mobilized from the posterior aspect of the ascending aorta and the superior vena cava. We have not mobilized, ligated, or divided the azygous vein to improve exposure of the right pulmonary artery because of the importance of the azygous vein as a collateral venous channel in patients undergoing inferior vena caval interruption.

Complete cardiopulmonary bypass is begun, and the water bath of the heat exchanger is kept at 10 to 15° C below the temperature of the patient. Ventricular fibrillation is less likely to occur with the ectothermic blood gas scheme.[8] Cooling and warming appears to be more rapid and uniform. Temperature is monitored in the esophagus and rectum. A needle temperature probe at the operative field is used to determine the temperature of the myocardium, diaphragm, and rectus abdominis muscle to assure uniform cooling. When the temperatures are all below 16° C, the aorta is clamped. Cold blood cardioplegia is infused into the aortic root, and the heart-lung machine is stopped. Blood is drained into the oxygenator, and the venous line is clamped. The circulation is arrested for 10 to 20 minutes, and the patient is reperfused with the heart-lung machine for 10 minutes, followed by another period of arrest. We have employed up to four periods of arrest totaling up to 60 minutes but have not observed any neurologic defects.

The first arteriotomy is made in the main pulmonary artery and extended into the left pulmonary artery. The main pulmonary artery is inspected for chronic thromboemboli attached to its wall. The fibrous plaque is dissected off the pulmonary artery wall using traction on the plaque with a dural elevator dissector. The dissection is carried distally until obstructions in all segmental branches of the lobar arteries are removed. One must be alert for possible fracturing of the plaque or penetration of the arterial wall.

The arteriotomy extends past the proximal upper lobe branches on the right and left. The proximal right pulmonary artery is inspected through an arteriotomy between the superior vena cava and aorta to detect mural thrombi.

Because of the extensive bronchial collateral circulation in these patients, circulatory arrest is necessary to eliminate blood from pulmonary circulation and to permit precise visualization of the distal arteries. The pulmonary arteries are closed with running sutures of 4-0 or 5-0 proline. We have not used patches to close the pulmonary artery. Usually, the artery is dilated, and closure does not narrow the vessel.

We performed a tricuspid annuloplasty in one patient, and in another we closed an atrial septal defect. The aortic clamp is removed. The heart-lung machine is used to warm the patient to 37° C, and the cardioplegia cannula is used as a needle vent in the ascending aorta to evacuate any air that may have entered the left heart. A left atrial pressure line is retained through the wall of the right superior pulmonary vein.

## POSTOPERATIVE MANAGEMENT

Hemodynamic instability has not been a significant problem in these patients, except in one patient in whom distal disease precluded complete endarterectomy, and pulmonary hypertension persisted. Volume is replaced to achieve the lowest left and right atrial pressures consistent with good cardiac output. The left atrial pressures are usually between 8 and 15 mm Hg.

Postoperative pulmonary dysfunction has been the most frequent problem in these patients. Pulmonary edema in the region of reperfusion has been observed in every patient. The edema is evident from chest x-rays. Hemorrhagic edema fluid may be suctioned from the endotracheal tube. The pathogenesis of the edema is undoubtedly multifactorial and related to diminished capillary integrity, pulmonary venule obstruction, and diminished plasma colloidal osmotic pressure due to hemodilution from cardiopulmonary bypass.[10] Increased blood flow to the edematous area is an obvious factor. The edema is usually transient and may clear completely within 48 hours of ventilation. In one patient, severe hemorrhagic edema from the right lung with total occlusion of the pulmonary artery preoperatively required placement of a double-lumen tube, differential tidal volume, and positive end-expiratory pressure to maintain gas exchange. The edematous lung appears extraordinarily susceptible to infection. Meticulous care in managing the intubated patient to avoid the introduction of organisms must be exercised. Also, the diminished immune response after cardiopulmonary bypass may be a factor in the susceptibility of the lung to infection.[9] Two patients developed late acid-fast pulmonary infections: In one patient, the organism was *Mycobacterium tuberculosis,* in the other it was *Mycobacterium fortuitum.* Two patients required tracheostomy for prolonged ventilatory support. One patient had transient phrenic nerve dysfunction. Other aspects of postoperative management are similar to those common to other types of cardiac surgery.

## RESULTS AND LONG-TERM MANAGEMENT

We experienced one operative death in a patient with severe distal obstruction from whom no significant amount of obstructive material could be removed. Another patient died in the second month postoperatively of respiratory insufficiency caused by reperfusion pulmonary edema. This patient demonstrated hemodynamic improvement postoperatively despite pulmonary insufficiency. The remaining patients improved by one to three functional classes according to the New York Heart Association classifications. Pulmonary artery systolic pressure decreased from 89.1 ± 16.4 (Std. Dev.) mm Hg preop-

Group 1: Excellent Results

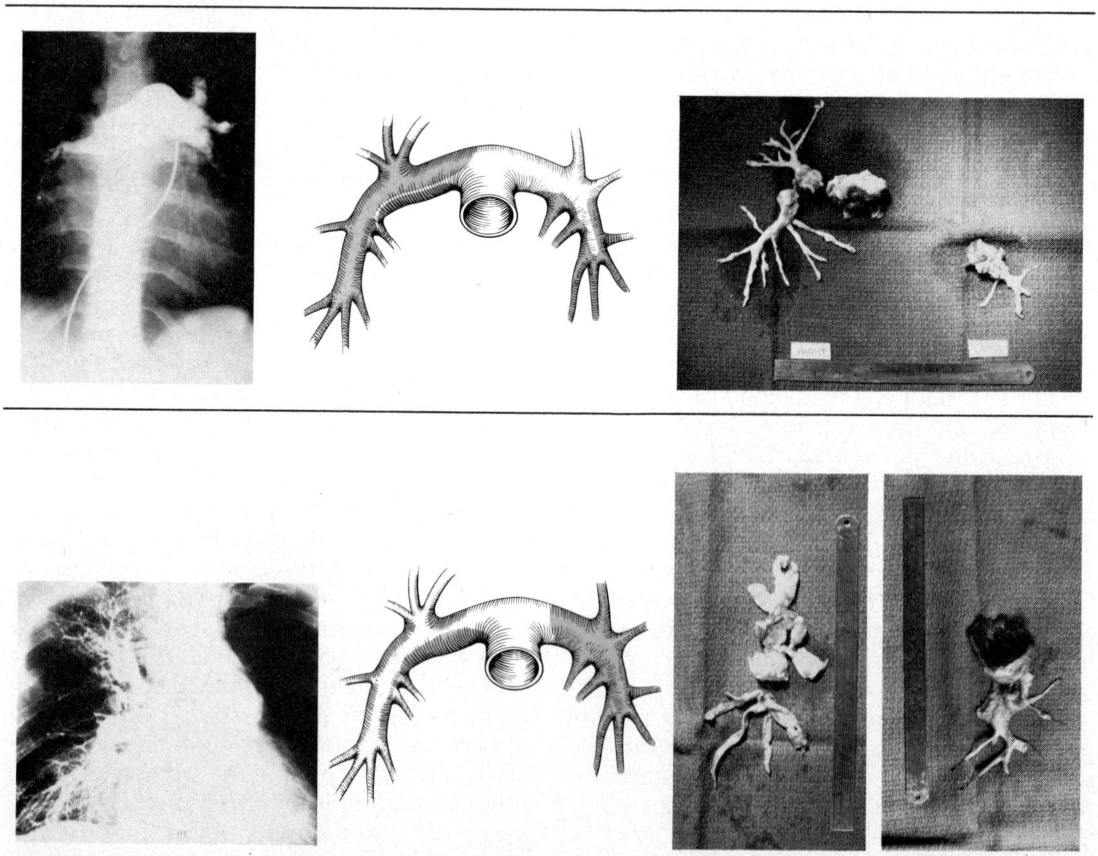

***Figure 15–1.*** The two patients with excellent results advanced from New York Heart Association functional class IV to functional class I. The material removed included large segments of chronic organized material. Cores of material were removed from the pulmonary arteries. Both patients had complete obstruction of one pulmonary artery.

# Group 2: Intermediate Results

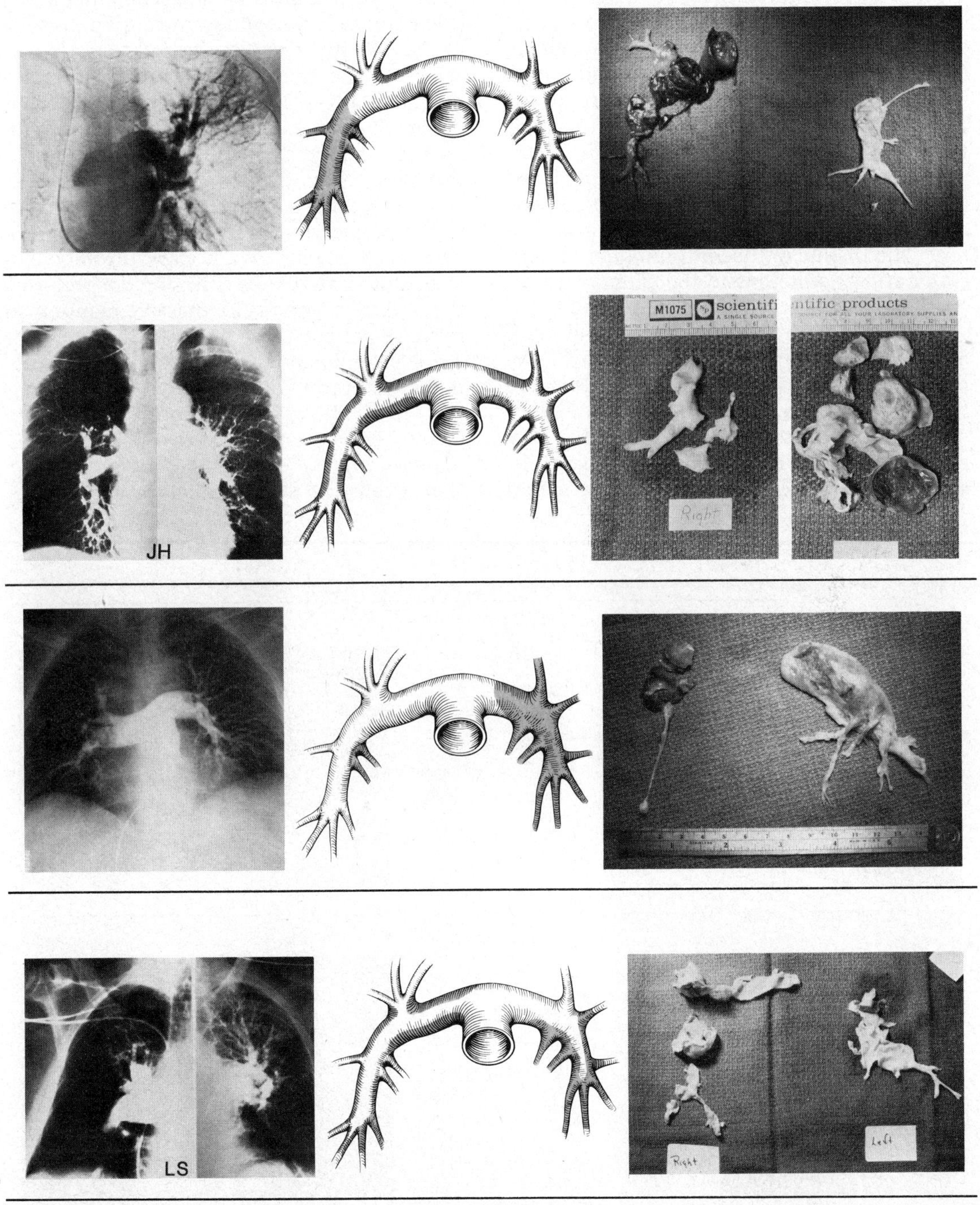


*Figure 15–2.* Examples of patients with intermediate results show that a large amount of material was often removed in smaller segments. Vascular obstruction in these patients was often incomplete.

eratively to 45.1 ± 15.5 mm Hg postoperatively ($p < 0.001$) in the entire group. Pulmonary vascular resistance fell from 12.1 ± 8.4 clinical units preoperatively to 4.0 ± 2.9 clinical units postoperatively. Radionuclide studies of right ventricular ejection fraction showed improvement postoperatively.

In one patient, closure of an atrial septal defect added to the improvement by closing an intracardiac right-to-left shunt and relieving cyanosis. In the patient with tricuspid valve insufficiency, improvement of tricuspid valve function by annuloplasty greatly improved right heart function. This patient had very longstanding (approximately 16 years) complete obstruction of the pulmonary artery. The plaque in the left pulmonary artery was densely adherent to the pulmonary artery wall and was removed piecemeal.

Figures 15–1 to 15–3 show the pulmonary angiogram, a graphic representation of the distribution of obstruction, and the specimen removed at operation in three groups of patients. In patients with poor results, only small amounts of material could be removed, or the material was densely adherent and friable and could only be removed piecemeal. In patients with excellent results, the chronic plaque was removed in large segments with cores from segmental arteries.

Chronic pulmonary embolism is an unusual cause of massive hemoptysis. In one patient with recurrent pulmonary emboli, the operation was performed during an episode of massive hemoptysis. The hemoptysis was relieved, and the patient has had no recurring hemoptysis following thromboendarterectomy.[3] Bronchial artery embolization for massive hemoptysis in these patients might carry the risk of pulmonary infarction, especially in patients with complete obstruction of the pulmonary artery on the side of bronchial embolization. Pulmonary thromboendarterectomy should be considered a preferred therapeutic approach for massive hemoptysis in these patients.

All patients are kept on life-long anticoagulation therapy with warfarin. Two patients had previous caval interruption. We performed caval interruption in one patient, but many of our patients refused caval interruption because of the potential for leg edema.

## Group 3: Poor Results

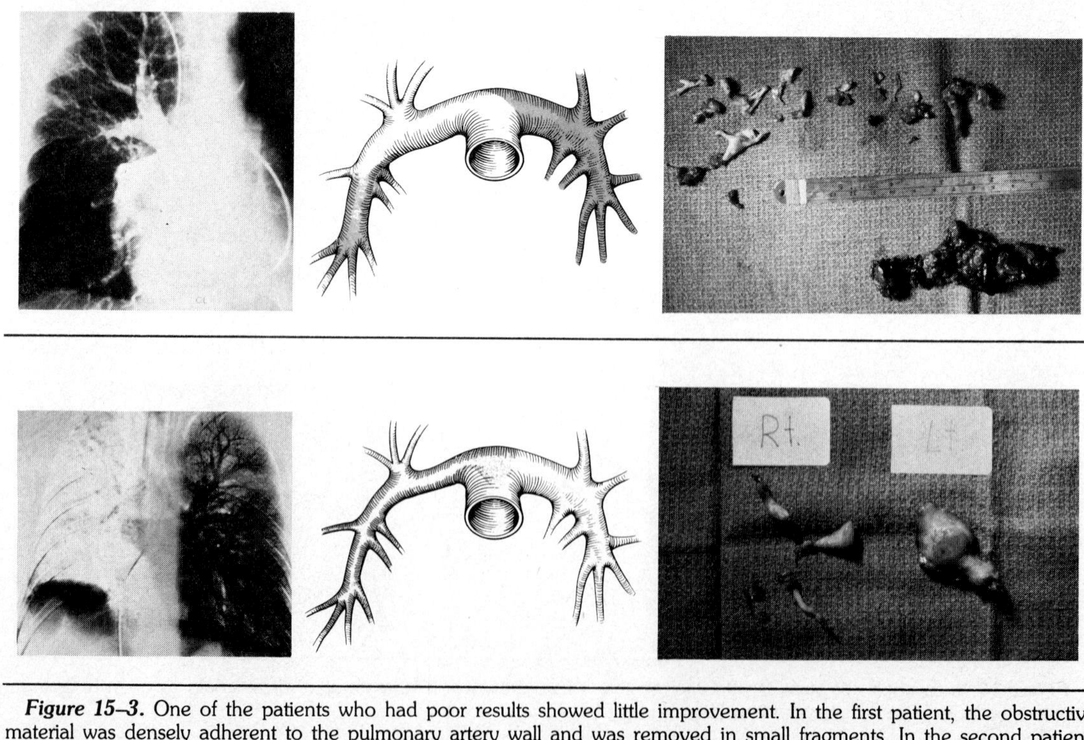


***Figure 15–3.*** One of the patients who had poor results showed little improvement. In the first patient, the obstructive material was densely adherent to the pulmonary artery wall and was removed in small fragments. In the second patient, reperfusion pulmonary edema contributed to lung failure, which was the cause of death two months postoperatively. The obstructed artery was small and contracted, and a small amount of chronic thrombus was present.

## REFERENCES


1. Cabrol, C., Cabrol, A., Acar, J., et al.: Surgical correction of chronic postembolic obstructions of the pulmonary arteries. J. Thorac. Cardiovasc. Surg., *76(5)*:620, 1978.
2. Daily, P. O., Johnston, G. G., Simmons, C. J., et al.: Surgical management of chronic pulmonary embolism. Surgical treatment and late results. J. Thorac. Cardiovasc. Surg., *79*:523, 1980.
3. Elliott, J. A.: Fatal massive haemoptysis after embolectomy for chronic pulmonary embolism. Thorax, *35*:705, 1980.
4. Moser, K. M., and Braunwald, N. S.: Successful surgical intervention in severe chronic thromboembolic pulmonary hypertension. Chest, *64(1)*:29, 1973.
5. Moser, K. M., Houk, V. N., Jones, R. C., et al.: Chronic, massive thrombotic obstruction of the pulmonary arteries. Circulation, *32*:377, 1965.
6. Nash, E. S., Shapiro, S., Landau, A., et al.: Successful thrombo-embolectomy in long-standing thrombo-embolic pulmonary hypertension. Thorax, *23*:121, 1968.
7. Sabiston, D. C., Jr., Wolfe, W. G., Oldham, H. N., Jr., et al.: Surgical management of chronic pulmonary embolism. Ann. Surg., *185(6)*:699, 1977.
8. White, F. N., and Weinstein, Y.: Carbon Dioxide Transport and Acid-base Balance During Hypothermia. *In* J. R. Utley (Ed.): Pathophysiology and Techniques of Cardiopulmonary Bypass, Vol. 2. Williams and Wilkins, Baltimore, 1983.
9. Utley, J. R.: The Immune Response to Cardiopulmonary Bypass. *In* J. R. Utley (Ed.): Pathophysiology and Techniques of Cardiopulmonary Bypass, Vol. 2. Williams and Wilkins, Baltimore, 1983.
10. Utley, J. R., and Stephens, D. B.: Fluid Balance During Cardiopulmonary Bypass. *In* J. R. Utley (Ed.): Pathophysiology and Techniques of Cardiopulmonary Bypass, Vol. 1. Williams and Wilkins, Baltimore, 1982.
11. Utley, J. R., Spragg, R. G., Long, W. B. III, et al.: Pulmonary endarterectomy for chronic thromboembolic obstruction: Recent surgical experience. Surgery, *92(6)*:1096, 1982.
12. Moser, K. M., Spragg, R. M., Utley, J. R., et al.: Chronic thrombotic obstruction of major pulmonary arteries: Results of thromboendarterectomy in 15 patients. Ann. Intern. Med. *99*:299, 1983.

CHAPTER 16

# VASOACTIVE HUMORAL FACTORS

JONAH MANNY, M.D.
HERBERT B. HECHTMAN, M.D.

Massive pulmonary embolus is associated with the abrupt onset of dyspnea, cyanosis, hypotension, jugular vein distention, extreme agitation of the patient, and on occasion with syncope and "sudden" death. The mortality is five- to sixfold greater in those patients in whom the diagnosis is not suspected and appropriate treatment is not instituted.[1] The primary mechanical consequence of embolism is reduction in the cross-sectional area of the pulmonary vascular bed. This increase in pulmonary vascular resistance leads to pulmonary hypertension and possible right ventricular failure manifest by increases in central venous pressure and fall in cardiac output. In addition, obstruction of the vascular bed results in regions that are ventilated but not perfused, that is, physiologic dead space ($V_D/V_T$). The degree of respiratory and hemodynamic compromise observed clinically and experimentally is not fully explained by mechanical obstruction. There is strong evidence that suggests that the difference in cardiorespiratory dynamics following simple pulmonary vascular ligation compared with thromboembolic obstruction is related to vaso- and bronchoactive substances released by either the embolus, the entrapped platelets, or the lung tissue itself. Vasoactive substances possibly responsible for the cardiopulmonary dysfunction are histamine, serotonin (5-hydroxytryptamine, 5HT) and the prostanoids.

An important role of histamine is unlikely, because injection of this amine does not evoke pulmonary hypertension, and experiments using $H_1$ and $H_2$ receptor antagonists have yielded conflicting results.[2, 3] Moreover, combined prostaglandin (PG) and histamine blockage does not abolish the pulmonary vascular response, which indicates that other vasoactive agents such as serotonin are important in accentuating the increased resistance to flow.

Serotonin is a potent neural and smooth muscle agonist. It is synthesized by neurons and enterochromaffin cells and is primarily stored in the dense bodies of platelets. In man, 5HT concentration is 390 ng/$10^9$ platelets. The normal plasma 5HT level of 150 ng/ml is maintained by an ongoing process of platelet uptake and release, as well as by endothelial clearance and catabolism via monoamine oxidase. A number of agents can trigger the platelet "release reaction." Thrombin activation of platelets and release of 5HT has been extensively studied. Platelets need not be destroyed or consumed by the process of activation, even when the event prompts 5HT release. The lungs, with their large endothelial surface area, play an important role in regulating circulating 5HT levels. About two-thirds of excess plasma 5HT is extracted by endothelial cell transport during a single passage through the pulmonary vascular bed.[4]

Following experimental pulmonary embolism, platelets are thought to interact with the clot, become entrapped in the lungs, and release 5HT into plasma. Thus, embolism results in a slight fall in circulating platelets, which have reduced concentrations of 5HT.[5]

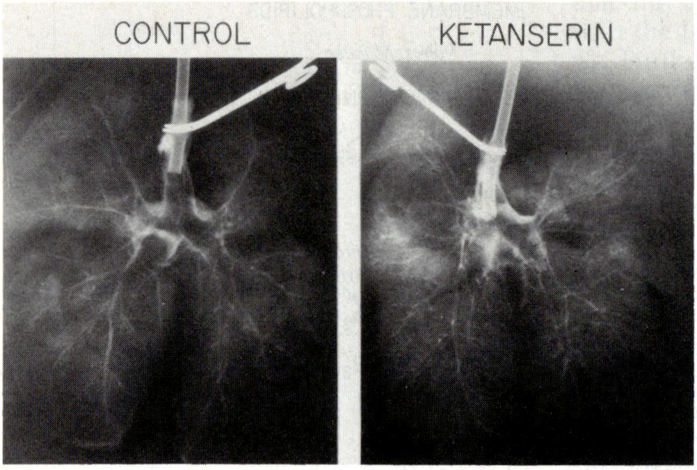


*Figure 16–7.* An angiogram following ketanserin therapy shows increased vascularity compared with a nontreated control dog. (From Huval, W. V., et al.: Therapeutic Benefits of 5-Hydroxytryptamine Inhibition Following Pulmonary Embolism. Ann. Surg., *197*:223, 1983.)

ment. This myocardial depression can be prevented by using $TxA_2$ synthetase inhibitors.

The pulmonary hypertension that accompanies embolization is also a consequence of both mechanical and vasospastic components. Inhibition of 5HT with ketanserin promptly lowers pulmonary arterial pressure. At least one-half of the rise in pulmonary pressure is due to vasoconstriction (Fig. 16–6).[9] This can also be seen angiographically, when ketanserin reverses vasoconstriction and leads to far better visualization of the pulmonary vasculature (Fig. 16–7).

These experimental data are derived from studies in animals, and their extrapolation to man must be done with some caution. Experimental clot is relatively freshly formed. Further, it is cut into small 3- × 5-mm fragments so that it can be infused into a large venous cannula. The freshness and large surface area of the injected clot emphasize platelet interactions. Finally, dog platelets are very rich in 5HT. Despite these cautions, it is thought that the conclusions regarding the possible actions of 5HT in man are qualitatively valid.

The role of the prostanoids is still unclear. For example, $PGI_2$ may directly dilate smooth muscle. It may also act indirectly by inhibition of 5HT transport as well as $TxA_2$ synthesis. Finally, $PGI_2$ causes the release of plasminogen activator, which stimulates clot lysis.[8, 10]

## SUMMARY

Following pulmonary embolism, potent vaso- and bronchoactive agents are released. Platelet-derived serotonin appears to be an important determinant of the resultant pulmonary hypertension and hypoxemia. The prostanoid $TxA_2$ plays a lesser role, particularly influencing $V_D/V_T$.

## REFERENCES

1. Sasahara, A. A., Sharma, G. V. R. K., Barsamian, E. M., et al.: Pulmonary thromboembolism, diagnosis and treatment. JAMA, *249*:2945, 1983.
2. Gilbert, R. P., Hinshaw, L. B., Kuida, H., et al.: Effects of histamine 5HT and epinephrine on pulmonary hemodynamics with particular reference to arterial and venous segment resistances. Am. J. Physiol., *194*:165, 1958.
3. Tucker, A., Weir, E. K., Reeves, J. T., et al.: Pulmonary microembolism: Attenuated pulmonary vasoconstriction with prostaglandin inhibitors and antihistamines. Prostaglandins, *11*:31, 1976.
4. Thomas, D. P., and Vane, J. R.: 5-Hydroxytryptamine in the circulation of the dog. Nature, *216*:335, 1967.
5. Utsunomiya, T., Krausz, M., Shepro, D., et al.: Prostaglandin control of plasma and platelet 5HT in normal and embolized animals. Am. J. Physiol., *241*:766, 1981.
6. Nadel, J. A., Colebatch, H. J. H., and Olsen, C. R.: Location and mechanism of airway constriction after barium sulfate microembolism. J. Appl. Physiol., *19*:387, 1964.
7. Utsunomiya, T., Krausz, M., Levine, L., et al.: Thromboxane mediation of cardiopulmonary effects of embolism. J. Clin. Invest., *70*:361, 1982.
8. Utsunomiya, T., Krausz, M., Valeri, C. R., et al.: Treatment of pulmonary embolism with prostacyclin. Surgery, *88*:25, 1980.
9. Huval, W. V., Mathieson, M. A., et al.: Therapeutic benefits of 5HT inhibition following pulmonary embolism. Ann. Surg., *197*:220, 1983.
10. Hechtman, H. B., Utsunomiya, T., et al.: Prostaglandin Mediation of Pulmonary Fibrinolytic Activity. *In* McConn, R. (Ed.): The Role of Chemical Mediators in The Pathophysiology of Acute Illness and Injury. Raven Press, New York, 1982, p. 253.

# INDEX

Numbers in *italics* refer to illustrations; numbers followed by a t refer to tables.